Differential diagnosis
of oral lesions

Differential diagnosis of oral lesions

NORMAN K. WOOD, D.D.S., M.S., Ph.D.

Professor and Chairman, Department of Oral Diagnosis,
Loyola University School of Dentistry, Maywood, Illinois;
Guest Lecturer, Northwestern University Dental School, Chicago, Illinois;
Consultant, Hines Veterans Administration Hospital, Hines, Illinois

PAUL W. GOAZ, B.S., D.D.S., S.M.

Professor, Department of Oral Diagnosis and Dental Radiology,
Baylor College of Dentistry, Dallas, Texas;
Consultant, Olin E. Teague Veterans Center,
Veterans Administration, Temple, Texas

SECOND EDITION

with **1318** illustrations, including **4** full-color plates

The C. V. Mosby Company

ST. LOUIS • TORONTO • LONDON   1980

SECOND EDITION

The C. V. Mosby Company
11830 Westline Industrial Drive, St. Louis, Missouri 63141

Library of Congress Cataloging in Publication Data

Main entry under title:

Differential diagnosis of oral lesions.

    Bibliography: p.
    Includes index.
    1. Stomatology. 2. Mouth—Diseases—Diagnosis.
I. Wood, Norman K., 1935-   II. Goaz,
Paul W., 1922-   [DNLM: 1. Mouth diseases—
Diagnosis. WU140 W877d]
RC815.D53   1980   616.3′1′075   80-18691
ISBN 0-8016-5617-6

GW/CB/B 9 8 7 6 5 4 3 2   02/D/294

Contributors

CHARLES C. ALLING III, D.D.S., M.S.

Professor and Chairman, Department of Oral and
Maxillofacial Surgery, University of Alabama School
of Dentistry, Birmingham, Alabama

GEORGE G. BLOZIS, D.D.S., S.M.

Professor and Chairman, Section of Oral
Pathology, Oral Diagnosis and Oral Medicine,
Ohio State University College of Dentistry,
Columbus, Ohio

HENRY M. CHERRICK, D.D.S., M.S.D.

Dean, School of Dental Medicine,
Southern Illinois University at Edwardsville,
Edwardsville, Illinois

THOMAS E. EMMERING, D.D.S., F.I.C.D.

Associate Professor and Chairman,
Department of Oral Radiology, Loyola University
School of Dentistry, Maywood, Illinois

STUART L. FISCHMAN, D.M.D.

Professor of Oral Medicine, State University
of New York at Buffalo School of Dentistry;
Director of Dentistry, Erie County
Medical Center, Buffalo, New York

RONALD E. GIER, D.M.D., M.S.D.

Professor and Chairman, Department of Oral
Diagnosis, University of Missouri, Kansas City,
School of Dentistry, Kansas City, Missouri

THOMAS M. LUND, D.D.S., M.S.

Professor and Head, Radiology Section,
Northwestern University School of Dentistry,
Chicago, Illinois

RUSSELL J. NISENGARD, D.D.S., Ph.D.

Professor of Periodontology and Microbiology,
State University of New York at Buffalo,
Schools of Dentistry and Medicine,
Buffalo, New York

**RAYMOND L. WARPEHA, D.D.S.,
M.D., Ph.D.**

Associate Professor, Department of Surgery;
Chairman, Division of Plastic Surgery,
Stritch School of Medicine, Loyola University,
Maywood, Illinois

Collaborators

DR. MANUEL REY GARCIA

Cirujano Dentista, Director de la Escuela
Nacional de Odontologiá, Ciudad Universitaria,
Mexico, D.F.

SOL GOLDMAN, D.D.S.

Assistant Professor of Oral Diagnosis,
Loyola University School of Dentistry,
Maywood, Illinois

MARIE C. JACOBS, D.D.S.

Associate Dean, Director of Clinical Affairs,
and Associate Professor, Department of
Oral Diagnosis, Loyola University
School of Dentistry,
Maywood, Illinois

ROGER H. KALLAL, D.D.S., M.S.

Associate Professor, Department of
Orthodontics, Northwestern University
Dental School; Attending Oral and
Maxillofacial Surgeon, Northwestern Memorial
Hospital; Private Practice of Oral Surgery and
Maxillofacial Surgery, Chicago, Illinois

LEON J. SCHWARTZ, D.D.S.

Associate Professor of Oral Diagnosis,
Loyola University School of Dentistry,
Maywood, Illinois

**ORION H. STUTEVILLE, D.D.S.,
M.D.S., M.D.**

Professor Emeritus of Surgery and
Former Chief, Section of Plastic Surgery,
Loyola University School of Medicine,
Maywood, Illinois

This effort is dedicated
to those who wage the battle against
oral disease in the private office,
clinic, and dental school—may it facilitate their
endeavors, as theirs have inspired ours.

Preface to second edition

The growth of knowledge may be compared to the ever-expanding ripples that are set in motion where a stone is dropped into a quiet body of water. Not surprisingly then, the interlude since the first edition of this book has witnessed the recognition of a significant number of new facts in the field of oral pathology. Such advances generate new concepts of etiology, differential diagnosis, and the behavior of lesions as well as their management. Hence the necessity for a new edition every few years is almost imperative.

A significant number of changes have been incorporated into this edition. The references with each chapter have been considerably expanded. Also the inventories of lesions with similar clinical and radiographic appearances have been amended and are now more complete. Significant reranking of lesions according to frequency was carried out on the basis of information from recent publications. Two hundred fifty new high-quality clinical and radiographic illustrations were added, as well as an additional color plate. Chapters 5, 6, 7, 9, 17, and 23 were extensively revised, and five new chapters were added. The earlier chapter on red lesions (oral mucositides) has been replaced by three new chapters in order to facilitate the differential diagnosis of these lesions. These are Chapter 10, "Solitary Red Lesions," Chapter 11, "Generalized Red Conditions," and Chapter 12, "Red Conditions of the Tongue." Chapter 23, "Mixed Radiolucent/Radiopaque Lesions Associated with Teeth" (peri-

apical and pericoronal), and Chapter 30, "Diseases of the Maxillary Sinus," are also new to this edition.

We are happy to acknowledge the help of the following people in efforts associated with this edition. Drs. Stuart L. Fischman and Russell J. Nisengard of the School of Dentistry at The State University of New York at Buffalo are contributors of the new chapter "Generalized Red Conditions." Mr. James Cockerill of the Visual Aids Department of Loyola University School of Dentistry very kindly provided us with excellent glossy prints. This group to which we are indebted also includes the considerable number of professional colleagues who very generously contributed excellent illustrations: courtesies are noted in the individual legends. We owe an expression of gratitude to Miss Sylvia Woodland and my wife Carole (N.K.W.) for the arduous and particular chore of typing the new manuscripts as well as the corrections and additions. In addition, Carole is responsible for the new line drawings.

We are particularly glad to have the opportunity to express our thanks to a number of our colleagues and students who have provided us with helpful criticisms of the first edition and for their suggestions on how to improve this effort. We hope that such helpful criticism will continue to flow.

Norman K. Wood
Paul W. Goaz

Preface to first edition

When one considers the many books presently catalogued as texts of oral diagnosis or oral medicine, the appearance of another effort in this area must surely be greeted with less than overwhelming enthusiasm. If one's survey of this situation, however, is slightly more analytical than a mere recitation of the titles of these textbooks, he is likely to conclude, as we did, that there is a need for another addition to this area of the literature.

The situation became apparent to us when we were faced with the responsibility of presenting two courses in oral diagnosis to the same class: an introductory course followed by a secondary endeavor of greater scope and depth. Little difficulty was encountered in selecting a text for the initial course, since several appeared to be well suited. For the second course in oral diagnosis, however, most of the available texts seemed unsuited to augment a course on the differential diagnosis of oral lesions. This dissatisfaction stemmed not only from the scope of the subjects covered in available texts but also from the organization of the material.

Consequently the preparation of this book was initially undertaken with the intention of filling a void in the instructive material for the "second course" in oral diagnosis for dental students, as well as for the general practitioner. While the work progressed, however, and as a result of comments from friends and colleagues, it also became apparent that our effort would be useful to the oral surgeon and to the oral pathology trainee.

The conception, implementation, development, and ultimately delivery of this book were achieved through the combined efforts of a large number of people. With any undertaking in an established field, present workers owe a great deal to the pioneers and developers who have gone before. We are no exception. We are deeply indebted to those giants who have developed oral diagnosis, oral medicine, oral pathology, and oral surgery to the disciplines they are today. In addition, we have benefitted greatly from many of the excellent textbooks and from papers published in several journals in these fields.

Nor should the immeasurable contributions of former teachers go unnoticed. Specifically, N. K. W. would like to express his deep thanks to four outstanding teachers under whom he has had the privilege of studying: Dr. Arthur Ham (Toronto, Ontario), Dr. H. M. Worth (Vancouver, British Columbia), Dr. Robert B. Shira (Boston, Massachusetts), and Dr. Orion H. Stuteville (Maywood, Illinois). He owes a particularly large debt to Dr. Stuteville, who has contributed so much to his understanding of oral lesions and their management.

Likewise, P. W. G. takes this opportunity to express the gratitude he feels for Dr. George W. Stuppy and Dr. J. Roy Blayney, who both played particularly important roles as teacher, advisor, confidant, and benefactor and who are directly responsible for the series of events that led to his participation in the composition of this book. He must also indicate his appreciation to N. K. W., who invited him to share this exciting and rewarding experience.

It is a pleasure to acknowledge our deep indebtedness to the contributors who have so freely given of their valuable time in authoring several of the chapters. Their contributions have given the book a much broader scope. These doctors are acknowledged in the list of contributors and also following the titles of the specific chapters.

We owe a large debt of gratitude to the many individuals who so kindly and generously provided illustrative materials from their personal collections. Acknowledgments have been made in the legends under each figure. Special thanks are due Dr. R. Goepp, Dr. E. Palacios, and Dr. O. H. Stuteville, who freely opened their files to us, from which we obtained a wealth of material.

Mrs. Danute Augius prepared some of the microscopic material that was used in the book, and we thank her for her fine work.

The line drawings were done by the careful and competent hands of Dr. Marie C. Jacobs and Mrs. Carole Wood. We are very much indebted to them for this important and difficult service.

A great debt of gratitude is owed the Visual Aids Department of Loyola University School of Dentistry. In particular we acknowledge our indebtedness to Mr. Robert Dienethal for his great service in the printing of the figures. Mr. Dienethal did an exceptional job in custom printing the radiographs. This is an especially particular and demanding chore, for which we thank him very much.

Special thanks also go to Miss Judy Napoleon and to Mrs. Phyllis Fine for typing the many rough drafts of the manuscript. Mrs. Carole Wood was responsible for the proofreading and the particularly arduous chore of typing the final manuscript. We owe a great deal to such a careful and willing worker.

Dr. Marshall H. Smulson carefully reviewed the chapter on periapical radiolucencies and offered many helpful comments. We thank him very much.

We wish to thank Dean A. Raffael Suriano and also former Dean William P. Schoen for doing everything possible to aid us in our task.

Many individuals have offered assistance in other ways and we gratefully acknowledge their help here.

Much of the logical sequence presented in this book evolved from intercourse with students over the years, and it illustrates that teaching is indeed a two-way street.

Of course, most of all, we owe the greatest gratitude to our wonderful wives, who patiently tolerated the last four years of neglect.

Norman K. Wood
Paul W. Goaz

Contents

xiii

COLOR PLATES

1, 2, 3, and 4

1

Introduction

The objective of this text is to present a systematic discussion of the differential diagnosis of oral lesions—based on a classification of lesions, which are grouped according to their similar clinical or radiographic appearances.

Part I consists of three *preparatory chapters:* Chapter 2 is devoted to a review of pertinent steps and modalities to follow in the examination of the patient. Chapter 3 explains on a functional and histologic basis the clinical and radiographic features of lesions discovered during the clinical examination. Chapter 4 outlines the diagnostic sequence preferred by us, commencing with the detection of the lesion and continuing progressively through intermediate steps until a final diagnosis is established.

Parts II and III make up the *differential diagnosis section* of the text, which deals with the specific disease entities: Part II is devoted primarily to the soft tissue lesions (Chapters 5 to 14), and Part III deals with lesions that originate in bone (Chapters 15 to 30). In each part the individual entities are classified into groups consisting of similar-appearing lesions, and each group forms the subject of a chapter.

Although our text is primarily for the clinician, the microscopic picture is also discussed; but the microscopic picture is stressed only when it contributes to the recognition and comprehension of the clinical or radiologic features. This approach evolved from our observation of dental students entering the clinic and encountering great difficulty as they attempted to relate their knowledge of histopathology to the clinical features of lesions. Apparently students experience this difficulty because of the following reasons. First, they are not adequately instructed in the simple but meaningful correlations between the histologic and clinical pictures. Second, they lack experience in the grouping of lesions according to clinical appearances, which is necessary before a usable differential diagnosis can be developed.

Of course, there are several excellent textbooks of oral pathology that might be expected to complement the clinical study of oral lesions; but these books classify and discuss lesions according to etiology, tissue of origin, microscopic nature, or areas of occurrence. Although such an approach has proved to be effective for presenting a course in pathology, in our experience it has been cumbersome for the fledgling clinician. In an attempt to alleviate this problem, we group and discuss lesions according to their clinical appearance. Regardless of etiology or area of occurrence, *all similar-appearing lesions are grouped together* and discussed in the same chapter. Not only has the usefulness of our approach been demonstrated in practice, but the efficiency of our effort might well be anticipated since the associations utilized for teaching the classification and recognition of clinical entities parallel the mental gymnastics one routinely employs in attempting to perceive and identify an unfamiliar object. Consequently the necessity of mentally reorganizing the material for effective recall is obviated.

The classic idea of the differential diagnosis seems to embody this natural ordering of information, and the same nature and sequential presentation of information may be successfully utilized in any endeavor to teach students to clinically apprehend and identify. We have attempted in the following chapters to arrange the presentation of what we consider the pertinent information in the same sequential manner.

Although our particular ranking of lesions in the ensuing pages may occasion the objection of some experts in various fields, no inerrant authority is claimed. We have attempted only to rank the entities in each category according to *frequency of occurrence*—with the discussion of the most common being first. The very rare lesions are simply listed. This particular arrangement is qualified as an impression that has developed from our personal experience and study as well as from our assessment of other authors' statistics.* It is not intended to be an authoritative statement but merely an aid to the clinician in the development of a differential diagnosis.

Our particular position regarding the ranking of lesions must be taken in the general context of this book since different frequency rates occur in different age groups and are modified by socioeconomics as well as by cultural and geographic factors. Also, when new cases are reported with each new issue of a journal, the rankings change; but we doubt that these changes will detract significantly from the usefulness of the arrangement presented here.

Those pathoses whose features are pathognomonic, and consequently do not generally present a problem in differential diagnosis, have not been included in this text since they do not, by their nature, fall within its objectives and are adequately discussed elsewhere.

Pathoses of the dental hard tissues, gingivitis, temporomandibular joint problems, and nonspecific facial and oral pain have been excluded since they also are adequately discussed elsewhere. In some cases entire books have been devoted to

---

*In this regard we are particularly indebted to Drs. Charles Halstead and Dwight Weathers of Emory University who have graciously made available to us statistical rankings from their extensive computerized study on the differential diagnosis of oral lesions.

these difficult and sometimes unresolved diagnostic problems.

At the same time it seems pertinent to point out that none of the discussions of entities included in this text are intended to be exhaustive descriptions of any disease but are intended only to present pertinent points that will help minimize confusion and contribute to the development of a differential diagnosis. Specifically we have not engaged in the detailed discussion of controversial questions concerning etiology and tissue origin when these subjects are in doubt since they likewise have been exhaustively discussed in other sources and contribute little that is clinically useful to the inexperienced clinician.

Also the discussions of the features of particular lesions have not been specifically subdivided on the basis of clinical, radiographic, and histologic characteristics. On the contrary, these have been blended together in an attempt to illustrate how the three disciplines interrelate and aid in the explanation of the features found in each.

Again the primary aim of this book is to provide the clinician with the pertinent features of relatively common oral diseases that we consider necessary to differentiate between similar-appearing lesions.

The diagnoses that appear in the descriptions of the reproduction of the clinical pictures and radiographs have been determined by microscopic examination in the vast majority of cases.

Part I

GENERAL PRINCIPLES OF DIFFERENTIAL DIAGNOSIS

2

History and examination of the patient

Charles C. Alling III

Industry's *decision seminar*, the law's *memorandum*, the military's *estimate of the situation*, and even an individual's *planning and budgeting* are all processes that are used to arrive at and then pursue a correct course of action. In the medical arts and sciences the process is *the history and examination*. These procedures embrace many inquiries and activities, including the physical and other examinations. Properly and conscientiously performed, the medical history and physical examination are the very best of the diagnostic aids. Without a comprehensive history and a properly performed examination of his patient, the doctor will become merely a hit-or-miss technician. These diagnostic procedures include the following:

History
    Identifying data
    Chief complaint
    Present illness
    Past medical history [if necessary]
        Family history
        Social history
        Occupational history
        Dental history
    Review of symptoms by systems
Physical examination
Radiologic examination
Differential diagnosis
Working diagnosis
    Medical laboratory studies
    Dental laboratory studies
    Biopsy
    Consultation
Final diagnosis
Treatment plan
Signature [of the physician]

HISTORY

For the majority of patients, a complete history is not necessary. In the case of any particular patient, however, and regardless of the complaint, the doctor must be aware of the great amount of useful information the history may produce. Only through the added advantage of a thorough history can the clinician most effectively correlate his learned facts, experience, and observations from the patient; and only then can he hope to achieve a consistency in arriving at the proper conclusion.

It should not be overlooked that during contact with the patient one will be able to identify useful indicators that will permit an assessment of mental status. While a proper history is being obtained and a physical examination is being performed, the doctor is usually provided with a rare and valuable insight into the patient's psyche. Certain mucosal lesions, many chronic maxillofacial pains, and some craniofacial myofascial problems may be related to motivational depressions. An accurate history will help to demonstrate the related psychic overtones and keep the doctor from prescribing a remedy that provides only transient relief and that may prove to be just another failure in a series of mutilating procedures.

A particularly important benefit from taking a history is the therapeutic effect that accrues to the patient in identifying the clinician as "his" or "her" doctor. Frequently a sincere rapport is established on which a meaningful doctor-patient relationship can be developed. A genuine sympathetic attitude on the part of the doctor is essen-

5

tial to the acquisition of an adequate history and to ensure that the patient will benefit from both the history and the therapy.

Identifying data

It may be useful, in the dynamics of patient management, to introduce the patient to your practice by having a courteous and personable receptionist obtain administrative and identifying data from him. This would include the following:

1. Name and address
2. Birth date
3. Sex
4. Principal racial or ethnic backgrounds
5. Occupation and address
6. Name and address of
   a. Informant, if other than the patient
   b. Referring source
   c. Family physician
   d. Family dentist or former dentist
   e. Third party health care provider
7. Other data (This may be tailored to a particular practice that will contribute to the health management of the patient. Medicolegal release and consent forms may be completed as the active therapy progresses.)

Some doctors and hospitals have the new patient sign a blanket consent for any procedure that may be determined necessary. However, it is recommended that the patient sign consent for only specific operations and that the consent be stated in terms that the patient understands, including the risks.

Chief complaint

The chief complaint should be recorded, if at all possible, in the patient's own words. It is the response to the doctor's question, "What problem brought you to see me?" Obviously in some instances, instead of the expression in the words of the patient, the notation will be made: "The patient was referred by Dr. John Doe for management of . . ."

If there are two or more chief complaints, number them on the history sheet and then pursue the applicable history of each complaint. If one complaint predominates in the patient's mind, and one usually will, it should be identified as such. The most successful management of the patient will result if his chief complaint is treated and corrected.

Present illness

Using the patient's own words when they are expressive and contributory, analyze the chief or primary complaints in the present illness sepa-

rately and, if possible, in the order of development according to a format.

Onset. State in terms of days or time before the appointment or admission when the current complaint was first noted. Use calendar dates. Do not write, "The patient noted a painful, bleeding gingivitis last Tuesday"; record instead, "Six days before admission or this appointment (which will be dated) the patient noted . . ." Include a notation of what the patient was doing at the time of onset and what, if anything, may have precipitated the signs and symptoms.

Course. A summary statement should be included that describes the progress of the entity since the initiation of the chief complaint. For example, symptoms may be described as intermittent, recurrent, constant, increasing, or decreasing in severity. Aggravating and alleviating factors should be identified. If pain is the major complaint, permit the patient to express it in familiar terms. Be very careful not to influence his description, but a number of terms may be suggested to permit adequate verbalization.

Adjectives that may be used to describe pain include the following:

throbbing	sharp	constricting
pounding	lancinating	squeezing
splitting	stabbing	gripping
bursting	cutting	tight
exploding	bright	scorching
heavy	boring	searing
dull	gnawing	hot
pressing	burning	
aching	cramping	

Previous treatment. Determine what was done, when, where, why, and by whom, and note the outcome of prior treatments.

The directed questions in the preceding suggested format should be employed if they are necessary to adequately describe the present illness. It may be that a spontaneous approach will be indicated in which the patient simply tells his tale with only an occasional remark by the doctor to encourage him to proceed and to direct him in providing certain pertinent information.

Past medical history

Past medical history may be handled in toto through a direct interview by the doctor, or forms may be used (Fig. 2-1) on which the patient initially supplies the indicated information and the doctor subsequently expands those areas that require amplification by direct questioning. Some-

CHARLES C. ALLING, DDS

PATIENT'S NAME: _____ AGE: _____ SEX: _____ RACE: _____

INFORMANT: _____ DATE: _____ CLINIC NO.: _____

CLOSEST RELATIVE: _____ PHONE _____

PAST MEDICAL HISTORY

NO	YES	COMMENTS
☐ Care of physician? (who, why)	☐	
☐ Serious illnesses?	☐	
☐ Serious injuries?	☐	
☐ Hospital admissions?	☐	
☐ Operations? (what, when, where)	☐	
☐ Transfusions? (why, when)	☐	
☐ Pregnancies? (past, present)	☐	
☐ Allergies? (food, drugs, other)	☐	
☐ Present medications (kinds, dosage)	☐	
☐ Illicit drugs (quality, quantity)	☐	
☐ Alcohol (quality, quantity)	☐	
☐ Tobacco (quality, quantity)	☐	

LAST PHYSICAL EXAMINATION: _____ DATE: _____ WHY: _____

REVIEW OF SYSTEMS

NEG		POS	COMMENTS
CARDIOVASCULAR:			
☐	Angina pectoris	☐	
☐	Myocardial infarction	☐	
☐	Congenital heart defect	☐	
☐	Rheumatic fever	☐	
☐	Rheumatic heart disease	☐	
☐	Murmurs	☐	
☐	Hypertension	☐	
☐	Stroke	☐	
☐	Other:	☐	
RESPIRATORY			
☐	Tuberculosis	☐	
☐	Emphysema	☐	
☐	Asthma	☐	
☐	Shortness of breath	☐	
☐	Dyspnea on exertion	☐	
☐	Orthopnea	☐	
☐	Edema	☐	
☐	Other:	☐	
GASTROINTESTINAL/LIVER			
☐	Ulcers	☐	
☐	Bleeding	☐	
☐	Hepatitis	☐	
☐	Jaundice	☐	
☐	Cirrhosis	☐	
☐	Other:	☐	

NEG		POS	COMMENTS
ENDOCRINE:			
☐	Diabetes	☐	
☐	Adrenal disorders	☐	
☐	Thyroid disorders	☐	
☐	Parathyroid disorders	☐	
☐	Steroids	☐	
☐	Other:	☐	
GENITOURINARY:			
☐	Kidney Infections	☐	
☐	Venereal disease	☐	
☐	Other:	☐	
HEMATOPOIETIC			
☐	Anemia	☐	
☐	Bleeding disorders	☐	
☐	Anticoagulants	☐	
☐	Leukemia	☐	
☐	Other:	☐	
NEUROLOGIC:			
☐	Epilepsy	☐	
☐	Convulsions	☐	
☐	Psychiatric treatment	☐	
☐	Faints/Spells	☐	
☐	Tranquilizers	☐	
☐	Other:	☐	

Fig. 2-1. Health questionnaire form.

times the past medical history is combined with a review of systems (Fig. 2-1).

The past medical history should include the following assessments:

1. General health of the patient before the chief complaint
2. Previous history and results of physical examinations
3. Idiosyncrasies to pharmacotherapeutic agents
4. Allergies, including sensitivities and reactions to antibiotics, analgesics, anesthetics, sedatives, tranquilizers, and topical agents
5. Previous operations and results
6. Previous injuries and results
7. Previous hospitalizations and results
8. Other histories (family, social, occupational, dental)

FAMILY HISTORY

The family history is important in the case of patients who are suspected or known to have diabetes, tuberculosis, hemophilia, cancer, one of the anemias, allergic diseases, cardiovascular-respiratory diseases, and diseases of the nervous, renal, digestive, and musculoskeletal systems.

SOCIAL HISTORY

The social history will help to identify psychosomatic imbalances that otherwise would be recognized only as somatic symptoms.

Practically all the maxillofacial maladies are reflected, to a greater or lesser degree, in the patient's psyche; and the patient usually strongly identifies the mouth and face as *his* image. Although he may be going to a dentist for somatic treatments, during the taking of the history, he may well make statements and nuances indicating whether psychic depressions are significant factors contributing to his complaint. The following physiologic symptoms are indicative of many actual psychic maladies and may, of course, help identify depressions: sleep disturbance, appetite disturbance, constipation or diarrhea, low back pain, fatigue, decreased pleasure, oral mucosal inflammations and ulcerations, burning tongue, xerostomia, altered taste.

As the history and physical examination proceed, if the patient shows signs of sadness, of considering himself worthless, or of having a negative outlook on life, then the identification of a depression becomes more certain. On the other hand, a patient may display either no evidence of depression or a low order of depression, may have a "can-do" attitude, and may actually do many things well—including describe his chief complaint(s) of oral lesions and maladies. He may also regard his chief complaints of oral lesions and maladies in a more balanced and rational context, which will in turn simplify their treatment.

Of course, active dental or oral therapy for an imagined or magnified complaint in a psychosomatically disabled patient will probably be doomed to failure. Consultation with the family physician, psychiatrist, or psychologist is usually indicated when such psychologically troubled patients are encountered.

OCCUPATIONAL HISTORY

The occupational history is important whenever the physical environment may have produced oral or skeletal lesions, as in the mining industry. Furthermore, if the occupation produces emotional strains and stresses, these may be reflected in the oral cavity by a variety of mucosal and gingival inflammations.

DENTAL HISTORY

As the patient interprets it, the dental history will reveal the success of previous dental treatments and the treatment plans that have been undertaken on his behalf.

Review of symptoms by systems

There are a number of approaches that may be employed for the review of symptoms by systems. One approach is to review the symptoms on a regional basis, actually cutting across the major body systems; but this is not recommended. Such a review may lump together the head and neck, chest, abdomen, and limbs and then consider the heart and lungs, digestive tract, and genitourinary and other systems.

A more logical approach is to review the symptoms system by system. This method in essence is based on the patient's responses to questions (either verbal or written) relative to the condition of, or complaints about, the following:

Weight
Amount and date of maximum and minimum weights
Reasons for changes
Optimum weight
Present weight

Strength
Unusual fatigue and when it occurred
Change in physical activity

Eyes
Presence or absence of glasses and contact lenses

Recent changes in vision
Recent inflammation or lacrimation

Ears, nose, and throat
Pain
Hearing changes
Tinnitus
Sinus disease
Mucous discharge
Bloody discharge
Nasal obstructions
Voice change
Sore throat
Tonsillitis

Oral cavity
Inflammations
Neoplasms
Cystic lesions
Developmental or congenital deformities
Occlusal changes
Masses in the upper neck
Habits that might affect lips, tongue, and oral soft and
   hard tissues

Heart and blood vessels
Peripheral vessels

Respiratory system

Stomach and intestines
Usual diet and unusual substitutions (alcohol, candy,
   starches)
Appetite
Nausea and vomiting
Unusual eructation
Diarrhea and constipation
Color and consistency of stools
History of jaundice
Amount of water consumed per day

Genitourinary organs

Hematopoietic system

Skin
Bruises
Itching and rashes

Extremities and joints
History of arthritis
Spontaneous fractures

Nervous system
Tremors
Convulsions
Anesthesias, paresthesias, and paralyses
Muscular pains

Endocrine system

Psyche

PHYSICAL EXAMINATION

The examination of any portion of the body consists of four modalities: inspection, palpation, percussion, and auscultation. These four words and the procedures that they represent have stood the test of time. They are words that doctors around the world can use for communicating with clarity. They describe every type of examination. Even as a hammer is the extension of an arm, an automobile is an extension of the legs, and computers are extensions of the brain, so laboratory studies and tests, consultations, biopsies, and radiographic examinations are extensions of these four basic modalities of performing a physical examination.

The regional physical examination of the oral and maxillofacial tissues and contiguous regions may be recorded in any of several different formats. For simplicity, as well as completeness, standardized forms are used by many doctors (Fig. 2-2). After the usual identifying data has been gathered, the initial signs are recorded, and then a routine is followed of appropriate inspection, palpation, percussion, and auscultation of the various regions and structures of the oral and maxillofacial regions.

In recent years the dental profession has become aware of the importance of taking blood pressure readings. This is particularly necessary when examining new patients as well as when examining or treating patients who are currently under treatment for hypertension. Table 2-1 gives the generally accepted normal range for systolic and diastolic blood pressure within various patient groups.

Table 2-1. Normal range for systolic and diastolic blood pressure

	Prepuberty female (5-15 yr)	Adult female	Prepuberty male (5-15 yr)	Adult male
Blood pressure	105 ($\pm$16)/57 ($\pm$9)	120 ($\pm$18)/75 ($\pm$14)	105 ($\pm$16)/57 ($\pm$9)	126 ($\pm$17)/79 ($\pm$13)
Pulse (per min)	75-100	60-90	75-100	60-90
Respiration (per min)	18-20	12-15	18-20	12-15
Oral temperature (F)	97.8-98.6	97-99	97.8-98.6	97-99
Oral temperature (C)	36.6-37	36.1-37.2	36.6-37	36.1-37.2

CHARLES C. ALLING, DDS

PHYSICAL EXAMINATION

PATIENT'S NAME:_____ REG. NO._____

INFORMANT (if other than patient)_____

A. General appearance and findings _____

B. Prostheses, health aids or appliances_____

C. Vital signs: BP_____ , P_____ , R _____ , Wgt_____ , Hgt_____ , Age _____

NORMAL D. Craniofacial skeleton	ABNORMAL	COMMENT		NORMAL F. Intraoral tissues	ABNORMAL	COMMENT
1. ☐ Cephalic index	☐		1. ☐ Breath	☐	
2. ☐ Orthognathic relations	☐		2. ☐ Saliva	☐	
3. ☐ TMJ	☐		3. ☐ Lips	☐	
4. ☐ Other	☐		4. ☐ Commissures	☐	
			5. ☐ Buccal mucosa	☐	
			6. ☐ Retromolar areas	☐	
NORMAL E. Extraoral tissues	ABNORMAL	COMMENT	7. ☐ Pharynx	☐	
			8. ☐ Soft palate	☐	
1. ☐ Cutaneous tissues	☐		9. ☐ Hard palate	☐	
2. ☐ Auricular structures	☐		10. ☐ Tongue	☐	
3. ☐ Ocular structures	☐		11. ☐ Floor of mouth	☐	
4. ☐ Nasal structures	☐		12. ☐ Gingiva	☐	
5. ☐ Sinal structures	☐		13. ☐ Occlusal relations	☐	
6. ☐ Thyroid cartilage	☐		14. ☐ Other	☐	
7. ☐ Thyroid gland	☐				
8. ☐ Trachea	☐				
9. ☐ Cervical chains	☐				
10. ☐ Parotid space	☐				

G. Preventive dentistry

  1. Oral hygiene
       ___ Poor   ___Average   ___Excellent
  2. Dental health motivation
       ___ Poor   ___ Average   ___ Excellent
  3. Previous dental care
       ___ Poor   ___ Average   ___ Excellent
  4. Nutrition
       ___ Poor   ___ Average   ___ Excellent

E. Extraoral tissues (continued)		
11. ☐ Submandibular spaces	☐	
12. ☐ Submental triangle	☐	
13. ☐ Salivary glands	☐	
14. ☐ Myofascial tissues	☐	
15. ☐ Neurological	☐	
16. ☐ Other	☐	

Fig. 2-2. Physical examination form.

RADIOLOGIC EXAMINATION

All too often, even before the history and physical examination have been obtained, a radiograph is the first procedure completed for a patient in the dental office. Although many unsuspected pathoses are discovered by routine radiography, the primary role of radiographs is to confirm clinical impressions. (See discussion of features obtained by palpation, Chapter 3.) Consequently the radiographic examination should follow the completion of the history and physical examination so only the views that will contribute to the recognition of the malady will be secured. In addition, the following strict admonition should be noted: Radiographs should never be accepted as the sole criterion for an operation.

Views that are appropriate for the study of oral and perioral lesions and that may be made with a dental radiographic unit include the following:

1. High-definition intraoral views, commonly called periapical films
2. Occlusal views
3. Extraoral views of the jaws
   a. Transparietal projection
      (1) Temporomandibular joint (Fig. 2-3, A)
   b. Transpharyngeal projection
      (1) Head and neck of the condyle (Fig. 2-3, B)
   c. Oblique lateral projections
      (1) Posterior body and ramus of the mandible (Fig. 2-3, C)
      (2) Body of the mandible (Fig. 2-3, D)
      (3) Anterior body of the mandible (Fig. 2-3, E)
      These views can be made as the head is rotated toward the cassette until the nose touches the plate.
4. Skull and facial bone series
   a. Cephalometric projections
      (1) Anteroposterior (or posteroanterior)
      (2) Lateral
   b. Anteroposterior (or posteroanterior) projection
      (1) Mandible, paranasal sinuses, and lateral facial bones
      With simple accessories to position the film and the head of the x-ray machine, these views can be readily obtained.

Many dental offices are equipped with x-ray machines that provide panoramic views of the mandible and lower portions of the maxilla. Care must be taken with the interpretation of these views, however, because they have a laminagraphic effect and only a given plane may be recorded with clarity. Thus structures or objects not in this plane may be distorted and only partly seen. Also the panoramic machines are calibrated for a given facial size and follow a predetermined course; adjustments are possible, but distortions may occur.

DIFFERENTIAL DIAGNOSIS

After the foregoing procedures the differential diagnosis should be arranged in the doctor's mind

Fig. 2-3. Grouped photographs illustrating positions of the x-ray tube and patient necessary for the various views and resultant radiographic pictures. **A,** Transparietal projection for the temporomandibular joint in closed and open positions. *Continued.*

Fig. 2-3, cont'd. B, Transpharyngeal projection for the temporomandibular joint. **C,** Posterior body of the mandible and ramus. **D,** Body of the mandible. **E,** Incisor region of the mandible.

and listed in his records on a priority basis, with the most probable lesion listed first (Chapter 4).

In many if not most instances, there will be only one clear-cut diagnosis and the treatment plan can be based on this conclusion without any additional diagnostic procedures. If the final diagnosis is not absolutely clear, however, the possibilities must be considered further through medical laboratory studies, dental laboratory studies, biopsy, consultation, and a renewed consideration of the chief complaint, present illness, histories, review of symptoms, and findings from the physical examination.

WORKING DIAGNOSIS

After completion of these procedures, approaches, and techniques, the accumulated data should permit the clinician to narrow the range of his differential diagnosis and arrive at a no. 1 choice, his working or tentative diagnosis.

Medical laboratory studies

Indicated tests are performed after the history has been secured and the physical examination has been completed. Frequently values obtained from such tests are helpful in establishing the final diagnosis. The summaries and interpretation of the laboratory tests discussed next will provide an overview of the information that can be obtained from these procedures.

Complete blood count. The complete blood count usually includes tests that have the potential of revealing a vast number of abnormal systemic conditions, some of which may be related to oral lesions. A stained smear of a blood sample can be prepared for a differential leukocyte count and for an examination of the erythrocyte and platelet morphology. Alterations in the size, shape, and hemoglobin content of erythrocytes can be determined, and an estimate of the platelet number can be made from the microscopic examination of the smear.

Total leukocyte count. Leukocytes are important in the defense of the body against invading microorganisms, since they combat most harmful bacteria. An increase (leukocytosis) is the most common alteration in the count and is usually interpreted to indicate the presence of a systemic infection. It may also be observed after general anesthesia and in such conditions as emotional upsets and blood dyscrasias. A decrease in the number of leukocytes (leukopenia) may also be seen in blood dyscrasias, overwhelming infections, and drug and chemical toxicoses.

Differential leukocyte count. The several types

of leukocytes can be identified microscopically. Each of these cell types normally makes up an average percentage of the total leukocyte count. The normal range of the count is 5000/ml to 10,000/ml. The normal percentages of the individual leukocytes in the differential count range as follows: neutrophils, 54% to 62%; lymphocytes, 25% to 33%; monocytes, 3% to 7%; eosinophils, 1% to 3%; and basophils, 0% to 1%. It is often helpful to know whether the proportions of these cells in the blood have changed, inasmuch as the changes may be indicative of a particular group of diseases. For instance, neutrophils are increased in most bacterial infections. Eosinophils may be increased in parasitic infestations and allergic conditions. Basophils may be increased in some blood dyscrasias. Lymphocytes may be increased in measles and in most chronic bacterial infections. Monocytes may be increased during recovery from severe infections, Hodgkin's disease, and lipid storage diseases.

Often the type of infectious agent and the course of the disease may be determined by studying the leukocyte count and differential values taken on successive days. It is recognized that a leukocytosis caused only by a moderate increase in the neutrophil fraction indicates an acute bacterial infection. On the other hand, a leukocytosis accompanied by a moderate increase in the lymphocyte fraction (lymphocytosis) suggests a chronic infection, either bacterial or fungal. A leukocytosis of over 20,000/ml strongly suggests the presence of leukemia.

The following method is useful for determining the course of patients with acute bacterial infections. As described, such patients may have a leukocytosis caused mainly by an increase in the neutrophil fraction:

1. There will usually be an increase in the percentage of immature neutrophils, and such a picture is described as a *shift to the left*. If serial values are determined, daily changes in the leukocyte count and differential will be apparent.

2. If the total leukocyte count is found to increase along with a concomitant rise in the neutrophil fraction, which shows an increase in the percentage of juvenile (immature) forms, the change is referred to as a *regenerative shift to the left*. Such a patient is said to be responding favorably because his marrow is able to produce an increased number of leukocytes to combat the infection.

3. If the total leukocyte count is decreasing

along with an increase in the immature forms, however, this is referred to as a *degenerative shift to the left*. Such a patient's condition is deteriorating because the infectious process is destroying the leukocytes faster than his marrow can produce them.

Platelet count. The number of platelets normally ranges between 150,000/ml and 450,000/ml of blood. They have many functions that are still undergoing investigation and definition. Mature effective platelets are necessary for coagulation of the blood and for clot retraction to be effective. Consequently, when the platelet count is low, the bleeding time can be expected to be prolonged. On the other hand, a platelet count provides information only about the quantity of platelets in the blood, and hemostatic disturbances may in fact be caused by a defect in the quality of the platelets. Although there are a number of blood disorders of dental interest in which the platelet count is normal, an increase may be the result of polycythemia vera, fractures, hemolytic anemia, or chronic myelocytic leukemia; and a decrease may be the result of thrombocytopenic purpura, pernicious anemia, aplastic anemia, or acute and chronic leukemias.

Hemoglobin concentration. Hemoglobin is the essential oxygen carrier of the blood, and in adults the normal range is 12 to 18 g/100 ml. Women usually have slightly lower values than men. The hemoglobin is decreased in hemorrhage and anemias and is increased in hemoconcentration (increase in the erythrocyte content of the blood or decrease in the water content of the blood). Polycythemia is an example of an excess of erythrocytes in the blood.

The hemoglobin concentration and erythrocyte count do not always rise or fall equally. This fact is often important in the differential diagnosis of anemias. In iron deficiency (microcytic) anemia the hemoglobin concentration is reduced more than the erythrocyte count; and in pernicious anemia the erythrocyte count is reduced more than the hemoglobin concentration. Most elective general anesthetics are not administered to patients with a hemoglobin concentration of less than 10 g/100 ml.

Hematocrit. This test measures the percentage volume occupied by the packed erythrocytes in relation to the total volume of the blood. The normal range is 40% to 54% in men and 37% to 47% in women. The percentages are raised in polycythemia, oxygen deficiency states, and dehydration.

• • •

In the usual dental setting the hematocrit, the hemoglobin concentration, and the erythrocyte count are used as measures of the oxygen-carrying capacity of the blood. Consequently only one of these tests is usually ordered.

Bleeding time. The bleeding time is the measure of the ability of capillary blood vessels to contract, or retract, after cutting and to retain a plug of coagulated blood. Thus, when there is an injury to bone or an injury in tissue with a great amount of collagen, there may be a prolonged bleeding time since there will be a lack of soft tissue into which the blood vessel can retract.

In general, the time required for bleeding to stop is related to the manner in which the wound was produced, the caliber of the vessel involved, the amount of tissue damage adjacent to the wound, and the systemic blood pressure. Consequently, although an abnormal bleeding time is not necessarily diagnostic of any particular type of hemostatic disorder, a dental patient with an abnormal bleeding time is going to require a more detailed hematological workup than usual. In a patient with hemophilia, the bleeding time may be within the normal range because of normal contraction and retraction of the blood vessels; but the lack of the ability of the patient's blood to clot would prevent formation of a mature coagulum, and hemorrhage would persist from a wound.

The upper limit of the normal bleeding time, determined by the Ivy technique, is 4 minutes. With other procedures, such as the Duke earlobe method, values as high as 7 to 8 minutes are regarded as normal.

Clotting time. The potential of the blood to form a mature coagulum within an appropriate time frame indicates a normal clotting time. A coagulation time of 6 to 17 minutes, determined by the Lee-White method, is considered normal. Abnormal values from this test may be indicative of a number of blood dyscrasias, such as (1) deficiencies of antihemophilic globulin, plasma thromboplastin component, or plasma thromboplastin antecedent and (2) fibrinogenemia. It is now possible for the hematologist to pinpoint the missing or deficient factors in the clotting mechanism by utilizing various tests; and the clinician can thereby frequently correct some of these coagulation disorders by administering the deficient factors.

Prothrombin time (PT). The PT test is an indirect measure of the capacity of the blood to clot. In the clotting process prothrombin is converted to thrombin. When the prothrombin level of the blood is lower than normal, the clotting tendency of the blood within the blood vessels is believed to be diminished. An abnormal PT may be indicative of deficiencies in the following blood factors: prothrombin, fibrinogen, and stable and labile factors. The prothrombin content of the blood is lowered in liver diseases, hypoprothrombinemia of infants, and vitamin K deficiency and after therapy with some drugs. The majority of cases of low blood prothrombin result from the administration of Dicumarol and similar drugs. These substances are given to reduce the clotting tendency of the blood and thus avoid thromboembolic phenomena. The PT test is often ordered daily during the acute stages of myocardial infarction, when accurate results are needed promptly to enable the physician to determine the size of the next dose of anticoagulant. The normal PT is usually reported as 11 to 13 seconds, with a normal control of 12 seconds.

Partial thromboplastin time (PTT). Since the PT test bypasses the intrinsic clotting system and the whole blood–clotting time is insensitive to all but gross deficiencies of coagulation, there is need for a simple procedure to detect mild to moderate deficiencies of the intrinsic clotting factors. When a crude phospholipid test extract (partial thromboplastin) is mixed with plasma, the mixture normally clots in 60 to 90 seconds, as compared with the normal PT of 11 to 13 seconds. A patient with factor VII deficiency will have a normal partial thromboplastin time (PTT) and a prolonged PT. Another use for the PTT is to demonstrate a circulating anticoagulant in plasma. Since variations in technique are widespread, the normal range for the PTT varies somewhat between laboratories; and results are usually expressed in seconds (e.g., "as compared with a normal of . . . seconds").

• • •

The PT and PTT tests examine the *extrinsic* and *intrinsic* clotting systems. They do not detect platelet disorders but merely screen for a possible bleeding diathesis. If the history warrants, a platelet count and bleeding time should be obtained to complete the initial evaluation.

Blood glucose. This test is performed to discover whether there is a disorder in glucose metabolism. The glucose concentration in whole blood is normally between 50 and 150 mg/100 ml; 10% to 15% higher in plasma. An increase in the blood glucose level is found in uncontrolled diabetes, chronic liver disease, and overactivity of a number of the endocrine glands. In mild diabetes there may be a normal glucose level; so if diabetes is suspected, more sensitive tests, such as the glucose tolerance test, must be performed. There may be a decrease in blood glucose in the case of tumors of the islets of Langerhans, underfunctioning of various endocrine glands, glycogen storage disease (von Gierke's), and overtreatment with insulin.

Blood urea nitrogen (BUN). The BUN test is a test of kidney function. Ordinarily the kidneys readily excrete urea, the end product of protein metabolism. Thus the blood urea concentration is usually fairly low. In certain kidney disorders, however, the ability of the kidneys to excrete urea may be impaired and the concentration of urea nitrogen in the blood then increases. Normal range for urea nitrogen is 9 to 20 mg/100 ml of blood. Though commonly used as a screening test for kidney function, the BUN test is not specific; if renal disease is suspected, evaluation of serum creatinine and the ratio of BUN to creatinine (normally 10:1) offer a more reliable assessment of renal status.

Serology. The serologic tests for syphilis measure the antibodies and other substances in the serum that increase in concentration after infection with *Treponema pallidum*. There are several varieties of these tests: Wasserman, Kolmer, Kahn, Hinton, Mazzini, reactive plasma reagin, and Venereal Disease Research Laboratory (VDRL) tests.

These serologic tests are quite sensitive and are dependable as screening procedures. Because of their nonspecific nature, however, they sometimes give positive results for diseases other than syphilis. Interpretation of the results from these tests therefore usually requires considerable skill and experience as well as correlation with the clinical findings and history. Positive reactions should be confirmed by the fluorescent treponemal antibody (FTA) test. In early primary syphilis the serologic tests are negative; but, as the lesions heal, the titer starts to rise. In secondary syphilis there is a high serologic titer. After adequate treatment of early syphilis, the titer will usually become nonreactive; but after adequate treatment of late syphilis, it will remain active indefinitely or will decrease slowly over a period of years, even though the lesions have healed and no further damage is occurring.

Urinalysis. A routine urinalysis will include a description of the macroscopic appearance of the urine, a microscopic examination, and a determination of the pH, specific gravity, sugar, albumin, and acetone content of the urine.

Normally samples of freshly voided urine are clear. Less acid urines may become cloudy on standing, however, because of the precipitation of phosphates. The odor of normal urine is characteristically faintly aromatic, and there is a wide variation in color. Highly dilute urine is a light straw color, whereas concentrated urine may be reddish yellow.

The microscopic examination of the urinary sediments may reveal important information about the condition of the urinary tract. There may be few erythrocytes per high-power field. Menstrual blood may be found in the urine of women. A specimen from a catheterized patient may contain erythrocytes because of urethral bleeding from the trauma of inserting the catheter. When an unusual number of unexplainable erythrocytes are encountered, further studies should be undertaken to determine the exact source of the blood. Leukocytes in the urine of men or in specimens from catheterized women suggest infection of the urinary tract. Casts in the urine suggest some disorder of the kidney tubules. The casts are formed by the precipitation of protein in the lumen of the distal portion of the nephron. These casts may be of variable composition; a hyaline precipitate may be mixed with blood cells or their debris, lipid, hemoglobin, or other cellular debris.

Normally there are not more than two or three erythrocytes per high-power field and very few leukocytes in the urine of men. In the urine of women of menstrual age, however, substantial quantities of both erythrocytes and leukocytes may be found. A few casts may be present normally, but a large number of casts suggest kidney disease.

Blood in the urine. Macroscopically apparent blood in the urine may appear as intact erythrocytes (hematuria) or dissolved hemoglobin derived from destroyed erythrocytes (hemoglobinuria). Since the hematuria can be the result of bleeding anywhere along the urinary tract between glomeruli and urethra, the site and cause of bleeding must be determined by more precise testing methods. Hemoglobinuria usually arises from conditions outside the urinary tract. The red cells are hemolyzed, and the dissolved hemoglobin in the plasma is excreted by the kidney. It is seen in severe burns, transfusion reactions, severe malaria, poisoning, and paroxysmal hemoglobinuria.

A normal finding would be no blood in the urine.

pH of the urine. pH is a measure of the degree of acidity or alkalinity of the urine. The kidneys maintain the blood at the correct pH by excreting into the urine any excess ions that might alter the pH of the blood. The urinary pH therefore varies widely, and changes do not indicate an abnormality. The kidneys may excrete urine with a pH value as low as 4.5 and as high as 8.2 under extreme conditions. The mean pH of the normal mixed 24-hour specimen, however, is about 6.0. Sometimes it is desirable to have an acid or alkaline urine; and in such cases the pH measurement is important.

For instance, when certain sulfa drugs are administered or when there is a marked hemolysis or destruction of muscle tissue, an alkaline urine is desirable since the sulfa drugs and products of hemolysis and muscle destruction are quite soluble in alkaline urine. In contrast, when the patient is being treated with certain urinary tract antiseptics, an acid urine is needed; but in bladder infections the urine may become highly alkaline because the bacteria transform urea into ammonia.

Specific gravity of the urine. The specific gravity urine test measures the ability of the kidneys to concentrate and dilute urine and thus gives an indication of their functional capacity. The specific gravity of urine normally varies between 1.015 and 1.025 but is subject to wide fluctuations under various conditions. Ordinarily the specific gravity rises when the fluid intake is low and falls when the intake is high. Inadequate concentration or dilution of urine indicates some disorder involving the kidney tubules.

Sugar in the urine. In some disorders sugar is found in the urine. This occurs most often in diabetes mellitus but may also occur in other metabolic disorders of varying importance. Because of its simplicity the sugar test is often used as a screening procedure to discover diabetes. Urine normally contains a variety of substances that reduce sugar reagents and thus give false-positive reactions.

If the reduction test is positive, other tests should be ordered to determine how much of the material giving the positive reaction is actually sugar. In normal nonfasting individuals the quantity of glucose present averages 140 mg/24-hour specimen, but there may be considerable variation. Normally there is no glucose in the urine of fasting individuals.

Albumin in the urine. Ordinarily the albumin in the blood does not pass through the glomerular walls into the urine. In several conditions, however, such as kidney disease, hypertension, severe heart failure, and drug toxicosis, albumin appears in the urine. In 5% to 15% of normal individuals, small amounts of albumin are sometimes found in the urine. This has been termed orthostatic or postural albuminuria. Since the test is not specific, a positive result indicates that more precise tests are needed.

Acetone in the urine. The acetone test is important in the diagnosis of ketosis, a type of acidosis produced by faulty metabolism. Normally there is no acetone in the urine. In a condition such as diabetes, however, sugar is not utilized properly and an excess of body fat is metabolized. The fatty acids are broken down into acetoacetic acid and β-hydroxybutyric acid; and because these cannot be completely disposed of by the tissues in the presence of impaired carbohydrate metabolism, they are converted to acetone—which is then excreted by the kidneys. Acetone in the urine indicates a general disorder of metabolism. The patient may exhibit symptoms of depression of the central nervous system.

Chest radiograph and electrocardiogram (ECG). A chest radiograph and an ECG should be ordered for any patient with a history of pulmonary or cardiovascular disease, especially if he has not been examined within the last 6 months. In addition, symptoms or physical findings may indicate that these tests should be obtained. Any patient over age 40 should have a chest radiograph and an ECG annually.

Dental laboratory studies

The fabrication and analysis of articulated models of the dental arches and the attendant records are an integral part of the examination of many patients. Metabolic diseases, neoplasms, odontogenic diseases, congenital deformities, developmental malformations, and acquired maladies affecting the configurations of the oral cavity are often well visualized in properly prepared models.

Biopsy

Variations on the theme "The best surgeon is a clinical pathologist who performs operations" are repeated throughout the surgical literature. It is obvious that the surgeon who appreciates the fundamental morphologic and biochemical changes in the tissues of his patients is likely to devise and perform better operations. Through the medium of biopsy, the doctor in clinical practice has an opportunity to learn and relearn important basic scientific facts. Thus he can gain a better understanding of the pathoses of the soft and hard tissues by establishing a two-way communication with his pathologist and by personally reviewing the microscopic findings.

Obtaining a biopsy specimen of an area in the oral cavity may be carried out under regional block anesthesia, with appropriate sedation, in the outpatient setting. There will be occasions, however, when the location, nature, and extent of the lesion require the hospitalization of the patient for the biopsy.

Although the biopsy procedures may be divided into a number of types, they are either excisional or incisional in nature:

The *excisional* biopsy is accomplished by removing the entire lesion and submitting it for microscopic examination. This is the preferable approach in most cases, since only one surgical experience is necessitated and the diagnosis and treatment occur without a delay, thus saving time and resources for all concerned.

The *incisional* biopsy implies the acquisition and presentation of a representative section from the lesion. The incisional biopsy is usually completed with a scalpel although punch, aspiration, and needle techniques are also employed. In the case of readily accessible oral lesions, the required narrow deep section of representative tissue is usually best obtained with a scalpel under local anesthesia. The representative section must include, if possible, the junction with the surrounding normal tissues. Necrotic areas should be avoided since they are seldom diagnostic; also superficial sections may show only mucosal reactions and inflammation rather than the region of primary concern. The specimen must be handled carefully to avoid crushing the delicate tissues. The use of ligatures as holding devices is highly desirable.

The *needle biopsy* is a suitable method of obtaining representative tissue especially when the lesion is deep to the surface. Frable and Frable (1979) recommended this technique as a useful method to diagnose lesions of the lymph nodes and salivary and thyroid glands as well as other soft tissue and bony lesions. They reported that in their study of 567 biopsies of head and neck lesions that the histopathologic results were 98% specific in cases of benign and malignant tumors. These authors recommended that this technique is simple to perform and saves time as well as hospital costs but requires the close cooperation of clinician and cytopathologist.

The majority of biopsy specimens are processed for permanent sections. The tissue is fixed for several hours and is then dehydrated and stained.

In this procedure the diagnosis is not available for at least 24 hours. If the diagnosis must be available immediately, however, *frozen sections* may be obtained. In the frozen section procedure the fresh specimen is subjected to extremely low temperatures and the sections are prepared and read within 30 minutes.

An adequate history should accompany the biopsy specimen, preferably on a standardized form. Too often the pathologist will receive a small piece of tissue in a bottle of fixative with a cryptic legend that the patient was a "25-year-old male." Obviously a more accurate diagnosis can be made if the pathologist has the benefit of an adequate history. The clinical history of the lesion should include a single word, a phrase, a sentence, or a paragraph for each of the following categories: duration, rapidity of growth, symptoms, previous involvement, other lesions, lymph involvement, and probable etiologic factors.

A description of the appearance of the lesion is very important; the following characteristics should be included: location, size, color, shape, attachment, consistency, mobility, and secondary changes.

Commentary on the overall management of biopsy specimens would include the following pertinent points:

1. Do not delay in the submission of the tissue to the pathologist.
2. When appropriate, submit radiographs with the specimen. Pathologists are extremely reliable in returning radiographs, which often provide additional important diagnostic information; the same comment could be made relative to clinical photographs, and these would be appreciated by the pathologist.
3. If possible, do not use coloring agents on incisional biopsy specimens because they may affect the various stains employed in preparing the histologic sections. If coloring agents are used to help outline the incision, be sure to advise the pathologist so he can protect his solutions.
4. When employing local anesthetics, attempt to inject around the lesion instead of directly into it since direct injection will distort the tissue.
5. Use sharp instruments. Electrosurgery causes severe alteration at the margins of the specimen so it usually is not recommended for this procedure.
6. Immediately place the specimens in an adequate volume of fixative (a minimum of ten times the volume of the specimen). Use widemouthed jars to avoid the possibility of a specimen's drying out on the neck of the jar. Often the pathologist will provide you with the fixative that is most desirable for his procedures. If he does not provide the fixative, consult with him to see whether the usual 10% buffered formalin will be appropriate.
7. In the event there are calcified or foreign bodies in the specimen, be sure to warn the pathologist so he can effect the proper decalcification prior to sectioning. It is possible that the presence of calcific or other hard substances will damage his microtome or ruin the remaining specimen during the sectioning procedure.

Exfoliative cytology. Smear techniques have been immensely successful as a screening procedure for diseases of the uterine cervix, in part because of two factors: (1) the cervix is small enough that a couple of passes with a cotton swab will assure contact with the entire surface, and (2) the mucosa of the cervix is normally nonkeratinized. Neither of these two factors is present in the oral cavity, however; hence oral exfoliative cytology is of limited use and should be considered only as a screening procedure. Furthermore, it is not as accurate for identifying malignant lesions as is the biopsy.

Indications for the use of intraoral exfoliative cytology include the following:

1. A diffuse lesion that covers a large area of mucosa where many incisional biopsies would be necessary to determine the range of pathologic change in the lesion
2. Surface lesions in a patient who has received cancericidal levels of radiation in which biopsies may cause persistent ulceration and possibly osteoradionecrosis
3. Patients who decline biopsy for various psychologic reasons (Such patients will frequently submit to exfoliative cytology, often agreeing to a standard biopsy later.)

Contraindications for the use of smear techniques to evaluate an oral lesion include:

1. Deep lesions covered with normal mucosa
2. Keratotic lesions
3. Lesions with grossly necrotic surfaces

Definitive treatment is never predicated on the basis of a cytology report.

Toluidine blue staining. Recently the toluidine blue staining technique has been recommended for the routine screening of suspicious oral lesions that may be malignant. There are important limitations to the accuracy of the technique, however. The toluidine blue dye stains the acidic groups (phosphoric, sulfuric, and carboxylic) present in normal and inflamed tissues as well as in benign and malignant tumors so that the results of the staining are equivocal. Any suspicious-looking lesion therefore should be submitted for a biopsy and an accurate diagnosis should be established (Fullmer, 1975).

In 1978 Baugman reported the results of an extensive study that was undertaken in order to determine the efficacy of toluidine blue in cancer screening. He applied toluidine blue to 30 oral lesions, of which biopsy specimens were then made to establish the final diagnosis. The following list illustrates the wide range of lesions that Baugman included in his study: pyogenic granuloma, 6; peripheral fibroma with calcification, 1; peripheral giant cell granuloma, 2; nonspecific ulcer, 6; squamous cell carcinoma, 4; carcinoma in situ, 1; severe epithelial dysplasia, 1; lichen planus (ketatotic), 1; erosive lichen planus, 3; benign mucous membrane pemphigoid, 1; lateral lingual tonsil, 1; and mucoepidermoid carcinoma, 1. Baugman reported that 23 of these 30 lesions stained positive. Interestingly he found that each ulcerated lesion stained while those with intact surfaces did not. This study strongly suggests that toluidine blue is not useful as a screening modality for oral cancer.

Consultation

Referral to a colleague should include two major elements:
1. A summation of the patient's history
2. An exact statement of what is requested of the doctor to whom the referral is being made

The exact statement should pinpoint whether advice, treatment of the patient, or transfer of the patient is requested.

It is quite apparent that strengthening the referral and consultation patterns between dentists and physicians would be in the best interest of the patients and the professions.

FINAL DIAGNOSIS

Chapter 4 is devoted to a suggested diagnostic sequence that the clinician may follow for each patient. The squence is initiated with the examination of the patient described in this chapter. It continues through the development of the differential diagnosis and working diagnosis. The final diagnosis is the proved diagnosis for a particular case—as determined by the pathology report, the descriptive manifestations, and the patient's response to treatment.

TREATMENT PLAN

If the diagnosis is correct, the right treatment is more certain to follow. Armed with the sure knowledge of the diagnosis, the doctor can formulate a rational treatment plan—which must take into account the strengths and limitations of the doctor himself, his operating team, the facilities, and the equipment. When all aspects of the case and the capabilities of the doctor have been considered, referral may be in order. The preoperative preparations and the operation are obvious; but if the treatment is to go forward in an intelligent manner, the responsible clinician must also consider long-range follow-up care and the monitoring that is often necessary.

SIGNATURE

If all the preceding have been performed correctly, the doctor will, with pride and responsibility, sign the history and the workup.

SPECIFIC REFERENCES
Baugman, R.: Toluidine blue staining. Paper presented to the Annual Meeting of the American Academy of Oral Pathology, Fort Lauderdale, Fla., April 1978.
Baugman, R.: Personal communication, Sept. 1979.
Frable, W. J., and Frable, M. A.: Thin-needle aspiration biopsy: the diagnosis of head and neck tumors revisited, Cancer **43**(4):1541-1548, 1979.
Fullmer, H. M.: Questions and answers, J. Am. Dent. Assoc. **91**:495, 1975.

GENERAL REFERENCES
Bánóczy, J.: Exfoliative cytologic examinations in the early diagnosis of oral cancer, Int. Dent. J. **26**:400, 1976.
Bernstein, M. L.: Biopsy technique: the pathological considerations, J. Am. Dent. Assoc. **96**(3):438-443, 1978.
Bernstein, M. L., and Miller, R. L.: Oral exfoliative cytology, J. Am. Dent. Assoc. **96**(4):625-629, 1978.
Jolly, M.: Minimizing biopsy error, Int. J. Oral Surg. **5**:41-51, 1976.
Sabes, W. R.: The dentist and clinical laboratory procedures, St. Louis, 1979, The C. V. Mosby Co.
Zegarelli, D. J.: Common problems in biopsy procedure, J. Oral Surg. **36**:644-647, 1978.

3

Correlation of gross structure and microstructure with clinical features

Norman K. Wood
Paul W. Goaz
Manuel Rey Garcia

IMPORTANCE OF NORMAL ANATOMY AND HISTOLOGY TO THE DIAGNOSTICIAN

The diagnosis of oral lesions is fundamentally an exercise in clinical pathology—which, in turn, is a study of changes. Usually such changes are precipitated by pathogenic or disease-producing agents. If the clinician is going to recognize and describe these changes, however, he must have a reference by which the altered states can be measured and compared.

In the case of the clinical oral diagnostician, this reference state is, of course, the state of oral health; so it follows that a thorough and basic knowledge of the normal oral cavity and surrounding regions is fundamental to the detection of oral disease.

In addition, it is quite apparent that the physical characteristics of a tissue cannot be appreciated without an awareness of the tissue's microstructure. This is because the microanatomy of the tissue correlates extremely well with the clinical features on which the diagnostician bases his judgments. The low-magnification photomicrograph of a tissue quite adequately illustrates the tissue architecture and so clearly provides a basis for the interpretation of the tissue's physical features that the conscientious clinician cannot afford to ignore.

Oral and perioral systems

The mucous membrane that lines the oral cavity consists of a layer of stratified squamous epithelium and a subepithelial layer, the lamina propria, which consists of a fibrous connective tissue and contains capillaries, nerves, and the minor salivary glands (Fig. 3-1).

The skin, like the mucous membrane, also possesses two layers—the epidermis and the underlying corium with its associated appendages, the sweat and sebaceous glands and the hair follicles (Fig. 3-2).

The remaining glandular systems of the perioral region of direct concern to the clinician are the major salivary glands and the thyroid and parathyroid glands. Either these glands are directly identified by the examiner, or the effects of their pathologic involvement come to his attention when he completes an adequate examination of the head and neck.

The bones of the region include the maxilla, the mandible, the zygoma and vomer, and the palatine, sphenoid, hyoid, and temporal bones as well as the cervical vertebrae. Inasmuch as these become especially apparent in any radiographic examination of their areas, the examiner must know their morphology and their relationship to each other and must be able to anticipate and interpret the bizarre forms their shadows may assume on the radiograph.

Other systems with which the oral examiner must be well informed are the teeth, larynx, trachea, and esophagus and the blood and lymphatic systems. Aberrations of these also occur in his area of responsibility and must be recognized.

The muscle systems with which the oral diagnostician must be familiar are those of facial expression, mastication, and swallowing as well as

Fig. 3-1. A, Diagram of the oral tissues, illustrating the component tissues and their relative positions: *1,* stratified squamous epithelium; *2,* lamina propria; *3,* loose connective tissue; *4,* mucous glands; *5,* serous glands (occasionally); *6,* sebaceous glands (Fordyce's granules); *7,* nerve; *8,* bone; *9,* cartilage; *10,* skeletal muscle. Fortunately a firm platform of muscle, bone, or cartilage is present beneath the superficial tissues. This facilitates examination and palpation of oral lesions.

Continued.

those involved in movements of the head. Not only do these muscles, along with the bony and cartilaginous structures and vessels, provide landmarks that facilitate an effective examination; they also, with the fascial planes, tend to mechanically obstruct or guide invading and spreading disease processes such as infections and neoplasms. Consequently the examiner must be aware of the exact location and plane of each muscle and the extent of its normal movements during function.

Oral and perioral tissues

The epithelial tissues of the oral and perioral region include the following:

1. Stratified squamous epithelial lining
2. Mucous, serous, and sebaceous glandular units
3. Enamel

The connective tissues, located beneath the surface epithelium, including the following:

1. Fibrous, adipose, and loose connective tissue
2. Muscle (skeletal and smooth) and nerves
3. Cartilage and bone
4. Dentin, cementum, and dental pulp

A well-defined layer of loose connective tissue is usually present beneath the skin or mucous membrane and permits these superficial layers to move over the deeper, firmer tissues such as

Fig. 3-1, cont'd. B, Composite photomicrographs of tissue components diagrammed in **A.**

muscle and bone. If this loose connective tissue layer is absent, the superficial layer is bound to the deep layer and cannot be moved separately from the underlying structures. Such a situation is normally found on the anterior hard palate and on the attached gingivae. Loose connective tissue contains blood and lymphatic vessels, nerves, adipose tissue, myxomatous tissue, sparse fibrous tissue, reticular fibers (precollagen fibers), elas-

tic fibers, undifferentiated mesenchymal cells, and blast cells of many varieties.

Only through a thorough understanding of these tissues, their specific natures, their physical relationships to each other, how they support or fail to support each other when subjected to the deforming pressures of the examiner's fingers, and even the characteristic sensations that the examiner can feel when palpating them will a

Fig. 3-2. A, Diagram of the skin and deeper tissues, illustrating the component tissues and their relative positions: *1,* keratinizing stratified squamous epithelium; *2,* corium; *3,* loose connective tissue; *4,* hair follicle; *5,* sebaceous glands; *6,* sweat glands; *7,* bone; *8,* cartilage; *9,* skeletal muscle. The firm platform below the oral tissues is also present beneath these dermal structures.

Continued.

full appreciation of the precepts of a physical examination be obtained.

EXPLANATION OF CLINICAL FEATURES IN TERMS OF NORMAL AND ALTERED TISSUE STRUCTURE AND FUNCTION
Features obtained by inspection

The examiner can only visualize the surface tissue and its topography, including contours, color, and texture. For a more critical evaluation of irregularities, he must rely on other procedures.

Contours. The diagnostician must, of course,

be familiar with the normal tissue contours in and around the oral cavity to be able to detect any disorder that might alter the usual configuration of the area. Changes in contour per se, however, are not in themselves specifically diagnostic since so many vastly different types of pathoses can produce similar alterations in contour.

Color. The examiner must be familiar with the normal characteristic color of each region in the oral cavity. He must be aware of the normal variations in color and shadings these tissues can assume, and certainly he must be able to recognize the color changes that signal abnormal conditions in a particular area.

Fig. 3-2, cont'd. B, Composite photomicrographs of tissue components diagrammed in **A.**

Pink. The normal color of the oral mucosa in whites is pink, because healthy stratified squamous epithelium is semitransparent and hence the red color of the blood in the extensive capillary bed beneath, although somewhat muted, shows through. The oral mucosa is *not* uniformly pink throughout, however, but has a deeper shade in some regions and a lighter shade in others. This is illustrated by the contrast between the darker red vestibular mucosa and the lighter pink gingiva.

Certain normal variations in the tissue that are

Fig. 3-3. Light pink region of oral mucosa. Photomicrograph of mucosa taken from the hard palate. Note the generous keratin layer, *1*, combined with the dense fibrous and quite avascular lamina propria, *2*. This combination accounts for the lighter coloration seen clinically on the hard palate and attached gingivae.

Fig. 3-4. This clinical picture illustrates the darker color of vestibular mucosa as contrasted with the lighter color of the attached gingivae. The histology of the two regions explains the basis of these color differences.

related to function are known to influence this spectrum of pink and thus to shift the color toward the red or, in the opposite direction, toward a lighter pink. One of the two main factors that induce a transition to a whiter appearance is an increase in the thickness of the epithelial layer, which makes the epithelium more opaque and is normally the result of an increased retention of keratin (Fig. 3-3). The other modification responsible for a more blanched appearance of the

mucosa is a less generous vascularity of the subepithelial tissues concomitant with a denser collagen component. These two modifications are often found simultaneously (Fig. 3-3), and the effective clinician must be able to correlate them with observed variations in microstructure as well as be able to interpret them as alterations caused by function, variations in function, or trauma.

For example, regions in the oral cavity that receive the greatest mechanical stimulation from mastication (the *masticatory mucosa*) react by developing a thicker layer of keratin for protection and also a denser less vascular lamina propria and so appear a light pink in color. These regions are the hard palate, the dorsal surface of the tongue, and the attached gingivae. On the other hand, regions such as the buccal mucosa, vestibule, floor of the mouth, and ventral surface of the tongue are not normally subjected to vigorous masticatory stimulation so they require only a thin layer of stratified squamous epithelium, which retains little keratin and consequently permits the very vascular submucosa to show through and impart the redder color (Fig. 3-4). These areas are said to be covered with *lining mucosa*.

White. Because of the many white lesions that may occur in the oral cavity, not only must the clinician inspect the color of the soft tissues very carefully but he must also become intimately familiar with the normal color variations from region to region. These pathologic white lesions are discussed in detail in Chapter 5.

For example, although a chronic mild irritation may act as a stimulus and induce the changes necessary to cause the mucosa to take on a lighter pink color, a more acute intense irritation will produce a thinning of the stratified squamous epithelium and a consequent inflammation of the subepithelial tissues. Thus such an involved area of the mucosa changes from pink to red because of (1) a thinning of the epithelial covering combined with (2) an increased vascularity and (3) a dissolution of part of the collagen content of the subepithelial tissue.

Yellow. A yellowish cast is frequently seen in areas of the oral mucosa. The soft palate in many persons appears quite yellow. The explanation for this can be readily found in the histology of the area, which will reveal a moderate distribution of adipose tissue contained in the connective tissue just beneath the basement membrane. Fordyce's granules, occurring in the buccal mucosa of most adults, are yellow—colored directly by the sebaceous material within the glandular units just beneath the epithelium.

Brownish, bluish, or black. Lesions of these colors will be discussed in detail later. It is appropriate to point out here, however, that the basis for the apparent clinical color of these lesions is frequently well demonstrated by histologic study whether the color is induced by melanin, hemosiderin, or heavy metals.

Surfaces. Normal mucosa is smooth and glistening except for the area of the rugae and the attached gingiva, which frequently demonstrates stippling and pebbling.

The surface of a pathologic mass may be smooth, papillomatous, ulcerated, eroded, keratinized, necrotic, or bosselated.

Masses that arise in tissues *beneath* the stratified squamous lining are, almost without exception, smooth surfaced. They may originate from mesenchyme, the salivary glands, a purulent infection, or an embryonic rest. As the nest of cells enlarges below and presses against the stratified squamous epithelium, the epithelium responds by a combination of stretching and minimal mitotic activity. Hence, as the mass becomes larger and bulges into the oral cavity, it is covered with a smooth epithelial surface. Examples of such masses are fibromas, osteomas, chondromas, hemangiomas, intradermal and compound nevi, many of the minor salivary gland tumors, cysts, retention phenomena, lipomas, myomas, schwannomas, neurofibromas, space abscesses, subepithelial bullae of erythema multiforme, bullous lichen planus, and bullous pemphigoid (Fig. 3-5).

Even the malignant counterparts of such tumors often have smooth surfaces, especially in their early phases; but when these lesions are situated in a region that is subjected to repeated trauma, they will, of course, become ulcerated and necrotic and their smooth surfaces will become roughened. Some exceptions to the rule that smooth-surfaced elevations originate below the epithelium are the intraepithelial vesicles and blebs seen in pemphigus and certain viral lesions.

As a general rule, however, masses that originate *in* the stratified squamous epithelium almost invariably have corrugated or papillomatous surfaces. Examples of these are papillomas, verrucae vulgari (warts), seborrheic keratoses, keratoacanthomas, verrucous carcinomas, and exophytic and ulcerative squamous cell carcinomas (Fig. 3-6). Exceptions would be the less than rough but pebbly surfaces sometimes seen overlying a granular cell myoblastoma and a lymphangioma. The granular cell myoblastoma often induces a pseudoepitheliomatous hyperplasia in the overlying epithelium, and this sometimes is severe enough to produce a pebbly surface (Fig. 3-7). The superficial lymphangioma frequently has dilated lymphatic spaces that extend right to the basement membrane, and these produce folds in the surface epithelium (Fig. 3-8).

The smooth-surfaced and rough-surfaced masses are categorized in Table 3-1.

Flat and raised entities. A macule is the result of a localized color change produced by the deposition of pigments or slight alterations in the local vasculature or other minimal local changes. This is a nonelevated lesion since there is usually no significant increase in the number (hyperplasia) or size (hypertrophy) of the cells. Hyperplasia and hypertrophy always result in an elevation, which may take the shape of a papule, a nodule, a polypoid, or a papillomatous mass.

For example, an ephelis or freckle is a brownish macule that histologically represents only an increased production of melanin by the normal number of melanocytes. On the other hand, an intradermal or intramucosal nevus histologically shows a significantly increased number of nevus cells producing melanin and an increased amount of collagen in the subepithelial area.

Fig. 3-5. Smooth-surfaced masses usually arise in tissues beneath the surface epithelium. **A,** Fibroma. **B,** Adenoid cystic carcinoma.

Hence both hypertrophy and hyperplasia are present and the lesion appears clinically to be pigmented and elevated (Fig. 3-9).

ASPIRATION

Aspiration is considered by some clinicians to be an extension of the visual examination, so its discussion is included here. Its primary value is to investigate the fluid contents of soft, cheesy, or rubbery masses whose characteristics suggest that they may contain fluid. An awareness therefore of the nature of the material contained in a mass will contribute significantly to the formulation of the appropriate differential diagnosis.

To aspirate masses indiscriminately, however, is generally considered unwise. Most clinicians recommend that a mass not be subjected to aspiration until just before surgery because of the danger of introducing bacteria from the surface flora and thus secondarily infecting the mass. If the mass does contain fluid, the fluid may be an excellent medium for the growth of bacteria; and if the mass does become infected, it may be necessary to delay surgery until the infection has resolved. Even then the tissue in the immediate area that was infected will prove difficult to dissect because of poor texture and postinflammatory fibrosis. If the mass is aspirated immediately

Fig. 3-6. Rough-surfaced masses usually arise within the surface epithelium. **A,** Papilloma. **B,** Seborrheic keratosis.

Fig. 3-7. Pebbly surfaced mass (granular cell myoblastoma). Note the presence of the pseudoepitheliomatous hyperplasia, which is often severe enough in these lesions to produce a pebbled surface.

Fig. 3-8. Pebbly surfaced mass (lymphangioma). Note the numerous lymphatic channels throughout the tissue and especially those extending into the surface epithelium. A roughened surface frequently results from such extensions.

Table 3-1. Smooth-surfaced and rough-surfaced masses

Lesions	Exceptions
Smooth surface*	
Benign and malignant mesenchymal tumors	Highly malignant varieties
	Late stages of less malignant varieties
	Traumatized lesions
	Superficial lymphangiomas
Embryonal nests	Draining cysts with sinuses
Cysts and nevi	Some raised nevi with roughened surfaces
Space abscesses	Draining abscesses and parulides
Subepithelial bullae	
Erythema multiforme, bullous lichen planus, bullous pemphigoid, and epidermolysis bullosa	Ruptured bullae
Inflammatory hyperplasias	
Hormonal tumors, epulides fissurata, epulides granulomatosa, papillary hyperplasias, and fibrous hyperplasias	Pyogenic granulomas Epulides fissurata occasionally
Benign minor salivary gland tumors	Traumatized lesions
Early malignant salivary gland tumors	
Retention phenomena	Traumatized lesions
Mucoceles and ranulas	
Rough surface†	
Papillomas	None
Verrucae vulgari	None
Seborrheic keratoses	None
Keratoacanthomas	None
Verrucous carcinomas	None
Exophytic carcinomas	None
Ulcerative carcinomas	None
Condyloma lata	None

*All smooth-surfaced lesions, with the exception of intraepithelial bullae, originate *beneath* the surface epithelium.
†All rough-surfaced lesions, with the exception of those that were smooth surfaced and became roughened because of trauma, infection, or malignancy, originate *in* the surface epithelium.

Fig. 3-9. Raised lesion (intradermal nevus). The large number of nevus cells present in the dermis produces the elevation of the lesion above the surface.

before surgery, then the introduction of organisms will not pose such a problem since the mass will have been enucleated before the potential bacterial infection could attain clinical significance.

The preoperative aspiration of a fluid-filled mass is a worthwhile precautionary procedure, however, because, if carried out properly, it eliminates the unpleasant surprise of opening an innocuous-appearing lesion that proves to be a dangerous vascular tumor.

Aspirate. Examination of the fluid withdrawn at aspiration is the essential, indeed the only, step in this aspect of the visual examination.

A straw-colored fluid may be yielded on aspiration of odontogenic and some fissural cysts (e.g., midpalatal cysts) and occasionally from cystic ameloblastomas. These generally have cholesterol crystals in their walls that are frequently shed into the lumen of the cyst and may be seen as small shiny particles when the syringe containing the aspirated fluid is transilluminated (Fig. 3-10). The crystals, which have a characteristic needlelike shape, may be studied in more detail under the microscope by placing a few drops of fluid on a slide under a coverslip.

Other types of cysts, such as epidermoid, sebaceous, and dermoid, which feel firmer on palpation than do odontogenic and fissural cysts, yield more viscous aspirates and thus require at least a 15-gauge needle for successful aspiration:

1. The lumina of the epidermoid cyst and the keratocyst are filled with exfoliated keratin, and the aspirate will be a *thick, yellowish-white, granular fluid* (Fig. 3-11).
2. The sebaceous cyst will yield sebum, which is *thick, homogeneous,* and *yellowish to gray.*
3. The walls of the dermoid cyst may contain most of the dermal appendages, including stratified, squamous, keratinizing epithelium with sebaceous and sweat glands and hair follicles. Thus the aspirate from this cyst will be the *thickest of all, a yellowish, cheesy substance that can be aspirated only with difficulty* because it consists of keratin, sebum, sweat, and exfoliated squamous cells.

A dark amber-colored fluid on aspiration may indicate a thyroglossal duct cyst (Fig. 3-12).

Lymph fluid may be aspirated from cystic hygromas and lymphangiomas. It is colorless, has a high lipid content, and thus appears cloudy and somewhat frothy.

Bluish blood is aspirated from early hematomas, hemangiomas, and varicosities, whereas the blood from an aneurysm or an arteriovenous shunt will be brighter red, reflecting the higher ratio of oxygenated to reduced hemoglobin of arterial blood (Fig. 3-13).

When a vascular lesion is suspected, care must be taken to utilize a needle of as small a gauge

Fig. 3-10. Cholesterol clefts. The cholesterol crystals that occupy these clefts migrate to the lumen surface, are suspended in the cyst fluid, and may be subsequently discovered in the aspirate.

Fig. 3-11. Thick yellowish-white cyst aspirate. Note the large quantity of keratin that fills the lumen of this epidermoid cyst and produces a viscous yellowish cystic fluid that would require a large-gauge needle for aspiration.

as possible to minimize postaspiration hemorrhage.

The aspiration of painful, warm, fluctuant swellings will usually yield pus. If the infectious organism is staphylococcal, and a significant percentage of pyogenic infections of odontogenic origin are, the color of the pus will usually be yellow or yellowish white. Also a superinfection with *Pseudomonas aeruginosa* will produce greenish blue pus.

Usually aspirating a streptococcal infection, such as Ludwig's angina, will be futile because most streptococcal organisms are not pyogenic and do not localize. Instead they produce spreading factors (e.g., the enzymes hyaluronidase, streptokinase, streptodornase, and coagulase),

Fig. 3-13. Aspiration of a deep cavernous hemangioma of the face.

Fig. 3-12. Aspiration of a thyroglossal duct cyst. Note the unusual displacement of this particular cyst to the right of the midline.

which facilitate their rapid dispersal through the tissues. Streptococcal organisms produce a red serosanguineous fluid, but usually not in large enough quantities to pool or be aspirated or to demonstrate fluctuance. Also, in contrast to staphylococcal infections, the streptococcal variety is more often associated with painful regional lymphadenitis.

Actinomycosis in its early stage is indicated by firm red swellings. Later pus pools under the surface and produces fluctuance. At this intermediate stage, aspiration will often yield a yellowish white pus with a few firm yellow granules in it. These are the sulfur granules, thought to be composed of mycelia and material produced as a byproduct of the natural defenses of the host. Any aspirate from an infection should be sent to the laboratory for routine bacterial culture and sensitivity tests. If actinomycosis is suspected, special anaerobic cultures should be requested.

A sticky, clear, viscous fluid will be yielded on aspiration of retention phenomena (mucoceles and cysts of the glands of Blandin and Nuhn and of the sublingual gland [ranula]) and sometimes from tumors of the minor salivary glands. This pooled liquid is a concentrated mucous secretion from which water is resorbed by the cells lining the cyst. Occasionally a low-grade mucoepidermoid tumor will produce enough mucus to clinically resemble a mucocele and will yield mucus on aspiration.

The papillary cyst adenoma and papillary cystadenoma lymphomatosum (their names indicate they are cystic) are often fluctuant and contain a thin straw-colored liquid that can be aspirated.

Subcutaneous emphysemas and laryngoceles are soft masses that are filled with air, as are the rare pockets of carbon dioxide and hydrogen produced by *Clostridium perfringens* in gas gangrene. The former two entities can be completely deflated by aspiration.

NEEDLE BIOPSY

Needle biopsies can be done using a special biopsy needle; this procedure can be advantageous in the biopsy of deeper structures such as the lymph nodes. The needle biopsy technique has the disadvantage of yielding a small-sized sample; and there is the added danger of lacerating some large blood vessels in the area.

Features obtained by palpation

The knowledgeable examiner is able to distinguish the various tissues encountered in and around the oral cavity by palpation. He is able to do this because, first, he is familiar with the normal gross anatomy of the structures and knows where these tissues and organs are situated, their extent, in which plane they lie, and their anatomic relationship to each other. Second, he can visualize the microscopic structures of these tissues, which correlate so well with the tactile sensations elicited by his palpation of these structures and tissues.

Palpation is actually a "third eye"—the most informative method of clinically examining the tissues lying beneath the surface. Fortunately for the examiner, the soft tissues of the body lie over bones, cartilages, or skeletal muscles, and hence the superficial tissues can be palpated against a sturdy base.

Surface temperature. Before he attempts to make a judgment relative to the level of the surface temperature of a region or part, the examiner should first establish what the patient's systemic temperature is as indicated on an oral thermometer. A rise in surface temperature of the skin is simple to detect. The examiner merely places the fingers of one hand on the skin in the area of concern and the fingers of the other hand on the skin on the contralateral spot of the body. Thus relatively subtle differences in temperature may be rapidly and comfortably detected and can frequently contribute significantly to arriving at the diagnosis.

The skin will generally have an increased temperature when it is inflamed or when it overlies an inflamed or infected region. The increased metabolic rate of the inflamed tissue, together with the increased vascularity of the area, is responsible for the increased local temperature of the part. The surface temperature of the skin overlying superficial aneurysms, arteriovenous shunts, and relatively large recent hematomas may also be elevated since the higher deep body temperature is carried by the blood to the skin overlying these areas. The estimation of normal surface temperature is a useful test on the skin; but trying to transfer such a reference to the oral cavity is of little value since the oral mucosa has a higher normal temperature than the skin. Although the examiner may be able to detect slight variations in temperature with his fingers over his own skin surface (being the same as that in the normal reference area on the patient), when the reference temperature to be evaluated is somewhat greater than the skin temperature of his fingers (as it is in the oral cavity), he is unable to detect subtle differences.

Anatomic regions and planes involved. In addition to knowing the microscopic anatomy of a region he is inspecting, the examiner must be thoroughly familiar with the gross anatomy of the region. Since many of the structures in the head and neck region can be at least partly palpated through the skin and/or oral mucosa, it becomes imperative that normal structures be anticipated and recognized.

For example, if the diagnostician locates a firm mass high in the submandibular space, he must be aware that the submaxillary gland is peculiar to that area and he must then establish whether or not the mass is discrete from the salivary gland. If he can determine that the mass is separate from the gland, he will deemphasize pathoses of this gland in the differential diagnosis. If he cannot, then he must consider salivary gland pathoses as a probable diagnosis.

Although it is important for the examiner to know what organs and tissues occur in an involved anatomic space, it is also essential that he be able to detect, identify, and evaluate their condition by manual examination. The acquisition of such a capability requires not only the basic anatomic knowledge but also considerable experience examining the area.

Sometimes, however, the information gained by palpation is very limited and the palpation itself may be very difficult—especially if the area is swollen, because the swelling will tend to obscure the definitive structures. Furthermore, if the area is painful, the patient will not permit a thorough palpation of the region and the mass. The clinician must keep in mind that sometimes a complete palpation will not be possible until the patient is anesthetized.

Initially the examiner must determine whether a mass in question is located superficially or deep. If it is superficial, he must then verify whether it involves the skin over the subcutaneous or fascial layer and also whether it involves a muscle or a muscle layer. If it involves a muscle layer, he must ascertain which muscles and whether regional organs (glands, vessels) or bones are associated with the mass.

Mobility. Once he has defined a mass in terms of its location in an anatomic plane and the tissue and organ involved, the examiner will determine whether the mass is mobile or fixed with regard to its neighboring tissues. By palpation he can establish whether the mass is freely movable in all directions. If it is freely movable, it is most likely a benign, possibly encapsulated, process originating in the loose subcutaneous or submucosal tissue (e.g., epidermoid or dermoid cyst or lymph node) (Fig. 3-14).

The mobility can be illustrated by fixing the

Fig. 3-14. Diagram of a freely movable mass. An epidermoid cyst would be an example of this type of mass —which could be moved freely in all directions by digital pressure. *A*, Stratified squamous epithelium; *B*, mucosa or skin; *C*, loose connective tissue layer; *D*, skeletal muscle.

Fig. 3-15. Diagram of a mass attached to the skin. A sebaceous cyst would be an example of this type of mass—which could not be moved independently of the skin but would not be attached to the deeper structures. This type of cyst thus can be moved as a unit with the skin.

mass with the fingers of one hand while moving the skin or mucosa over the mass with the other hand. Next an attempt is made to move the mass independently of its underlying tissue. This will demonstrate whether it is freely movable in all directions. If the mass is found to be fixed to the skin, that is, the skin cannot be moved independently of the mass, but is not fixed to the underlying tissue, this is an important clue and would limit the differential diagnosis.

For instance, epidermoid and dermoid cysts would be regarded as unlikely alternatives because, although they are not fixed to the underlying tissues, they are not bound to skin but are freely movable in all directions (unless fibrosis has resulted from a previous infection). These two cysts originate in nests of epithelium that have been trapped in the subcutaneous layer either during embryonic formation or as a result of a traumatic incident in which surface epithelial fragments were driven deep to the subepithelial layer.

On the other hand, sebaceous cysts would be high on the list of possibilities since they are freely movable over underlying tissues but are bound to the skin. This diagnosis is logical if one considers that sebaceous cysts form when sebaceous units of the skin become blocked but retain their continuity with the cystic glandular elements and the skin (Fig. 3-15).

A contrary set of circumstances might be observed when the skin is found to be freely movable over the mass but the mass is bound to the

deeper structures. This situation then poses a question relative to the structures to which the mass is bound. It could be attached to muscle, bone, cartilage, fat, salivary gland, or thyroid gland. The tissue or organ to which the mass is most intimately attached will most often prove to be the tissue of origin (Fig. 3-16). For example, if the mass is located in or bound to the parotid gland, the most likely possibility is that it is of salivary gland origin.

If the mass is bound to the skin or mucosa and also to the underlying structures, however, there are only four possibilities:

1. Fibrosis after a previous inflammatory episode
2. An infiltrating malignant tumor that originated in the skin or mucous membrane and has invaded the deep structures (Fig. 3-17)
3. A malignancy that originated in a deep structure and has invaded the subcutaneous or submucosal tissue and the skin or mucosa
4. A malignancy that originated in the loose connective tissue and has invaded both the superficial and the deep layers

When examining the oral cavity, the diagnostician should remember that under normal conditions the mucosa covering the hard palate and the gingivae is bound tightly to the underlying bone. In addition, the loose submucosal layer under the papillated, keratinized, stratified squamous epithelium of the dorsal surface of the tongue is very thin and frequently nonexistent;

Fig. 3-16. Diagram of a mass attached to muscle. A rhabdomyoma would be an example of this type of mass—which could not be moved independently of the involved muscle but would not be fixed to the skin or mucous membrane.

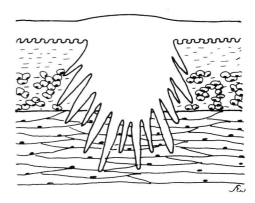

Fig. 3-17. Diagram of an epithelial mass—fixed to all layers of tissue. An invasive squamous cell carcinoma at this stage would fix the skin or mucous membrane to the deeper tissues.

and the epithelial layer is therefore actually bound closely to the underlying tongue musculature. Hence the mucosa of the dorsal surface cannot normally be moved independently of the deeper muscular part. In the remaining regions of the oral cavity, however, there is a substantial loose submucosal layer, which, in the absence of disease, permits the surface epithelial layer to be moved independently of the deeper tissues and structures.

The palpation of a mass during function will frequently aid in determining whether the mass is fixed to deeper structures—and if so, which ones. The mass in question is palpated while the patient demonstrates the normal movements of the region. For example, if a fluctuant mass in the anterior midline of the neck moves up and down as the patient swallows, it may be diagnosed as part of, or attached to, the hyoid bone, larynx, trachea, thyroid or parathyroid gland, or intervening muscles. If it elevates when the patient protrudes his tongue, the examiner may suspect that it is a thyroglossal cyst and that a persistent epithelial or fibrous cord or a fistula is leading to the tongue. (These are not always present in patients with thyroglossal cysts, however; so if a mass does not elevate on protrusion of the tongue, a thyroglossal duct cyst is not necessarily ruled out.)

In some cases a mass may encroach on adjacent moving structures and impair or limit movement. For example, a chondroma or hyperplasia of the condyle may produce deviation and limitation of jaw movements.

Extent. The determination of the foregoing characteristics by palpation is important not only for masses located below the surface but also for visible superficial lesions.

Clinicians must always bear in mind that what is visible may represent just the "tip of the iceberg." Consequently it is important that the tissue surrounding and underlying the bases of these apparent surface lesions be carefully palpated to determine the maximum extension of the lesion into adjacent tissues. Of course, positive identification of small cellular areas of penetration into the surrounding tissue can be made only by microscopic examination; but the surgeon must grossly estimate the extent of penetration of the surrounding tissue by palpation before surgery.

Whether a mass will have poorly defined, moderately defined, or well-defined borders, as determined by palpation, will depend on four factors:

1. Border characteristics of the mass
2. Relative consistency of the surrounding tissues
3. Thickness and nature of the overlying tissue
4. Sturdiness of the underlying tissue

Borders of the mass. Malignancies usually have ill-defined borders that are extremely difficult to detect by palpation. This observation is readily evident if we consider two features characteristic of these disorders:

1. Malignant tumors often infiltrate adjacent tissue by extending many *processes of tumor* into the surrounding normal tissue.
2. Malignant tumors also produce a *scirrhous reaction* in the infiltrated tissue.

The processes of the tumor are irregular in size, shape, and distribution. The result is an irregular and vague outline. These extensions also anchor the neoplasm to neighboring tissue and thus preclude the possibility that the tumor may be moved manually independent of its surroundings.

The tumor, with its extensions, elicits an inflammatory reaction in the adjacent tissue that is somewhat similar to an allergic or foreign body reaction. This inflammatory reaction results in the sequela of fibrosis. The fibrosis develops in the irregular and diffuse areas that are inflamed and results in a more tenacious binding of the tumor to the adjacent tissues, by an ill-defined fibrous attachment whose limits are impossible to perceive by manipulation of the mass.

Some early low-grade malignancies, however, such as the verrucous carcinoma, may be exceptions to the foregoing generalizations. Such neoplasms occur usually as exophytic masses on the mucous membrane or the skin and, by virtue of this position, possess well-defined borders. The result is a minimum of direct contact between the tumor and the subcutaneous connective tissue, which precludes an extensive inflammatory response and a resulting fibrosis of vague outline.

Another exception involves some of the slow-growing malignancies that develop fibrous borders. The borders are composed of (1) connective tissue from the stroma of the dislodged normal tissue and (2) fibrous tissue newly formed in response to the tumor. These masses have borders that may be detected and delineated by palpation.

Inflammation occurs much more frequently as a response to other insults than as a response to malignant tumors, and it usually has poorly defined borders regardless of etiology.

Inflammation in a nonencapsulated organ or tissue seldom develops a smooth well-defined border; and the subsequent scarring in the areas of resolved inflammation will duplicate the limits of the inflammatory process, which are vague and irregular. On the contrary, if the inflammation of an encapsulated organ or tissue is confined within the capsule, the margins of the affected tissue will possess the well-defined characteristics of the encapsulated organ.

Also the resolution of the inflammation as well as reparative scarring within the capsule (e.g., a lymph node, the parotid gland) will result in a mass with a well-defined detectable border. This, of course, is a consequence of the enclosing and restricting action of the capsule. If the inflammation breaks through the capsule and involves the surrounding tissue, however, the resultant extracapsular fibrosis will render the mass fixed to the surrounding tissue and the borders may then be ill defined. The postinflammatory fixed lymph node would be an example of such a process.

Whether the limits of a pathologic process can be well defined by palpation will depend significantly on the shape of the lesion as well as on the nature of its borders. Of course, to determine the exact extent of a thin lesion or any lesion with a flattened, feather-edged border is difficult. On the other hand, the limits of a plump lesion (e.g., spherical mixed tumor) are relatively easy to detect.

Consistency of surrounding tissue. The consistency or the degree of firmness of a lesion, in contrast to that of its surrounding tissue, will also affect the ease with which the lesion itself or its borders may be identified by palpation.

For example, the borders of a firm dermoid cyst occurring in loose subcutaneous tissue can be readily determined, whereas to ascertain the borders of a relatively soft lipoma when it occurs in the same type of loose connective tissue is difficult, if not impossible.

The same relative situation often pertains in the case of a firm mass occurring on or around the borders of a muscle. If the surrounding normal tissue is of the same consistency as the pathologic mass, the borders cannot be determined. Again the determination of the exact proportions of firm masses or lesions in the oral cavity that are situated over bone, and especially where mobility over the bone cannot be demonstrated, will prove to be extremely difficult by palpation. Regardless of the physical circumstance attending the palpation of a lesion in or over bone, determining the extent of bony involvement without a roentgenogram is impossible.

When a roentgenogram indicates some degree of bone loss, identifying the site of origin as being soft tissue or bone itself without a biopsy may be difficult and often impossible. Even when the microscopic diagnosis is fibrosarcoma, the clinician still cannot be certain of the origin of the mass. If an adequate radiographic examination does not reveal a radiolucency in the bone, the clinician can proceed on the assumption that the lesion in question most likely has originated in the soft tissue.

Thickness of overlying tissue. Clearly, to determine by palpation the physical characteristics of a superficial mass is much easier than to make a similar determination of a deep mass. Also it is apparent that overlying dense fibrous tissue or tensed muscle tissue will obscure and may even obliterate the characteristic features of a lesion.

As an example, the borders of a branchial cleft

cyst lying superficial to the sternocleidomastoid muscle may be readily delineated and the mass will be soft and fluctuant. In contrast, if the cyst lies beneath the sternocleidomastoid muscle, its borders may not be defined by palpation and the cystic mass will feel firm and nonfluctuant. A covering of bone or cartilage, of course, will preclude the palpation of an underlying mass, although if the mass has expanded the bone or cartilage its presence may be suspected.

Sturdiness of underlying tissue. If the tissue underlying a mass is bone, cartilage, dense fibrous tissue, or tensed muscle, the true physical characteristics of the mass will be more readily determined and the margins, if discrete, easier to delineate by palpation. On the other hand, soft tissue platforms that fail to support a mass for adequate manipulation may confuse the examiner concerning the characteristics of the mass. Fortunately, firm platforms for palpation are present in most regions of the body.

Size and shape. Size and shape may be determined for a lesion that protrudes through or above the skin or mucous membrane surface by inspection and the use of a millimeter rule. In addition, a careful history will frequently indicate the duration of the growth; and on the basis of the present size, the growth rate can be approximated, which information may be of significant value. Likewise, the history will help to establish whether a lesion is increasing in size at a steady rate, whether it is paroxysmal and predictable (like a ranula, which will enlarge just prior to eating), or whether it drains intermittently (like a rupturing abscess, which will periodically decrease in size).

When masses are located within a tissue, however, palpation is necessary to determine their approximate size and shape. Round or ovoid masses are generally cysts, early benign tumors, or enlarged lymph nodes. Primary malignant tumors of lymph nodes and also early metastatic tumors of lymph nodes are usually round or ovoid with a smooth border. As indicated, irregularly shaped masses are most likely to be inflammatory fibrotic conditions or malignant tumors.

Consistency. Consistency provides one of the most important clues to the identification of the tissue, organ, or pathosis that the examiner may encounter during the physical examination. Since he must be equally familiar with the texture and compressibility of normal tissue as well as with those of abnormal tissue, a description of the normal is given in Table 3-2.

The following terms are commonly used to de-

Table 3-2. Consistency of normal tissues and organs*

Consistency	Tissues or organs
Soft	Adipose tissue
	Fascia
	Veins
	Loose connective tissue
	Glandular tissue, minor salivary glands, and sublingual salivary gland
Cheesy	Brain tissue
Rubbery	Skin
	Relaxed muscle
	Glandular tissue with capsule
	Arteries and arterioles
	Liver
Firm	Fibrous tissue
	Tensed muscle
	Large nerves
	Cartilage†
Bony hard	Bone
	Enamel
	Dentin
	Cementum
	Cartilage†

*NOTE: Many normal tissues and organs, e.g., dental pulp, thyroid and parathyroid glands, lymph nodes, and lymphatic vessels, usually cannot be palpated under normal conditions, so they have not been categorized here.
†Cartilage is difficult to classify; it seems to fall into an intermediate category, being too firm to be included in the firm group and not firm enough to be placed in the bony hard group.

fine the consistency of tissue: soft, cheesy, rubbery, firm, and bony hard. The term *soft* is associated with tissue that is easily compressible, such as a lipoma or a mucocele. Cysts filled with thin fluid would generally be soft; but if they were under tension, they would be rubbery. *Cheesy* indicates a somewhat firmer tissue that gives a more granular sensation but no rebound. *Rubbery* describes a tissue that is firm but can be compressed slightly and rebounds to its normal contour as soon as the pressure is withdrawn, such as skin. *Firm* identifies a tissue, such as fibrous tissue, that cannot be readily compressed. *Bony hard* is self-explanatory.

Needless to say, there are examples in each category that are borderline and appear to overlap adjacent categories, so it may not always be possible to explicitly describe a consistency with one of these terms. However, they are universally employed and, in general, connote a similar meaning to most individuals.

At least three different factors can modify the consistency of a tissue or mass as perceived by palpation:

1. A thick layer of overlying tissue, especially muscle or fibrous tissue, will appreciably modify or mask the true nature of a mass.
2. Soft glandular tissue surrounded by a dense connective capsule will be perceived firmer than it otherwise would be and is.
3. The depth in the tissue will alter the consistency sensed by palpation; that is, a soft mass will seem firmer if it is deeper in the tissue than it would feel if it were situated more superficially.

Each tissue's consistency correlates so well with its microstructure that the examiner should at least be familiar with the microstructure as revealed by histology. To demonstrate the close correlation between texture and histology, the microscopic anatomies of examples from each group of consistencies are shown together in Fig. 3-18 for comparison.

Once the examiner has familiarized himself with the location and consistency of normal tis-

Fig. 3-18. Normal tissues categorized according to consistency. The general appearance of the following normal tissues at low magnification reflects the consistency of the tissue to palpation. **A,** Tissues with soft consistency: *1,* adipose tissue; *2,* unencapsulated mucous glands; *3,* loose connective tissue; note the presence of thin-walled vessels. **B,** Tissue with cheesy consistency: brain tissue. **C,** Tissues with firm consistency: *1,* fibrous tissue; *2,* skeletal muscle; tensed muscle feels firm whereas relaxed muscle feels rubbery.

sues and organs, he will be quite capable of differentiating between normal and abnormal tissue when he detects a consistency that contrasts with the expected consistency of the tissue he is palpating.

The consistency of abnormal tissue can be described with the same terms as those used for characterizing normal tissue: soft, cheesy, rubbery, firm, and bony hard. Representative segments of pathologic masses have been selected and categorized according to consistency in Table 3-3. Again, in an effort to underscore the correlation between microstructure and physical consistency, photomicrographs of pathologic tissues with similar consistencies have been grouped together in Fig. 3-19.

Fluctuance and emptiability. All soft, cheesy, or rubbery lesions or masses over 1 cm in diameter should be tested for fluctuance. This done by placing the sensing fingers of one hand on one side of the mass and gently pressing on the mass with the probing fingers of the other hand. If the sensing fingers can detect a wave or force passing through the lesion, the mass is said to be fluctuant (Fig. 3-20). The following four factors determine whether fluctuance can be perceived in a soft, cheesy, or rubbery lesion (Table 3-4):

1. *The mass must contain liquid or gas in a relatively enclosed cavity* (Fig. 3-20). Examples of such fluctuant masses are cysts, mucoceles, ranulas, pyogenic space abscesses, early hematomas, subcutaneous emphysemas, varicosities, Warthin's tumors, papillary cyst adenomas, lipomas, and plexiform neurofibromas (Fig. 3-21). Although a lipoma and a plexiform neurofibroma do not have a true lumen containing a fluid, the high liquid content of the cells and interstitial tissue is apparently sufficient to produce fluctuance in these tumors.

2. *The mass must be located in a superficial plane.* If it is covered by a deep layer of relatively inflexible tissue or a structure such as a muscle, the mass cannot be palpated in a manner that might demonstrate fluctuance. An example would be a branchial cleft cyst situated under the sternocleidomastoid muscle. In this position its fluctuance would be obscured, as might most of its other characteristics that could be determined by palpation (Fig. 3-22).

3. *The mass must be in a fluctuant stage.* Many
(Text continued on p. 44.)

D

Fig. 3-18, cont'd. D, Tissues with bony-hard consistency: *1,* bone; *2,* cementum; *3,* dentin; *4,* cartilage.

Table 3-3. Consistency of pathologic masses

Lesions	Exceptions
Soft	
Cysts	Cysts under tension—rubbery
	Infected and fibrosed cysts—firm
	Sebaceous cysts, keratocysts, and dermoid cysts—cheesy
Warthin's tumors and papillary cyst adenomas	Occasionally sclerosed types firm in some areas
Vascular tumors and phenomena	Sclerosing types—firm
Hemangiomas, lymphangiomas, varicosities, and cystic hygromas	Hemangioendotheliomas—firm
	Hemangiosarcomas—firm
Fatty tumors	Sclerosing types of liposarcoma—firm
Lipomas, hibernomas, xanthomas, and liposarcomas	
Myxomas	None
Plexiform neurofibromas	None
Inflammatory hyperplasias (granulomatous types)	Fibrosed types—firm
Emphysemas	None
Laryngoceles	None
Retention phenomena	If high tension, rubbery
Mucoceles and ranulas	If fibrosed, firm
Cheesy	
Cysts	Infected and fibrosed types—firm or alternate areas of cheesiness and firmness
Sebaceous, dermoid, and epidermoid	
Tuberculous nodes	Early or late tuberculosis nodes—firm
Rubbery	
Cysts with contents under tension	None
Lymphomas	None
Myomas	None
Myoblastomas	Those with severe pseudoepitheliomatous hyperplasia—firm
Aneurysms	None
Pyogenic space infection	Early stages—firm
Edematous tissue	None
Early hematomas	If not much tension, soft

Table 3-3. Consistency of pathologic masses—cont'd

Lesions	Exceptions
Firm	
Infection	None
Streptococcus, early staphylococcus, early actinomycosis, and histoplasmosis	
Benign tumors of soft tissue	Fatty tumors, plexiform neurofibromas, myxomas, and hemangiomas
Fibromas, neurofibromas, schwannomas, and amputation neuromas	
Malignancies of soft tissues	None
Squamous cell carcinomas, melanomas, fibrosarcomas, and sclerosing liposarcomas	
Osteosarcomas	Occasionally bony hard
Chondrosarcomas	Occasionally bony hard
Metastatic carcinomas	Occasionally osteoblastic metastatic prostatic carcinomas bony hard
Benign and malignant salivary gland tumors	Warthin's tumors and papillary cyst adenomas—soft
	Occasionally mucoepidermoid tumors with alternate soft and firm areas
Inflammation and infection of parotid and submaxillary salivary glands	None
Inflammation and infection of lymph nodes	Caseous or liquefied nodes—soft and cheesy
Bony hard	
Osteomas	None
Exostoses	None
Osteogenic sarcomas	Undifferentiated—firm
Pleomorphic adenomas occasionally	Usually firm
Chondromas	Occasionally firm
Chondrosarcomas	Occasionally firm
Osteoblastic metastatic prostatic carcinomas, occasionally	Usually firm

Fig. 3-19. Pathologic tissues categorized according to consistency. The general appearance of each of the following pathologic tissues at low magnification reflects the consistency of the tissue to palpation. **A,** Soft consistency: *1,* myxoma; *2,* plexiform neurofibroma (low and high magnifications); *3,* ranula. **B,** Cheesy consistency: *1,* epidermoid cyst; note that the lumen is filled with keratin, which imparts the cheesy consistency; *2,* tuberculous node; the large amorphous area is caseation necrosis, which imparts the cheesy consistency. **C,** Rubbery consistency: *1,* rhabdomyoma; *2,* lymphoma; the lymph node capsule helps to impart the rubbery consistency to this entity.

Fig. 3-19, cont'd. Pathologic tissues. **D,** Firm consistency: *1,* squamous cell carcinoma; the keratin nests and surrounding fibrous tissue contribute to the firmness of this lesion; *2,* pleomorphic adenoma; the generous amount of hyaline in this tissue is responsible for the firmness; occasionally cartilage and bone are present in this type of tumor and impart a bony hardness to some areas; *3,* fibrosarcoma; the amount of dense fibrous tissue imparts the firmness to this lesion. **E,** Bony hard consistency: *1,* torus; *2,* osteogenic sarcoma; frequently new bone formation and the production of fibrous tissue will contribute to the consistency of this tumor; *3,* chondrosarcoma.

Fig. 3-20. Diagram illustrating fluctuance in a cystlike lesion.

Table 3-4. Characteristics of soft, cheesy, or rubbery masses

Lesions	Fluctuant	Emptiable
Cysts	Yes	No
Abscesses	Yes	No
Mucoceles	Yes	No
Ranulas	Yes	No
Early hematomas	Yes	No
Subcutaneous emphyse-mas	Yes	No
Lipomas	Yes	No
Plexiform neurofibromas	Yes	No
Myxomas	Yes	No
Papillary cyst adenomas	Yes	No
Warthin's tumors	Yes	No
Varicosities	Variable	Variable
Cystic hygromas	Variable	Variable
Laryngoceles	Variable	Variable
Capillary hemangiomas*	Variable	Variable
Lymphangiomas	Usually	Usually not
Cavernous hemangiomas	Usually not	Usually
Aneurysms	No	Yes
Draining cysts	No	Yes
Draining abscesses	No	Yes
Inflammatory hyperplasias	No	No

*Capillary hemangiomas are often less than 1 cm in diameter and are usually too small for fluctuance to be accurately detected.

clinical lesions represent a fluctuant stage in a multiphasic disease process. Earlier, in the development of the disorder, the fluid-filled cavity may not have formed, however; or later, during the resolution, the required architecture on which fluctuance depends may have become altered or obliterated. This may be either the natural history of the disease or the result of treatment. For example, an odontogenic staphylococcal infection that has broken through the cortical plates and commenced to involve the adjacent soft tissue is tender, red, and firm. As the process continues, the typical staphylococcal space infection results in a soft, fluctuant, painful, nonemptiable mass. As the abscess resolves, regardless of the treatment, the fluctuant stage will give way to a firm stage and the firm stage may either disappear completely or leave a small area of fibrosis. Actinomycosis will often demonstrate the same cycle, as will infected cysts to some extent.

4. *Developing fibrosis around the mass may obscure the fluctuance.* Chronically infected cysts that flare up from time to time often lose their fluctuance and become hard and tender. This is an example in which inflammation and the resulting fibrosis around a fluid-filled cavity can

mask fluctuance. Occasionally the epithelial lining and the lumen will be completely destroyed, so the basic requirement for fluctuance, a fluid-filled cavity, is lost.

Lesions demonstrating variable fluctuance. A large group of the soft and rubbery lesions demonstrate variable fluctuance. This is almost always related to the degree of emptiability that a particular lesion has. In other words, some lesions are fluctuant whereas others of the same variety are not. All soft, cheesy, or rubbery lesions can be classified according to emptiability.

1. Some cannot be emptied at all by digital pressure (Fig. 3-23).
2. Others, such as hemangiomas, cystic hygromas, lymphangiomas, and laryngoceles, may show fluctuance or emptiability, depending on the individual structural characteristics of the specific lesion.
3. Still others, including aneurysms, most cavernous hemangiomas, draining cysts, and draining space abscesses, are usually nonfluctuant and completely emptiable with ease. They almost never develop an architecture that would result in their being fluctuant.

A number of factors influence the emptiability of a mass: course, number, diameter, and position of exit vessels or channels. Also the width of the base of a lesion will relate to the ease with which the lesion can be emptied.

Fig. 3-24 shows a diagram of an aneurysm. Note that the aneurysm could be readily emptied by digital pressure. The usual cavernous hemangioma is similar in this respect. The cavernous spaces are large but few. The exit channels are large, and the base of the lesion sessile. Such a hemangioma would not demonstrate fluctuance, for it has all the features that permit rapid and complete emptying.

Fig. 3-25, by contrast, is a diagram representing a capillary hemangioma with many blood sinuses connected by small vessels. Note that the exit vessels are few and small and the base is somewhat pedunculated. A hemangioma of this type would probably not be readily emptied by digital pressure since the slight pressure that would deform the lesion would also tend to occlude the small exit vessels. Thus the lesion would consequently be partially fluctuant and partially emptiable.

Fig. 3-26 is also an illustration of a capillary hemangioma that probably could not be emptied at all. The laryngocele, a developmental pouch projecting from the larynx, is inflated with air

Fig. 3-21. Fluctuant pathologic masses. **A,** Radicular cyst. **B,** Mucocele. **C,** Papillary cyst adenoma. **D,** Warthin's tumor (papillary cystadenoma lymphomatosum).

Fig. 3-22. Diagram of muscle overlying a cyst and masking its characteristics.

Fig. 3-23. Diagram illustrating a nonemptiable cystlike lesion.

Fig. 3-24. Diagram illustrating complete emptiability in an aneurysmlike lesion.

Fig. 3-25. Diagram illustrating the difficulty encountered in attempting to completely empty a capillary hemangioma, which has many small channels and few exit vessels.

Fig. 3-26. Diagram illustrating a pedunculated capillary hemangioma, which would be nonemptiable by digital pressure.

Fig. 3-27. Diagram illustrating the importance of finger position when attempting to empty a lesion with this configuration. Careful pressure applied at point Y would readily empty the lesion, whereas rapid pressure applied at point X would tend to occlude the exit channel and render the lesion nonemptiable.

Fig. 3-28. Diagram illustrating the presence of a sinus draining a cyst or abscess. This causes a usually fluctuant lesion to become nonfluctuant and emptiable.

when the patient coughs. Frequently the connecting channel to the larynx is small and easily occluded; and although the laryngocele usually shows fluctuance, it can be slowly emptied by careful digital pressure. A cyst also would be fluctuant but not emptiable since a channel for the egress of the fluid is not a normal feature of this lesion.

Position or location of the examiner's finger or fingers is important in determining whether a lesion can be emptied or not. In Fig. 3-27 the examiner's finger at point X would block the efferent channel and mask the fact that the lesion is really emptiable. This lesion would empty readily, however, with digital pressure if the finger were positioned at point Y.

The reason for the emptiability of a draining cyst or abscess is obvious and is illustrated in Fig. 3-28. Such a lesion generally is not fluctuant unless the opening is quite small.

Painless, tender, or painful. During the digital examination it becomes apparent whether a mass is painless, tender, or painful; and this information will aid greatly in arranging a suitable list of diagnostic possibilities. In the development of a working diagnosis, it is helpful if the painful mass is evaluated on the basis of the following possible etiologies (Table 3-5):

1. *Pain because of inflammation.* The painful effect of an increase in the fluid content of a tissue by a pathologic agent is intensified when the tissue is confined within rigid or semirigid walls (dental pulp, lymph node, submaxillary or parotid salivary glands). The increased internal pressure that results from the interstitial accumulation of fluid is intensified by the external pressure of the examiner's fingers and is registered as pain or an increase in pain.

The most frequently encountered example is, of course, an inflammatory process resulting from mechanical trauma or infection. Occasionally a tumor, especially of the malignant variety, will indirectly cause pain by infiltrating a major duct of a major salivary gland—thereby inducing a retention phenomenon and an enlarged salivary gland that is tender or painful because of the markedly increased internal pressure. Occasionally also a tumor confined by adjacent normal tissue will become secondarily infected and thus change from a painless to an inflamed and painful lesion.

2. *Painful tumors.* Some neural tumors (e.g., the amputation neuroma, which actually is not a true neoplasm but represents an overexuberant misdirected repair process in a severed nerve) are frequently painful to palpation. As a general rule, however, benign and malignant tumors are painless masses unless they are traumatized or secondarily infected.

3. *Pain because of sensory nerve encroachment.* Masses otherwise painless but located near relatively large sensory nerves may elicit pain when they rapidly enlarge and encroach on the nerve space. This most frequently happens when the nerve pathway is bone as opposed to soft tissue; in soft tissue, especially when the process is slow growing, the nerve is pushed ahead of the mass and pain is not elicited until an unyielding tissue is encountered. Occasionally a rapidly growing malignant tumor, such as a chondrosarcoma growing within the bone, will cause pain because it expands more rapidly than the bone can be resorbed. Hence the pressure on the surrounding bone and nerve tissue evokes pain.

Usually, however, the pain produced by the encroachment of a malignant tumor on a sensory nerve is of short duration since the rapidly growing tumor causes its early destruction. An exception is the adenoid cystic carcinoma, which frequently spreads through the perineural space. Pain is usually of long duration with these untreated tumors because they may travel along the periphery of but seldom invade the nerve.

Tenderness in a mass usually indicates the presence of a low-grade inflammation and internal pressure, which in practice are frequently induced by the repeated manipulation of a pain-

Table 3-5. Painless, tender, and painful masses

Lesions	Exceptions
Painless	
Benign and malignant tumors	Amputation neuromas
	Adenoid cystic carcinomas
	Chondrosarcomas within bone occasionally
	Infected tumors
	Traumatized tumors
	Tumors pressing nerves
Cysts	Traumatized lesions
Benign hyperplasias	Traumatized lesions
Vascular phenomena, aneurysms, etc.	Traumatized lesions
Laryngoceles	Traumatized lesions
Late hematomas	Traumatized lesions
Sarcoidosis and tuberculosis	Traumatized lesions
Retention phenomena in nonencapsulated glands	Traumatized lesions
Tender	
Low-grade inflammations and/or infections	None
Mild physical trauma	
Retension phenomena in encapsulated glands	
Bacterial, viral, fungal, and rickettsial infections	
Mononucleosis	Occasionally nontender
Early hematomas	Occasionally nontender
Subcutaneous emphysemas	Occasionally nontender
Mikulicz's disease	Occasionally nontender
Sjögren's syndrome	Occasionally nontender
Painful	
Acutely inflamed tissue	None
Severe physical trauma and acute infections	
Infected cysts	Those with draining sinuses
Infected tumors	None
Tumors	
Amputation neuromas	Early stage
Adenoid cystic carcinomas	Early stage
Chondrosarcomas	Peripheral

less mass by a series of examiners. Frequently, however, a tender mass indicates the presence of a chronic infection.

The degree of pain that a mass produces often varies, depending on the stage of development of the mass or the type of infection that may have caused the pain. For example, a retention phenomenon of major glands may be tender in the early stages but become exquisitely painful as the situation worsens. Untreated bacterial infections are typically tender in the early stage, painful in the acute phase, and tender during resolution. Fungal, spirochetal, tuberculous, rickettsial, and viral infections, on the other hand, are more typically chronic in their nature and are tender only throughout the course of their development

and resolution. Hence an infection of a node that demonstrates the same level of tenderness for a prolonged period is unlikely to be bacterial, especially if the patient has not received treatment. On the contrary, the tender node that becomes acutely painful and then resolves is probably an example of a bacterial infection.

The foregoing discussion notwithstanding, a bacterial infection of a tissue caused by a virulent resistant organism that is being unsuccessfully treated may remain tender for a prolonged period.

Unilateral or bilateral. Whether a lesion is unilateral or bilateral can be determined by inspection and/or palpation. When a clinician encounters pathosis, he should investigate the contralateral region of the body for the purpose of determining whether the condition is bilateral or not. As a general rule, if similar masses are present bilaterally and in the same locations, they are most likely normal anatomic structures. The carotid bulb in the bifurcation of the artery, the mastoid process, the lateral processes of the cervical vertebrae, and the wings of the hyoid bone are such bilaterally occurring anatomic structures that are frequently mistaken for pathologic masses. Bilateral palpation coupled with a knowledge of anatomy is obligatory if these normal structures are to be differentiated from pathologic masses.

Solitary or multiple. A solitary lesion nearly always indicates a local benign condition or an early malignancy. Multiple lesions, on the other hand, must alert the examiner to the following possibilities:

Addison's disease
Blood dyscrasias
Hodgkin's disease
Infectious mononucleosis
Multiple fungal infections
Multiple metastases
Paget's disease
Reticuloendotheliosis

The syndromes with multiple lesions should also be considered:

Albright's syndrome
Basal cell nevus syndrome
Gardner's syndrome
Peutz-Jeghers syndrome

Syndrome of multiple neuromas, carcinoma of the thyroid, and pheochromocytoma
von Recklinghausen's disease

Features obtained by percussion

Percussion is the act of tapping a part of the body to evaluate the quality of the echo produced. The physician routinely percusses the chest to determine the outline of the heart and also to evaluate the lung fields. The dentist frequently percusses teeth to determine whether they have adequate bone support and also to determine whether they are sensitive. Percussion is not particularly useful, however, for the examination of the lesions discussed in this text.

Features obtained by auscultation

Auscultation is the act of listening with or without the aid of a stethoscope to sounds produced inside the body. The physician routinely auscultates the chest to evaluate heart and lung sounds. The dentist may auscultate the temporomandibular joint to detect crepitus. Auscultation of pathologic masses is to be encouraged because this method will detect the presence of bruits, which are a characteristic of aneurysms and arteriovenous shunts.

GENERAL REFERENCES

Dolby, A. E.: Oral mucosa in health and disease, Oxford, England, 1975, Blackwell Scientific Publications.
Whitten, J. B.: Cytologic examination of aspirated material from cysts or cystlike lesions, Oral Surg. **25**:710-716, 1968.

4

The diagnostic sequence

Norman K. Wood
Paul W. Goaz

It is of paramount importance that the clinician initiate a precisely formulated diagnostic sequence when he is confronted by a lesion. Such an established approach to the perception, examination, and conception of a set of circumstances helps to assure two safeguards: first, when a definite and methodical diagnostic procedure is formulated and followed, *all the pertinent features* will be identified; and second, by adapting and following a routine, the dentist accomplishes the total procedure *rapidly as well as effectively.*

Some authorities argue that the experienced diagnostician does not rely on such a cumbersome and formal procedure since he is apparently able to diagnose a lesion after only a brief inspection. This is seldom if ever the case, however, because generally his expertise is based not on instant recognition but on the rapid and effective use of a diagnostic sequence he has perfected through experience. Of course, the astute diagnostician has seen many lesions on numerous occasions and is thus able to anticipate the nature of a familiar disorder and still maintain an excellent "batting average."

We have found the following diagnostic sequence to be both effective and practical:

Detection and examination of the patient's lesion
Examination of the patient
    Chief complaint(s)
    Onset and course
Reexamination of the lesion
Classification of the lesion
Listing the possible diagnoses
Developing the differential diagnosis
Developing the working diagnosis (operational diagnosis, tentative diagnosis, clinical impression)
Formulating the final diagnosis [proved by biopsy, culture, and/or response to treatment]

DETECTION AND EXAMINATION OF THE PATIENT'S LESION

Obviously a lesion will be detected before it is examined. Most lesions are discovered during routine examination; but in some cases, and especially when pain or discomfort is a symptom, the patient is the first to become aware of the disorder and he initiates its examination.

Once the clinician has recognized or at least suspects that an abnormal change is at hand, he then proceeds to examine it using the modalities described in Chapters 2 and 3. These include visual examination in combination with palpation, percussion, and auscultation. The findings are noted and mentally evaluated. As a matter of personal preference, he may elect to do a cursory or a thorough examination of the lesion at this time although the situation may dictate a thorough examination immediately. The importance of examining the lesion is that the clinician can gain information that will alert him to look especially for possible related findings in the remainder of the patient examination.

EXAMINATION OF THE PATIENT

Patient examination has been discussed in considerable depth in Chapters 2 and 3. Although the specific steps of examination of the patient will not be detailed here, the sections of the interview dealing with the patient's chief complaint(s) and the onset and course of his present problem should be emphasized because they often yield particularly helpful diagnostic clues.

Chief complaint(s)

Common chief complaints related to oral diseases include the following: pain, sores, burning sensation, bleeding, loose teeth, recent occlusal problems, delayed tooth eruption, dry mouth, too much saliva, a swelling, and bad taste.

Pain. The patient should be encouraged to describe the main characteristics of his pain, its nature (sharp or dull), its severity, duration, and location, and the precipitating circumstances.

The following disturbances may be the cause of oral pain:

1. Inflammation from any cause
2. Mechanical pressure on sensory nerve endings
3. Infected or traumatized tumors
4. Other tumors that characteristically cause pain (central malignant tumors of bone, adenoid cystic carcinoma, amputation neuroma)

Sores. When a patient uses the term "sore" or "a sore" to describe his complaint, this may indicate the presence of mucosal inflammations or ulcers from any cause except early ulcerative malignancies (which are usually painless).

Burning sensation. A burning sensation is usually felt in the tongue and is often caused by a thinning or erosion of the surface epithelium. The following disease states may produce a burning sensation:

1. Geographic tongue
2. Erosive lichen planus
3. Avitaminosis
4. Anemia
5. Neuroses

A generalized burning sensation in the mouth is also frequently found to be associated with an increased interalveolar space.

Bleeding. Intraoral bleeding may be caused by these disturbances:

1. Gingivitis and periodontal disease
2. Traumatic incidents, including surgery
3. Inflammatory hyperplasias
4. Allergies
5. Tumors (traumatized tumors and tumors that are very vascular, e.g., hemangiomas)
6. Diseases that cause or are associated with deficiencies in hemostasis

Loose teeth. Loss of supporting bone or the resorption of roots may result in loose teeth and may indicate the presence of any of the following:

1. Periodontal disease
2. Trauma
3. Normal resorption of deciduous teeth
4. Pulpoperiapical lesions
5. Malignant tumors
6. Benign tumors that may induce root re-

sorption (chondromas, myxomas, hemangiomas)

7. Histiocytosis X
8. Hypophosphatasia
9. Familial hypophosphatemia
10. Papillon-Lefèvre syndrome

Recent occlusal problem. When a patient complains that "recently the teeth don't bite right" or "recently some teeth are out of line," the clinician must consider overcontoured restorations or the following diseases:

1. Periodontal disease
2. Traumatic injury (fracture of bone or tooth root)
3. Periapical abscess
4. Cysts or tumors of tooth-bearing regions of the jaws
5. Fibrous dysplasia

Delayed tooth eruption. Delayed eruption of a tooth may be related to any of the following:

1. Malposed or impacted teeth
2. Cysts
3. Odontomas
4. Sclerosed bone
5. Tumors
6. Maldevelopment

If there is a generalized delay, the clinician should consider the possibilities of anodontia, cleidocranial dysostosis, or hypothyroidism.

Dry mouth. A dry mouth may result from the following disorders:

1. Local inflammation
2. Infection or fibrosis of the major salivary glands
3. Dehydration states
4. Atropine therapy
5. Autoimmune diseases
6. Psychosomatic problems

Too much saliva. The complaint of excessive saliva may be related to psychosomatic problems. It may be associated with the insertion of new dentures; and if it continues, it may indicate a decreased or an increased vertical dimension.

A swelling. When a patient's chief complaint is a swelling, all of the following entities must be considered as a probable cause:

1. Inflammations and infections
2. Cysts
3. Retention phenomena
4. Inflammatory hyperplasias
5. Benign and/or malignant tumors

Bad taste. A complaint of bad taste may result from any of the following:

1. Periodontal disease

2. Acute necrotic ulcerative gingivitis
3. Intraoral malignancies

Onset and course

The following classification of onsets and courses related to the growth rate of specific masses has proved helpful to us:

1. Masses that increase in size just prior to eating
   a. Salivary retention phenomena
2. Slow-growing masses (duration of months to years)
   a. Reactive hyperplasias
   b. Chronic infections
   c. Cysts
   d. Benign tumors
3. Moderately rapid growing masses (weeks to about 2 months)
   a. Chronic infections
   b. Cysts
   c. Malignant tumors
4. Rapidly growing masses (hours to days)
   a. Abscesses (painful)
   b. Infected cysts (painful)
   c. Aneurysms (painless)
   d. Salivary retention phenomena (painless)
   e. Hematomas (painless but sting on pressure)
5. Masses with accompanying fever
   a. Infections
   b. Lymphomas

REEXAMINATION OF THE LESION

At this point in the examination, unanswered questions frequently occur to the clinician; and he may want to reexamine the lesion to reevaluate his original findings or to complete more detailed observations. For example, if the lesion is found to be soft, he may wish to determine whether it (1) is fluctuant, (2) can be emptied, (3) blanches on pressure, (4) pulsates, or (5) produces a gas or liquid on aspiration and what the nature of the aspirate is. On the other hand, if the lesion is firm, he may want to determine its extent, whether it is freely movable, whether it is fixed to the mucosa or the underlying tissue, and so on.

CLASSIFICATION OF THE LESION

By the time the clinician has reached this point in the diagnostic sequence, he should be able to classify the lesion according to whether it has originated in soft tissue or bone. Having arrived at a conclusion, he must next describe the lesion in terms of its clinical or radiographic appearance.

For example, the soft tissue lesions will be subclassified as white, exophytic, ulcerative, and so on, whereas the bony lesions may be categorized as periapical radiolucencies, cystlike radiolucencies, multiple radiopacities, and so on. Since the lesions in the ensuing pages of this text have been classified and the chapters organized on the basis of similar clinical or radiographic appearances, the clinician can use the same scheme to describe the lesion he encounters and thus facilitate his reference between patient and book.

LISTING THE POSSIBLE DIAGNOSES

When most of the available appropriate data have been collected, a list of all the lesions that may produce a similar clinical or radiographic picture should be compiled. Initially the order of the list will not be important since the primary objective of this preliminary step is merely to include every entity that is clinically and/or radiographically similar to the condition under study.

At this point in the diagnostic exercise, the clinician may find it convenient to refer to the list at the beginning of each chapter. These previews are compilations of the entities that could possibly fit into the general descriptive category of each chapter; and they form, in turn, the chapter titles.

DEVELOPING THE DIFFERENTIAL DIAGNOSIS

The process of developing a differential diagnosis may be defined briefly in the context of this discussion as the rearranging of the list of possible diagnoses, with the most probable lesion ranked at the top and the least likely at the bottom.

The actual process of ranking the lesions may become very complicated as the clinician attempts to match the features of the lesion being examined with the usual (or characteristic) features of the specific lesions in his list. To become competent in the art of differential diagnosis, therefore, not only must he be familiar with the signs and symptoms produced by a great many diseases but he must also possess some statistical knowledge relative to the incidence of each disease entity. It is particularly important that he be aware of the relative incidences of individual lesions because in the completed differential diagnosis the most commonly occurring lesion will usually be ranked above the least commonly occurring unless other specific features prompt a modification of this ranking.

Consequently, we strongly recommend that in developing the differential diagnosis, the clinician first rank the lesions in order of their *relative frequency of occurrence,* as they are in the list at the beginning of each chapter; however, he must realize that many conditions will modify the general frequency: age, sex, race, country of origin, and anatomic location.

Age. The age of a patient will greatly modify the rankings. For example, an ulcer occurring in the floor of a 50-year-old man's mouth would indicate a high probability of squamous cell carcinoma; but such a diagnosis would be very unlikely if an ulcer occurred in a 10-year-old boy's mouth. Tables 4-1 and 4-2 group the soft tissue and bony lesions that show a tendency for occurring in patients within particular age spans.

Sex. The fact that certain lesions occur more frequently in males or in females will also contribute to the listing of the lesions in the differential diagnosis. As an example, squamous cell carcinoma affects males two to four times more often than females. On the other hand, about 80% of periapical cementomas occur in women over 30 years of age. Tables 4-3 and 4-4 group the soft tissue and bony lesions that show a predilection for occurring in female or male patients.

Race. The importance of racial (and hereditary) influences on the incidence of some diseases is illustrated by the well-known fact that a preponderance of patients afflicted with sickle cell ane-

Table 4-1. Predilection of soft tissue lesions for special age groups

Infants	Children	Persons under age 40	Persons over age 40
Candidiasis*	Albright's disease (6-10 yr)	Albright's disease (ages 6-10)	Benign mucous membrane pemphigoid
Eruption cyst	Childhood infectious diseases	ANUG (ages 15-35; rare below age 12)	Candidiasis†
Hemangioma (85% by end of first year)	Eruption cyst	Benign salivary gland tumor (ages 30-39)	Denture stomatitis
Lingual thyroid	Infectious mononucleosis	Branchial cyst	Desquamative gingivitis
Lymphangioma	Juvenile melanoma	Candidiasis	Epulis fissuratum
Neuroectodermal tumor (before 6 mo)	Pulp polyps	Childhood infectious diseases	Hemochromatosis
White sponge nevus	White sponge nevus	Cystic hygroma	Inflammatory papillary hyperplasia
		Dermoid or epidermoid cyst	Keratoacanthoma
		Eruption cyst	Leukoedema
		Erythema multiforme	Leukoplakia (90%)
		Hemangioma (85% by end of first yr)	Lichen planus
		Hodgkin's disease (ages 20-40)	Lipoma
		Infectious mononucleosis	Lymphoma
		Juvenile melanoma	Malignant salivary gland tumors (ages 40-60)
		Lingual thyroid	Melanoma
		Lymphangioma (88% before age 3)	Metastatic carcinoma
		Mucocele (65% before age 30)	Metastatic carcinoma to cervical nodes
		Neuroectodermal tumor (before 6 mo)	Pemphigus (seldom under age 30)
		Palatal tori (peak before age 30)	Radiation mucositis
		Papilloma	Squamous cell carcinoma
		Peripheral giant cell granuloma (over age 30)	Verrucous carcinoma (ages 60-80)
		Peripheral fibroma with calcification (peak at age 25)	
		Plasma cell gingivitis	
		Pulp polyps	
		Pyogenic granuloma (60%)	
		Recurrent aphthous ulcer	
		Thyroglossal cyst	
		White sponge nevus	

*Also common in persons over age 40.
†Also common in infants.

Table 4-2. Predisposition of bony or calcified lesions for special age groups

Infants	Children	Persons under age 30	Persons over age 30	Persons over age 40
Caffey's disease (birth to 2 yr)	Acute leukemia	Acute leukemia	Ameloblastoma (ages 20-50, peak at age 40)	Artery calcification
Letterer-Siwe disease (ages 1-3)	Basal cell nevus syndrome (ages 5-30)	Adenomatoid odontogenic tumor (peak at age 16)	Cementoma	Calcified node
Osteopetrosis (malignant)	Burkitt's tumor (ages 2-14)	Ameloblastic fibroma (peak at age 16)	Chondrosarcoma (ages 20-60, peak in 50s)	Cancer
Rickets	Central hemangioma (ages 10-20)	Aneurysmal bone cyst (under age 20)	Osteopetrosis (benign)	Chondrosarcoma (ages 20-60; peak in 50s)
Stafne's cyst?	Cherubism	Basal cell nevus syndrome (ages 5-30)	Pindborg tumor (ages 28-48)	Metastatic carcinoma
Thalassemia major	Fibrous dysplasia (ages 10-20)	Burkitt's tumor (ages 2-14)	Primary hyperparathyroidism (ages 30-60)	Minor salivary tumor
	Follicular cyst (ages 10-20)	Caffey's disease (birth to 2 yr)	Residual cyst (peak at age 52)	Multiple myeloma (ages 40-70)
	Garré's osteomyelitis (ages 5-12)	Cancer	Sclerosing cemental masses	Squamous cell carcinoma (peripheral)
	Hand-Schüller-Christian disease (ages 1-10)	Ewing's sarcoma (peak at ages 14-18)		Osteomalacia
	Multilocular cyst (over age 15)	Osteogenic sarcoma of jaws (ages 10-40, peak at age 27)		Osteomyelitis
	Osteoid osteoma	Reticulum cell sarcoma of bone (70% under age 40)		Paget's disease
	Osteopetrosis (malignant)	Cementifying and ossifying fibroma (young adults)		Postextraction sockets
	Rickets	Cementoblastoma (under age 25)		Secondary hyperparathyroidism (ages 50-80)
	Stafne's cyst	Central giant cell granuloma (60% under age 20)		Sialolith
	Thalassemia major	Central hemangioma (ages 10-20)		
		Cherubism		
		Developing tooth crypt (under age 20)		
		Eosinophilic granuloma		
		Fibrous dysplasia (ages 10-20)		
		Follicular cyst (ages 10-20)		
		Garré's osteomyelitis (under age 25)		
		Hand-Schüller-Christian disease (ages 1-10)		
		Letterer-Siwe disease (ages 1-3)		
		Multilocular cyst (over age 15)		
		Mural ameloblastoma (ages 18-30)		
		Odontogenic fibroma (under age 25)		
		Odontogenic keratocyst (ages 10-20)		
		Odontoma in developing stages (under age 20)		
		Osteoblastoma (75% under age 20)		
		Osteoid osteoma		
		Osteopetrosis (malignant)		
		Parulis		
		Primordial cyst (ages 10-30)		
		Rickets		
		Sickle cell anemia		
		Stafne's cyst		
		Thalassemia major		
		Thalassemia minor		
		Traumatic bone cyst (under age 25)		

Table 4-3. Sex predilection of soft tissue lesions (ratios or percents are given in parentheses)

Male	Female
Cancer (except minor salivary gland tumors)	Benign mucous membrane pemphigoid (2:1)
Lymphoma (2:1)	Desquamative gingivitis
Melanoma (2:1)	Geographic tongue (2:1)
Metastatic carcinoma to cervical nodes	Hemangioma
Squamous cell carcinoma (4:1 to 2:1)	Lichen planus (2:1)
Buccal (10:1)	Lipoma (7:1 or equal)
Floor (93%)	Palatal tori (2:1)
Lip (98%)	Peripheral giant cell granuloma (2:1)
Tongue (75%)	Peripheral fibroma with calcification
Verrucous carcinoma (3:1)	Plasma cell gingivitis
Erythema multiforme	Pyogenic granuloma (3:1)
Hemochromatosis	Ranula
Keratoacanthoma (2:1)	Recurrent aphthous ulcers
Leukoplakia	Salivary gland tumors (2:1)
Lymphoepithelial cyst (3:1)	
Median rhomboid glossitis	
Mucocele	
Radiation mucositis	

Table 4-4. Sex predisposition of bony lesions

Male	Female
Cancer	Cancer
Chondrosarcoma	Metastatic carcinoma
Ewing's sarcoma (2:1)	Minor salivary gland tumors
Lymphoma (2:1)	Cementoma
Melanoma (2:1)	Central giant cell granuloma (2:1)
Multiple myeloma (2:1)	Central hemangioma (2:1)
Osteogenic sarcoma	Osteoporosis
Squamous cell carcinoma	Primary hyperparathyroidism (7:1)
Central (2:1)	Sclerosing cemental masses
Peripheral (4:1 to 2:1)	Secondary hyperparathyroidism (2:1)
Cherubism	Stafne's cyst
Eosinophilic granuloma (2:1)	
Hand-Schüller-Christian disease (2:1)	
Incisive canal cyst (3:1)	
Osteoblastoma	
Osteoid osteoma (2:1)	
Osteomyelitis (5:1)	
Residual cyst (2:1)	
Traumatic bone cyst	

mia are black. Also diffuse cementosis (sclerosing cemental masses) occurs predominately in black women over 30 years of age.

Country of origin. Information concerning the country of origin or residence may be an important clue for identification of the disease. Burkitt's lymphoma seldom affects people of non-African origin. Also the greater use of chewing tobacco and snuff in the southeastern section of

the United States is related to the increased incidence of intraoral verrucous carcinoma observed in that region.

Anatomic location. The extent to which the anatomic location of the lesion may affect the lesion's ranking in the differential diagnosis is illustrated by the following examples:

1. Although the lower lip is a common site for the development of a mucocele but a rare

location for a minor salivary gland tumor, both these lesions may be in the same list of possible diagnoses.

2. The posterior region of the hard palate is a characteristic location for a minor salivary gland tumor but is an uncommon location for a mucocele.
3. Although the posterior hard palate is a characteristic site for a salivary gland tumor, this lesion is almost never found in the anterior hard palate and gingivae.

Table 4-5 groups the various bony lesions that show a preference for either the maxilla or mandible and also for specific sites within these bones.

• • •

It is important to emphasize that the preceding pertinent facts are just a few examples from a large body of general information concerning the natural behavior of lesions that the clinician will learn from his clinical experience in addition to the knowledge provided by formally structured courses.

After the ranking has been adjusted for incidence, the next step is to compare the pertinent information, signs, symptoms, or other findings gained from the examination of the patient with the usual features of the lesions in the list. The lesion showing the greatest amount of correlation with the present findings should be ranked highest, and the lesion showing the least correlation should be ranked lowest. Thus the earlier rank-

Table 4-5. Jawbone and regional predilection of bony lesions

Mandible and predominant region	Maxilla and predominant region	Rare in maxilla
Ameloblastic fibroma (molar, premolar)	Adenomatoid odontogenic tumor (canine)	Caffey's disease
Ameloblastoma (80%; posterior, 70%)	Chondrosarcoma (2:1)	Cementifying and/or ossifying fibroma
Aneurysmal bone cyst (much more common in molar)	Compound odontoma	Ewing's sarcoma
Benign nonodontogenic tumors (molar, ramus)	Fibrous dysplasia (4:3)	Garré's osteomyelitis
Caffey's disease	Paget's disease (20:3)	Osteomyelitis
Calcifying odontogenic cyst (70%)	Residual cyst (65%)	Reticulum cell sarcoma
Cancer		Traumatic bone cyst
Acute leukemia (molar)		
Ewing's sarcoma		
Metastatic carcinoma (95%; molar, premolar)		
Osteogenic sarcoma (body)		
Reticulum cell sarcoma (molar, angle, ramus)		
Squamous cell carcinoma		
Peripheral (3:1; molar)		
Central (2:1)		
Cementifying and/or ossifying fibroma (molar, premolar)		
Cementoblastoma (first molar, premolar)		
Cementoma (90%; incisor)		
Central giant cell granuloma (65%; two thirds are anterior to molar)		
Central hemangioma (65%; ramus, premolar)		
Cherubism (ramus, third molar)		
Complex odontoma		
Condensing osteitis		
Eosinophilic granuloma		
Follicular cyst		
Garré's osteomyelitis		
Odontogenic fibroma		
Odontogenic keratocyst (65%)		
Odontogenic myxoma (molar, premolar)		
Osteomyelitis (7:1; body)		
Pindborg tumor (2:1; molar, premolar)		
Postextraction sockets		
Primordial cyst (third molar)		
Sclerosing cemental masses		

ing on a frequency basis is modified at this time.

Two or more lesions present. From time to time clinicians examine patients with various combinations of lesions. Perhaps one patient will present with two lesions in the oral cavity. Another patient may have a lesion in the oral cavity and another in the neck. In still another patient the examination may reveal a lesion in the oral cavity and another in a more distant site, for example, the lung. After some thought, it becomes obvious that it is necessary to develop the differential diagnosis along distinctly contrasting lines in each of these cases.

Basically when two or more lesions are present, seven possibilities or propositions must be considered (modified from Mitton et al., 1976):

1. Lesions are related.
   a. Lesion A and lesion B are identical (two aphthous ulcers).
   b. Lesion B is secondary to lesion A (metastatic tumor and primary tumor).
   c. Lesion A is secondary to lesion B (metastatic tumor and primary tumor).
   d. Lesion A and lesion B are both secondary to a third lesion, which may be occult (metastatic tumors and primary tumor).
   e. Lesion A and lesion B are manifestations of systemic disease (infections, histiocytosis X, disseminated malignancy).
   f. Lesion A and lesion B form part of a syndrome (café-au-lait spots and multiple neurofibromas in von Recklinghausen's disease).
2. Lesions are completely unrelated to each other and occur together only as a matter of chance.

DEVELOPING THE WORKING DIAGNOSIS (OPERATIONAL DIAGNOSIS, TENTATIVE DIAGNOSIS, CLINICAL IMPRESSION)

Although the clinician has completed a differential diagnosis, he is not yet completely prepared to treat the lesion. He must now recheck the *credibility* of his top choices. This is done by further examination of the lesion, by asking the patient more definitive questions to expand the history, by perhaps ordering additional tests, and finally by reevaluating all the assembled pertinent data. Once their validity has been supported, the top choices will be referred to as the working diagnosis or clinical impression. The clinician may, in some cases, be so confident of his no. 1 ranked entity that he excludes all the others from his working diagnosis.

The *working diagnosis* must indicate the proper management, especially if the management is to include surgery, because it will aid the surgeon in planning his operation—how long to schedule the operating room for, what instrument setups to have prepared, whether to do an incisional or an excisional biopsy or a frozen section, whether to have blood available and, if so, how much and what type.

Before the surgery commences, the surgeon may choose to do one last test, such as aspiration of the lesion. This is an excellent precaution in certain instances and will rule out or identify vascular tumors, thereby avoiding the dangerous surprise that awaits the unsuspecting surgeon who encounters an unrecognized vascular tumor at surgery.

FORMULATING THE FINAL DIAGNOSIS

The final diagnosis in most cases of oral pathoses is provided by the oral pathologist who evaluates a biopsy in the light of all the available clinical data. In some instances the microscopic picture is quite diagnostic. In other cases, however, the microscopic picture may be so equivocal that the pathologist must depend heavily on the accompanying clinical symptoms in establishing the final diagnosis. In still other cases (e.g., an empty traumatic bone cyst) the clinician must establish the final diagnosis at the time of the surgery since there may not be a specimen available for microscopic examination.

SPECIFIC REFERENCE

Mitton, V. A., Eversole, L. R., Kramer, H. S., and Stern, M.: Clinical-Pathological Conference: case 16, part 1 and part 2. Stafne's bone cyst of the mandible and concurrent pulmonary coccidioidomycosis, J. Oral Surg. **34:**616-617, 715-716, 1976.

PART II

SOFT TISSUE LESIONS

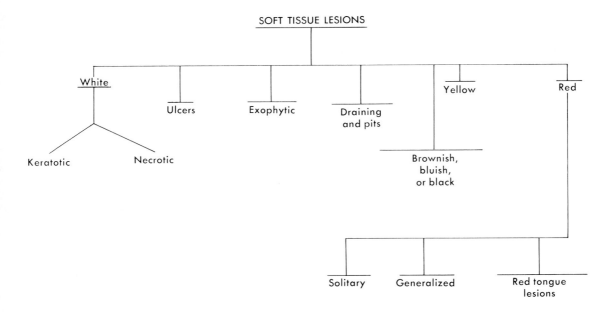

5

White lesions of the oral mucosa

Norman K. Wood
Paul W. Goaz

Following is a list of white lesions of the oral mucosa:

Keratotic white entities
Leukoedema
Linea alba buccalis
Leukoplakia
    Nicotinic stomatitis or smoker's palate
    Snuff dipper's lesion
    Cigarette smoker's lip lesion
Benign migratory glossitis and mucositis
Peripheral scar tissue [not keratotic]
Lichen planus
White hairy tongue
Papilloma
Verruca vulgaris
Verrucous carcinoma
Chronic keratotic candidiasis
White sponge nevus
Skin grafts
Rarities
    Acanthosis nigricans
    Bohn's nodule (Epstein's pearl)
    Condyloma acuminatum
    Condyloma latum
    Darier's disease
    Dermatitis herpetiformis
    Dyskeratosis congenita
    Focal epithelial hyperplasia
    Focal palmoplantar and marginal gingival hyperkeratosis
    Grinspan's syndrome
    Hereditary benign intraepithelial dyskeratosis
    Hypersplenism and leukoplakia oris
    Hypovitaminosis A
    Inverted papilloma
    Koplik's spots
    Lupus erythematosus
    Molluscum contagiosum
    Pachyonychia congenita
    Pityriasis rubra pilaris
    Porokeratosis
    Pseudoepitheliomatous hyperplasia
    Psoriasis
    Scleroderma (nonkeratotic)
    Squamous acanthoma
    Submucous fibrosis (nonkeratotic)

    Superficial sialolith of minor glands (nonkeratotic)
    Syndrome of dyskeratosis congenita, dystrophia, unguium, and aplastic anemia
    Syphilitic interstitial glossitis leukoplakia
    Verruciform xanthoma
    Warty dyskeratoma

Sloughing, pseudomembranous, necrotic white lesions
Plaque
Traumatic ulcer
Pyogenic granuloma
Chemical burns
Acute necrotizing ulcerative gingivitis
Candidiasis
Necrotic ulcers of systemic disease
Diffuse gangrenous stomatitis
Rarities
    Diphtheria
    Heavy metal mucositis
    Noma
    Superficial abscess
    Syndrome of familial hypoparathyroidism, candidiasis, and retardation
    Syndrome of idiopathic hypoparathyroidism, Addison's disease, and candidiasis
    Syphilitic chancre and mucous patch
    Tuberculosis
    Verruciform xanthoma

Vesicles and bullae [discussed in Chapter 11]

White lesions of the oral mucosa may be conveniently divided into two groups: those that cannot be scraped off with a tongue blade (most are keratotic) and those that can be scraped off with a tongue blade (sloughing, pseudomembranous necrotic types). This chapter is likewise divided into two such parts—the first dealing with the keratotic entities (which as a group are the more commonly encountered white lesions) and the second reviewing the sloughing types.

A third type, the vesiculobullous lesion, almost

61

Fig. 5-1. A, Benign mucous membrane pemphigoid; arrow indicates white bullous lesion. Two ulcers are present on each side of the bullous lesion and were produced when previous bullae ruptured. Although vesicular and bullous lesions are white they are more suitably grouped with generalized reddish conditions (see Chapter 11). **B,** Recurrent herpetic lesion on the buccal gingiva. Note that in this case the predominant clinical change is white although careful scrutiny will reveal pinpoint ulcers in the center of the white areas.

invariably has a white or grayish-white appearance and so must be considered as white lesions particularly during the examination process (Fig. 5-1).

However, when the clinician advances to the differential diagnosis process, he finds it much more suitable to group these lesions by themselves or as generalized reddish conditions (see Chapter 11). We introduce this information at the onset of this chapter particularly to alert students to the fact that such lesions are white both when the blisters are intact and also for a day or two after they rupture.

Keratotic white entities

To the inexperienced clinician the oral mucosa may appear only pink.

As his experience increases and his observation becomes more acute, however, he will discover the wide spectrum of pinks that are char-

Fig. 5-2. The attached gingiva is a paler pink than the vestibular mucosa due to the keratinized surface and less vascularity.

acteristic of the normal oral mucosa, varying from a dark pink (reddish) to a very pale pink (almost white). In addition, he will become familiar with the mucosal locations in the oral cavity where these different shades may normally be found. Furthermore, he will be able to comprehend the variations on the basis of microscopic structure and function.

The various colors and hues as well as the morphologic structure of the oral mucous membrane are related, in part, to the mechanical influences of mastication.

Surfaces exposed to vigorous stimulation by the mastication of hard and rough foods respond by forming a thicker epithelium with perhaps a heavier keratin covering and usually a denser, fibrous, less vascular subepithelial connective tissue. These surfaces compose the masticatory mucosa and appear white in color—the mucous membrane on the hard palate, the fixed gingiva, and the dorsal surface of the tongue (Fig. 5-2).

On the other hand, protected surfaces form very little keratin, have a less fibrous, more vascular subepithelial layer, and are of a darker pink or more reddish hue—the vestibule, floor of the mouth, ventral surface of the tongue, and retromolar regions. These surfaces are said to be *lining* mucosa.

Individual variations in the color of the oral mucosa will be apparent and are probably an expression of one or more genetically controlled factors; that is, some people readily form keratin as a result of minor stimuli whereas others require a strong stimulus to produce minimal keratinization. The clinician must also be cognizant of the fact that a patient's hemoglobin concentration will affect the shade of pink. For example,

Fig. 5-3. Leukoedema. **A,** Note the white wrinkled appearance of the buccal mucosa, present bilaterally, in a 45-year-old black man. **B,** Photomicrograph showing acanthosis, ballooning in the prickle cells, and parakeratosis.

the patient with polycythemia will have a redder mucosa than will the patient with anemia.

In some regions normal keratinization and/or epithelial thickening may be so marked as to appear pathologic. Leukoedema and linea alba are such examples.

LEUKOEDEMA

Leukoedema is a quite common variation of the normal oral mucosa. It appears as a diffuse, filmy, milky opalescence on the buccal mucosa. Although its etiology is unknown, leukoedema may develop as a result of masticatory function and has been shown to be related to poor oral hygiene

(Martin and Crump, 1972). Studies have failed to demonstrate that its formation is related to tobacco use, syphilis, or malocclusion; but an increased incidence and severity have been shown to occur with age. Martin and Crump (1972) reported that about 50% of black teenagers and children have this normal variation, and it is a common observation in 90% of black adults. Although the percentage of whites affected is reported to be approximately 45%, Durocher and co-workers (1972) showed that under good lighting conditions leukoedema could be found in 93% of the whites they examined. Current consensus holds that the lesion does not undergo malignant changes.

FEATURES

Leukoedema is totally asymptomatic and is usually found during routine oral examination. Although frequently discovered on the buccal mucosa, it also occurs on the labial mucosa and soft palate. The degree of severity varies from a faint filmy appearance, which requires close inspection for detection, to a much denser opalescence with wrinkling or folding of the surface (Figs. 5-3 and 5-4). Leukoedema cannot be removed with a tongue blade.

Microscopically an increased thickness of the epithelium can be observed usually with marked intracellular edema (ballooning) in the prickle cell layer. A hyperparakeratosis (hyperkeratosis with retention of nuclei) of varying thickness may be present (Fig. 5-3).

DIFFERENTIAL DIAGNOSIS

The commonly occurring lesions that may be confused with leukoedema are *leukoplakia*, *cheek-biting lesion*, and *white sponge nevus*. A discussion of the differential diagnosis of these lesions is presented under the differential diagnosis of leukoplakia (p. 70).

MANAGEMENT

Since leukoedema is a normal variant, its recognition is important and no treatment is required.

LINEA ALBA BUCCALIS

Linea alba (white line) is a streak on the buccal mucosa at the level of the occlusal plane extending horizontally from the commissure to the most posterior teeth. It is usually seen bilaterally and may be quite prominent in some people (Fig. 5-5). Because it occurs at the occlusal plane and conforms to the space between the teeth, it is

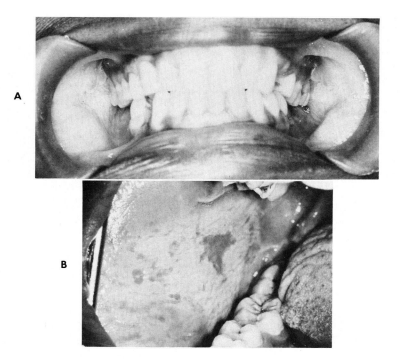

Fig. 5-4. Leukoedema. **A,** Milky wrinkled appearance was present bilaterally in this 52-year-old black woman. **B,** Red eroded areas in this example of leukoedema were caused by cheek biting. Stretching the tissue eliminated the white appearance in both cases. (**A** courtesy S. Smith, D.D.S., Chicago.)

Fig. 5-5. Linea alba. **A,** Prominent example in classic location. **B,** Unusual location and appearance of linea alba on mucosal surface of lower lip. Patient habitually sucked the tissue in against his anterior teeth.

thought to result from slight occlusal trauma to the buccal mucosa.

This impression is strengthened by the observation that a linea alba is frequently more prominent in people who have little overjet of the molars and premolars. The prominence of the linea alba varies greatly from one individual to another, being especially marked in some people and completely absent in others (Fig. 5-5).

Histologically an increased thickness or hyperorthokeratosis (hyperkeratosis without retention of nuclei) is seen.

Management requires only the recognition of linea alba as a normal variation.

LEUKOPLAKIA

Leukoplakia* is a keratotic plaque occurring on mucous membranes; its immediate cause is chronic irritation. As with other keratotic lesions, it cannot be scraped off with a tongue blade. Although definitive statements on the role of genetics and systemic conditions that predispose the oral mucosa to leukoplakia must await further investigations, much is already known about the local or direct causes of this condition. For example, a variety of local chronic irritations, acting alone or in combination, will produce leukoplakial lesions in certain individuals.

The following have been suggested to be of etiologic importance in leukoplakia:

Tobacco products
Cold temperatures
Hot and/or spicy foods
Alcohol
Occlusal trauma
Sharp edges of prostheses or teeth
Actinic radiation
Syphilis
Candidia albicans

The fact that the presence of the above factors cannot be documented in approximately 20% of oral cancer patients (Ballard et al., 1978) has produced a search for additional causative factors. Recently Weaver and co-workers (1979) reported interesting findings from a study of 200 patients with squamous cell carcinoma of the head and neck. These investigators reported that 11 of these patients had never used alcohol or tobacco but all but one of these 11 had used mouthwash

---

*At one time a significant number of pathologists used the term "leukoplakia" to describe a specific histopathologic picture. Today most pathologists use "leukoplakia" only to describe a keratotic white patch that cannot be diagnosed as any other disease, caused by chronic irritation on a mucous membrane; and only thus is the term used in this book.

Fig. 5-6. Keratotic condition of the oral mucosa produced by holding Listerine mouthwash in the mouth for 15 minutes once a day. (From Bernstein, M. L.: Oral Surg. **46**(6):781-785, 1978.)

containing 25% alcohol many times daily for more than 20 years. In this context Bernstein (1978) reported and illustrated diffuse keratotic changes (leukoplakia type we would presume) in the oral mucosa due to the use of Listerine mouthwash (Fig. 5-6). These changes disappeared soon after discontinuation of the mouthwash.

The chronic irritation, regardless of type, must be intense enough to induce the surface epithelium to produce and retain keratin but not so intense as to cause a breakdown of the tissue with resulting erosion or ulcer formation. Obviously genetic and systemic factors play a role in preconditioning the mucosa, because some people develop a leukoplakial lesion as the result of a relatively minor insult whereas others either show no reaction to the same or more prolonged and severe stimulus or suffer tissue destruction and an inflammatory lesion.

Leukoplakia, then, likely commences as a protective reaction against a chronic irritant. This reaction produces a dense layer of keratin, which is retained for the purpose of insulating the deeper epithelial components from the deleterious effects of the irritant.

When clinical leukoplakial lesions are studied microscopically, they can be seen to embrace a whole spectrum of histologic changes ranging from an innocuous lesion that shows only increased keratosis to invasive squamous cell carcinoma. These differences cannot be detected clinically; so to establish the specific diagnosis every lesion must be examined microscopically.

Waldron (1970, p. 813) stated that leukoplakias may be histologically divided into two main categories (Fig. 5-7):

1. Those that show no atypia (dysplasia)
2. Those that show different degrees of atypia

In Bánóczy and Csiba's study of oral leukoplakia in Hungary (1976) 24% of their subjects showed dysplasia. Waldron and Shafer's study (1975) revealed a similar figure (20%). A lesion may show severe atypia with malignant change throughout the depth of the epithelial layer, but its basement membrane may still be intact. Such a lesion is identical with carcinoma in situ or intraepithelial carcinoma (Fig. 5-8).

When an intraepithelial carcinoma breaks through the basement membrane, it becomes a frank invasive squamous cell carcinoma. The investigator must study microscopic sections from various areas of a biopsy of leukoplakia, since the complete spectrum of histopathology from increased keratosis to invasive squamous cell carcinoma may be found in the surgical specimen from one lesion.

Leukoplakia may also be divided into two types according to whether or not it spontaneously dis-

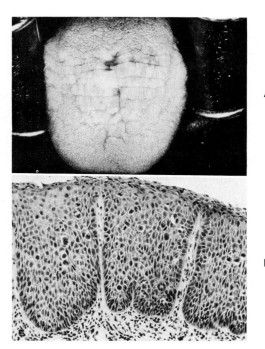

Fig. 5-7. Leukoplakia. **A,** Photomicrograph of a completely benign leukoplakic lesion showing acanthosis and hyperkeratosis but no dysplasia (atypia). **B,** Photomicrograph of a leukoplakic lesion that has undergone moderate dysplasia. Dysplastic cells are present in the lower portion of the epithelium. Arrow indicates the approximate superior extent of the dysplastic change.

Fig. 5-8. Leukoplakic lesions. **A,** The ulcer in the leukoplakic lesion on the dorsal surface of the tongue proved to be a carcinoma in situ. **B,** Photomicrograph of the ulcerated area in **A** showing malignant changes throughout the epithelium. The basement membrane is still intact.

appears after the chronic irritant has been eliminated. Those lesions that disappear are referred to as *reversible* leukoplakias, whereas the remaining lesions are termed *irreversible* leukoplakias.

Pindborg and co-workers (1968) reported that 20% of the leukoplakial lesions in their study disappeared completely, 18% diminished in size, and 45% did not decrease in size. On this basis 62% of the lesions could then be classified as complete or partially irreversible. Obviously reversible leukoplakias are not malignant; but a significant number of irreversible leukoplakias are premalignant or frankly malignant.

It has been tempting to speculate that reversible leukoplakia would not show dysplastic changes histologically. In this regard it is informative that both Pindborg and co-workers (1977) and Mincer and co-workers (1972) showed that some of these lesions that show dysplastic changes within the epithelium do regress spontaneously after elimination of the causative factor.

Concerning malignancy in leukoplakic lesions Waldron and Shafer reported in 1975 that 3.1% of their series were infiltrative squamous cell carcinomas. It is currently believed that there is an overall malignant transformation rate of 3% to 6% for oral leukoplakia (Kramer et al., 1978).

Bánóczy and Sugár (1972) stated that if the following features are present there is a higher risk of malignant transformation in oral leukoplakial lesions:

1. Persistence of the lesion for some years
2. Female patient
3. Lesion situated on the margin or base of the tongue
4. Combination of these first three factors
5. Erosive lesion

The consensus of pathologists is that the speckled variety of leukoplakia (with small red velvety areas dispersed through the white lesion, Figs. 5-9 and 5-10, *B*) is more likely to be malignant than the more homogeneous variety. Also, if the lesion has cracks or erosions or ulcers in the absence of mechanical trauma, this is an ominous sign (Fig. 5-11, *F*).

Recently it has been recognized that leukoplakias occurring in the floor of the mouth and ventral surface of the tongue have a much greater chance of undergoing malignant transformation. Kramer and co-workers, (1978) referring to this lesion as *sublingual keratosis*, reported that 27% of their lesions were carcinoma at the time of initial biopsy and that 24% showed malignant change in the follow-up period. Pogrel's study

Fig. 5-9. Speckled leukoplakia. **A,** Retromolar lesions. **B,** Palatal lesions. Both lesions proved to be squamous cell carcinoma. (**B** courtesy J. Lehnert, D.D.S., Minneapolis.)

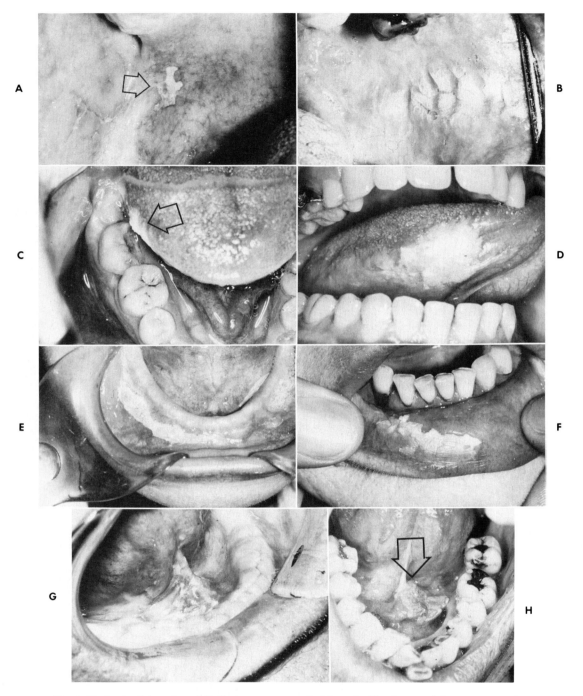

Fig. 5-10. Leukoplakia. **A** and **B,** Both patients smoked heavily. The lesions did not regress when smoking was stopped so they were excised. Neither showed dysplastic change. **C** and **D,** Lesion in 17-year-old white male due to irritation from sharp edges of second molar. Lesion regressed after tooth was restored. **E,** Lesion in vestibule caused by denture irritation. **F,** Prominent lesion on lower lip caused by biting habit and sharp incisal edges of lower anterior teeth. **G** and **H,** Microscopy showed squamous cell carcinoma. **G,** Speckled sublingual leukoplakia or speckled erythroplakia. **H,** Elevated firm mass with induration of the base. (**G** courtesy J. Lehnert, D.D.S., Minneapolis. **H** courtesy S. Smith, D.D.S., Chicago.)

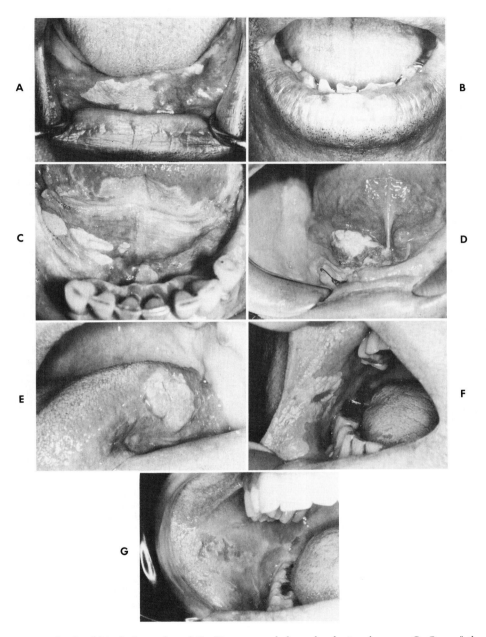

Fig. 5-11. Leukoplakic lesions. **A** and **B,** Biopsy revealed no dysplastic changes. **C,** One of the prominent white areas showed moderate dysplastic changes whereas the remainder showed only acanthosis and hyperkeratosis. **D** to **F,** These lesions proved to be squamous cell carcinoma. **G,** Although this lesion on the buccal mucosa appears suspicious because of the ulcerations, it is a benign condition caused by cheek biting. (**D** courtesy E. Kasper, D.D.S., Maywood, Ill.; **E** and **F** courtesy O. H. Stuteville, D.D.S., M.D., St. Joe, Ark.)

(1978) corroborated this trend; he reported that 16% of the leukoplakias he studied from this region showed malignant transformation within 5 years. Waldron and Shafer (1975) reported that 42% of the floor of the mouth leukoplakias they studied showed dysplasia as compared to 20% of all the leukoplakias studied.

Leukoplakial lesions are characteristically asymptomatic and are most often discovered during a routine oral examination. Leukoplakia is a very common lesion as shown by the fact that 6.2% of all tissue specimens submitted to two large oral pathology laboratories were leukoplakia (Waldron and Shafer, 1975). The greater percentage of patients with these lesions are between 40 and 70 years of age, and the lesions are seldom found in individuals under 30 years of age. Although they may occur anywhere in the oral mucosa, their most frequent sites are the tongue, floor of the mouth, lower lip, commissures, palate, mucobuccal fold, alveolar ridge, retromolar area, and buccal mucosa (Figs. 5-10 and 5-11). The lesions may vary greatly in size, shape, and distribution. The borders may be either distinct or indistinct and smoothly contoured or ragged. Lesions may be homogeneous with a fine grainy texture or mottled and rough in appearance. Early lesions are macules and nonpalpable. Later the surface may become rough and raised, thus becoming a speckled or verrucous type of leukoplakia (Fig. 5-9). If the lesion is malignant, enlarged cervical nodes may signal the occurrence of metastatic spread. The lesions may be solitary, or there may be multiple plaques scattered through the mouth.

The cause may be obvious from the location of the lesion (e.g., a white patch on an edentulous ridge directly beneath an occluding maxillary molar, in direct line with the course of the smoke from a pipe held in the smoker's favorite position, or in the area where the individual prefers to hold his quid of tobacco or dip of snuff).

DIFFERENTIAL DIAGNOSIS

When a white lesion is encountered, the clinician should determine whether it can be easily removed by scraping. If it cannot, all the sloughing pseudomembranous types can be eliminated and the following keratotic varieties should especially be considered: cheek-biting lesion, lichen planus, verrucous carcinoma, verruca vulgaris, leukoedema, and white sponge nevus.

White sponge nevus is the most uncommon of the group. In addition, it occurs soon after birth or at least by puberty and is usually widely distributed over the oral mucous membrane. In contrast, leukoplakia is seen mostly in patients over 40 years of age and usually is not disseminated throughout the oral cavity. White sponge nevus, furthermore, will show a familial pattern not so characteristic for leukoplakia.

Leukoedema is usually easily differentiated from leukoplakia because it classically occurs on the buccal mucosa, frequently covering most of the oral surface of the cheeks and extending onto the labial mucosa with a faint milky opalescence. Thus the definite whiteness that characterizes the leukoplakial lesion is not a feature of the mild case of leukoedema. The characteristic folded and more prominent wrinkled pattern (eliminated by stretching) of the leukoedema, furthermore, distinguishes it from the leukoplakial lesion.

Verruca vulgaris must be differentiated from the verrucous type of leukoplakia; and this is usually possible because the verruca vulgaris, which does not commonly occur in the oral cavity, is a small raised white lesion seldom more than 0.5 cm in diameter. Verrucous leukoplakia, on the other hand, tends to be much larger and is always circumscribed by a border of inflamed mucosa, a feature not usually found in the verruca vulgaris. In addition, if chronic trauma to the area can be identified, the diagnosis of leukoplakia is further favored.

Since *verrucous carcinoma* may develop from a leukoplakial lesion, the clinician must decide whether this lesion is elevated (exophytic) enough to be suspected as a verrucous carcinoma.

Lichen planus may appear as a plaquelike lesion, and in such instances it may be confused with leukoplakia. In contrast to leukoplakia, however, which is more often a solitary lesion, lichen planus usually occurs as several lesions distributed throughout the oral cavity. Also the lesions of lichen planus may develop several different configurations simultaneously in the same mouth (e.g., white plaques, Wickham's striae,* bullae, erosions). When such a variety of lesions is present, distinguishing between these two diseases is greatly facilitated. If reddish-white skin lesions accompany the oral lesions, this also favors a diagnosis of lichen planus.

Identifying the *cheek-biting lesion* may be a problem for the clinician. In the chronic cheek chewer the buccal mucosa takes on a whitish cast because of the increased thickness of the epithelium and keratin. In special periods of height-

---

*Fine grayish-white lines arranged in a lacelike pattern.

ened stress, the patient may actually chew away small bits of tissue, producing a plaquelike whitish lesion with a ragged eroded surface that may cause the inexperienced clinician to suspect squamous cell carcinoma (Fig. 5-11, *G*). Careful questioning of the patient will usually elicit the cause and promote the proper diagnosis. Careful follow-up will reveal the regression of the erosions when the habit is modified or eliminated.

MANAGEMENT

When a leukoplakial lesion is discovered on the oral mucosa, the clinician must make every effort to identify the local chronic irritants that may have induced its development. All these irritants must then be eliminated and the patient reexamined every week to determine whether the lesion is regressing. If evidence of regression is not detectable within 2 weeks (color photographs are useful as records for comparison), the lesion should be completely excised. This is a simple procedure for small lesions but is a relatively complicated operation if the lesions are large or involve many surfaces.

If the lesions are large or widespread, stripping procedures must be used—in stages with free grafts or else with allowance for the denuded surface to epithelialize by secondary healing. Since longitudinal studies by Silverman and Rosen (1968) and Bánóczy and Sugár (1972) showed that approximately 6% of the irreversible leukoplakial lesions underwent malignant transformation to squamous cell carcinoma, there seems to be little doubt that all irreversible leukoplakial lesions should be completely excised. At the same time, however, these authors did not always advocate that a lesion be observed for 2 weeks after the irritants had been eliminated; rather they insisted that if the clinician were unduly wary of a particular lesion it should be immediately and completely excised.

In any case careful postsurgical follow-up is essential. If the microscopic diagnosis is squamous cell carcinoma, the patient should be referred to a clinician who is competent in treating oral cancers. The management of intraoral squamous cell carcinoma is discussed in more detail in Chapter 6.

Nicotinic stomatitis or smoker's palate

Nicotinic stomatitis is a specific type of leukoplakia seen mostly in men who are pipe smokers. It occurs on the palate, and in most cases the whole mucosal surface of the hard palate is affected. It begins as a reddish stomatitis of the

palatal mucosa; and as the irritation is continued, leukoplakic changes occur and the lesion becomes slightly opalescent and finally white in color. Classically it is described as having a parboiled appearance because of its many transecting wrinkles and fissures, which divide the white mucosal surface into small nodular areas (Fig. 5-12). A red dot is usually situated in the middle of each nodule and represents the inflamed orifice of a minor salivary gland duct. The lesion usually disappears rapidly after the habit is discontinued. Nicotinic stomatitis seldom, if ever, becomes malignant.

Nicotinic stomatitis must be differentiated from all the other conditions of the oral cavity that produce multiple papules: papillary hyperplasia, Darier's disease (Fig. 5-13), focal epithelial hyperplasia, Goltz's syndrome, Cowden's syndrome, acanthosis nigricans, multiple neuroma syndrome, multiple oral fibromas in tuberous sclerosis, multiple papillomas and verrucae (no syndrome), and multiple condylomas (modified from Buchner and Sandbank, 1978).

Papillary hyperplasia and nicotinic stomatitis are the only entities that have a marked predilection for the palate. The small centrally placed dots in nicotinic stomatitis differentiate this condition

Fig. 5-12. Nicotinic stomatitis. Both patients were pipe smokers. **B,** Close-up view. (**B** courtesy P. D. Toto, D.D.S., Maywood, Ill.)

Fig. 5-13. Darier's disease. These multiple firm papules were present on various oral surfaces and the skin. (Courtesy M. Bernstein, D.D.S., Louisville.)

Fig. 5-14. Snuff dipper's leukoplakia. **A,** Note the parboiled appearance of the white lesion in the vestibule where the patient held his snuff. **B,** The lesion disappeared 2 weeks after discontinuance of the habit.

from papillary hyperplasia, which occurs under an acrylic denture.

Snuff dipper's lesion

Snuff dipper's lesion is most frequently encountered in areas of the world where the habit is prevalent. This leukoplakia-type lesion occurs on the mucosal surface where the snuff is habitually held. The mandibular vestibule, in both the incisor and the molar regions, is the most prevalent site. The resultant leukoplakic lesion usually has a wrinkled appearance (Fig. 5-14). If the habit is eliminated, the majority of the lesions completely disappear in about 2 weeks. Those that remain should be completely excised and examined microscopically. Roed-Petersen and Pindborg (1973) were unable to demonstrate a statistical difference between the percentage of snuff dipper's lesions that showed atypias and the percentage of other leukoplakias that showed atypias. Long exposure to snuff is usually required, however, to induce malignant changes; and when carcinoma does develop, the lesions are usually low-grade malignancies.

Cigarette smoker's lip lesion

Cigarette smoker's lip lesion is an interesting entity that has only recently been recognized. Berry and Landwerlen (1973) reported it in about

11% of the inpatients at a neuropsychiatric hospital. Early lesions showed increased redness and stippling of the lip in a localized area and were typically flat or slightly raised with elliptical, circular, irregular, or triangular borders. More advanced lesions appeared pale to white and were slightly elevated with a nodular or papillary shape. Berry and Landwerlen reported that 62% of the patients affected had lesions on both lips and most showed associated finger burns. The authors theorized that the sedation these psychiatric patients received increased their pain threshold and consequently they repeatedly suffered low-grade thermal damage to the lips and fingers. Berry and Landwerlen did not observe malignant change in any of the lesions biopsied.

BENIGN MIGRATORY GLOSSITIS AND MUCOSITIS (GEOGRAPHIC TONGUE, ECTOPIC GEOGRAPHIC TONGUE)

Geographic tongue occurs in 1% to 2% of children and adults. Although its cause is unknown,

Fig. 5-15. Geographic tongue. (Courtesy P. Akers, D.D.S., Chicago.)

Fig. 5-16. Fibrosed areas appearing as white lesions. **A,** Posttraumatic scar on the lateral border of the tongue. **B,** Scar at the site of a root resection incision.

psychologic influences are suspected. Clinically, irregularly shaped red patches and white patterns resembling a map are distributed over the dorsal and ventral surfaces and borders of the tongue (Fig. 5-15). The red patches are initially quite small and surrounded by a small white rim. These red patches, which are areas of desquamated filiform papillae, enlarge and regress—thus changing the pattern from week to week. Eventually they disappear entirely for a time.

The condition is usually asymptomatic; but occasionally a patient will complain of a burning sensation, tenderness, and pain. In our experience, instituting a bland diet and coating the denuded surface with triamcinolone in Orabase at bedtime relieve the discomfort until the painful desquamated areas regress.

Benign migratory glossitis is usually not a diagnostic problem, although some atypical cases have been diagnosed as *leukoplakia* by inexperienced clinicians. The differential diagnosis of benign migratory glossitis is discussed in greater detail in Chapter 12.

Recently situations have been described in which the condition also affected other regions of the oral mucosa. These cases have been referred to under different names, one of which is ectopic geographic tongue (Weathers et al., 1974).

PERIPHERAL SCAR TISSUE

Peripheral scar tissue (a nonkeratotic lesion) involving the subepithelial layer and/or epithelium has been observed in the oral cavity. The condition is not common because oral tissue is so vascular that the superficial tissue destroyed by a pathologic process is usually completely re-

placed by normal tissue. In some instances, however, the healing of surgical wounds, large traumatic ulcers, giant aphthae in Sutton's disease, or other conditions may result in the formation of dense scar tissue; and although the scar tissue does not become as light in color as most keratotic lesions, it does appear very pale and may not be recognized by the student, especially if the lesion is plaquelike (Fig. 5-16).

Usually scars may be identified by relating to pertinent points in the patient's history or by the location of the entity (e.g., a linear pale mark on the labial alveolus that corresponds to an incision for root resection, Fig. 5-16). Some patients show a tendency toward keloid formation on the skin, and a few patients are also prone to oral keloid formation although the oral cases are usually not so pronounced.

Oral scars may be solitary entities but will be multiple in cases of Sutton's disease and submucous fibrosis.* The area of the scar will be quite firm to palpation, and in some cases the deeper

---

*Submucous fibrosis is a chronic disease affecting any part of the oral and sometimes the pharyngeal mucosa. It is considered to be precancerous and may simulate scleroderma inasmuch as ultimately there is a stiffening of certain areas of the oral mucosa. The mucosa eventually becomes blanched and opaque.

layers will be bound to the mucosa. Intraoral scar tissue is usually not a diagnostic or management problem although adhesions after major surgery may have to be excised.

LICHEN PLANUS

Lichen planus is a complex mucocutaneous disease of the oral cavity of unknown etiology. It occurs with a variety of different-appearing lesions, some of which are white. There are three basic types of lesions: keratosis, bullae, and erosions. The disease affects less than 1% of the population, does not appear to be related to the use of tobacco, and is not restricted to any particular ethnic groups; a familial pattern has not been identified. The disease affects primarily nervous people, particularly when they are experiencing psychologic disturbances. These patients frequently have exacerbations of lichen planus during periods of deep emotional strain and remissions after the personal crisis has been resolved.

Within the past decade or so several reports have indicated that oral lichen planus may be associated with diabetes mellitus (Grinspan et al., 1966; Howell and Rick, 1973; Smith, 1977). It is interesting that Christensen and co-workers (1977) found no difference in glucose tolerance test results between lichen planus patients and patients without lichen planus.

Various reports have indicated that there is an increased incidence of oral squamous cell carcinoma in patients with oral lichen planus. In a recent review of this subject, Krutchkoff and co-workers (1978) concluded that at the present time there is insufficient evidence to conclusively show that oral lichen planus represents a premalignant state in itself. On a related subject Neumann-Jensen and Pindborg (1977) studied the smoking habits of 611 oral lichen planus patients. These authors reported that daily smokers showed a higher prevalence of plaque-type lesions than of reticular and atrophic types. They

Fig. 5-17. Lichen planus. **A,** Wickham's striae on the right and left buccal mucosa of a 45-year-old woman. **B,** Photomicrograph of lichen planus showing the sawtooth rete ridges and chronic inflammation, which is limited to the upper segment of the lamina propria. Note the early formation of microbullae just beneath the epithelium on the left side of the photomicrograph.

speculated that perhaps smoking changed the reticular and atrophic types into plaque types and asked the question, "Could the plaque lesions then be regarded as leukoplakia?"

The characteristic microscopic picture reveals a hyperparakeratosis or hyperorthokeratosis with an acanthosis. The rete ridges are often sawtoothed in appearance, and there is a bandlike distribution of dense chronic inflammation below the basement membrane, which is usually restricted to the lamina propria. The basal cell layer frequently undergoes liquefactive degeneration and may be entirely missing (Fig. 5-17).

If liquefaction is severe and restricted to small foci, bullae may form; but if the process is severe and more disseminated, erosions will develop because of the loss of surface epithelium.

FEATURES

Most cases of lichen planus are of the keratotic type and are asymptomatic. The bullous types, however, and especially the erosive types, may cause burning and intense pain. About 65% of the patients with lichen planus are women, and approximately 80% are 40 years or older. In Tyldesley's series (1974) 98.4% of the patients were over 30 years old. The average age of those affected is 52 years. The initial lesions of lichen

planus may appear on either the skin or the oral mucous membrane. In a series studied by Silverman and Griffeth (1974), about 25% of the patients with oral lesions had accompanying skin lesions. Thirty-five percent of Tyldesley's intraoral cases also had skin lesions. Intraoral lesions may be of the keratotic (white), bullous, or erosive type.

The keratotic lesions occur in a variety of different forms. The reticular pattern with a lacework of fine white lines (Wickham's striae) is the most widely recognized appearance and is practically pathognomonic for lichen planus (Fig. 5-17). Many other shapes and patterns of white lesions are seen, however, such as plaques, annular shapes, streaks, circles, and flower petal formations (Fig. 5-18).

The bullous lesions and the erosive types are included with the other generalized reddish lesions in Chapter 11. It has been our experience that, even when these other types of lesions are present, a careful examination of the oral mucosa and lips will almost invariably reveal at least a small area of Wickham's striae usually at the periphery of one of the other lesions. Such a discovery essentially identifies the pathosis as lichen planus. Although there does not seem to be any area of the oral mucosa that is immune, Silver-

Fig. 5-18. Lichen planus. **A** and **B,** Annular lesions on the tongue and vestibular mucosa, respectively. **C,** Extensive involvement of the dorsal surface of the tongue. **D,** Three types of lesions on the buccal mucosa: *1,* bullous type; *2,* erosion; *3,* Wickham's striae. (**B** courtesy P. D. Toto, D.D.S., Maywood, Ill.)

man and Griffeth (1974) reported that the following sites were most often involved (listed in descending order of frequency):

Buccal mucosa (85%)
Gingiva
Tongue
Palate
Floor of the mouth
Vermilion border

The skin lesions are small flat papules that may coalesce to form larger flat plaques or nodules (Fig. 5-19). The borders are smoothly contoured

Fig. 5-19. Skin lesions of lichen planus. (Courtesy N. Thompson, D.D.S., Maywood, Ill.)

and sharply demarcated from the surrounding skin. They are reddish purple in color and are often covered with a semitransparent thin scale. Fine grayish lines (Wickham's striae) may be present on their surfaces.

DIFFERENTIAL DIAGNOSIS

Leukoplakia, lichenoid drug reactions, unusual examples of linea alba, cheek-biting lesions, leukoedema, ectopic geographic tongue, lupus erythematosus, and white sponge nevus must all be differentiated from the keratotic lesions of lichen planus.

The differential diagnosis of the *bullous* and *erosive types* is taken up with the discussion of the other mucositides in Chapter 11. As with the other keratotic lesions in this group, the fact that the white lesions cannot be removed with a tongue blade eliminates all the sloughing white lesions, which are discussed in the latter half of this chapter (p. 87).

White sponge nevus can be eliminated from consideration because it is usually manifested at birth or at the latest by puberty, whereas 98% of the lichen planus lesions occur in patients over 30 years of age.

Lupus erythematosus may be indicated by keratotic white lesions with or without a surrounding area of erythematous oral mucosa. However, these keratotic lesions are not in a thin linear reticular pattern but have a much broader dimension. In addition, the characteristic flaky or feathery appearance of these lupus lesions is helpful for diagnosis (Fig. 5-20). In systemic lupus the characteristic blood changes will be diagnostic.

Ectopic geographic tongue may be distinguished by the fact that its lesions have a red

A   B

Fig. 5-20. Lupus erythematosus. Note characteristic feathery edges of keratotic patches.

center with a slightly raised white border that is rapidly altered, producing a noticeable change in pattern within a few days. Although the white lesions of lichen planus may occur in a variety of shapes and distributions and these characteristics may change, such changes take place relatively slowly and usually require a few weeks before they become apparent.

Leukoedema is easily recognized; but if wrinkles are present, these may be interpreted as Wickham's striae by the inexperienced clinician. Stretching the tissue, however, will eliminate the wrinkles or folds in leukoedema and permit the distinction between it and lichen planus.

Cases in which *cheek biting* is superimposed on a leukoedema may be easily confused with lichen planus, and a biopsy may be necessary to correctly identify the condition. The fact that the whiteness of leukoedema can be made to completely disappear by stretching the buccal mucosa is a helpful differentiating test.

Unusual examples of *linea alba* may mimic lichen planus. Some patients suck their cheeks into tight contact with their teeth, and this may produce linea alba patterns that resemble Wickham's striae on the buccal mucosa where the mucosa contacts the crowns of the teeth (Fig. 5-5, *B*).

Lichenoid drug reactions have recently been reported. Apparently in such cases drugs have induced changes that resemble the Wickham's striae of lichen planus.

Various degrees of severity occur, ranging from painless keratotic lesions to painful, severely erosive cases (Fig. 5-21). The following drugs have been implicated: thiazides, methyldopa, bismuth, chloroquine, gold derivatives, mepro-

Fig. 5-21. Lichenoid drug reaction in 64-year-old white woman on antihypertensive medication. Patient had a diffuse stomatitis. Distinct small regions of white reticular patterns could be seen.

bamate, para-aminosalicylic acid, and quinicrine.

Apparently the best way to differentiate between painful cases of lichen planus and lichenoid drug reaction is to initiate a course of systemic administration of cortisone. If no improvement is observed within 2 weeks lichenoid drug reaction should be considered the working diagnosis. Then under the physician's direction the drugs that the patient is taking should be discontinued or substituted for. Using such an approach lichenoid drug lesions will slowly heal, but 4 to 6 months may be required before complete remission occurs (Burry and Kirk, 1974). Severe cases of lichenoid drug reaction could appear very similar clinically to allergic manifestations such as erythema multiforme. As with bona fide lichen planus one would expect rapid improvement of allergic states after the systemic administration of cortisone.

Leukoplakia is frequently the lesion that is the most difficult to differentiate from lichen planus. When skin lesions of lichen planus are present, the distinction is easy; or if the white intraoral lesions of lichen planus take the form of Wickham's striae, the diagnosis is also readily discernible. If, however, as sometimes happens, the lichen planus is a solitary plaquelike lesion, the disturbance may be incorrectly diagnosed as leukoplakia since leukoplakia most often occurs as a solitary plaquelike lesion. The differentiation is rendered more difficult by the fact that both diseases usually affect patients over 40 years of age. The fact that leukoplakia affects more men whereas lichen planus occurs more in women will provide a hint as to the nature of the lesion. If, after a thorough investigation, a chronic irritant cannot be identified and an area characteristic of Wickham's striae is discovered, no matter how small, the probability that the lesion is lichen planus is increased. Cases such as these, however, frequently must be identified by a biopsy. In addition, cases of disseminated intraoral leukoplakia in which several areas of the oral mucosa are involved may be easily mistaken for lichen planus; but again biopsy will usually distinguish between the two.

Bánóczy and co-workers (1979) in an interesting report described keratotic lesions that mimic leukoplakia and lichen planus and are apparently caused by electrogalvanic currents.

MANAGEMENT

The majority of cases of lichen planus (particularly those of the keratotic type) require no treatment other than their identification and reassurances to the patient. In light of a recent report by Silverman and Griffeth (1974), however, which seemed to suggest an increased risk of the development of squamous cell carcinoma in oral lesions of lichen planus, such patients should be reexamined periodically. Patients who complain of small localized burning, tenderness, or soreness of the oral mucosa will find relief from applications of triamcinolone in an emollient (e.g., Kenalog in Orabase) before retiring. Severe cases respond to the systemic administration of a sedative and cortisone.

WHITE HAIRY TONGUE

White hairy tongue is a condition that occurs on the dorsal surface of the tongue and is of little clinical significance. Its cause is still unknown. It results from an elongation of the filiform papillae because of the increased retention of keratin. It is much more common in men and seldom produces symptoms or causes clinical problems. On occasion, a patient may become alarmed when he suddenly detects its presence. The length of the papillae may vary from short to relatively long (Fig. 5-22). When the papillae are extremely long, the patient may complain of gagging. Under the influences of a varying diet, this lesion may take on different colors. Farman (1977) reported that patients with malignant neoplasia are much more prone to develop this condition.

White hairy tongue does not present a diagnostic problem, and careful frequent brushing of the dorsal surface of the tongue is the preferred treatment for milder cases. When the papillae have reached an extreme length, clipping fol-

Fig. 5-22. White hairy tongue.

lowed by tongue brushing is an effective control measure.

PAPILLOMA

The papilloma is classified as a benign tumor of epithelium. Its cause is not known. It is a relatively infrequent lesion of the oral cavity. If it is subjected to chronic irritation, its surface will be covered by a layer of keratin and the lesion will be white. If it is not chronically irritated, the lesion will have a pink color.

FEATURES

The patient may complain of a small tab or mass on the mucosa, or the papilloma may be an incidental finding during an oral examination. It is an exophytic lesion with a characteristic papillomatous shape; that is, the lesion is almost always pedunculated and has a rough, cauliflowerlike, pebbly surface caused by the presence of deep clefts that extend well into the lesion from the surface (Figs. 5-23 and 5-24). The intraoral papilloma is seldom larger than 1 cm in diameter but may occasionally grow to several centimeters.

In a review of 110 lesions, Greer and Goldman (1974) reported that, although it may occur anywhere on the mucosa, the papilloma is most frequently seen on the tongue; these authors found 33% of the lesions in their study at this site. In descending order of frequency, the following were sites where a papilloma was found:

Tongue	Lips
Palate	Mandibular ridge
Buccal mucosa	Floor of the mouth
Gingiva	

Greer and Goldman also reported that most of the cases occurred in persons aged 21 through 50 years and that the average age was 38 years. The majority of tumors in their study varied in size from 2 × 2 mm to 1.0 × 1.5 cm, with a few measuring as large as 2.5 to 3 cm in diameter. A narrow stalk was characteristic of these lesions.

Because no dysplastic areas were found in any of the 110 papillomas in their series, Greer and Goldman concluded that malignant change in oral papillomas must be very rare, if indeed it occurs at all.

Microscopically a narrow connective tissue core extends from the tissue beneath the lesion and branches into numerous folds; the folds are covered by epithelium that characteristically shows acanthosis. A surface layer of keratin may or may not be present, depending on the amount

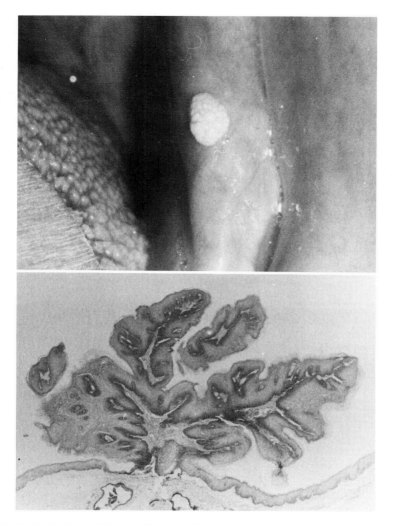

Fig. 5-23. Papilloma. This papilloma is white because of its keratotic surface.

A

B

Fig. 5-24. Papillomas. Both lesions were pedunculated. (**B** courtesy S. Smith, D.D.S., Chicago.)

of irritation to the surface, and this determines whether the lesion is white or pink.

DIFFERENTIAL DIAGNOSIS

The following lesions must be differentiated from the papilloma: verruca vulgaris, papillary squamous cell carcinoma, verrucous carcinoma, condyloma acuminatum, condyloma lata, and pseudoepitheliomatous hyperplasia.

The *verruca vulgaris,* although common on the skin, is not frequent in the oral cavity. It almost always has a relatively sessile base, whereas the papilloma is pedunculated. Microscopically the verruca vulgaris often has round eosinophilic bodies in the cells of the upper part of the prickle cell layer and in the granular cell layer; these are thought to be viral inclusion bodies and are not found in papilloma. Actually the clinical distinction between verruca vulgaris and papilloma is not critical since both are managed identically. Some pathologists do not even distinguish between verruca vulgaris and papilloma.

The *papillary squamous cell carcinoma* is a "garden-variety" exophytic squamous cell carcinoma that possesses basically a polypoid shape and a surface that is white and pebbly or relatively smooth (Fig. 5-25). In contradistinction to the papilloma its base is not as pedunculated, the lesion grows much more rapidly and soon exceeds the usual 0.5 to 2.0 cm size of the papilloma. Its rapid growth and narrower base differentiate the papillary squamous cell carcinoma

Fig. 5-25. Papillary squamous cell carcinomas.

from the verrucous carcinoma, which has a very broad base and usually achieves much less vertical growth into the oral cavity.

Verrucous carcinoma characteristically is seen in patients in their 60s and 70s and is mostly associated with smoking or chewing tobacco or snuff. It usually covers a much wider surface area, has a base that is almost as wide as the lesion, and does not achieve much vertical height (Fig. 5-26).

Condyloma lata and *condyloma acuminata* (Fig. 5-27) may look identical to the papilloma clinically. However, they are much less common and a careful history would frequently reveal that the patient has experienced oral sex with an infected individual.

Pseudoepitheliomatous hyperplasias are surface epithelial changes that may occur in lesions such as fungal infections, syphilis, granular cell myoblastomas, and peripheral ameloblastomas. The papillary changes may be severe enough to produce a pebbly surface usually of a broad nature but sometimes they occur as a smaller lesion (Fig. 5-28). However, in almost every case these epithelial proliferations have a sessile base. Thus the lesion should not be confused with a papilloma.

The *verruciform xanthoma* is a white keratotic

Fig. 5-26. Verrucous carcinomas. (**A** from Claydon, P. J., and Jordan, J. E.: J. Oral Surg. **36**:564-567, 1978. Copyright by the American Dental Association. Reprinted by permission. **B** courtesy R. Lee, D.D.S., Findlay, Ohio.)

Fig. 5-27. Condyloma acuminatum at the angle of the mouth. (Courtesy E. Seklecki, D.D.S., Tucson, Ariz.)

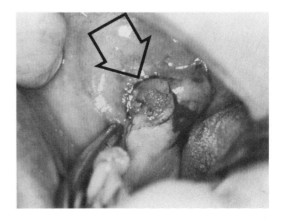

Fig. 5-28. Pseudoepitheliomatous hyperplasia on the surface of a peripheral ameloblastoma in the edentulous third molar region. Photograph was taken after initial incision was made for removal of hyperplasia. (Courtesy R. Latronica, D.D.S., Albany, N.Y.)

Fig. 5-29. Verruciform xanthoma. **A,** Intraoral view showing white lesion in buccal mucosa. **B,** View of surgical specimen showing corrugated surface. (From Graff, S., et al.: Oral Surg. **45:** 762-767, 1978.)

lesion that occurs with some frequency on the skin but rarely occurs in the oral cavity. Its whitish, corrugated surface is illustrated in Fig. 5-29. It is similar to the verrucous carcinoma in that it has a broad base and vertical projection into the oral cavity is minimal. However, it has a much softer consistency than verrucous carcinoma because there is much less keratin in the former lesion. Also the corrugations are much more shallow and more regular in the verruciform xanthoma.

MANAGEMENT

The papilloma must be excised by means of an elliptic incision in the tissue underlying the lesion. Excision through the stalk will usually result in recurrence. The excised tissue must always be examined microscopically to assure the final diagnosis.

VERRUCA VULGARIS

Verruca vulgaris is an exophytic growth of the epithelium that is a very common lesion of the skin but seldom occurs orally. It has been convincingly shown to be caused by a virus (Wysocki and Hardie, 1979).

FEATURES

The verruca vulgaris has been found on the skin, on the vermilion border, and infrequently on the labial or buccal mucosa or tongue. It is a mass with a rough, coarse, pebbly surface and a broad base. Although it cannot always be differentiated from papilloma, its surface clefts and depressions are characteristically much more shallow and the mass more sessile. It will vary in whiteness according to the degree of surface

Fig. 5-30. Small verruca vulgaris on the border of the tongue.

keratinization (Fig. 5-30). Multiple lesions may occur, and these most likely represent examples of autoinoculation.

Microscopically the verruca has a broad base, usually only slightly narrower than the greatest diameter of the lesion, with a relatively thicker connective tissue core than is found in the papilloma. The core ramifies into the epithelium-covered papillae. The connective tissue branches of the core tend to slant upward and outward from the center of the base. Eosinophilic viral inclusion bodies are frequently seen in the superficial part of the prickle cell layer and in the granular cell layer. The degree of surface keratinization varies from lesion to lesion.

DIFFERENTIAL DIAGNOSIS

The differentiating aspects of verruca vulgaris are discussed under the differential diagnosis of papilloma (p. 80).

MANAGEMENT

Complete excision with microscopic study of the specimen is the proper treatment for a solitary oral lesion of verruca vulgaris. Dermatologists frequently use fulguration for the removal of multiple verrucae on the skin.

VERRUCOUS CARCINOMA

The verrucous carcinoma is an exophytic type of low-grade squamous cell carcinoma that has a considerably better prognosis than do other types of carcinomas. It usually occurs in persons who smoke or who use snuff or chewing tobacco. Verrucous carcinoma was first defined as a separate entity by Ackerman in 1948.

FEATURES

Verrucous carcinoma occurs most often in the buccal mucosa, alveolar ridge, and gingiva of elderly patients. In Shafer's study (1972) males and females were approximately equally affected with the average age for males being 63 and for females the average age was 73. In Jacobson and Shear's paper (1972) ten were females and five were males.

Clinically the mature lesion will cover a wide area of the mucosal surface but will show minimal elevation. The base is sessile and usually approximately equal to the greatest dimension of the lesion. The surface is rough, pebbly, and mamillated, perhaps with deep crevices separating distinct mamillated folds (Fig. 5-26). The surface may be white, red, or red and white depending on the degree of surface keratinization present. The mass is moderately firm on palpation but noticeably less firm than the invasive types of squamous cell carcinoma. It is usually only superficially invasive, and metastasis is uncommon.

Microscopically there is generally an abrupt transition at the junction from normal epithelium to tumor. The tumor epithelium is considerably thickened and shows papillary projections outward while there are also downward projections of broad blunt rete ridges, which are delimited by an intact basement membrane. Usually differentiation is orderly, but a minor degree of atypia may be present. A considerable amount of surface keratin will usually be present, and this will dip down with the invaginating epithelial pegs (Jacobson and Shear, 1972).

DIFFERENTIAL DIAGNOSIS

The differential diagnosis of verrucous carcinoma is discussed under the differential diagnosis of papilloma (p. 81).

Fig. 5-31. Chronic keratotic (hyperplastic) candidiasis of long standing on the dorsal surface of the tongue. It could not be scraped off.

MANAGEMENT

Five-year survival rates as high as 75% have been reported after wide excision of the verrucous carcinoma lesion. These patients should be observed carefully, however, because there is a tendency for multifocal tumors to develop after excision. Treatment by radiation has not proved to be uniformly successful, primarily because the tumor is low grade. In fact, radiation has actually been suspected of inducing a higher degree of malignancy in these lesions. The management of invasive carcinoma is discussed in detail under squamous cell carcinoma in Chapter 6.

CHRONIC KERATOTIC (HYPERPLASTIC) CANDIDIASIS

Chronic hyperplastic candidiasis (moniliasis) is a keratotic lesion that has been described by some pathologists as differing from the usual picture of candidiasis insofar as it cannot be scraped off. In cases of very low-grade chronic infections by *Candida albicans,* the yeast products may not be sufficiently concentrated to coagulate the surface epithelium but rather may stimulate the production or retention of keratin. The resultant lesion in such cases is then actually a type of leukoplakia (Figs. 5-31 and 5-32).

Microscopically the pseudohyphae of *C. albicans* can be identified in the superficial layers of the keratin. Whether the *Candida* organisms initiated the hyperkeratosis or were secondary invaders of a leukoplakial lesion is not positively known. In our experience some of these lesions have seemed to result primarily from the *Candida* because they disappeared after repeated topical applications of nystatin cream. The more com-

Fig. 5-32. Hyperplastic candidiasis of the dorsal surface of the tongue.

Fig. 5-33. White sponge nevus. The lesions are easily seen bilaterally in the buccal mucosa. The patient stated they had been present all his life. (Courtesy J. Jacoway, D.D.S., Chapel Hill, N.C.)

mon pseudomembranous type of candidiasis is discussed in the section on sloughing pseudomembranous white lesions later in this chapter.

WHITE SPONGE NEVUS

White sponge nevus is a hereditary condition in which white lesions occur on various mucous membranes of the body (e.g., the mucosa of the oral cavity, vagina, and pharynx). It has an autosomal dominant inheritance pattern, and the lesions may be present at birth or may begin or become more intense at puberty.

FEATURES

White sponge nevus is a mucous membrane abnormality that varies considerably in its severity of involvement. Sometimes the white lesions, which have a rough, wrinkled surface, occur only on the buccal mucosa; other times they may be widespread and include almost the entire oral mucosa (Fig. 5-33). The lesions are asymptomatic and do not show a tendency toward malignant change.

Microscopically the epithelium is greatly thick-

ened because of an acanthosis and a hyperparakeratosis. Marked spongiosis (intracellular edema) occurs throughout the prickle cell layer.

DIFFERENTIAL DIAGNOSIS

Clinically the white sponge nevus must be differentiated from leukoedema, leukoplakia, lichen planus, pachyonychia congenita, and hereditary benign intraepithelial dyskeratosis.

If the clinician is able to establish that the lesions have been present since birth or at least since early life, this will almost completely eliminate *lichen planus* and *leukoplakia* because these lesions are quite unusual in patients under 30 years of age.

Leukoedema is found with some regularity in children although it usually is not pronounced and will be only a milky opalescence whereas white sponge nevus will have a rough granular somewhat leathery surface. Furthermore, stretching the tissue will frequently obliterate leukoedema but will not affect the appearance of white sponge nevus.

The intraoral picture of *pachyonychia congen-*

Fig. 5-34. Pachyonychia congenita. **A,** Intraoral view showing keratotic lesions on the tongue that had been present from infancy. Skin lesions were also present. **B,** Characteristic malformation of the nails. (From Maser, E. D.: Oral Surg. **43:**373-378, 1977.)

ita might be easily confused with white sponge nevus because the keratotic white lesions may look quite similar and may be present from birth in both diseases (Fig. 5-34). However, the presence of the nail anomalies as well as the skin lesions in pachyonychia congenita distinguish this entity from white sponge nevus.

Hereditary benign intraepithelial dyskeratosis (HBID) may be indicated by similar whitish keratotic oral lesions, but this entity is seen only in a triracial population in North Carolina.

Microscopically there may be a tendency toward confusing the white sponge nevus with leukoedema, hereditary benign intraepithelial dyskeratosis, and pachyonychia congenita; however, further discussion of this problem is beyond the scope of this text.

MANAGEMENT

Usually proper identification is all that is required since the white sponge nevus is benign. Occasionally a raw surface will result from the desquamation of the thickened epithelium, and various palliative procedures will be necessary to relieve the burning and tenderness.

SKIN GRAFTS

Although intraoral skin grafts are easily recognized by most clinicians who have seen them, they may be misdiagnosed as leukoplakic lesions by the uninitiated (Figs. 5-35 and 5-36). This is especially true with white patients because the skin graft will appear white, and after some months its borders may not be clearly defined. In black patients the abundance of melanin in the

Fig. 5-35. Intramucosal skin grafts. **A,** White man. **B,** Black man. (Courtesy P. Akers, D.D.S., Chicago.)

skin graft will usually preclude confusion with leukoplakia (Fig. 5-35, *B*). Mistaking a skin graft for a lesion is not very likely because the nature of the area becomes evident during the patient interview (history).

Fig. 5-36. Intraoral skin grafts. **A,** Two small skin grafts (arrow) placed in treatment for periodontal disease. **B,** Large skin graft on ventral surface of the tongue placed in ridge-deepening procedure. (Courtesy P. O'Flaherty, D.D.S., Downers Grove, Ill.)

Fig. 5-37. Superficial keratin-filled cyst in the sublingual area of an infant.

Fig. 5-38. Small epidermoid cyst attached to the uvula. The keratin-filled lumen in this very superficial cyst produces the white color.

RARITIES

The following diseases may occur rarely as white lesions of the oral mucosa that cannot be removed by scraping with a tongue blade (Figs. 5-37 to 5-39):

Acanthosis nigricans
Bohn's nodule (Epstein's pearl)
Condyloma acuminatum
Condyloma latum
Darier's disease
Dermatitis herpetiformis
Dyskeratosis congenita
Focal epithelial hyperplasia
Focal palmoplantar and marginal gingival hyperkeratosis
Grinspan's syndrome
Hereditary benign intraepithelial dyskeratosis
Hypersplenism and leukoplakia oris
Hypovitaminosis A
Inverted papilloma
Koplik's spots
Lupus erythematosus
Molluscum contagiosum
Pachyonychia congenita
Pityriasis rubra pilaris
Porokeratosis
Pseudoepitheliomatous hyperplasia
Psoriasis
Scleroderma (nonkeratotic)
Squamous acanthoma
Submucous fibrosis (nonkeratotic)
Superficial sialolith of minor glands
Syndrome of dyskeratosis congenita, dystrophia unguium, and aplastic anemia
Syphilitic interstitial glossitis leukoplakia
Verruciform xanthoma
Warty dyskeratoma

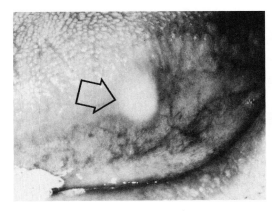

Fig. 5-39. Granular cell myoblastoma. This lesion had a yellowish-white cast.

Fig. 5-40. Arrow indicates white plaque (materia alba) that can be easily removed.

Sloughing, pseudomembranous, necrotic white lesions

The sloughing, pseudomembranous, necrotic white lesions, in contrast to the keratotic lesions, *may be scraped off the mucosa* with a tongue blade, leaving a raw bleeding surface. The white material may be necrotic or coagulated surface epithelium or a mixture of necrotic epithelium, plasma proteins, and microorganisms.

PLAQUE (MATERIA ALBA)

Plaque, or materia alba, is included in this group for completeness and because it may be mistaken for a lesion. In some mouths exhibiting particularly poor hygiene a mixture of food debris and bacteria may be seen as white plaques on the gingiva and alveolar mucosa and on the teeth (Fig. 5-40).

The clinician may notice a slightly inflamed mucosal surface beneath the plaque after the plaque has been removed with a gauze.

TRAUMATIC ULCER

On occasion, oral mucosa that has been crushed by mechanical trauma will appear as a sloughing white lesion (Fig. 5-41). A history of such a traumatic event is diagnostic. Clinicians must learn that a patient whose resistance is lowered by systemic disease may develop secondary infections or gangrene in these injured areas. Thus, if the severity of a traumatic lesion seems to be out of proportion to the intensity of the precipitating trauma, underlying systemic disease should be suspected.

PYOGENIC GRANULOMA

The pyogenic granuloma is discussed in considerable detail in Chapter 7 with the other exophytic lesions. We make brief mention of it here because this particular variety of inflammatory hyperplastic lesion almost invariably has a white area of varying size on its surface (Fig. 5-42). This white material is necrotic tissue that can be removed easily with a gauze or a tongue blade.

Fig. 5-41. Sloughing traumatic lesions. **A,** Traumatic lesion on the tip of the tongue caused by neonatal incisors. **B,** Sloughing white lesion on the palate produced during a traumatic orotracheal intubation. (Courtesy G. MacDonald, D.D.S., Belleville, Ill.)

Fig. 5-42. Pyogenic granuloma. **A,** On labial gingiva. **B,** On buccal mucosa. Note the white necrotic material on the surfaces of both lesions. (Courtesy A.C.W. Hutchinson collection, Northwestern University Dental School Library, Chicago.)

The necrosis is produced by recurrent mechanical trauma to this exophytic lesion.

CHEMICAL BURNS

Chemical burns most often result from the patient applying analgesics, such as aspirin or acetaminophen, to the mucosa adjacent to an aching tooth. Other cases may result, however, from the dentist's inadvertently applying caustic medicaments to the mucosa.

We have frequently seen an interesting mild white filmy desquamation on the oral mucosa of new patients who apply for dental care in the dental school clinic. Invariably, when questioned, these patients admit to the vigorous use of mouthwash and dentifrice just prior to coming to the clinic. Evidently they are trying to cover up their neglect of dental hygiene with a concentrated last-minute effort. It seems to us that the strong concentration of various agents have caused a superficial "burn" to the mucosa. Kowitz and co-workers (1976) and Rubright and co-workers (1978) reported this type of mild sloughing precipitated by the use of mouthwashes and dentifrices, respectively.

The clinical appearance of these burns in most cases depends on the severity of the tissue damage. Mild burns will cause a localized mucositis, whereas more severe burns will coagulate the surface of the tissue and produce a diffuse white lesion. If the coagulation is severe, the tissue can be scraped off—leaving a raw, bleeding, painful surface (Fig. 5-43).

The identification of these lesions is best accomplished by determining, through the history, that medicaments or drugs have been applied to the oral mucosa.

The sloughing of the surface mucosa caused

Fig. 5-43. Chemical burns. Both lesions were caused by the topical use of aspirin to relieve tooth-ache. The white material could be removed.

by excessive use of mouthwashes or dentifrice would be much milder and more disseminated than the more localized reaction to an analgesic tablet.

The treatment for chemical burns is the application of a protective coating, such as Orabase, and the initiation of a bland diet.

Systemic analgesics may be administered if pain is a problem. The patient should be advised that analgesic tablets are to be swallowed and not to be used topically.

ACUTE NECROTIZING ULCERATIVE GINGIVITIS (VINCENT'S INFECTION, TRENCH MOUTH)

Acute necrotizing ulcerative gingivitis (ANUG) is a moderately common inflammatory disorder of the gingiva, which produces a necrotic ulcerative destruction of the free margin, crest, and interdental papillae. Since a discussion of gingivitis and periodontitis has not been included in the text, we have accordingly abbreviated the description of ANUG and include it here only because it complements the group of white lesions that are the subject of this section of the chapter.

The untreated lesions are almost always covered by a grayish-white membrane that can be readily scraped off, leaving a raw bleeding surface. The etiology of ANUG is complex. There seems to be little doubt that predisposing conditions are essential for the development of this disease and that the most important predisposing condition is a decreased resistance to infection. Some presumptive evidence exists that gingivitis and periodontitis (poor oral hygiene) may predispose an individual to ANUG. The lowered resistance could, in turn, be the result of one or a combination of stress-producing conditions that would permit the overgrowth of or superinfection by components of the normal oral flora. Such a synergistic combination of anaerobic oral fusiform bacilli and spirochetes is usually incriminated.

FEATURES

The patient with ANUG frequently complains of tenderness, discomfort, or increasingly intense pain in the gingiva. Lassitude, bad taste, a fetid odor, and an inability to eat properly are also frequent symptoms. A patient may state that this problem has recurred several times. Clinical examination will often disclose that one or more, or all, of the crests—or perhaps the complete interdental papilla—have been destroyed by an ulcerative process and are covered by a necrotic grayish white pseudomembrane (Fig. 5-44).

Although removal of the pseudomembrane may be painful for the patient, this maneuver is usually easily accomplished and leaves a raw bleeding surface. In severe cases the process may spread, causing destruction of the marginal gingivae between the papillae and producing extensive ulcers.

The ANUG patient may have an increased temperature and usually a painful regional lymphadenopathy. The disease can occur at any age, but the majority of cases affect patients between 17 and 35 years of age. ANUG does not show a predilection for either sex.

DIFFERENTIAL DIAGNOSIS

The picture of destructive lesions that have produced punched-out defects of the interdental papillae is practically pathognomonic for ANUG, so long as the process has not affected other areas of the mucous membrane.

Somewhat similar lesions may occur in *sickle cell anemia;* but this disease may be readily identified by a special sickle cell blood preparation or by the electrophoretic examination of the hemoglobin.

If the necrotic gangrenous process has involved other regions of the oral mucosa in addition to the interdental papillae and marginal gingivae, then the diagnosis is *diffuse gangrenous stomatitis*—whose presence is suggestive of an underlying debilitating systemic disease.

MANAGEMENT

Treatment of ANUG is directed toward the three features of the etiology: (1) superinfection by the anaerobic fusiforms and spirochetes and other oral microorganisms, (2) the underlying gingival or periodontal problem, and (3) the patient's lowered resistance to infection.

Fig. 5-44. Acute necrotic ulcerative gingivitis. **A,** The tips of the interdental papillae are destroyed first. **B,** Severe case in which necrotizing process has extended to the remaining marginal gingiva and to the alveolar mucosa. (**B** courtesy J. Keene, D.D.S., Downers Grove, Ill.)

The acute phase may be managed by any of the following procedures, either singly or in combination:

1. Administration of penicillin (500 mg q.i.d.) for at least 5 days
2. Careful scaling, curettement, and debridement (NOTE: This can be accomplished with considerably less discomfort to the patient if it is postponed 24 to 48 hours after the institution of antibiotic therapy.)
3. Oral rinsing with a solution of 3% hydrogen peroxide in saline (1:3) 12 times a day (It is important that the patient understand the role his lowered resistance has played in gum infection.)

Recontouring of the gingiva after regression of the disease may be necessary.

CANDIDIASIS (CANDIDOSIS, MONILIASIS, THRUSH)

Candidiasis is an infection by a dimorphic yeastlike fungus, *Candida albicans*. The saprophytic yeast phase of this microorganism is a component of the normal oral flora of most if not all people. *Candida* exists in a probable antipathetic symbiotic relationship* with many of the other oral microorganisms.

Because *C. albicans* has such low virulence in the yeast phase, some changes must take place in the local environment to produce conditions favorable to its relative overgrowth and tissue invasion. Several such changes have been identified:

1. A reduction or a proportional change in the competitive flora will predispose a person to candidiasis.
2. A drastic reduction in the resistance of the tissues also favors this infection.

These alterations may be effected by either local or systemic factors and may be related to age, hormonal status, and genetics.

Changes in the physical nature of the local tissue surfaces that permit penetration and afford a compatible medium for the growth of the organism are frequently present. Thrush in infants and candidiasis in patients on long-term broad-spectrum antibiotic therapy are examples of candidiasis caused by an altered oral flora.

Secondary *Candida* infections in angular cheilosis, denture mucositis, erythema multiforme, leukoplakia, and ruptured bullous lesions are examples of a candidiasis resulting from a lowered

---

*An association between dissimilar groups of organisms that is advantageous to one but disadvantageous to the other.

resistance of the local tissues as well as from the altered epithelial surface—providing the proper soil for proliferation of the organism. In such instances the candidiasis may mask the initial disease process. Candidiasis in terminal patients or in patients who are suffering from leukemia or other severe and often debilitating diseases is probably an example of a *Candida* infection resulting from lowered systemic resistance.

FEATURES

The patient with candidiasis may complain of a burning sensation, tenderness, or sometimes pain in the area of the affected mucosa. Spicy foods will cause occasional discomfort due to the increased sensitivity of the affected mucosa. The patient may report that he has been on a prolonged course of broad-spectrum antibiotics for a sore throat or other infection.

The oral infection may show as fine whitish deposits on an erythematous patch of mucosa or as more highly developed small, soft, white, slightly elevated plaques bearing a remarkable resemblance to milk curds (Figs. 5-45 and 5-46). The disease may range in severity from a solitary region to a diffuse whitish involvement of several or all the mucosal surfaces. The mucosa adjacent to, or between, these whitish plaques appears dark and moderately swollen. The plaques or pseudomembranes may be stripped off the mucosa, leaving a raw bleeding surface. When solitary restricted sites are involved, the buccal mucosa and vestibule are the most frequent regions affected—followed by the tongue, palate, gingivae, floor of the mouth, and lips.

A convincing diagnosis can be made by microscopically examining some of the pseudomembrane or plaque material. In cases of candidiasis, several species of oral flora will be present in the scrapings along with coagulated surface epithelium and significantly great masses of both yeast forms and mycelial filaments. Culturing *C. albicans* is a less sensitive diagnostic procedure, however, since this microorganism can be obtained from a large percentage of healthy mouths; thus its isolation is of little pathologic significance.

DIFFERENTIAL DIAGNOSIS

As a rule all the keratotic lesions discussed in the first part of this chapter may be readily eliminated by the fact that they cannot be easily removed by scraping with a tongue blade.

The following necrotic white lesions must be considered in the differential diagnosis: chemical

Fig. 5-45. Candidiasis. **A,** Typical milk-curd lesion on the soft palate of a man on prolonged broad-spectrum antibiotic therapy. **B,** Lesions on the palate of a leukemic patient.

Fig. 5-46. Candidiasis on the dorsal surface of the tongue.

Fig. 5-47. Syphilitic lesions. **A,** Chancre on the anterolateral border of the tongue. It is unusual for a chancre to have a white necrotic surface. **B,** Mucous patch on the tongue of a patient with secondary syphilis. (**A** courtesy T. Wall, D.D.S., Chicago. **B** courtesy R. Gorlin, D.D.S., Minneapolis.)

burns, gangrenous stomatitis, superficial bacterial infections, traumatic ulcers, necrotic ulcers of systemic disease, and the mucous patch.

The *mucous patch* of syphilis is usually a discrete, small, white necrotic lesion on the tongue, palate, or lips (Fig. 5-47), while candidiasis is usually much more diffuse. The accompanying skin lesions of secondary syphilis in addition to the positive serology readily differentiates the mucous patch from candidiasis.

Necrotic ulcers and *gangrenous stomatitis* of debilitating systemic disease may be very difficult to differentiate from candidiasis because the latter entity is usually also found in patients with debilitating secondary disease. These lesions are discussed in Chapter 6 (see Fig. 6-11). As a general rule if the ulcer is deep then candidiasis would not be the primary cause although such an ulcer could indeed be secondarily infected with *Candida albicans.*

Traumatic ulcers with necrotic surfaces can in almost all instances be related to a history of specific trauma.

Superficial bacterial infections may occur in patients with debilitating disease and indeed may mimic pseudomembranous candidiasis. Tyldesley and co-workers (1979) described such lesions

occurring in renal transplant patients who were receiving combined steroid and immunosuppressive drug therapy. Previously some of these lesions were believed to be antibiotic-resistant candidiasis. Culture of these lesions yielded abundant bacteria such as staphylococci, *Neisseria,* coliforms, and lactobacilli. On the other hand, if removable white plaques filled with yeast form and pseudohyphae are present, then the diagnosis is either primary or secondary candidiasis.

Because its oral lesions are also covered by pseudomembranes, *gangrenous stomatitis* may be confused with candidiasis. Its plaques or pseudomembranes are not raised above the mucosa, however, but cover an ulcerating lesion that may extend to bone. Also its pseudomembranes are usually a dirty gray color, in contrast to the whiteness of those that develop in candidiasis. Gangrenous stomatitis may carry a much graver prognosis than does candidiasis, since the patient may be seriously ill with an uncontrolled debilitating disease; however, candidiasis also affects terminally ill patients.

Chemical burns in some instances may closely mimic candidiasis. The distinction is usually made by an accurate history, disclosing that a medicament has been applied to the mucosa.

MANAGEMENT

If the candidiasis seems to have been caused by an extended course of a broad-spectrum antibiotic, the drug should be discontinued and if possible a more selective antibiotic with a narrower spectrum substituted. Nystatin suspension, an antifungal agent used as a mouthwash, is helpful. Goebel and Duquette (1974) reported encouraging results with the oral use of vaginal troches of nystatin and the topical application of nystatin ointment. They suggested that the success with this regimen resulted from the longer direct contact of higher concentrations of these preparations with the organisms. Systemic administration of antifungal agents is usually not effective for the treatment of oral candidiasis because the organisms are protected within the necrotic tissue.

It is important to remember that any oral lesion with surface debris may harbor candidal organisms even to the extent that a secondary candidiasis may become established. Nystatin treatment in cases such as these would produce some improvement but full remission must await successful treatment for the primary lesion.

NECROTIC ULCERS OF SYSTEMIC DISEASE AND DIFFUSE GANGRENOUS STOMATITIS

Necrotic ulcers may occur in debilitating systemic diseases such as leukemia, sickle cell anemia, and uremia. The ulcers are usually deep craters with a white necrotic surface (Fig. 5-48). In most instances they commence as small mucosal injuries that become chronically infected because of the decreased resistance of the patient. These lesions are discussed and illustrated in Chapter 6.

DIFFUSE GANGRENOUS STOMATITIS

Diffuse gangrenous stomatitis is also an oral disease in which a pseudomembrane is formed. Its cause is almost identical to that of ANUG, but it occurs in extremely debilitated patients. It must be differentiated from localized gangrenous stomatitis (cancrum oris or noma), a single localized and very destructive lesion (Fig. 5-49) seldom encountered in the United States.

FEATURES

Diffuse gangrenous stomatitis is usually found in patients with severe debilitating diseases, such as advanced diabetes, uremia, leukemia, blood dyscrasias, malnutritional states, or heavy metal poisoning. The patient complains of sensitive or painful oral lesions and a very unpleasant odor. The lesions are multiple, affecting several mucosal surfaces, and are surrounded by a thin inflamed margin. The lesions themselves are covered by a dirty gray to yellow pseudomembrane that can be readily removed—leaving a raw, bleeding, painful surface. They may be elliptic, linear, or angular in shape. A tender to painful cervical lymphadenopathy is invariably present.

DIFFERENTIAL DIAGNOSIS

Differential aspects of diffuse gangrenous stomatitis are discussed under the differential diagnosis of candidiasis (p. 93).

Fig. 5-48. Necrotic ulcer on the palate of a patient with mycosis fungoides. (Courtesy M. Sneed, D.D.S., Chicago.)

Fig. 5-49. Noma on the buccal mucosa of a patient terminally ill with acute myelogenous leukemia. (From Weinstein, R. A., et al.: Oral Surg. **38**:10-14, 1974.)

MANAGEMENT

Local treatment of diffuse gangrenous stomatitis is similar to the regimen described for ANUG, systemic penicillin and hydrogen peroxide rinses many times a day. This condition has a much graver prognosis than does ANUG because of the serious predisposing systemic conditions present. Unless the systemic problems can be improved, the oral lesions may be difficult to eliminate completely.

RARITIES

The following either are rare disease entities or seldom occur as white sloughing lesions of the oral mucosa:
Diphtheria
Heavy metal mucositis
Noma
Superficial abscess
Syndrome of familial hypoparathyroidism, candidiasis, and retardation
Syndrome of idiopathic hypoparathyroidism, Addison's disease, and candidiasis
Syphilitic chancre and mucous patch (Fig. 5-47)
Tuberculosis
Although these are rare lesions, the examining clinician must be cognizant of them while developing a differential diagnosis. Unless specific characteristics of the lesion in question indicate otherwise, however, they will be assigned a low rank on his list of probable entities.

SPECIFIC REFERENCES

Ackerman, L. V.: Verrucous carcinoma of the oral cavity, Surgery **23**:670-678, 1948.

Ballard, B. R., Sues, G. R., Pickren, J. W., et al.: Squamous cell carcinoma of the floor of the mouth, Oral Surg. **45**:568-579, 1978.

Bánóczy, J., and Csiba, A.: Occurrence of the epithelial dysplasia in oral leukoplakia, Oral Surg. **42**:766-774, 1976.

Bánóczy, J., Roed-Petersen, B., Pindborg, J. J., and Inovay, J.: Clinical and histologic studies on electrogalvanically induced oral white lesions, Oral Surg. **48**:319-323, 1979.

Bánóczy, J., and Sugár, L.: Longitudinal studies in oral leukoplakia, J. Oral Pathol. **1**:265-272, 1972.

Bernstein, M. L.: Oral mucosal white lesions associated with excessive use of Listerine mouthwash, Oral Surg. **46**:781-785, 1978.

Berry, H. H., and Lanwerlen, J. R.: Cigarette smokers lip lesion in psychiatric patients, J. Am. Dent. Assoc. **86**:657-662, 1973.

Buchner, A., and Sandbank, M.: Multiple fibroepithelial hyperplasias of the oral mucosa, Oral Surg. **46**:34-39, 1978.

Burry, J. N., and Kirk, J.: Lichenoid drug reaction from methyldopa, Br. J. Dermatol. **91**:475-476, 1974.

Christensen, E., Holmstrup, P., Wiberg-Jørgesen, F., et al.: Glucose tolerance in patients with oral lichen planus, J. Oral Pathol. **6**:143-151, 1977.

Clayton, J. R., and Jordan, J. E.: Verrucous carcinoma, J. Oral Surg. **36**:564-567, 1978.

Durocher, R. T., Thalman, R., and Fiore-Donno, G.: Leukoedema of the oral mucosa, J. Am. Dent. Assoc. **85**:1105-1109, 1972.

Farman, A. G.: Hairy tongue (lingua villosa), J. Oral Med. **32**:85-91, 1977.

Goebel, W. M., and Duquette, P.: Mycotic infections associated with complete dentures: report of three cases, J. Am. Dent. Assoc. **88**:842-844, 1974.

Graff, S. G., Burk, J. L., and McKean, T. W.: Verruciform xanthoma, Oral Surg. **45**:762-767, 1978.

Greer, R. O., and Goldman, H. M.: Oral papillomas, Oral Surg. **38**:435-440, 1974.

Grinspan, D., Diaz, J., Villapol, L. O., et al.: Lichen ruber planes de la muquese buccale son association a un diabete, Bull. Soc. Fr. Dermatol. Syphiligr. **72**:721, 1966.

Howell, F. V., and Rick, G. M.: Oral lichen planus and diabetes: a potential syndrome, J. Calif. Dent. Assoc. **1**:58-59, July 1973.

Jacobson, S., and Shear, M.: Verrucous carcinoma of the mouth, J. Oral Pathol. **1**:66-75, 1972.

Kowitz, G. M., Lucatorto, F. M., and Cherrick, H. M.: Effects of mouthwashes on the oral soft tissues, J. Oral Med. **31**:47-50, 1976.

Kramer, I. R. H., El-Labbon, N., and Lee, K. W.: The clinical features and risk of malignant transformation in sublingual keratosis, Br. Dent. J. **144**:171-180, 1978.

Kramer, I. R. H., Lucas, R. B., Pindborg, J. J., and Sobin, L. H.: Definition of leukoplakia and related lesions: an aid to studies on oral precancer. WHO Collaborating Centre for Oral Precancerous Lesions, Oral Surg. **46**:518-539, 1978.

Krutchkoff, D. J., Cutler, L., and Laskowski, S.: Oral lichen planus: the evidence regarding potential malignant transformation, J. Oral Pathol. **7**:1-7, 1978.

Martin, J. L., and Crump, E. P.: Leukoedema of the buccal mucosa in Negro children and youth, Oral Surg. **34**:49-58, 1972.

Mincer, H. H., Coleman, S. A., and Hopkins, K. P.: Observations on the clinical characteristics of oral lesions showing histologic epithelial dysplasia, Oral Surg. **33**:389-399, 1972.

Neumann-Jensen, B. J., and Pindborg, J. J.: Smoking habits of 611 patients with oral lichen planus, Oral Surg. **43**:410-415, 1977.

Pindborg, J. J., Daftary, D. K., and Mehta, F. S.: A follow-up study of sixty-one oral dysplastic precancerous lesions in Indian villagers, Oral Surg. **43**:383-390, 1977.

Pindborg, J. J., Jolst, O., Renstrup, G., and Roed-Petersen, B.: Studies in oral leukoplakia, a preliminary report on the period prevalence of malignant transformation in leukoplakia based on a follow-up study of 248 patients, J. Am. Dent. Assoc. **78**:767-771, 1968.

Pogrel, M. A.: Sublingual keratosis and malignant transformation, J. Oral Pathol. **8**:176-178, 1978.

Roed-Petersen, B., and Pindborg, J. J.: A study of Danish snuff-induced oral leukoplakia, J. Oral Pathol. **2**:301-313, 1973.

Rubright, W. C., Walker, J. A., Karlsson, U. L., and Diehl, D. L.: Oral slough caused by dentifrice detergents and aggravated by drugs with antisialic activity, J. Am. Dent. Assoc. **97**:215-220, 1978.

Shafer, W. G.: Verrucous carcinoma, Int. Dent. J. **22**:451-459, 1972.

Silverman, S. J., and Griffeth, M.: Studies on oral lichen planus. II. Follow-up on 200 patients, clinical characteristics, and associated malignancy, Oral Surg. **37**:705-710, 1974.

Silverman, S. J., and Rozen, R. P.: Observations on the clinical characteristics and natural history of oral leukoplakia, J. Am. Dent. Assoc. **76**:772-777, 1968.

Smith, M. J. A.: Oral lichen planus and diabetes mellitus: a possible association, J. Oral Med. **32:**110-112, 1977.

Tyldesley, W. R.: Oral lichen planus, Br. J. Oral Surg. **11:**187-206, 1974.

Tyldesley, W. R., Rotter, E., and Sells, R. A.: Oral lesions in renal transplant patients, J. Oral Pathol. **8:**53-59, 1979.

Waldron, C. A.: Oral epithelial tumors. In Gorlin, R. J., and Goldman, H. M., editors: Thoma's oral pathology, ed. 6, St. Louis, 1970, The C. V. Mosby Co.

Waldron, C. A., and Shafer, W. G.: Leukoplakia revisited, Cancer **36**(4):1386-1392, 1975.

Weathers, D. R., Baker, G., Archard, H. O., and Burkes, E. J.: Psoriasiform lesions of the oral mucosa (with emphasis on "ectopic geographic tongue"), Oral Surg. **37:**872-888, 1974.

Weaver, A., Fleming, S. M., and Smith, D. B.: Mouthwash and oral cancer: carcinogenic or coincidence? J. Oral Surg. **37:**250-253, 1979.

Weinstein, R. A., Choukas, N. C., and Wood, W. S.: Cancrum oris-like lesion associated with acute myelogenous leukemia, Oral Surg. **38:**10-14, 1974.

Wysocki, G. P., and Hardie, J.: Ultrastructural studies of intra-oral verruca vulgaris, Oral Surg. **47:**58-62, 1979.

GENERAL REFERENCES

Abbey, L. M., Sawyer, D. R., and Syrop, H. M.: Oral squamous acanthoma, Oral Surg. **45:**255-260, 1978.

Andreasen, J. O.: Oral lichen planus. I. A clinical evaluation of 115 cases, Oral Surg. **25:**31-42, 1968.

Archard, H. O., Carlson, K. P., and Stanley, H. R.: Leukoedema of the human oral mucosa, Oral Surg. **25:**717-728, 1968.

Arwill, G. H., and Gisslen, H.: Histochemical studies on lichen planus, Oral Surg. **37:**239-248, 1974.

Aufdemorte, T. B., and McPherson, M. A.: Refractory oral candidiasis, Oral Surg. **46:**776-780, 1978.

Birkholz, H., Sills, A. H., and Reid, R. A.: Peripheral ameloblastoma, J. Am. Dent. Assoc. **97:**658-660, 1978.

Bruum, J. P.: Time lapse by diagnosis of oral cancer, Oral Surg. **42:**139-149, 1976.

Cawson, R. A.: Chronic oral candidiasis and leukoplakia, Oral Surg. **22:**582-591, 1966.

Dolby, A. E.: Oral mucosa in health and disease, Oxford, England, 1975, Blackwell Scientific Publications.

Fischman, S. L., Barnett, M. L., and Nisengard, R. J.: Histopathologic, ultrastructural, and immunologic findings in an oral psoriatic lesion, Oral Surg. **44:**253-260, 1977.

Gardner, D. G.: Peripheral ameloblastoma, Cancer **39:**1625-1633, 1977.

Garfunkel, A. A., Pisanty, S., and Michaeli, Y.: Familial hypoparathyroidism, candidiasis and mental retardation—a histopathologic study of the dental structures, J. Oral Med. **34:**13-17, 1979.

Gorlin, R. J.: Genetic disorders affecting mucous membranes, Oral Surg. **28:**512-525, 1969.

Hamner, J. E., Looney, R. D., and Chused, T. M.: Submucus fibrosis, Oral Surg. **37:**412-421, 1974.

Hamner, J. E., Mehta, F. S., Pindborg, J. J., and Daftary, D. K.: An epidemiologic and histopathologic study of leukoedema among 50,915 rural Indian villagers, Oral Surg. **32:**58-65, 1971.

Hayward, J. R., and Regezi, J. A.: Oral dysplasia and in situ carcinoma: clinicopathologic correlations of eight patients, J. Oral Surg. **35:**756-762, 1977.

Jayant, K., Balakrishnan, V., Sanghui, L. D., and Jussawalla, D. J.: Quantification of the role of smoking and chewing tobacco in oral, pharyngeal, and esophageal cancers, Br. J. Cancer **35:**232-235, 1977.

Jones, J. H., and Russel, C.: Candidial infection and leukoplakia, Br. J. Oral Surg. **11:**177-180, 1973.

Ju, D. M. C.: On the etiology of cancer of the lower lip, Plast. Reconstr. Surg. **52:**151-154, 1973.

Kapstad, B., and Bang, G.: Verrucous carcinoma of the oral cavity treated with Bleomycin, Oral Surg. **42:**588-590, 1976.

Kramer, I. R.: Precancerous lesions of the mouth, J. Laryngol. Otol. **90:**95-100, 1976.

Lehner, T.: Oral thrush, or acute pseudomembrane candidiasis, Oral Surg. **18:**27-37, 1964.

Lindgren, S., Enerback, L., and Freidberg, N.: Oral acantholytic itching disease responding to dapsone, Oral Surg. **42:**597-605, 1976.

Malaowalla, A. M., Silverman, S., and Bilimoria, K. F.: Oral cancer in 57,518 industrial workers of Gujarat, India, Cancer **37:**1882-1886, 1976.

Maser, E. D.: Oral manifestations of pachyonychia congenita: report of a case, Oral Surg. **43:**373-378, 1977.

Mashberg, A., and Meyers, H.: Anatomical site and size of 222 early asymptomatic oral squamous cell carcinomas, Cancer **32:**1436-1445, 1973.

McLeran, J. H., Hale, M. L., and Higa, L. H.: White sponge nevus, J. Oral Surg. **26:**338-341, 1968.

Mehta, F. S., Shroff, B. C., Gupta, P. C., and Daftary, D. K.: Oral leukoplakia in relation to tobacco habits, Oral Surg. **34:**426-433, 1972.

Miller, A. S., and Pullon, P. A.: Hard raised lesion in the right buccal mucosa (sialolith in minor salivary gland), Dent. Survey **57:**28, 1979.

Mosadami, A., Shklar, G., Loftus, E. R., and Chauncey, H. H.: Effects of tobacco smoking and age on the keratinization of palatal mucosa: a cytologic study, Oral Surg. **46:**413-417, 1978.

Myllarniemi, S., and Perheentupa, J.: Oral findings in the autoimmune polyendocrinopathy-candidosis syndrome (APECS) and other forms of hypoparathyroidism, Oral Surg. **45:**721-729, 1978.

Nakissa, N., Hornback, N. B., Shidnia, H., and Sayoc, E. S.: Carcinoma of the floor of the mouth, Cancer **42:**2914-2919, 1978.

Pindborg, J. J., Roed-Petersen, B., and Renstrup, G.: Role of smoking in floor of mouth leukoplakias, J. Oral Pathol. **1:**22-29, 1972.

Pisanty, S., and Garfunkel, A.: Familial hypoparathyroidism with candidiasis and mental retardation, Oral Surg. **44:**374-383, 1977.

Praetorius-Clausen, F.: Rare oral viral disorders (Mulluscum contagiosum, localized keratoacanthoma, verrucae, condyloma acuminatum, and focal epithelial hyperplasia), Oral Surg. **34:**604-618, 1972.

Rossi, E. P., and Hirsch, S. A.: A survey of 4,793 oral lesions with emphasis on neoplasia and premalignancy, J. Am. Dent. Assoc. **94:**883-886, 1977.

Saunders, I.: Bohn's nodules, Br. Dent. J. **132:**457-458, June 1972.

Schiodt, M., Halberg, P., and Hentzer, B.: A clinical study of 32 patients with oral discoid lupus erythematosus, Int. J. Oral Surg. **7:**85-94, 1978.

Schiodt, M., and Pindborg, J. J.: Histologic differential diagnostic problems for oral discoid lupus erythematosus, Int. J. Oral Surg. **5:**250-252, 1976.

Shafer, W. G.: Oral carcinoma in situ, Oral Surg. **39:**227-238, 1975.

Silverman, S., Bhargava, K., Marri, N. J., et al.: Malignant transformation and natural history of oral leukoplakia in 57,518 industrial workers in Gujarat, India, Cancer **38:**1790-1795, 1976.

Stiff, R. H., and Ferraro, E.: Hereditary keratosis, Oral Surg. **28:**697-701, 1969.

Tenzer, J. A, and Gold, L.: Recurrent snuff dipper's lesion treated by excision and skin graft, Oral Surg. **28:**691-695, 1970.

Tyldesley, W. R., and Appleton, J.: Observations on the ultra-structure of the epithelium in oral lichen planus, J. Oral Pathol. **2:**46-57, 1973.

Whitten, J. B.: The electron microscopic examination of congenital keratosis of the oral mucous membranes. I. White sponge nevus, Oral Surg. **29:**69-84, 1970.

Young, L., and Lenox, J. A.: Pachyonychia congenita, Oral Surg. **36:**663-666, 1973.

Zegarelli, D. J.: Red and white intraoral lesions, Dent. Survey **55:**34-42, 1979.

6

Oral ulcers and fissures

Norman K. Wood
Paul W. Goaz

Ulcers and fissures of the oral cavity include the following:

Ulcers
Traumatic ulcer
Recurrent aphthous ulcer and intraoral recurrent ulcer of
    herpes simplex
Ulcers from odontogenic infections
Sloughing, pseudomembranous ulcers
Generalized mucosities and vesiculobullous diseases
Squamous cell carcinoma
Syphilis
    Chancre
    Gumma
Ulcers secondary to systemic disease
Traumatized tumors (types usually not ulcerated)
Minor salivary gland tumors
Rarities
    Actinomycosis
    Adenoid squamous cell carcinoma
    Basal cell carcinoma
    Botryomycosis
    Cancrum oris
    Food-and-mouth disease
    Fungal infections (blastomycosis, coccidioidomycosis,
        cryptococcosis, histoplasmosis, sporotrichosis)
    Gonococcal stomatitis
    Granulomatous disease of the newborn
    Hand-foot-and-mouth disease
    Herpes zoster
    Keratoacanthoma
    Lethal midline granuloma
    Leukemia
    Lymphoma
    Median rhomboid glossitis—ulcerative variety
    Metastatic tumor
    Mycosis fungoides
    Necrotizing sialometaplasia
    Neurotrophic ulcer
    Sarcoidosis
    Sutton's disease
    Tuberculosis
    Warty dyskeratoma

Fissures
Angular cheilosis
Congenital cleft

Epulis fissuratum
Fissured tongue
Median rhomboid glossitis—fissured variety
Squamous cell carcinoma—fissured variety
Syphilitic rhagades

Ulcers

Oral ulcers represent a variable and impressive group of lesions. A cursory examination of the foregoing list will reveal that some of these lesions are caused by local influences (e.g., traumatic ulcers) whereas others are manifestations of systemic problems (the oral ulcers in sickle cell anemia).

Also, when attempting to characterize this group of lesions, the clinician will be greatly aided by considering Spouge's (1973, p. 371) general description that some oral ulcers are *primary*—with early manifestations as erosions or ulcers, such as the traumatic ulcers, whereas others are actually *secondary*—because they are subsequent to other clinical forms which, after rupturing and sloughing, become ulcerated (e.g., vesicles and blebs).

Exophytic lesions frequently illustrate this secondary change when they become ulcerated from chronic mechanical injury or as the result of an incisional biopsy.

The terms "erosion" and "ulcer" are often confused and mistakenly used interchangeably. Spouge (1973, p. 371) defined an *erosion* as a shallow crater in the epithelial surface that appears clinically as a very shallow erythematous area and implies only superficial damage. He defined an *ulcer* as a deeper crater that extends through the entire thickness of surface epithelium and involves the underlying connective tissue.

Oral ulcers are unique inasmuch as they have

diverse etiologies but frequently show similar histologic changes and thus cannot be differentiated by routine microscopy. This microscopic uniformity derives from the fact that as soon as an ulcer is formed in the oral mucosa it is immediately subjected to irritating oral liquids and flora and consequently an acute or chronic inflammation is immediately initiated. The resultant inflammatory changes may mask the more characteristic and diagnostic histologic changes that are a feature of the basic pathosis.

The intraoral herpes simplex lesion is a good example of an oral ulcer that loses its microscopic picture because of secondary contamination. In its early vesicular stage there are pathognomonic features: ballooning of the epithelial cells and giant cells present in the vesicular fluid. After the vesicle ulcerates, these definitive features are soon lost and all that remains is the histologic picture of a nonspecific ulcer.

The following changes are inferred when the clinician encounters a microscopic diagnosis of "nonspecific" ulcer:

1. The complete thickness of the surface epithelium will be missing, and the exposed connective tissue will often be necrotic on the surface and covered by a fibrinous exudate (Fig. 6-1).
2. Depending on its age and the circumstances relating to its development, the ulcer will have acute inflammation with polymorphonuclear leukocytes in the connective tissue at its borders.
3. A less acute phase of the ulcer will show a greater concentration of chronic inflammatory cells, such as lymphocytes, plasma cells, and possibly macrophages with some fibroblastic proliferation.
4. In the healing phase of the ulcer, granulation tissue with fibroblastic proliferation will predominate; and a few macrophages, plasma cells, and lymphocytes may also be present.

In spite of the foregoing, it is possible to diagnose definitively some of the ulcers discussed in this chapter by routine light microscopy when they are stained with hematoxylin and eosin (H & E).

For example, histologic changes in squamous cell carcinoma and ulcerative mesenchymal minor salivary gland tumors will be diagnostic as long as the biopsy actually includes a section of tumor underlying the ulcer. It is true that lesions such as chancres, herpetic ulcers, and tuberculous, sarcoid, and fungal lesions may produce tis-

Fig. 6-1. Nonspecific ulcer. Photomicrograph reveals loss of the surface epithelium and the upper portion of the lamina propria. Note the abundance of inflammatory cells.

sue changes that indicate a definitive diagnosis; but usually special staining procedures, such as Gram's, silver, or PAS,* must be utilized to assist in making a definitive microscopic identification.

When attempting to complete a differential diagnosis of a clinical ulcer, the clinician should separate the oral ulcers into two groups: *short-term* ulcers (i.e., those that persist no longer than 3 weeks and regress spontaneously) and *persistent ulcers* (those that last for weeks and months).

The majority of traumatic ulcers, recurrent aphthous ulcers (except major aphthae), recurrent intraoral herpetic ulcers, and chancres fall into the category of short-term ulcers.

Occasional traumatic ulcers, major aphthae, ulcers from odontogenic infection, malignant ulcers, gummas, and ulcers secondary to debilitating systemic disease are classified as persistent ulcers and may remain for months and even years. Persistent ulcers should be considered malignant till proved otherwise.

TRAUMATIC ULCER

The traumatic ulcer is by far the most common oral mucosal ulcer. The cause may be mechanical, chemical, or thermal; and the traumatic incident may be accidentally self-inflicted or iatrogenic.

FEATURES

The patient with a traumatic ulcer will complain of tenderness or pain in the area of the lesion and usually will be able to identify its cause.

---

*The periodic acid–Schiff reaction is a widely used method that stains glycogen, epithelial mucus, neutral polysaccharides, and glycoproteins.

A variety of causes will come to the inquiring clinician's attention: lip, tongue, and cheek biting (sometimes after the administration of a local anesthetic), a toothbrush that slipped, a child who was running with an object in his mouth and fell, or a mouth burned by hot liquids or toothache drops.

Traumatic ulcers are most common on the tongue, lips, mucobuccal fold, gingiva, and palate. They may persist for just a few days or may last for weeks (especially ulcers of the tongue). They may vary greatly in size and shape but seldom are multiple or recurrent unless they result from ill-fitting dentures. Their borders are somewhat raised and reddish, and their bases have a yellowish necrotic surface that can be readily removed (Figs. 6-2 and 6-3). Ulcers on the vermilion border, unlike those on the oral mucosa, usually have a crusted surface because of the absence of saliva. In some instances the ulcers will conform nicely to the shape of a tooth cusp or a denture flange, or they may be positioned against a sharp edge of a tooth.

The clinician must be certain of the cause-and-effect relationship not only to make a definitive diagnosis of traumatic ulcer but also to identify and eliminate the traumatizing agent. Frequently there will be a tender or painful regional lymphadenitis from contamination of the ulcer by the oral flora.

DIFFERENTIAL DIAGNOSIS

The history of the traumatic injury in most cases will enable the clinician to identify the traumatic ulcer and establish a working diagnosis. The history of a traumatic incident may be misleading, however, and cause the true identity of a more serious lesion to be overlooked. Since traumatic ulcers may be either short-term or persistent, both varieties must be considered in the differential diagnosis. For a more thorough discussion, refer to the differential diagnosis section at the end of this chapter (pp. 116 and 118).

MANAGEMENT

Most traumatic ulcers become painless within 3 or 4 days after the injury-producing agent has been eliminated, and most heal within 10 days. Occasionally, however, a lesion will persist for some weeks because of continued traumatic in-

Fig. 6-2. Traumatic ulcers. **A,** Ulcer on the maxillary ridge due to a traumatic extraction. **B,** Ulcer on the maxillary alveolus due to trauma from the lower canine. **C,** Traumatic ulcer on the ventral surface of the tongue resulting from a self-inflicted bite. **D,** Ulcer caused by a sharp premolar root. This lesion, which appeared clinically to be a squamous cell carcinoma, proved on biopsy to be a traumatic lesion. (**A** courtesy D. Bonomo, D.D.S., Flossmoor, Ill. **B** courtesy P. D. Toto, D.D.S., Maywood, Ill.)

sults or continued irritation by the oral liquids or because of the development of a secondary infection. This last often indicates the presence of a lowered resistance from an underlying systemic disease.

In our experience, coating the ulcerated surface of the persistent traumatic ulcers, as well as of the less serious varieties, with triamcinolone acetonide in emollient (Kenalog in Orabase) before bedtime and after meals usually relieves the pain and hastens the healing. The Orabase protects the denuded connective tissue from continued contamination by the oral liquids, and the cortisone component tends to arrest the inflammatory cycle (which may become self-perpetuating).

Persistent ulcers not responding to the foregoing regimen should be surgically excised and closed primarily; and the excised tissue must always be microscopically examined since a persistent ulcer could very likely be a malignant lesion as well as one of the other benign lesions discussed in this chapter.

RECURRENT APHTHOUS ULCER (CANKER SORE) AND INTRAORAL RECURRENT ULCER OF HERPES SIMPLEX

Until the recent past much confusion has existed concerning recurrent aphthous ulcers (RAU)[*] and intraoral recurrent herpes simplex (IRHS) ulcers, despite many publications reporting research that described these entities. Some investigators consider that the lesions have a

---

[*]Sutton's disease, in contrast to the aphthous ulcers, was at one time considered to be a separate entity since the ulcers are larger and more persistent and characteristically cause scarring. Currently Sutton's disease is thought of as a more severe manifestation of RAU, and the lesions are frequently referred to as major aphthae (Stanley, 1973). In addition, the oral lesions of Behçet's and Reiter's syndromes may be identical with RAU although they frequently involve the whole mucosa. Consequently these are listed as mucositides in Chapter 11.

Fig. 6-3. Traumatic ulcers. **A,** Ulcer on the floor of the mouth caused by a rough temporary crown on the mandibular right second premolar tooth. **B,** Ulcerated and ecchymotic lesion on the posterior palate of a male who was holding a Popsicle stick in his mouth when he fell. **C,** Symmetric ulceration and hyperplastic reaction on the anterior palate that was caused by a suction cup on a denture. (**C** courtesy A. C. W. Hutchinson collection, Northwestern University Dental School Library, Chicago.)

Fig. 6-4. Recurrent aphthous ulcers. **A** to **C,** Typical lesions that disappeared within 14 days. **D,** Major aphtha (Sutton's disease) that persisted for several months.

common cause and are identical because both share the following characteristics:

1. They are recurrent, painful, superficial oral ulcers that persist 8 to 14 days.
2. They are associated with a tender regional lymphadenopathy.
3. They heal spontaneously usually without sequelae.

It is generally agreed now, however, that RAU and IRHS are distinct and separate entities.

Several hypotheses as to the etiology of RAU have been proposed; they include psychic, allergic, microbial, traumatic, endocrine, hereditary, and autoimmune mechanisms (Stanley, 1973). Currently it seems likely that the RAU develop as a result of several different mechanisms.

In addition, it is generally agreed that the usual IRHS ulcers are secondary lesions produced by the herpesvirus and are the counterpart of herpes labialis. This means that patients have been primarily infected with the herpesvirus and, although a small percentage may experience the more severe primary herpetic stomatitis, the majority of the initial infections must be subclinical or minor manifestations. Primary herpetic gingivostomatitis is discussed in Chapter 11.

FEATURES

The RAU and IRHS ulcers may be quite clearly differentiated on a clinical basis by utilizing the contrasting features summarized by Weathers and Griffin (1970) (Figs. 6-4 and 6-5 and Table 6-1).

DIFFERENTIAL DIAGNOSIS

Application of the criteria in Table 6-1 will enable the clinician to differentiate between RAU and IRHS in most cases. Of course, if other body surfaces are involved, the various syndromes mentioned earlier must be considered. A further discussion of the distinguishing features of similar-appearing intraoral ulcers is presented in the differential diagnosis section at the end of this chapter (p. 116). For a discussion of generalized oral ulcerations or mucositides, see Chapter 11.

MANAGEMENT

Except for the major aphthae, RAU and IRHS resolve in 8 to 14 days without treatment. For the treatment of aphthous ulcers, Stanley (1973) recommends a tetracycline mouthwash (an oral suspension of uncoated Achromycin crystals, 250 mg/tsp, in 5 ml H_2O) to be flushed over the affected region for at least 2 minutes. After debridement with the tetracycline mouthwash, the ulcer is coated by a thick layer of triamcinolone acetonide in emollient dental paste (Kenalog in Orabase) after meals and before going to bed. Systemic analgesics are administered if necessary. We have found this regimen to give very

Fig. 6-5. Secondary herpetic lesions on the palate. Note the several small punctate ulcers—some of which have coalesced to form larger ulcers. (Courtesy P. Akers, D.D.S., Chicago.)

Table 6-1. Comparison of features of recurrent aphthous ulcers (RAU) and intraoral recurrent herpes simplex (IRHS) ulcers

	RAU	**IRHS**
Age	Wide range	Any age but more common in middle and older age groups
Location	On freely movable mucosa (nonkeratinized), lips, buccal mucosa, tongue, mucobuccal fold, floor of mouth, soft palate (Fig. 6-4)	On fixed mucosa; tightly bound to periosteum (keratinized), hard palate, gingiva, and alveolar ridge (Fig. 6-5)
Initial lesion	Erythematous macule or papule; undergoes central blanching followed by necrosis and ulceration	Cluster of small discrete gray or white vesicles without red erythematous halo Vesicles quickly rupture, forming small punctate ulcers 1 mm or less in diameter
Mature lesion	Shallow ulcer 0.5 to 2 or 3 cm in diameter; yellow necrotic center; regular border; constant erythematous halo	Shallow ulcer no larger than 0.5 cm in diameter; several lesions may coalesce to form larger lesion, usually not larger than 0.5 cm in diameter
Number of lesions	Usually occur singly, but occasionally two or three widely distributed (Fig. 6-4)	Usually several small punctate ulcers in cluster in small localized area (Fig. 6-5); regular border, usually round in shape; variable erythematous halo
Histology	Mature lesion: nonspecific ulcer	Early lesion: vesicular fluid contains epithelial cells with balloon degeneration and multinucleated giant cells Mature lesion: after third day, nonspecific ulcer

satisfactory results but usually reserve the use of tetracycline for multiple ulcers or major aphthae.

Various procedures (e.g., cryotherapy, photochemical activation) have been used to treat herpetic lesions—with varying results. Currently photochemical activation is not recommended. From a theoretic point of view, Kenalog in Ora-base should not be applied to IRHS since the corticosteroid may contribute to the dissemination of the virus; but to date we have not observed any such sequelae, nor are we aware that any have been reported.

Recently two promising new agents have been introduced that have demonstrated success as anti–herpes simplex viral agents: vidarabine (Vira-A) and 2-deoxy-D-glucose (FDA Drug Bulletin December 1978-January 1979; Rowe et al., 1979). Vidarabine to date has been extremely successful in reducing the high mortality in herpes simplex viral encephalitis. Recent studies using this drug on herpes labialis lesions have reported encouraging results (Rowe et al., 1979).

ULCERS FROM ODONTOGENIC INFECTIONS

Ulcers resulting from the drainage of pus from odontogenic infections are easily recognized. Two rather similar clinical situations can cause them:

1. The ulcer may serve as the cloacal opening of a sinus draining a chronic alveolar abscess.
2. The ulcer may be the site of a superficial space abscess that has spontaneously ruptured.

FEATURES

In most cases of chronic alveolar abscess, the ulcer is on the alveolar ridge on either the buccal or the lingual surface, usually near the mucobuccal fold; but occasionally it will be on the palate (Figs. 6-6 and 8-6). The majority of chronic

A

B

Fig. 6-6. Odontogenic ulcers. **A,** A sublingual abscess from the infected lateral incisor ruptured to produce this ulcer. **B,** The ulcer represents the oral opening of a draining chronic alveolar abscess from the pulpless lower incisor.

alveolar abscesses are seen in children under 14 years of age. Such draining sinuses and similar pathoses are discussed in detail in Chapter 8 so they will not be considered here.

Other ulcers may represent the ruptured surface of an odontogenic space abscess situated on the palate or in the sublingual or vestibular areas (Fig. 6-6). Pressure on the adjacent soft tissue causing pus to exude from the ulcer will identify the condition. If odontogenic infection is suspected, a thorough clinical radiologic examination of the teeth and supporting structures will almost always provide enough information to enable the examiner to either identify or rule out an odontogenic infection.

Should the results of the examination be equivocal, a gutta percha point may be placed in the ulcer and passed into the tract as far as it will go without undue force. A radiograph may then be taken. If the ulcer is a cloaca of an alveolar abscess, the point will frequently be found to extend to the apex of an infected tooth.

DIFFERENTIAL DIAGNOSIS

The odontogenic ulcer can be misdiagnosed only as the result of a cursory or careless examination. When a small ulcer 0.2 to 1 cm in diameter is present on the mucosa of the palate, alveolus, or vestibule, an odontogenic ulcer must always be considered as a very likely possibility. Two other less likely possibilities are sinus openings from osteomyelitis or infected malignant tumors. A more thorough discussion may be found in the differential diagnosis section at the end of this chapter (p. 116).

MANAGEMENT

Endodontic therapy or extraction, which on occasion may have to be accompanied by the administration of antibiotics, will usually result in the healing of the ulcer.

SLOUGHING, PSEUDOMEMBRANOUS ULCERS

Sloughing, pseudomembranous ulcers have been described in detail in Chapter 5 and are mentioned here because they are shown to have an ulcerated surface when the membrane is removed. Such lesions include crushing types of traumatic ulcers, ANUG, candidiasis, and gangrenous stomatitis.

ANUG is the most common example of such lesions; and the fact that the necrotic and ulcerative process involves one or more of the tips of the interdental papillae is practically pathognomonic for the disease. Similar lesions may be seen on the gingivae accompanying other oral lesions, however, such as diffuse gangrenous stomatitis (Chapter 5).

GENERALIZED MUCOSITIDES AND VESICULOBULLOUS DISEASES

Generalized mucositides and vesiculobullous diseases have been included here because, even though singly the entities may themselves be uncommon to rare, as a group they are relatively common. Although the diseases produce oral ulcerations, the ulcerations are secondary to primary mucositides and/or vesicular and bullous lesions. Thus in most cases the whole mucosal surface of the oral cavity is a mass of ulcers, blebs, and erosive erythematous areas. A list of such diseases would include the following:

Behçet's syndrome
Erosive lichen planus
Erythema multiforme
Primary herpetic gingivostomatitis
Gangrenous stomatitis
Stevens-Johnson syndrome
Vesiculobullous lesions (benign mucous membrane pemphigoid, bullous lichen planus, cat-scratch disease, epidermolysis bullosa, herpangina, herpes zoster, pemphigus and its variants, foot-and-mouth disease, hand-foot-and-mouth disease)

Some of these more common diseases are discussed in detail in Chapter 11. Their usually wide dissemination in the oral cavity precludes their being misdiagnosed as one of the discrete frequently solitary ulcers discussed in this chapter, however. They are included here mainly because a solitary lesion may precede the more severe manifestations of the disease and thus be confused with the solitary ulcers that are the subject of this chapter.

SQUAMOUS CELL CARCINOMA

Squamous cell carcinoma is the most common oral malignancy and represents about 95% of all malignant tumors that occur in the mouth and jaws. It is discussed as a white lesion in Chapter 5, as an exophytic lesion in Chapter 7, and as a red lesion in Chapter 10. In this chapter the ulcerative variety will be stressed.

Although the cause of squamous cell carcinoma is unknown, chronic irritation from the use of tobacco products, alcohol, and other carcinogens either singly or in combination may trigger a malignant change in a genetically and systemically conditioned oral mucosa. Ionizing and actinic radiation will also induce such malignant changes. Shillitoe and Silverman (1979) reviewed the current knowledge concerning the association of herpes simplex virus and oral cancer. Weaver and co-workers (1979) offered evidence that pointed to the possible etiologic role of mouthwashes in the production of oral cancer.

At one time implicating chronic mechanical trauma (i.e., sharp teeth or denture flanges) as a cause of intraoral squamous cell carcinoma was fashionable; but statistical studies have failed to confirm a relationship between chronic mechanical injury and this type of ulcer (Spouge, 1973, p. 394). We have not observed a single case of squamous cell carcinoma in which mechanical trauma alone could be implicated. In septic mouths, however, we have developed the clinical impression that squamous cell carcinoma does occur more frequently.

FEATURES

Squamous cell carcinoma is the most common persistent ulcer to occur in the oral cavity or on the lips. Because it is almost always painless, the patient usually is not aware of its presence until it has become relatively advanced. Consequently the smaller ulcerative tumors are found during routine oral examinations.

Squamous cell carcinoma of the oral cavity and lips occurs approximately two times as frequently in men as in women. Although it may affect any age group, it is predominantly a disease of the middle aged and elderly. Classically the ulcerative squamous cell carcinoma is described as a craterlike lesion having a velvety red base and a rolled indurated border (Figs. 6-7 and 6-8). If situated on the vermilion border, it may be covered with a crust because of the absence of saliva (Fig. 6-7, *A*). The intraoral ulcer is usually devoid of necrotic material.

It is the authors' opinion that a greater percentage of ulcerated oral carcinomas tend to be of the infiltrative type than of the exophytic or verrucous types, and thus as a group they have a poorer prognosis since they are more invasive.

Sometimes the tumor will expand partly by infiltration and partly by exophytic growth, and in such cases the surface often becomes ulcerated from a diminished blood supply or chronic trauma.

The granular reddish (velvety) appearance of the base is the result of a lack of keratin and a thinner than normal prickle cell layer. The absence of these masking layers permits the red

Fig. 6-7. Ulcerative squamous cell carcinoma. **F,** Photomicrograph of a poorly differentiated squamous cell carcinoma. (**A** courtesy R. Oglesby, D.D.S., Chicago.)

color of the vasculature to show through on the surface.

If the tumor has infiltrated the surrounding connective tissue, the base and borders of the lesion will be very firm to palpation. If it is situated on a normally freely movable mucosal surface and it has infiltrated the deeper tissues, the mucosa will be fixed to the deeper structures. When this occurs in specific locations, such as the lateral border and undersurface of the tongue, the function of the organ may be impaired and there will be a detectable alteration in speech.

The lower lip (95% of labial lesions are on the lower lip) and the tongue (especially the lateral borders and ventral surface) are the most frequent sites of oral squamous cell carcinoma. (A large percentage of tongue carcinomas, however,

are not ulcerative but are leukoplakial or erythroplakial.) The floor of the mouth, alveolar gingivae, retromolar area, buccal mucosa, and palate (soft palate or the region at the junction of the hard and soft palates) are also fairly frequently involved. The anterior hard palate appears to be immune to squamous cell carcinoma.

Lesions are usually solitary but in some cases have been multifocal. Approximately 7% of patients with oral carcinoma develop one or more additional tumors.

Intraoral carcinomas spread characteristically to the regional cervical lymph nodes—where the submaxillary, superficial, and deep cervical nodes are the most commonly affected. In some cases contralateral nodes may be involved. In an interesting and extensive study of 898 cases of

Fig. 6-8. Ulcerative squamous cell carcinoma. **A,** Lateral border of tongue associated with leuko-plakia. **B,** Median region of vermilion border. **C,** Posterior to tuberosity in the left maxilla. **D,** Floor of the mouth and anterior ridge in the right incisor region. The ulcerated lesion is associated with a large erythroplakic patch on the floor of the mouth. (**A, B,** and **D** courtesy J. Lehnert, D.D.S., Minneapolis.)

oral and oropharyngeal squamous cell carcino-mas, Shear and co-workers (1976) reported sta-tistics concerning lymph node metastasis. These investigators illustrated that poorly differentiated tumors have a markedly higher metastasis rate than well-differentiated or moderately differen-tiated tumors. In addition, their study showed that lesions of the posterior third of the tongue or oropharynx have a higher tendency to metas-tasize than those that occurred on the anterior two thirds of the tongue. In turn this latter group showed a higher tendency to metastasize than tumors that occurred on the lips, oral floor, cheek mucosa, hard palate, and gingiva.

The bloodstream is not considered to be a fre-quent route of metastasis. Distant metastases have been observed mostly in the lungs, liver, and thoracic lymph nodes and are generally found in patients who have survived relatively long periods.

Microscopically the intraoral squamous cell carcinoma may vary in degree of malignancy from a low grade, with excellent differentiation,

to a very anaplastic high grade of malignancy, with poor or no differentiation.

The low-grade malignancy will demonstrate a high degree of normal maturation of the basal cells up through the stratum corneum. Project-ing fingers and nests of epithelium will be seen at the borders of the ulcer infiltrating the sub-epithelial connective tissue. The fingers of epi-thelial tissue will show malignant changes that may include increased numbers of mitotic fig-ures, hyperchromatism, prominent and/or mul-tiple nucleoli, an increased ratio of nucleus size to cell size, pleomorphism of the cells in size and shape, individual cell keratinization, keratin pearls deep to the epithelial surface, and a dimi-nution or loss of intercellular bridges (Fig. 6-7, *F*).

The very anaplastic high-grade malignancy, on the other hand, will show no maturation of the cells. Identifying the tissue of origin may be dif-ficult or even impossible. The malignant charac-teristics just mentioned in connection with the well-differentiated type will be more prominent and severe, except that intracellular keratinization and keratin pearls may not be present.

Varying degrees of malignancy may be present in the same tumor. Oral pathologists usually identify the degree of malignancy by characterizing the tumor as well-differentiated, moderately differentiated, poorly differentiated, or anaplastic.

DIFFERENTIAL DIAGNOSIS

Ulcerative squamous cell carcinoma is classified as a persistent ulcer; a discussion of its distinguishing features may be found under the differential diagnosis of persistent ulcers at the end of this chapter (p. 117).

MANAGEMENT

Early detection and early treatment of oral cancer are mandatory. Unfortunately much valuable time is lost before these two processes are accomplished. Bruun's study (1976) on 34 patients with oral cancer indicated the magnitude of the problem. This investigator reported that the average time delay between the onset of symptoms and when the patient came for professional examination was 4.9 months. The second statistic was even more alarming: the additional delay experienced between detection and correct diagnosis (treatment) was 5.6 months.

When a suspicious ulcer is discovered on the oral mucosa, it should be observed carefully to determine whether or not it is transient. If it does not show signs of regressing within 2 weeks, a biopsy should be done. Of course if the suspicion index is high during the initial visit, immediate arrangements should be made to do a biopsy of the lesion.

Preferably an excisional biopsy should be done, including a generous border of normal tissue. If the size of the lesion precludes excisional biopsy and the clinician is highly suspicious that the lesion is cancerous, the patient should be referred to a tumor board or a surgeon who is competent to undertake the complete management of the case. Also, if the clinician is highly suspicious of the lesion when it is first discovered, the period of observation should be eliminated and he should refer the patient without delay.

As a rule an incisional biopsy of a highly suspicious lesion should not be done until the patient has been prepared for resection. A frozen section should then be taken and examined to determine whether the lesion is malignant and the extent of the resection that should immediately follow the biopsy, depending on the proved nature of the lesion. This approach will help to eliminate a prolonged waiting period between the incisional biopsy and the resection.

The tumor board may decide that the particular lesion should be treated by surgical excision (with possibly a complete or partial neck dissection), by radiation, or by a combination of these procedures. The current status of radiotherapy in the treatment of oral cancer has been reviewed by Vermund and his co-workers (1974).

Cryosurgery has been utilized for the treatment of intraoral carcinoma and may in some instances be the method of choice for the patient whose poor physical health precludes surgery (Gage, 1971). More recently Gage (1976) reported that cryosurgery was an acceptable method of treatment of stage I or stage II cancers but was inadequate for stage III and stage IV cancers. Webster and Reid (1976) reported that their results were disappointing and detailed some of the problems resulting from cryotherapy for oral cancer. Sonkodi's study (1979) indicated that cryosurgery is especially applicable for treating benign and malignant lesions of the anterior third of the oral cavity where healing is good, complications are few, and inspection is fairly easy. Patterson (1979) reported the use of electrocoagulation (disk electrode) in the treatment of intraoral cancer. Of his 25 cases treated in this manner 11 survived more than 5 years, 8 died of other disease, and only 6 died of recurrent tumor.

Management of the posttreatment period is very important. Spouge (1973, p. 401) recommends the removal of any local irritation, with specific attention to the five "S's": smoking, spirits, spices, sepsis, and syphilis. A complete examination is necessary every 4 to 6 months to detect the recurrence of the tumor at the earliest possible date.

Close cooperation between the physician, dentist, and patient is necessary so that radiation caries will be minimized. The combination of meticulous oral hygiene, frequent dental examination, and self-administered daily application of topical fluoride has given gratifying results (Carl et al., 1972).

If extractions are necessary before radiation therapy is initiated, a generous alveolectomy should be completed in the extraction site so that a good mucosal coverage may be accomplished. This will help to reduce the incidence of osteoradionecrosis (osteomyelitis) after radiation therapy.

A statistical 5-year survival rate may be predicted for a certain carcinoma, and this average expectancy can be anticipated to be altered by specific therapeutic modes. The prognosis of an individual lesion of ulcerative squamous cell carcinoma, however, can be forecast only on the basis of the distinctive features of that particular tumor.

The assessment of a particular lesion has been referred to as "clinical staging" (Shafer et al., 1974, p. 111). The staging of an individual lesion is determined by such considerations as the following:

1. Size and extent of the primary lesion
2. Degree of infiltration by the primary lesion
3. Presence or absence of metastases to regional lymph nodes
4. Whether or not distant metastases are present
5. Whether contralateral or ipsilateral nodes are involved
6. Whether or not nodes are fixed

In addition to providing a better insight as to the prognosis of an individual lesion, clinical staging provides a systemized basis for selecting the most appropriate mode of treatment—whether surgery, radiotherapy, radium, or a combination of irradiation and surgery.

Furthermore, the anatomic site of the lesion modifies the prognosis (staging) markedly, as does the degree of histologic differentiation.* For instance, in regard to anatomic location, a lesion on the lower lip has the best prognosis whereas a lesion on the posterior third of the tongue has the poorest. Also, to illustrate the fact that the importance of the degree of differentiation must be modified on the basis of the lesion's other features, it can be pointed out that a poorly differentiated carcinoma that is restricted to a primary site has a better prognosis than does a well-differentiated lesion that has already metastasized to a lymph node. Langdon and co-workers (1977) reported on the study of 131 cases of intraoral cancer, corroborating that site and histodifferentiation are indeed important factors in prognosis. As a result of their study they suggested a new classification for oral cancer, that is, the STNMP system, in which "S" stands for site and "P" stands for histopathology.

SYPHILIS (CHANCRE AND GUMMA)

Syphilis is a venereal disease caused by the motile spirochete *Treponema pallidum;* it may

---

*Histologic classification of a lesion is not one of the features involved in clinical staging.

be congenital or acquired. The untreated acquired form has three easily recognizable stages:

1. The primary lesion is the *chancre,* which is usually solitary.
2. The secondary lesions are numerous *macules, papules, mucous patches,* and/or *condylomas.*
3. The tertiary (oral) lesions are *gummas* and *interstitial glossitis.*

The mucous patch is a grayish-white sloughing lesion and has been included in the list of rarities under sloughing, pseudomembranous, nonkeratotic white lesions in Chapter 5. Both the chancre and the gumma are ulcerated lesions, so they are included here; but because they are completely different lesions from the standpoint of pathogenic sequence and clinical appearance, they are described separately.

Chancre

Chancres are found on the genitalia in 90% of syphilis patients, but they may occur on the oral mucous membrane. They develop at the site of inoculation, where there is a defect in the surface continuity of the skin or mucosa. The *T. pallidum* organisms are transferred by direct contact with primary or secondary lesions of an infected individual. The chancres develop about 3 weeks after inoculation and persist for 3 weeks to 2 months.

FEATURES

Chancres on the genitalia are characteristically painless.

Oral lesions, on the other hand, almost invariably become painful soon after they ulcerate because of contamination by the oral fluids and flora. A cervical lymphadenitis is almost always present and is usually tender and painful because of the contamination.

The primary oral lesions occur most often on the lips, on the tip of the tongue, in the tonsillar region, or on the gingivae—commencing as small erythematous macules that become papules or small nodules and then ulcerate. Mature chancres measure from 0.5 to 2 cm in diameter and have narrow, copper-colored, slightly raised borders with a reddish-brown base (center) (Figs. 6-9 and 6-10). The lesions are ulcerated over nearly their entire surface with a base that is shiny and usually clear of necrotic material and debris. Occasionally chancres will retain white sloughy material (Fig. 5-47, *A*) and then will need to be differentiated from the other white pseudomembranous ulcers. Chancres occurring on the vermilion border are usually crusted.

Fig. 6-10. Chancre of the lower lip. (Courtesy R. Gorlin, D.D.S., Minneapolis.)

Fig. 6-9. Chancre. **A,** Two lesions on the dorsal surface of the tongue. **B,** Lesion at the junction of the hard and soft palates.

The chancres are very contagious. They are teeming with spirochetes, which may be detected by means of dark-field or phase microscopy—the usual methods for examining material from the lesions. These methods are not diagnostic for oral lesions, however, because of the probable contamination of the ulcers by nonpathogenic oral spirochetes; the *T. pallidum* can be positively identified if immobilized by syphilis antiserum.

The serologic reaction is usually negative until 1 or 2 weeks after the chancre appears if there has been no treatment.

Screening tests (e.g., Kahn, Wassermann, reactive plasma reagin) are used routinely; and, although not very specific, they are quite sensitive. Consequently, if one of these tests gives a positive result, another test specific for the diagnosis of syphilis should be performed—for example, the fluorescent treponemal antibody (FTA) test or the microhemagglutination antibody test (MHA), both of which are usually available from the state department of health.

Since the lesions are contaminated by the oral flora, the microscopic picture of a mature oral chancre is seldom specific enough to identify the chancre. Hence the microscopic diagnosis is usually "nonspecific" ulcer. Sometimes, however, the characteristic obliterative endarteritis and perivascular cuffing by lymphocytes are apparent deep in the tissue. Silver stain will also reveal the presence of numerous spirochetes in the inflamed areas of the biopsy specimen.

DIFFERENTIAL DIAGNOSIS

Because chancres may be present for a period of 3 weeks to 2 months, they must be classified as both short-term and persistent ulcers. The distinguishing features are discussed in the differential diagnosis section at the end of this chapter (p. 117).

MANAGEMENT

When systemic penicillin is initiated during the primary stage of the disease, over a period of several days it will successfully eliminate syphilis in the vast majority of cases.

The multiple secondary lesions of syphilis appear 5 to 6 weeks after the disappearance of the chancres and undergo spontaneous remission within a few weeks, but recurrences may be manifested periodically for months or several years.

Gumma

Although a variety of lesions may occur in different locations during the tertiary stage of untreated syphilis, gummas develop in 33% to 66% of such cases. They are the most common syphilitic lesion seen in the oral cavity (Meyer and Shklar, 1967) and appear to be the result of a type of sensitivity reaction since the severity of the lesion is vastly out of proportion to the few *Treponema* organisms present.

FEATURES

Intraoral gummas occur most often in the midline of either the palate or the tongue, starting as small, firm, painless, nodular masses and often growing to become several centimeters in diameter. Necrosis commences within the nodules and produces an ulceration of the surface epithelium. The lesions are sharply demarcated; and the necrotic tissue at the base of the ulcers may slough away, leaving a punched-out defect. The semifirm type of necrosis imparts a rubberlike consistency to the nodular ulcerative masses. On occasion the necrosis will be very destructive, causing perforation of the palate and the formation of a persistent oronasal fistula. The nodular ulcers heal after some months.

Microscopically the picture of a nonspecific ulcer with an extraordinary amount of necrosis is seen, and occasionally a few giant cells are present. The serology at this stage is usually reactive and often at a high titer.

DIFFERENTIAL DIAGNOSIS

Gummas may be easily confused with *tubercular lesions, sarcoidosis, granulomatous fungal (mycotic) infections, oral malignancies, necrotizing sialometaplasia,* and the *rare lethal midline granuloma.* The differential features will be discussed in the differential diagnosis section at the end of this chapter (p. 117).

MANAGEMENT

For the following two reasons, patients suffering from gummas should be managed by clinicians who have been specially trained in all aspects of syphilitic disease:

1. Intraoral gummas imply the presence of additional gummas in other locations, which will cause more serious complications.
2. Treatment must be tailored to minimize the possibility and intensity of the Jarisch-Herxheimer reaction.

ULCERS SECONDARY TO SYSTEMIC DISEASE

The frequency of ulcers occurring secondary to a particular systemic disease is not sufficiently high to warrant the assignment of separate categories to the individual ulcers. When all the ulcers resulting from such systemic diseases are considered as a group, however, their combined incidence is high enough to avoid their being included among the rarities.

Such ulcers most often occur in uncontrolled diabetes, uremia, and blood dyscrasias (e.g., pancytopenia, leukemia, cyclic neutropenia, sickle cell anemia).

With the exception of sickle cell anemia and uremia, the pathogenesis of ulcer formation is similar. The resistance of the host tissue and the leukocytic defense is so diminished that a small break in the integrity of the mucosa becomes superficially infected by the oral flora and an ulcer results. Although a diffuse gangrenous stomatitis may also occur in these diseases (Chapter 5), the discrete ulcers are emphasized in this chapter.

FEATURES

The ulcers are tender or painful, usually well demarcated, and shallow with a narrow erythematous halo; and they may contain some yellowish or gray necrotic material. They may vary in size from 0.5 to 2 or 3 cm in diameter. A painful regional cervical lymphadenitis is almost invariably present.

In sickle cell anemia the ulcers form in regions of ischemic infarcts caused by the plugging of small blood vessels by sickle cell thrombi occurring during the sickle cell crisis. Such ulcers are usually painless and frequently involve the marginal gingivae and interdental papillae (Fig. 6-11).

Ulcers occurring in patients with uremia may also involve the marginal gingivae (Fig. 6-11) or other regions of the oral mucosa. These ulcers are related to (1) the bacterial breakdown of urea (present in high concentrations in the saliva) to ammonia, (2) mouth breathing in acidosis, (3) dehydration, (4) bacterial or fungal infection.

It has been well recognized that oral candidiasis, usually of the pseudomembranous type, is a frequent complication of systemic diseases that decrease the resistance of the patient. However, Tyldesley and co-workers (1979) drew attention to superficial oral bacterial infections in renal transplant patients who were taking immunosuppressive drugs. These authors stress that these superficial bacterial infections look almost identical to pseudomembranous candidiasis and that only culturing the lesions revealed their true nature.

DIFFERENTIAL DIAGNOSIS

For the distinguishing features of these ulcers secondary to systemic disease, refer to the differential diagnosis section at the end of this chapter (pp. 116-117).

Fig. 6-11. Ulcers in systemic disease. **A,** Gingival ulcer in a patient with sickle cell anemia. **B,** Gingival ulcer in a patient with acute leukemia. **C** and **D,** Ragged sloughing gingival ulcers in a uremic patient. (**D** was taken 2 weeks after **C.** The uremia had been corrected and hydrogen peroxide mouthwashes instituted.) (**A** courtesy R. Dixon, D.D.S., Chicago. **B** courtesy G. MacDonald, D.D.S., Belleville, Ill.)

MANAGEMENT

In the management of oral ulcers secondary to a systemic disease, it is most important that the dental clinician recognize the possibility of a predisposing condition and realize that the condition is basic to the oral problem.

When the patient's history indicates that the suspected systemic disease has not been detected by his physician, it is especially important that the dentist seek medical consultation. The dentist and the physician together will be able to manage the problem as a team, for the oral condition is not likely to respond satisfactorily to local treatment alone. While the physician is treating the systemic disease, the dental clinician will initiate procedures to assure the establishment of the best possible oral hygiene. Toward this end, the use of hydrogen peroxide mouth rinses many times a day is recommended (Fig. 6-11). The hydrogen peroxide will debride the ulcerated tissues. In addition, the systemic administration of antibiotics (i.e., penicillin) will compensate for the patient's diminished defenses and help control the oral ulcers. It is critical at this juncture

to determine whether the pseudomembranous ulcerative lesions are infected with bacteria or *Candida albicans.*

TRAUMATIZED TUMORS (TYPES USUALLY NOT ULCERATED)

As described in Chapter 3, exophytic growths *originating in tissues separate from and beneath the surface epithelium* characteristically have smoothly contoured nonulcerated surfaces. Such lesions would include the following:

Benign and malignant mesenchymal tumors
Inflammatory hyperplasias
Metastatic tumors (situated deep to the surface epithelium)
Most types of minor salivary gland tumors
Odontogenic tumors

These entities are discussed in detail in Chapter 7 as exophytic lesions. The fact that some of them become ulcerated prompts their inclusion as a group in this chapter. The cause of the ulceration is usually obvious but should always be identified so the lesion will not be confused with a primarily ulcerative lesion.

Fig. 6-12. Ulcerated tumors. **A** and **B,** Chondrosarcoma. (**B** was taken 2 weeks after an incisional biopsy of the lesion in **A.**) **C,** Ameloblastoma with an unusual surface ulceration inflicted by an upper molar. (**A** courtesy R. Nolan, D.D.S., Waukegan, Ill.)

The ulceration is often the result of mechanical trauma from mastication with ill-fitting dentures. Fig. 6-12, *C,* illustrates a case in which a central ameloblastoma became ulcerated when an extruded upper third molar repeatedly traumatized the posterior mandibular swelling produced by the ameloblastoma. In our experience even malignant mesenchymal tumors almost always have a smooth surface until some traumatic episode causes a surface erosion or ulceration. Such a surface ulceration is frequently the result of an incisional biopsy. Fig. 6-12, *A* and *B,* showed a smooth-surfaced exophytic chondrosarcoma of the maxilla that became necrotic and ulcerated after an incisional biopsy.

In other instances masses of tumor cells will interfere with the blood supply of the surface epithelium to such an extent that the epithelium becomes necrotic and ulcerative. Then too, occasionally, a tumor mass will extrude from a recent extraction wound; and since the growth does not have an epithelial covering, it soon becomes necrotic and ulcerated because of the irritating nature of the oral environment.

It is important to recognize that these ulcerated lesions are primarily exophytic in nature; and their classification as such will facilitate their identity.

MINOR SALIVARY GLAND TUMORS

The majority of salivary gland tumors are firm exophytic lesions that seldom ulcerate except under conditions described in the preceding discussion. Some types of salivary gland tumors, however, *contain quantities of pooled liquid and are relatively soft and fluctuant.* Such lesions would include the following:

Low-grade mucoepidermoid tumor

Mucous adenocarcinoma

Papillary cyst adenoma

Papillary cystadenoma lymphomatosum (Warthin's tumor)

If the collection of fluid is near the surface, the pool will eventually rupture and cause the formation of an ulcerated surface. These tumors may ulcerate at a relatively early stage even before they have attained sufficient mass to produce an exophytic lesion. They therefore appear as shallow persistent ulcers that can easily be mistaken for a squamous cell carcinoma (Fig. 6-13). Their

Fig. 6-13. Ulcerated minor salivary gland tumors. **A,** Low-grade mucoepidermoid tumor. **B,** Pleomorphic adenoma 1 week after incisional biopsy. Prior to the biopsy, the surface was smooth and nonulcerated. (**A** courtesy D. Bonomo, D.D.S., Flossmoor, Ill.)

discussion is included in the differential diagnosis section at the end of this chapter (p. 117).

DIFFERENTIAL DIAGNOSIS

The following lesions need to be considered in the differential diagnosis with ulcerated minor salivary gland tumors of the posterior hard palate: squamous cell carcinoma, necrotizing sialometaplasia, midline lethal granuloma, chancre, gumma, leukemic ulcer, malignancy of the maxillary sinus, neurotrophic ulcer, traumatic ulcer, and major aphthous ulcer (Fig. 6-4, *D,* and 6-14).

RARITIES

A multitude of rare lesions may occur as oral ulcers. A partial list, arranged in alphabetical order, would include the following (Fig. 6-15):

Actinomycosis
Adenoid squamous cell carcinoma
Basal cell carcinoma
Botryomycosis
Cancrum oris
Foot-and-mouth disease
Fungal infections (blastomycosis, coccidioido-
mycosis, cryptococcosis, histoplasmosis, sporotrichosis)
Gonococcal stomatitis
Granulomatous disease of the newborn
Hand-foot-and-mouth disease
Herpes zoster
Keratoacanthoma
Lethal midline granuloma
Leukemia
Lymphoma
Median rhomboid glossitis—ulcerative variety
Metastatic tumor
Mycosis fungoides
Necrotizing sialometaplasia
Neurotrophic ulcer
Sarcoidosis
Sutton's disease
Tuberculosis
Warty dyskeratoma

DIFFERENTIAL DIAGNOSIS OF ORAL ULCERS

Since oral ulcers may be conveniently divided into two groups: short-term (those that usually disappear within 3 weeks) and persistent (those usually lasting longer than 3 weeks), it is equally advantageous to discuss the differential diagnosis of these two groups separately. The following important points, however, are common to both groups:

1. The complaint of *pain in an oral ulcer does not* permit a definite conclusion concerning the identity of the ulcer since the majority of oral ulcers, regardless of their cause, soon become painful from contamination by the oral liquids and flora.
2. Likewise, because of contamination by oral fluids, a *painful regional lymphadenitis almost always accompanies* oral ulcers.

Thus the presence or absence of pain in the ulcer or the associated enlarged nodes is not a conclusive diagnostic feature. Exceptions to this rule are squamous cell carcinoma and other peripheral malignancies—which are characteristically painless early in their course because most of the peripheral sensory nerve endings are destroyed or their surfaces are covered by tumor epithelium. These malignant lesions often do not become painful until they have attained a large size. When metastatic spread to regional lymph nodes has occurred, the enlarged nodes are likewise characteristically painless, as well as quite firm.

Again, it should be emphasized that these characteristics are not diagnostic because such enti-

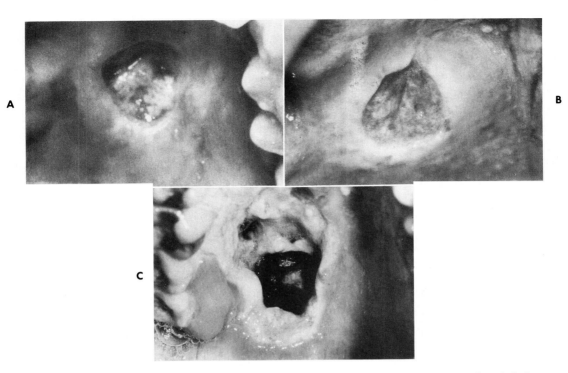

Fig. 6-14. A and **B,** Two cases of necrotizing sialometaplasia on the palate. **C,** Midline lethal granuloma. (**A** courtesy A. Abrams, D.D.S., Los Angeles. **B** courtesy C. Dunlap, D.D.S., and B. Barker, D.D.S., Kansas City, Mo. **C** courtesy S. Goldman, D.D.S., Maywood, Ill.)

Fig. 6-15. Rare oral ulcers. **A,** Metastatic carcinoma from squamous cell carcinoma of the esophagus in a 46-year-old man. **B,** Benign mucous membrane pemphigoid. **C,** Palatal lesion of psoriasis. (**A** courtesy E. Robinson, D.D.S., Toledo, Ohio. **B** courtesy P. D. Toto, D.D.S., Maywood, Ill. **C** courtesy D. Bonomo, D.D.S., Flossmoor, Ill.)

ties as benign lymph node hyperplasias and enlarged fibrosed nodes are usually firm and painless.

Short-term ulcers are shallow lesions; they are not raised above the mucosal surface. In contrast, persistent ulcers are frequently somewhat exophytic; in other words, they are situated over a slight nodular, dome-shaped, or plateaulike mass (Fig. 6-7).

Short-term ulcers

The more common short-term ulcers, ranked according to their approximate frequency of occurrence in the general population, are as follows:

Traumatic ulcer

Recurrent aphthous ulcer and intraoral recurrent herpes simplex lesion

Ulcer occurring as a result of odontogenic infection

Ulcer occurring with generalized mucositis or vesiculobullous disease

Ulcer secondary to systemic disease

With *ulcers secondary to systemic disease*, the clinician usually determines this circumstance from the patient's history if the disease has been previously detected. If the patient is not aware of the predisposing disease, however, a careful history should reveal information that will suggest the possibility of a specific disease or group of diseases. For instance, the patient may complain of fatigue, dizziness, and nausea in some of the anemias or of polydipsia and polyuria in diabetes. The patient may have a fever and/or a paleness of the mucosa, which should alert the clinician to the possibility of one of the anemias, leukemias, or pancytopenias. Appropriate laboratory procedures will be invaluable in helping to identify the specific disease. Since there is nothing specific in the appearance of these oral ulcers, the clinician must obtain a complete history and rely on it in every case.

The *single ulcer* heralding the arrival of any of the *generalized mucositides or vesiculobullous diseases* will appear perhaps a few days or weeks before the diffuse nature of the disease manifests itself. A discussion of the differential diagnosis of the oral mucositides is included in Chapter 12.

Ulcers resulting from odontogenic infection are easily diagnosed if the clinician remembers to include them in the differential diagnosis. Although there will not be a fluctuant painful swelling at this stage, a careful systematic approach will identify the involved tooth from which the infection is draining. The clinician should suspect any small ulcer on the alveolus or palate

of being associated with an odontogenic infection. He should then attempt to demonstrate the presence of a sinus with a gutta percha cone; and if successful, he should radiograph the area with the cone in place to determine whether the tract leads to the apex of a tooth. Sometimes digital pressure on the involved tooth or on the alveolus will cause a drop of pus to be expressed from the opening in the ulcer, which will aid in arriving at the correct diagnosis.

The *recurrent aphthous ulcers* and *intraoral recurrent herpes simplex lesions* can be differentiated, in most cases, by the criteria listed in Table 6-1. As a general rule a cluster of small punctate ulcers not over 0.5 cm in diameter and occurring on mucosa that is fixed to periosteum is intraoral recurrent herpetic lesions (hand-foot-and-mouth disease would show these small ulcers in the three locations). On the other hand, a yellowish ulcer measuring between 0.5 and 2 cm in diameter with a narrow erythematous halo and occurring on a loose mucosal surface is a recurrent aphthous ulcer. This conclusion is made if trauma cannot be implicated and the patient does not have an underlying systemic disease associated with a stomatitis or if an odontogenic infection cannot be identified.

Traumatic ulcers are easily recognized if the clinician can establish the cause of the physical injury. In some cases the origin or nature of the trauma is obscure and consequently the diagnosis will be quite difficult. Occasionally traumatic lesions, especially those occurring on the tongue, may persist for some weeks; the discussion of these is included in the differential diagnosis of persistent ulcer.

Persistent ulcers

The most common persistent ulcers, ranked according to their approximate incidence in the general population, include the following:

Traumatic ulcer

Ulcer from odontogenic infection

Squamous cell carcinoma

Chancre

Gumma

Ulcer secondary to systemic disease

Traumatized tumor that does not usually ulcerate

Low-grade mucoepidermoid tumor

Metastatic tumor

In addition, if it is situated on the palate, the recently recognized, necrotizing sialometaplasia must be considered. *Necrotizing sialometaplasia* is an uncommon, benign, inflammatory condition of the minor salivary glands usually of the posterior hard palate (Samit et al., 1979) (Fig. 6-14, *A* and *B*). The cause is unknown. Infarction has been suggested, although the underlying predisposing factors are not clear. The lesion is usually a nodule of slight elevation and the surface may be ulcerated or not. These lesions, although uncommon, mimic minor salivary gland tumors in appearance and location and so must always be considered as a possible diagnosis when a soft tissue mass is observed in the posterior hard palate.

Metastatic tumors to the oral soft tissues are quite uncommon and occur usually in the lower half of the oral cavity. In the absence of a primary tumor elsewhere or symptoms of such, secondary tumors would be assigned a very low rank on the differential list.

If a cystic area in a *low-grade mucoepidermoid tumor* ruptures, the resemblance to a squamous cell carcinoma may be striking since both tumors may appear as deep ulcers with firm, raised, rolled borders (Fig. 6-13, *A*). Although the squamous cell carcinoma is a much more common oral malignancy, if the questionable lesion is situated in the posterolateral region of the hard palate, it is most likely to be a minor salivary gland tumor, such as a mucoepidermoid tumor, since the hard palate is an unlikely site for a squamous cell carcinoma. If a mucocelelike lesion was reported to be in the same location a few days earlier, then mucoepidermoid tumor must be given a high priority in the differential diagnosis. If the lesion in question is painless, the possibility that it is a traumatic ulcer, a chancre, an ulcer secondary to systemic disease, or major aphthae will be eliminated. If an odontogenic infection cannot be found, the probability that it is an odontogenic ulcer is lessened. Intraoral gummas occur most often in the midline of the palate or tongue and are not as common as the mucoepidermoid tumor.

Tumors and *growths* originating in tissues separate from and beneath the stratified squamous epithelial surface do not characteristically ulcerate; but they may do so because of a mechanical injury or as the result of an incisional biopsy. If such ulcers are the result of an incisional biopsy, they should be easily identified from the history; on the other hand, if they have resulted from mechanical trauma, a careful intraoral examination will disclose the cause. The differential diagnosis of exophytic lesions is covered in detail in Chapter 7.

Ulcers secondary to systemic disease are usually short term, but they may persist if the predisposing systemic disease is not detected and controlled. They may be confused with any of the shallow persistent ulcers—traumatic ulcer, early squamous cell carcinoma, chancre, early mucoepidermoid tumor. Usually the systemic problem will become apparent through the history or clinical examination and prompt the proper diagnosis. These ulcers secondary to systemic disease are usually painful, in contrast to early squamous cell carcinoma or early mucoepidermoid tumors. A traumatic ulcer can generally be ruled out by establishing the absence of physical injury. Although a patient who appears to have an ulcer secondary to a systemic disease may have positive serologic findings, a chancre can be ruled out if a smear of the lesion does not provide spirochetes that are immobilized by syphilitic antiserum.

Gummas are not common oral lesions and occur mostly in the midline of the palate or the midline of the dorsum of the tongue. Similar-appearing pathoses rarely develop at these sites. A traumatic ulcer on a palatal torus or a midline lethal granuloma might be considered; but the ulcerated torus should be recognized, and the malignant midline granuloma is so rare as to be an unlikely diagnosis. Also the rubbery consistency of the gumma would eliminate both the torus and the midline lethal granuloma. The serologic findings will usually be strongly positive in the case of gummas, but only incidentally so in the case of a torus or the very rare midline lethal granuloma.

Chancres usually result in positive serologic findings, especially after the lesion has been present for 2 or more weeks. If the patient states that he was recently in contact with a person who may have had syphilis, this establishes a high priority for chancre in the differential diagnosis. If the ulcer is reddish brown, has a copper-colored halo, and is shallow and if there is no history of mechanical trauma, the diagnosis is strengthened; the impression may be additionally strengthened if the patient is under 40 years of age, because then the lesion is less likely to be an early squamous cell carcinoma or mucoepidermoid tumor. If spirochetes immobilized by syphilitic antiserum are found in the ulcer, the diagnosis of chancre is firmly established.

Squamous cell carcinoma is the most common malignant ulcer of the oral mucosa. The early lesion may be a painless shallow ulcer with a velvety red base. The healing traumatic ulcer may resemble this because its base may be filled

Fig. 6-16. Oral fissures. **A,** Fissured tongue. **B,** Very large epulis fissuratum. **C,** Angular cheilosis. **D,** Squamous cell carcinoma. **E,** Fissured type of median rhomboid glossitis.

with reddish-pink granulation tissue. The questionable lesion is most likely a squamous cell carcinoma, however, if the following are true: (1) the patient is over 40 years of age, is a male, and smokes or drinks heavily; (2) there is no evidence that the lesion is related to trauma or systemic disease; (3) the serologic findings are negative, and the presence of spirochetes cannot be demonstrated; (4) the lesion is not located on the posterolateral region of the hard palate.

Ulcers from odontogenic infection are discussed under the differential diagnosis of short-term ulcers.

Traumatic ulcers, especially on the tongue, may in some cases persist for several weeks after the traumatic factor has been eliminated. Such ulcers cannot be differentiated from malignancies on a clinical basis alone and often require complete excision before they resolve. This procedure

is recommended because it permits the microscopic examination of the ulcerated tissue.

Fissures

Fissures represent a separate clinical entity in contrast to the ulcers and should be grouped separately. The more common fissures occurring in the oral region, ranked according to approximate frequency, include the following (Fig. 6-16):

Fissured tongue
Epulis fissuratum
Angular cheilosis
Congenital cleft
Squamous cell carcinoma—fissured variety
Median rhomboid glossitis—fissured variety
Syphilitic rhagades

The differential diagnosis for these entities has not been included in this text.

SPECIFIC REFERENCES

Bruun, J. P.: Time lapse by diagnosis of oral cancer, Oral Surg. **42:**139-149, 1976.

Carl, W., Schaaf, N. G., and Chan, T. Y.: Oral care of patients irradiated for cancer of the head and neck, Cancer **30:**448-453, 1972.

Food and Drug Administration: FDA Drug Bulletin: Vidarabine approved for Herpes Simplex virus encephalitis, F.D.A. Drug Bull. **8:**36, December 1978-January 1979.

Gage, A. A.: Cryosurgery for oral and pharyngeal tumors, Panminerva Med. **13:**488-493, 1971.

Gage, A. A.: Five year survival following cryosurgery for oral cancer, Arch. Surg. **11:**990-994, 1976.

Langdon, J. D., Rapidis, A. D., Harvey, P. W., and Patel, M. F.: STNMP—A new classification for oral cancer, Br. J. Oral Surg. **15:**49-54, 1977.

Meyer, I., and Shklar, G.: The oral manifestations of acquired syphilis: a study of eighty-one cases, Oral Surg. **23:**45-57, 1967.

Patterson, W. B.: Treatment of intraoral cancer by electrocoagulation, Cancer **43**(3):821-824, 1979.

Rowe, N. H., Brooks, S. L., Young, S. K., et al.: A clinical trial of topically applied 3 percent vidarabine against recurrent herpes labialis, Oral Surg. **47:**142-147, 1979.

Samit, A. M., Mashberg, A., and Greene, G. W.: Necrotizing sialometaplasia, J. Oral Surg. **37:**353-356, 1979.

Shafer, W. G., Hine, M. K., and Levy, B. M.: A textbook of oral pathology, ed. 3, Philadelphia, 1974, W. B. Saunders Co.

Shear, M., Hawkins, D. M., and Farr, H. W.: The prediction of lymph node metastasis from oral squamous cell carcinoma, Cancer **37:**(4):1901-1907, 1976.

Shillitoe, E. J., and Silvermann, S.: Oral cancer and herpes simplex virus—A review, Oral Surg. **48:**216-223, 1979.

Sönkodi, I.: Cryosurgery in stomato-oncology, Int. J. Oral Surg. **8:**95-101, 1979.

Spouge, J. D.: Oral pathology, St. Louis, 1973, The C. V. Mosby Co.

Stanley, H. R.: Management of patients with persistent recurrent aphthous stomatitis and Sutton's disease, Oral Surg. **35:**174-179, 1973.

Tyldesley, W. R., Rotter, E., and Sells, R. A.: Oral lesions in renal transplant patients, J. Oral Pathol. **8:**53-59, 1979.

Vermund, H., Rappaport, I., and Nethery, W. J.: Role of radiotherapy in the treatment of oral cancer, J. Oral Surg. **32:**690-695, 1974.

Weathers, D. R., and Griffin, J. W.: Intraoral ulcerations of recurrent herpes simplex and recurrent aphthae: two distinct clinical entities, J. Am. Dent. Assoc. **81:**81-87, 1970.

Weaver, A., Fleming, S. A., and Smith, D. B.: Mouthwash and oral cancer: carcinogenic or coincidence? J. Oral Surg. **37:**250-253, 1979.

Webster, M. H. C., and Reid, W. H.: Problems following cryotherapy for oral cancer, Br. J. Oral Surg. **14:**72-75, 1976.

GENERAL REFERENCES

Ah Moo, E. W.: Lethal midline granuloma of the face, Oral Surg. **23:**578-585, 1967.

Alexander, W. N.: Venereal disease and the dentist, J. Acad. Gen. Dent. **23**(2):14-18, 1975.

Ballard, B. R., Suess, G. R., Pickern, J. W., et al.: Squamous cell carcinoma of the floor of the mouth, Oral Surg. **45:**568-579, 1978.

Barton, R. T.: Monoblock resection for carcinoma of the floor of the mouth, Laryngoscope **79:**1307-1311, 1969.

Bays, R. A., Hamerlinck, F., and Cormane, R. H.: Immunoglobulin-bearing lymphocytes and polymorphonuclear leukocytes in recurrent aphthous ulcers in man, Arch. Oral. Biol. **22:**147-153, 1977.

Birkholz, H., and Riegler, H. C.: Tuberculosis of the tongue, J. Am. Dent. Assoc. **98:**60-61, 1979.

Bruni, A., and Mahrt, D. H.: Carcinoma of the upper and lower lips: treatment with hyperbaric oxygenation, cobalt teletherapy and surgical reconstruction: report of case, J. Oral Surg. **30:**678-683, 1972.

Cawson, R. R.: Oral ulceration—clinical aspects, Oral Surg. **33:**912-921, 1972.

Challacombe, S. J., Barkhan, P., and Lehner, T.: Haematological features and differentiation of recurrent oral ulceration, Br. J. Oral Surg. **15:**37-48, 1977.

Christen, A. G.: The clinical effects of tobacco on oral tissue, J. Am. Dent. Assoc. **81:**1378-1382, 1970.

Dunlap, C. L., and Barker, B. F.: Necrotizing sialometaplasia, Oral Surg. **37:**722-727, 1974.

Dunley, R. E., and Jacoway, J. R.: Necrotizing sialometaplasia, Oral Surg. **47:**169-172, 1979.

Durrani, K. M.: Surgical repair of defects from noma (cancrum oris), Plast. Reconstr. Surg. **52:**629-634, 1973.

Eisenberg, E.: Intraoral isolated herpes zoster, Oral Surg. **45:**214-219, 1978.

Ferguson, M. M., Hart, D. M., Lindsay, R., and Stephen, K. W.: Progesterone therapy for menstrually related aphthae, Int. J. Oral Surg. **7:**463-470, 1978.

Freedman, G. L., and Hooley, J. R.: Median rhomboid glossitis, Oral Surg. **24:**621-622, 1967.

Forney, S. K., Foley, J. M., Sugg, W. E., and Oatis, G. W.: Necrotizing sialometaplasia of the mandible, Oral Surg. **43:**720-726, 1977.

Giles, H. V.: Local histoplasmosis: buccolingual form, Oral Surg. **25:**167-170, 1968.

Gormley, M. B., Marshall, J., Jarrett, W., and Bromberg, B.: Thermal trauma—a review of 22 electrical burns of the lip, J. Oral Surg. **30:**531-533, 1972.

Greer, J. L., Crine, J. D., and Tilson, H. B.: Malignant lymphomas of the oral soft tissues, J. Oral Surg. **36:**971-974, 1978.

Harris, B. C., Taylor, C. G., and Wade, W. W.: Miliary tuberculosis with oral manifestations: report of case, J. Oral Surg. **31:**305-307, 1973.

Horwitz, S.: Photochemical inactivation of herpes simplex: a practical dental service, Dent. Survey, pp. 30-31, April 1973.

Jamsky, R. J.: Gonococcal tonsilitis: report of a case, Oral Surg. **44:**197-200, 1977.

Jesse, R. H., Barkley, H. T., Lindberg, R. D., and Fletcher, G. H.: Cancer of the oral cavity, Am. J. Surg. **120:**505-508, 1970.

Ju, D. M. C.: On the etiology of cancer of the lower lip, Plast. Reconstr. Surg. **52:**151-154, 1973.

Kohn, M. W., and Eversole, L. R.: Keratoacanthoma of the lower lip: report of cases, J. Oral Surg. **30:**522-526, 1972.

Krashen, A. S.: Cryotherapy of herpes of the mouth, J. Am. Dent. Assoc. **81:**1163-1165, 1970.

Krolls, S. O., and Hicks, J. L.: Mixed tumors of the lower lip, Oral Surg. **35:**212-217, 1973.

Liroff, K. P., and Zeff, S.: Basal cell carcinoma of the palatal mucosa, J. Oral Surg. **30:**730-733, 1972.

Lynch, D. P., Crago, C. A., and Martinez, M. G.: Necrotizing sialometaplasia, Oral Surg. **47:**63-69, 1979.

Malaowalla, A. M., Silverman, S., and Bilimoria, K. F.: Oral cancer in 57,518 industrial workers of Gujarat, India, Cancer **371:**1882-1886, 1976.

Merchant, H. W., Gangarosa, L. P., Glassman, A. B., and Sobel, R. E.: Betamethasone-17-benzoate in the treatment of recurrent aphthous ulcers, Oral Surg. **45:**870-875, 1978.

Merchant, H. W., and Schuster, G. S.: Oral gonococcal infection, J. Am. Dent. Assoc. **95:**807-809, 1977.

Miller, A. S., and Pullon, P. A.: Mobile teeth and ulcerated soft tissue lesions, Dent. Survey **55**(4):71, 1979.

Miller, M. F., Garfunkel, A. A., Ram, C., and Ship, I. I.: Inheritance patterns in recurrent aphthous ulcers: twin and predigree data, Oral Surg. **43**:886-891, 1977.

Monoteleone, L.: Periadenitis mucosa necrotica recurrens, Oral Surg. **23**:586-591, 1967.

Najjar, T. A., Wilchins, S., Levy, M., and Hrycak, P.: Cryosurgical and thermal monitoring system for management of malignancy, Oral Surg. **47**:114-119, 1979.

Nakissa, N., Homback, N. B., Shidnia, H., and Sayoc, E. S.: Carcinoma of the floor of the mouth, Cancer **42**:2914-2919, 1978.

Nelson, J. F., and Ship, I. I.: Intraoral carcinoma: predisposing factors and their frequency of incidence as related to age at onset, J. Am. Dent. Assoc. **82**:564-568, 1971.

Nichols, R. T.: Bilateral radical neck dissection, Am. J. Surg. **117**:278-281, 1969.

Peters, R. A., Beltaos, E., Greelaw, R. H., and Shloesser, L. L.: Intraoral extranodal Hodgkin's disease, J. Oral Surg. **35**: 311-312, 1977.

Pindborg, J. J., Daftary, D. K., and Mehta, F. S.: A follow-up study of sixty-one oral dysplastic precancerous lesions in Indian villagers, Oral Surg. **43**:383-390, 1977.

Prabhu, S. R., Daftary, D. K., and Dholokia, H. M.: Tuberculous ulcer of the tongue. Report of case, J. Oral Surg. **36**: 384-386, 1978.

Pullon, P. A., and Miller A. S.: An ulcerated lesion of the tongue, Dent. Survey **55**(3):66, 1979.

Ratzer, E. R., Schweitzer, R. J., and Frazell, E. C.: Epidermoid carcinoma of the palate, Am. J. Surg. **119**:294-297, 1970.

Rauch, D. M., and Friedman, E.: Systemic tuberculosis initially seen as an oral ulceration: report of case, J. Oral Surg. **36**:387-389, 1978.

Ritchie, G. M., and Fletcher, A. M.: Angular inflammation, Oral Surg. **36**:358-366, 1973.

Robinson, E. R., and Stuteville, O. H.: Metastatic tumors to the tongue: review of the literature and report of a case, Oral Surg. **15**:980-985, 1962.

Rossi, E. P., and Hirsch, S. A.: A survey of 4,793 oral lesions with emphasis on neoplasia and premalignancy, J. Am. Dent. Assoc. **94**:883-886, 1977.

Russell, T. E., III: Toluidine blue—its role in oral cancer detection, J. Acad. Gen. Dent. **27**:22, March-April 1974.

Schmitt, C. K., and Folsom, T. C.: Histologic evaluation of degenerative changes of the lower lip, J. Oral Surg. **26**:51-56, 1968.

Schuler, S., McDonald, J. S., Strull, N. J., and Alpert, B.: Soft-tissue reticulum-cell sarcoma of the oral cavity, Oral Surg. **45**:894-901, 1978.

Sela, M. N., and Pisanti, S.: Early diagnosis and treatment of patients with leukemia. A dental problem, J. Oral Med. **32**: 46-50, 1977.

Sheridan, P. J.: Intraoral lesions of adults associated with herpes simplex virus, Oral Surg. **32**:390-397, 1971.

Ship, I. I.: Socioeconomic status and recurrent aphthous ulcers, J. Am. Dent. Assoc. **73**:120-123, 1966.

Ship, I. I.: Epidemiologic aspects of recurrent aphthous ulcerations, Oral Surg. **33**:400-406, 1972.

Shklar, G.: Lichen planus as an oral ulcerative disease, Oral Surg. **33**:376-388, 1972.

Sibulkin, D., and Cohen, H. J.: Oral mucosal erosions, Oral Surg. **34**:202-204, 1973.

Smith, E. B.: Management of herpes simplex infections of the skin, J. Am. M. A. **235**:1731-1733, 1976.

Spiro, R. H., and Frazell, E. L.: Surgical treatment of recurrent or multifocal mouth cancer. Evaluation of twenty-seven patients treated by a second "commando" operation, Am. J. Surg. **122**:50-52, 1971.

Stanley, H. R.: Aphthous lesions, Oral Surg. **33**:407-416, 1972.

Suckiel, J. M., Davis, H., Patakas, B. M., and Kaminski, R. M.: Early and late manifestations of necrotizing sialometaplasia, J. Oral Surg. **36**:902-905, 1978.

Svirskij, J. A., Freeman, P. D., and Lumerman, H.: Solitary intraoral keratoacanthoma, Oral Surg. **43**:116-122, 1977.

Terezhalmy, G. T., Bottomly, E. K., and Pelleu, G. B.: The use of water soluble bioflavonoid-ascorbic acid complex in the treatment of recurrent herpes labialis, Oral Surg. **45**:56-62, 1978.

Tiecke, R. W., Baron, H. J., and Casey, D. E.: Localized oral histoplasmosis, Oral Surg. **16**:441-447, 1963.

Tomich, C. E., and Hutton, C. E.: Adenoid squamous cell carcinoma of the lip. Report of cases, J. Oral Surg. **30**:592-598, 1972.

Turner, H., and Snitzer, J.: Carcinoma of the tongue in a child, Oral Surg. **37**:663-667, 1974.

Weitzner, S.: Adenoid squamous-cell carcinoma of vermilion mucosa of lower lip, Oral Surg. **37**:589-593, 1974.

Wesson, C. M.: Oral ulceration as the first symptom of diabetes, Oral Surg. **25**:686-690, 1968.

Whitaker, L. A., Lehr, H. B., and Askouitz, S. I.: Cancer of the tongue, Plast. Reconstr. Surg. **30**:363-370, 1972.

Wolf, J. E., and Ebel, L. K.: Chronic granulomatous disease: report of case and review of the literature, J. Am. Dent. Assoc. **96**:292-295, 1978.

Young, L. L., Dolan, T. C., and Sheridan, P. J.: Oral manifestations of histoplasmosis, Oral Surg. **33**:191-205, 1972.

Zagarelli, D. J., Tsukada, Y., Pickren, J. W., and Greene, G. W.: Metastatic tumor to the tongue, Oral Surg. **35**:202-211, 1973.

7

Peripheral oral exophytic lesions

Norman K. Wood
Paul W. Goaz

Peripheral exophytic structures and lesions of the oral cavity include the following:

Exophytic anatomic structures
Accessory tonsillar tissue
Buccal fat pads
Circumvalate papillae
Foliate papillae
Genial tubercles
Lingual tonsillar tissue
Palatal rugae
Palatine tonsils
Papilla palatinae
Stensen's papillae
Sublingual caruncles
Tongue
Uvula

Exophytic lesions
Tori and exostoses
Inflammatory hyperplasias
    Fibroma
    Pyogenic granuloma
    Hormonal tumor
    Epulis fissuratum
    Parulis
    Inflammatory papillary hyperplasia
    Peripheral giant cell granuloma
    Pulp polyp
    Epulis granulomatosum
    Myxofibroma
    Peripheral fibroma with calcification
Mucocele and ranula
Hemangioma, lymphangioma, and varicosity
Central exophytic lesions
Papilloma and verruca vulgaris
Exophytic squamous cell carcinoma
Verrucous carcinoma
Minor salivary gland tumors
Peripheral benign mesenchymal tumors
Nevus and melanoma
Peripheral metastatic tumors
Peripheral malignant mesenchymal tumors
Rarities
    Solitary lesions
        Actinomycosis

Ameloblastoma (peripheral)
Antral neoplasms
Blastomycosis
Bohn's nodule (Epstein's pearl)
Chondroma of soft tissue
Choristoma
Condyloma acuminatum
Condyloma lata
Congenital epulis of the newborn
Early chancre
Early gumma
Eruption cyst
Extraosseous odontogenic tumor
Focal hyperplasia of the minor salivary glands
Giant cell fibroma
Gingival cyst
Granular cell myoblastoma
Granulomatous fungal disease
Hamartoma
Histiocytosis X
Juvenile nasopharyngeal angiofibroma
Juvenile xanthogranuloma
Keratoacanthoma
Lead poisoning
Lethal midline granuloma
Leukemic enlargement
Lingual thyroid gland
Lymphoma
Median nodule of the upper lip
Median rhomboid glossitis (nodular variety)
Molluscum contagiosum
Myxoma of soft tissue or oral focal mucinosis
Necrotizing sialometaplasia
Neuroectodermal tumor of infancy
Nodular leukoplakia
Plasmacytoma of soft tissue
Pseudosarcomatous fasciitis
Sarcoidosis
Squamous acanthoma
Sialolith
Sturge-Weber syndrome
Teratoma
Tuberculosis
Verruciform xanthoma
Multiple lesions
    Acanthosis nigricans

Acrokeratosis verruciformis of Hope
Amyloidosis
Bohn's nodules
Chronic granulomatous disease
Crohn's disease
Condyloma acuminata
Condyloma lata
Cowden's disease
Cysticercosis
Darier's disease
Eruption cysts
Focal dermal hypoplasia (Goltz's syndrome)
Focal epithelial hyperplasia
Gardner's syndrome
Giant cell fibromas
Hereditary telangiectasia
Histiocytosis X
Idiopathic gingival fibromatosis
Kaposi's sarcoma
Lichenoides chronica
Lymphangiomas of neonates
Lymphomas
Lymphomatoid papulosis
Lymphoproliferating disease of the palate
Molluscum contagiosum
Multiple exostoses
Multiple fibroepithelial hyperplasias
Multiple gingival cysts
Multiple hamartoma neoplasia syndrome
Multiple lipomas
Multiple melanomas
Multiple mucoceles
Multiple myeloma
Multiple papillomas
Multiple expansile brown giant cell lesions (hyperparathyroidism)
Multiple peripheral metastatic carcinomas
Multiple verrucae
Noonan's syndrome
Orodigitofacial syndrome (multiple hamartomas of the tongue)
Oral florid papillomatosis
Phenytoin hyperplasia
Pyostomatitis vegetans
Sarcoidosis
Syndrome of multiple mucosal neuromas, pheochromocytoma, and carcinoma of the thyroid
Syphilitic papules
Thrombocytopenic purpura
Urticaria pigmentosa
von Recklinghausen's disease
Xanthoma disseminatum

The term "exophytic lesion" in the context of the following discussion means *any pathologic growth that projects above the normal contours of the oral surface.*

Hypertrophy, hyperplasia, neoplasia, and the pooling of fluid are four mechanisms by which exophytic lesions may be produced. "Hypertrophy" refers to an enlargement caused by an increase in the size but not in the number of cells. "Hyperplasia" is generally defined as an enlargement caused by an increase in the number of normal cells. "Neoplasia" is defined as the formation of a *neoplasm,* which is identical with a *tumor* and may be either benign or malignant.

In our opinion a sharp distinction as to whether a particular exophytic lesion is the result of hypertrophy or hyperplasia or a combination of these two processes cannot often be made. Hence this aspect will not be stressed in the discussion to follow and does not usually contribute to the clinical recognition of a lesion.

The terms that are used to describe the shapes of exophytic lesions are often confusing. The descriptive terms used in this discussion to identify the specific shapes are as follows: *papillomatous, verrucous, papule, nodule* (a papule more than 0.5 cm in diameter), *dome shaped, polypoid,* and *bosselated* (Fig. 7-1). As a general rule exophytic lesions with a papillomatous or verrucous shape originate in the surface epithelium (e.g., verrucae vulgari, papillomas, verrucous carcinomas, keratoacanthomas) whereas those with a smoothly contoured shape originate in the deeper tissues and are beneath and separate from the stratified squamous epithelium (e.g., tori, fibromas, lipomas, early malignant mesenchymal tumors).*

The surfaces of the lesions may become eroded (red), keratinized (white), or ulcerated, depending on the reaction of the epithelial surface to varying degrees of trauma. Mild trauma may cause the epithelial surface to become either eroded or keratinized, whereas severe trauma may cause the surface to become ulcerated.

When an exophytic lesion is found on an area of oral mucosa that is overlying bone, it must be identified as originating in either the soft tissues or the bone. Such a distinction will be extremely important in developing the differential diagnosis. A careful visual, digital, and radiographic examination will usually indicate whether the origin is in soft tissue or bone.

If the lesion and accompanying soft tissues can be moved over the underlying bone and a radiograph fails to show bony changes, the lesion probably originated in the soft tissue. The examiner must realize, however, that the mucosa over the anterior hard palate and alveolar gingivae cannot normally be moved independently of the underlying bone. Thus in these locations tissue mobility is of no help as far as identifying whether the lesion originated in tissue or in bone. The examiner may have difficulty in other locations identifying the tissue of origin when there are changes in both tissues. This circumstance

---

*This concept is discussed in detail in Chapter 3.

Fig. 7-1. Various shapes of exophytic lesions. **A,** Nodular. (A papular mass is a nodule measuring less than 0.5 cm.) **B,** Dome shaped. **C,** Polypoid. **D,** Papillomatous. **E,** Verrucous. **F,** Bosselated.

Fig. 7-2. Buccal fat pads.

prompts the inclusion of a large number of possibilities in the differential diagnosis as well as multiple entities in the working diagnosis.

Lesions originating centrally (in bone) may become exophytic lesions, but these will not be detailed in this chapter since they are discussed in Part III of the text.

Exophytic anatomic structures

Although there is little doubt that they will be confused with pathologic lesions, the following exophytic anatomic oral structures are listed to complete the series:

Accessory tonsillar tissue
Buccal fat pads (Fig. 7-2)
Circumvalate papillae
Foliate papillae
Genial tubercles
Lingual tonsillar tissue
Palatal rugae
Palatine tonsils
Papilla palatinae
Stensen's papillae

Sublingual caruncles
Tongue
Uvula

Occasionally some of these structures attain such a size that they are not recognized by the student but are mistaken for pathoses. The anatomic location of the structures, however, will usually enable the experienced clinician to immediately recognize them. Nevertheless, since some normal structures are occasionally mistaken for exophytic lesions, the location and appearance of the following will be described: foliate papillae, genial tubercles, lingual tonsillar tissue, and accessory tonsillar tissue.

The *foliate papillae* are located on the posterolateral borders of the tongue. They vary greatly in size, being absent in some patients and quite prominent in others. Frequently they are nodular with deep vertical fissures appearing to divide them into several closely associated exophytic projections (Fig. 7-3). They are normally pink in color unless traumatized, and they have about the same consistency as the rest of the tongue. The great variation in size and occasionally appearance is frequently troublesome for the inexperienced clinician. Furthermore, lingual tonsillar tissue is also frequently seen in the area of the foliate papillae and may be confused with the foliate papillae as well as with other pathoses.

The *genial tubercles* may become exophytic in patients who have experienced extreme resorption of their edentulous mandibular ridges. In some cases the genial tubercles project into the anterior floor of the mouth under the mucosa just posterior to the lingual surface of the mandible; in others they project superiorly above the level

of the anterior portion of the ridge. If an exophytic mass is bony hard to palpation and is attached to the lingual surface of the mandible in the midline, it should be recognized as the genial tubercles; and if the genial tubercles interfere with the construction of dentures, they should be surgically reduced.

Lingual tonsillar tissue forms part of Waldeyer's ring, which is composed of the pharyngeal tonsil (adenoids), the palatine tonsil, and the lingual tonsil. These larger aggregates of lymphatic tissue are linked together by isolated tonsillar nodules, and thus they encircle the entrance to the oropharynx. The lingual tonsillar tissue is on the pharyngeal surface of the tongue and frequently extends over the posterolateral borders into, or just posterior to, the location of the foliate papillae (Fig. 7-4, *A*).

The portion of the lingual tonsil that is apparent in the area of the foliate papillae may vary greatly in size. It may be just a small deposit of tonsillar tissue appearing as a single discrete pink papule or nodule with a smooth yellowish-pink glossy surface; or it may be larger accumulations of tonsillar tissue giving the appearance of an aggregation of papules and thus recognizable as a nodular or dome-shaped mass with a coarse, pebbly (papular) surface (Fig. 7-4). In some cases the grooves between the individual papules will be quite deep and will impart a papillomatous appearance to the structure (Fig. 7-4). Lingual tonsillar tissue is usually moderately firm to palpation.

Accessory tonsillar tissue may occur in various locations in the oral cavity (e.g., floor of the mouth, ventral surface of the tongue, soft palate, and most often posterior pharyngeal wall) (Fig. 7-5). Some patients seem to have a relative abundance of lymphoid tissue; and these are the people in whom the small usually smooth-surfaced papules and nodules are most commonly found, in various sites throughout the oral cavity. The glossy yellowish-pink sheen will often permit the ready identification of tonsillar tissue.

Recent studies indicate a higher prevalence of accessory oral tonsil tissue than was previously believed (Adkins, 1973; Knapp, 1970a). Knapp examined 503 randomly selected young men for the presence of oral tonsil tissue. He reported that 21% of the patients had tonsil aggregates on the soft palate, 12% had tonsil aggregates on the floor of the mouth, and 5% had them on the ventral surface of the tongue. These nodules varied from 1 to 3 mm in size and their number in individual patients ranged from 1 to 25.

Fig. 7-3. Foliate papillae.

Fig. 7-4. Lingual tonsillar tissue. **A,** Classic position for the tonsil (arrow). **B,** Unusually large tonsil located more anterior than usual.

Fig. 7-5. Accessory tonsillar tissue. **A,** Several nodules on the posterior pharyngeal wall.
Continued.

Fig. 7-5, cont'd. B, Small deposit of tonsillar tissue on the ventral surface of the tongue (arrow).

Concerning pathosis of oral tonsil tissue Adkins described in some detail the changes observed in lymphoid hyperplasia. In a more comprehensive study Knapp (1970b) described three types of pathosis most commonly found in these aggregates: (1) hyperplasia—pink, (2) pseudocyst—yellow (lymphoepithelial cyst), and (3) hyperemia—red. Knapp stressed the importance of including these entities in the differential diagnosis of exophytic, yellow, and red lesions.

• • •

Although each of the exophytic anatomic structures can undergo pathologic change, a discussion of every possibility is beyond the scope of this text.

Exophytic lesions

TORI AND EXOSTOSES

Tori and exostoses are the most common oral exophytic lesions and are discussed in detail in Chapters 26 and 27 as radiopacities of the jaws. They are readily recognizable, peripheral, benign, slow-growing bony protuberances of the jaws. They usually appear symmetrically as nodular or bosselated lesions having smooth contours and covered with normal mucosa. They are bony hard to palpation and are attached by a broad, bony base to the underlying jaw. Growth occurs mainly during the first 30 years of life.

Palatal tori are located on the hard palate usually in the midline (Fig. 7-6). They are seen in approximately 42% of females and 25% of males (King and Moore, 1976). Mandibular tori are found in about 12% of adults and are located on the lingual aspect of the mandible above the mylohyoid ridge, most often bilaterally in the premolar region (Fig. 7-6). No differences in occurrence between the sexes have been noted. King and Moore (1976) reported the very interesting findings that patients from London have a markedly lower incidence and smaller-sized tori than do patients in the United States.

Similar bony protuberances that occur in other locations around the jawbones are termed "exostoses" (Fig. 7-6).

DIFFERENTIAL DIAGNOSIS

Tori and exostoses are usually so readily identifiable that it does not seem necessary to discuss their distinguishing features. Ulcerated mucosa over these bony protuberances may pose a diagnostic problem. In almost all cases, however, the ulcers are traumatic in origin and the history and clinical examination will disclose the cause.

Despite the foregoing, occasionally the following lesions may closely resemble a torus or exostosis both clinically and radiologically: (1) a mature cementifying or ossifying fibroma that has caused a bulge on the cortical palate (Fig. 27-2), (2) an ossified subperiosteal hematoma, (3) a nonresolved bony callus, (4) an osteoma, and (5) an early osteosarcoma and early chondrosarcoma.

MANAGEMENT

Removal is usually considered to be unnecessary unless prompted by psychologic, prosthetic, phonetic, or traumatic considerations.

Fig. 7-6. A, Palatal tori and lingual exostoses. **B,** Mandibular tori. **C,** Buccal exostoses.

INFLAMMATORY HYPERPLASIAS

Inflammatory hyperplasias include a relatively large group of lesions that have an identical basic pathogenesis: chronic trauma. This spectrum of lesions is usually divided into separate entities according to the specific traumatic agent involved. Following is a list of these lesions, in the approximate descending order of frequency of occurrence:

Fibroma (inflammatory fibrous hyperplasia)
Pyogenic granuloma
Hormonal tumor
Epulis fissuratum
Parulis
Inflammatory papillary hyperplasia (palatal papillomatosis)
Peripheral giant cell granuloma
Pulp polyp (chronic hyperplastic pulpitis)
Epulis granulomatosum
Myxofibroma
Peripheral fibroma (with calcification)

FEATURES

The initiating chronic injury, regardless of type, produces an inflammation, which in turn stimulates the formation of granulation tissue that consists of proliferating endothelial cells, a very rich patent capillary bed, chronic inflammatory cells, and a few fibroblasts (Fig. 7-7). The granulation tissue (granuloma) soon becomes covered with stratified squamous epithelium.

Clinically at this stage the lesion will be asymptomatic and smoothly contoured or lobulated with a very red appearance because of the rich vascularity and transparency of the nonkeratinized epithelial covering. It will be moderately soft and spongy and will blanch on careful digital pressure. Most lesions are sessile (broad based).

If the recurring insult is eliminated at this stage, the lesion will shrink markedly as the inflammation subsides and the vascularity is reduced. If the insult is permitted to continue, however, the granulomatous lesion will continue to increase in size although some fibrosis may occur in the regions farthest removed from the areas being irritated. These fibrotic areas will appear as pale pink patches on the reddish surface of the lesion. In time the complete lesion may fibrose, resulting in a pale pinkish smooth or lobulated firm lesion (a fibroma).

If the instigating factor is eliminated at the mixed stage, the decrease in size of the lesion will be directly proportional to the amount of inflammation present—in other words, if the lesion is composed mostly of fibrous tissue, there will not be much shrinkage; but if there is considerable granulation tissue and inflammation present, there will be marked regression in size. Usually

Fig. 7-7. Inflammatory hyperplasia. **A,** This lesion is composed of mostly granulation tissue and inflammatory components. **B,** Photomicrograph of granulation tissue showing the inflammatory components. **C,** This inflammatory hyperplastic lesion has some fibrosed regions that appear clinically as pale patches in the red lesion. (**A** courtesy P. D. Toto, D.D.S., Maywood, Ill.)

these lesions show a fairly consistent pattern of injury, healing, and reinjury.

DIFFERENTIAL DIAGNOSIS

The inflammatory hyperplasias are not usually confused with other lesions because their locations are suggestive of the cause and the causative traumatic factors are easily identified.

Certain *benign* and *malignant tumors* may mimic these lesions, however, and this aspect will be discussed when the specific lesions are described.

MANAGEMENT

Management of the inflammatory hyperplastic lesions is prescribed on the basis of the clinical appearance of the specific lesion, which in turn is governed by the microstructure.

Basically, if the lesion is red and soft and the irritating cause can be eliminated, the clinician may expect to observe a significant reduction in size, perhaps even to the point of eliminating the need for excision. If excision is required, however, the procedure will be much easier and less blood will be lost if the lesion is permitted to regress (sclerose) before it is removed.

If, on the other hand, the lesion is pale pink and quite firm, almost no reduction can be expected because its bulk is probably fibrous tissue. Excision of such a lesion with microscopic examination of the specimen is the procedure indicated.

Fibroma (inflammatory fibrous hyperplasia)

The great majority of fibromas of the oral mucosa are not generally believed to be true neoplasms but to represent end-point inflammatory hyperplastic lesions, such as any of the ten other types listed on p. 127. Thus they are really aggregates of scar tissue covered with a smooth layer of stratified squamous epithelium (Fig. 7-8).

The lesions are most often sessile or slightly pedunculated with a smooth contour, pale pink, and firm to palpation—occurring on the gingiva, tongue, buccal mucosa, and palate. A careful excisional biopsy is the indicated treatment.

DIFFERENTIAL DIAGNOSIS

The fibroma may be confused with such benign tumors as lipofibroma, myxofibroma, minor salivary gland tumors, neurofibroma, neurilemmoma, rhabdomyoma, and leiomyoma.

The *lipofibroma* and *myxofibroma* may feel softer on palpation than the fibroma, but the *other benign tumors* noted here possess no distinguishing characteristics that would permit a differential diagnosis.

The giant cell fibroma is a small, firm, papular or polypoid lesion that occurs on the gingiva, tongue, buccal mucosa, and palate and is not more than 1 cm in diameter. These should be in-

Fig. 7-8. Inflammatory fibrous hyperplasia (fibroma). **A,** This lesion represents a fibrosed pyogenic granuloma or hormonal tumor. **B,** Fibrosed lesion of inflammatory hyperplasia on the buccal mucosa. **C,** Photomicrograph of a fibroma. Note the dense avascular collagen.

cluded in the differential diagnosis of fibroma (Weathers and Callihan, 1974).

The fibroma would be ranked above any of these lesions, however, because of its relatively high incidence in the oral cavity.

Pyogenic granuloma

The pyogenic granuloma is a special type of inflammatory hyperplasia. Its surface becomes ulcerated, usually because of trauma during mastication, and this granulomatous lesion then becomes contaminated by the oral flora and liquids. As a result an acute inflammatory response occurs.

Clinically the necrotic ulcerated surface often appears to be composed of a white sloughy material. The fact that this necrotic material clinically resembles pus prompted early clinicians to refer to the lesion as a pyogenic granuloma; however, there is no pus in the lesion.

Microscopically clusters of polymorphonuclear leukocytes are present in some areas of the granuloma, especially areas adjacent to the necrotic or ulcerated surface (Fig. 7-9).

A pyogenic granuloma may also be produced by such chronic irritants as calculus, overhanging margins of crowns or other restorations, implantation of foreign bodies, and chronic biting of soft tissue.

FEATURES

Clinically the pyogenic granuloma is an asymptomatic papule, nodule, or polypoid mass usually with a rough, ulcerated necrotic surface (Figs. 5-42 and 7-9). In the granulomatous stage it will appear red, feel moderately soft, and bleed readily. If the lesion is of the mixed variety (granuloma with fibrous areas), it will appear red with pink areas. If it is completely fibrosed, it will be light pink and firm to palpation (a fibroma).

Angelopoulos (1971), reviewing a large series of pyogenic granulomas, reported that 65% to 70% occurred on the gingivae—with the following sites being involved in decreasing order of frequency: lips, tongue, buccal mucosa, palate, vestibule, and alveolar mucosa in edentulous regions. He found that the maxillary labial gingiva was the most common region involved. The lesions occurred at all ages, but 60% were in patients between 11 and 40 years of age. Females were affected more often than males. The average size of the lesions was 0.9 × 1.2 cm.

Eversole and Rovin (1972), reporting on a series of 166 pyogenic granuloma–gingival fibro-

Fig. 7-9. Pyogenic granuloma. **A,** Clinical view. **B,** Photomicrograph. Note the polymorphonuclear leukocytes distributed throughout the granulation tissue.

matoid lesions, found that 56% involved the anterior segment of the dental arch. These authors found a female-to-male ratio of 4:1, with an average age of 35.1 years.

DIFFERENTIAL DIAGNOSIS

We consider any of the other inflammatory hyperplastic–type lesions with ulcerated surfaces to be examples of pyogenic granuloma. This would include traumatized fibromas, hormonal tumors, epulis fissuratum and epulis granulomatosum, parulis, pulpitis aperta, myxofibroma, peripheral giant cell granuloma, and peripheral fibroma with calcification. Thus it is not necessary to discuss the distinguishing features of these lesions.

The pyogenic granuloma may be confused with an exophytic capillary hemangioma and small benign and malignant mesenchymal tumors that have become ulcerated because of trauma.

Small benign and malignant mesenchymal tumors with ulcerated surfaces may appear clinically identical to the pyogenic granuloma, although the much higher incidence of the granuloma should prompt the clinician to rank this

lesion no. 1 in his differential diagnosis. However, if absolutely no evidence can be established to show the existence of a chronic irritant either present or past this should prompt the diagnostician to deemphasize the inflammatory hyperplasia lesions. This aspect is covered more fully in Chapter 10, p. 229.

An *exophytic capillary hemangioma* likewise may be indistinguishable from the pyogenic granuloma both clinically and microscopically, especially when the surface of the former lesion is ulcerated. Actually the acquired (noncongenital, traumatic) capillary hemangioma may represent a type of inflammatory hyperplasia.

If its surface is ulcerated, a *peripheral giant cell granuloma* may also appear clinically identical to a gingival pyogenic granuloma. If the lesion is more bluish, however, there is a greater probability that it is a peripheral giant cell granuloma than if it is red to pink—in which case the diagnosis of pyogenic granuloma would take precedence.

The *peripheral fibroma with calcification,* which characteristically displaces the interdental papilla, will also mimic the fibrosed pyogenic granuloma occurring on the gingiva (Fig. 7-18). If a slightly underexposed radiograph shows small radiopaque foci within the shadow of the growth, then the lesion is most likely a peripheral fibroma with calcification.

MANAGEMENT

Elimination of the causative trauma and the removal and microscopic study of the lesion itself are all that is required in most cases. If the lesion is small and reddish, elimination of the chronic irritating factor will usually result in its regression to a point at which excision will not be required.

Hormonal tumor

Some pathologists include hormonal tumors with the pyogenic granuloma. On the basis of the circumstances influencing their development, however, we are inclined to treat hormonal tumors as a somewhat different entity. They are inflammatory hyperplastic-type lesions of the gingivae (usually involving the interdental papillae) observed in patients who are experiencing the hormonal imbalances that occur during puberty, pregnancy, and menopause. The hormonal changes are thought to be responsible for an exaggerated response of the gingivae to local irritation. The causative irritants are usually calculus or overhanging margins of dental restora-

Fig. 7-10. Hormonal tumor. This inflammatory hyperplastic lesion was present in a girl at puberty. Poor hygiene was evident.

tions (Fig. 7-10). The development of a differential diagnosis is the same as is described for the pyogenic granuloma.

Epulis fissuratum

Epulis fissuratum is an inflammatory hyperplastic type of lesion observed at the borders of ill-fitting dentures. In most instances the dental flanges are overextended usually as a result of alveolar bone resorption.

FEATURES

The exophytic, often elongated, epulis usually has at least one cleft into which the denture flange fits, with a proliferation of tissue on each side (Fig. 7-11).

Cutright (1974), reviewing a large series of these lesions, reported that most were asymptomatic, that there was a greater incidence in the maxilla than in the mandible, and that the anterior regions of both jaws were more often affected than were the posterior regions. He also found that the lesions occurred most often under the buccal and labial flanges and were seen predominantly in female patients. Epulides fissurata were found in patients from childhood to old age but were seen more often in patients in their 40s and 50s.

DIFFERENTIAL DIAGNOSIS

The frequency of occurrence of the epulis fissuratum so far exceeds that of any other exophytic lesion at the periphery of dentures that a differential diagnosis discussion is not particularly helpful.

The slight possibility that a concurrent *malignant tumor* could be arising in the epulis fissuratum must be appreciated, however, and the microscopic examination of excised tissue is al-

Fig. 7-11. Epulis fissuratum.

ways imperative. In addition, on rare occasions squamous cell carcinomas, verrucous carcinomas, and malignant salivary gland tumors have arisen around denture flanges (Fig. 7-12) where there was no preexisting epulis fissuratum; hence, this slight possibility must always be borne in mind.

MANAGEMENT

If the lesion is small and composed mostly of inflamed tissue and if the denture flange is reduced, the hyperplastic growth may subside in 2 or 3 weeks without further treatment. When there are larger more fibrosed lesions, excision combined with perhaps a sulcus-deepening procedure will be necessary. In either case a new well-adapted denture should be fabricated, or at least the current appliance should be adjusted and rebased.

Parulis

A parulis is a small inflammatory hyperplastic type of lesion that develops on the alveolar mucosa at the oral terminal of a draining sinus (Fig. 7-13). This lesion usually accompanies a draining chronic alveolar abscess in children. We have noted that the maxillary labial and buccal alveolar mucosa is the most frequent site, but the man-

Fig. 7-12. Palatal growths posterior to denture flanges. **A,** Epulis fissuratum. **B,** Malignant salivary gland tumor.

Fig. 7-13. Parulis. These inflammatory hyperplastic-type lesions occur at the mucosal draining site of a chronic alveolar abscess.

dibular alveolar mucosa and palate may also be involved (Fig. 7-13).

Slight digital pressure on the periphery of a parulis may force a drop of pus from the sinus opening, and this is almost pathognomonic.

The lesion usually regresses spontaneously after the chronic odontogenic infection has been eliminated. If it is of considerable size and there

is a substantial amount of fibrosis, however, the lesion will regress somewhat and then persist as a fibroma.

Very rarely a draining osteomyelitis or infected malignant tumor may produce a similar appearance.

Inflammatory papillary hyperplasia (palatal papillomatosis)

Inflammatory papillary hyperplasia occurs almost exclusively on the palate beneath either a complete or a partial removable denture. We have noted that it is more commonly associated with a flipper-type partial or a full denture. Approximately 10% of the people who wear dentures have this condition, and most of them wear their dentures continually. Although its cause is not well understood, palatal papillomatosis appears to be related to the frictional irritation produced by loose-fitting dentures on the palatal tissue.

FEATURES

A small region in the vault or perhaps the whole palatal mucosa under the denture may be covered with numerous small painless polypoid masses that are seldom over 0.3 cm in diameter (Fig. 7-14). As with all the other inflammatory hyperplastic lesions, these masses are red and soft and bleed easily in the inflammatory or granulomatous stage. If they become fibrosed, however, they will be firm and pale pink in color.

DIFFERENTIAL DIAGNOSIS

Since inflammatory papillary hyperplasia occurs almost exclusively on the palate under a full or partial removable denture, it can seldom be confused with other lesions.

Fig. 7-14. Inflammatory papillary hyperplasia.

Fig. 7-15. Peripheral giant cell granuloma. The significant amount of hemosiderin in this lesion produced a bluish color. (Courtesy S. Svalina, D.D.S., Maywood, Ill.)

Nicotinic stomatitis may also feature small multiple nodules on the palate, which will be reddish before a hyperkeratosis develops. The following observations will aid in the differentiation of this condition from inflammatory papillary hyperplasia:

1. Nicotinic stomatitis on the hard palate occurs almost exclusively in pipe smokers who are not wearing maxillary full dentures.
2. The lesions in nicotinic stomatitis are more nodular and broader but less elevated.
3. The nodules in nicotinic stomatitis have a characteristic red dot in their approximate center, which is not seen in papillary hyperplasia.

In unusual cases the clinician may feel he should consult the list of entities catalogued at the end of this chapter, in the column of rare multiple lesions.

MANAGEMENT

The patient must be persuaded to remove his denture at night to rest the tissues.

If the case is in the granulomatous stage, the placement of a soft tissue–conditioning liner in the denture may curb the inflammatory response and effect a reduction in the size and extent of the polypoid masses—possibly to such a degree that surgery will not be necessary.

In fibrosed cases surgical removal is usually required, and the denture containing a surgical dressing may be utilized as a stent. Miller (1977) reviewed the suggested methods of removal: (1) surgical curettage, (2) electrosurgery, (3) cryosurgery, and (4) mucobrasion. A new denture well adapted to the oral tissues should then be fabricated.

Uohara and Federbusch (1968) described an interesting procedure that utilizes a modified razor blade attached in a bow shape to a holder. The cutting edge is drawn from posterior to anterior in continuous strokes, removing strips of hyperplastic tissue with clean incisions.

Although inflammatory papillary hyperplasia does not tend to undergo malignant change, any excised tissue should be examined microscopically.

Peripheral giant cell granuloma

There may be some authors who object to including peripheral giant cell granuloma with the inflammatory hyperplastic group of lesions; but it seems appropriate in this context because they share several similar clinical characteristics. Although the cause of peripheral giant cell granuloma is considered unknown, trauma appears to play a role in a significant number of cases.

FEATURES

Microscopically multinucleated giant cells are scattered throughout the granulation tissue. Extravasated erythrocytes and varying amounts of hemosiderin are observed. If a sufficient amount of hemosiderin exists near the periphery, the lesion will be bluish in color. Otherwise it is red to pale pink, depending on the relative proportions of collagen and vascular component present.

The peripheral type occurs as an exophytic lesion exclusively on the gingivae and edentulous alveolar mucosa (Eversole and Rovin, 1972) (Fig. 7-15). The peripheral giant cell granuloma is most often nodular in shape, but sometimes it will be polypoid (base pedunculated rather than sessile). It may feel soft to hard, depending on the relative proportions of collagen and inflammatory component present.

Bhaskar and Cutright (1971), reviewing a series of peripheral giant cell granulomas, reported that the lesions occurred most often in patients over 20 years of age (average age approximately 45). These authors observed, furthermore, that the lesions were found predominantly in whites and on the mandible much more than on the maxilla.

In a series of 720 peripheral giant cell granulomas reviewed by Giansanti and Waldron (1969) a significantly greater number of women were affected, especially in the 20- to 60-year range. The mean age was 31.3 years; 45% occurred on the maxillary gingiva or mucosa, and 55% were located on the mandibular gingiva or mucosa. This lesion accounted for 0.5% of all surgical accessions to their laboratory.

DIFFERENTIAL DIAGNOSIS

The differential diagnosis of pink or red lesions of the peripheral giant cell granuloma is identical with that detailed for the *gingival pyogenic granuloma* (p. 130). The differential diagnosis for the bluish variety is discussed in Chapter 9 (p. 193).

MANAGEMENT

All the tumors clinically identified as peripheral giant cell granulomas should be excised with a border of normal tissue, and the specimen should be examined microscopically. Since there is some inclination to suspect the role played by chronic trauma in the formation of this lesion, all chronic irritants should be eliminated.

Pulp polyp (chronic hyperplastic pulpitis, pulpitis aperta)

Chronic hyperplastic pulpitis proliferates from the pulp when gross caries have destroyed part or all of the tooth crown covering the pulp chamber (Fig. 7-16). It is an uncommon lesion observed mostly in the deciduous and permanent first molars of children and young adults. The lesion acquires a stratified squamous covering apparently as the result of a fortuitous grafting of vital exfoliated epithelial cells from the adjacent oral mucosa. Its histologic characteristics are identical with those of the other types of inflammatory hyperplasias.

DIFFERENTIAL DIAGNOSIS

Occasionally a flap of *adjacent gingiva* will extend into a large proximal carious lesion and appear to be a chronic hyperplastic pulpitis. Careful

Fig. 7-16. Pulp polyp.

examination, however, will disclose that the exophytic growth is continuous with the gingiva rather than the pulp. The occurrence of any other type of lesion growing from the pulp is much too rare to be considered in this text.

MANAGEMENT

There are two ways of treating a pulp polyp:
1. Conservation of the tooth through endodontic procedures followed by a full coverage type of restoration
2. Extraction of the tooth

Epulis granulomatosum

Epulis granulomatosum is the specific inflammatory hyperplastic type of lesion that grows from a tooth socket after the tooth has been lost (Fig. 7-17). The precipitating cause in almost every case is a sharp spicule of bone in the socket. The growth may become apparent in a week or two after the loss of the tooth; and the clinical characteristics are similar to those of the other inflammatory hyperplasias.

DIFFERENTIAL DIAGNOSIS

The two other lesions that might be confused with an epulis granulomatosum are an antral polyp protruding into the oral cavity through a maxillary molar or premolar socket and a malignant tumor growing from a recent extraction wound (Fig. 7-17). In most cases a radiograph will provide information enabling the clinician to identify either of these two entities.

In the case of a *malignant mesenchymal lesion* growing out of a recent extraction wound, a radiograph will usually show either bony destruction or a combined radiolucent-radiopaque lesion.

The oroantral fistula that permits the extrusion of an *antral polyp* quite often will be evident as a well-defined loss of bone from the antral floor.

Fig. 7-17. Epulis granulomatosum. **A,** A retained deciduous root was the irritating factor in this case. **B,** Sharp bony spicules remaining in an extraction socket caused this lesion. **C,** This lesion proved to be an antral polyp that had extruded through a socket with an oroantral fistula. (**B** courtesy P. Akers, D.D.S., Chicago. **C** courtesy P. D. Toto, D.D.S., Maywood, Ill.)

If antral polyps are present, the patient should be referred to a surgical specialist for management and to ensure that the "polyp" is not an antral malignancy.

MANAGEMENT

Careful inspection of the socket and removal of any bony spicules at the time the tooth is extracted will prevent the formation of epulides granulomatosa. Treatment of an epulis granulomatosum requires the excision of the lesion and a careful curettement of the alveolus to assure the elimination of irritating bony spicules. Because the growth might be malignant, the tissue removed should be examined microscopically.

Myxofibroma (fibroma with myxomatous change)

A myxofibroma is generally considered to be a variety of inflammatory fibrous hyperplasia in which some myxomatous tissue has developed or some area of the fibroma has undergone myxomatous degeneration. Microscopically regions of dense fibroblastic tissue are interspersed with pale myxomatous-appearing tissue.

FEATURES

A myxofibroma may occur anywhere in the oral cavity or on the lips. It is most common on the palate and gingiva and usually feels significantly softer than the fibroma and often is less pale.

DIFFERENTIAL DIAGNOSIS

A myxofibroma may be confused with a lipofibroma, a plexiform neurofibroma, or some other inflammatory hyperplastic lesion.

Both the *lipofibroma* and the *plexiform neurofibroma* are soft, spongy, and fluctuant. The myxofibroma is usually not so soft and occurs more commonly in the oral cavity than does the lipofibroma or the plexiform neurofibroma; so it would be assigned a more prominent rank in the list of possible diagnoses.

An exception might occur in the case of a patient with a moderately soft nodular or polypoid exophytic oral lesion who has von Recklinghausen's disease. In this case the plexiform neurofibroma (the only soft, fluctuant, peripheral neural tumor) would be assigned the no. 1 rank in the differential diagnosis. Tomich (1974) discussed some of the rare lesions that need to be differentiated from the myxofibroma.

MANAGEMENT

Complete excision with microscopic study of the tissue is the indicated treatment for myxofibroma.

Peripheral fibroma with calcification, peripheral odontogenic fibroma, peripheral ossifying fibroma

The peripheral fibroma with calcification is a benign overgrowth of gingival tissue that most oral pathologists consider to be a type of inflammatory hyperplastic lesion. It is believed to involve the periodontal ligament superficially; and it often contains odontogenic epithelial nests as well as deposits of cementum, bone, and dystrophic calcification scattered throughout a background of fibrous tissue. If the calcified element is significant, radiopaque foci will be observed within the soft tissue tumor mass on radiographs (Fig. 7-18).

Recently King and co-workers (1979) reported that gingival tissue possesses unusually thin stringy rete ridges (usually formed by two rows of basal cells) that extend a considerable distance into the underlying connective tissue. They reported seeing the same phenomenon in peripheral fibromas with calcification. These interesting findings raise the probability that the nests and strands of epithelial cells in the lesion in question represent isolated sections of this unique rete ridge system rather than representing examples of odontogenic epithelium. This lesion is also included with the mixed radiolucent-radiopaque lesions in Chapter 24.

A

B

Fig. 7-18. Peripheral fibroma with calcification. **A,** The lesion (arrow) is causing the lateral incisor and canine to separate. **B,** Radiograph. The arrow indicates calcification within the mass.

FEATURES

The peripheral fibroma with calcification occurs exclusively on the free margin of the gingiva and usually involves the interdental papilla (Fig. 7-18). The lesion frequently causes a separation of the adjacent teeth, and occasionally minimal bone resorption can be seen beneath the lesion. Cundiff (1972) reviewed a series of 365 cases and found that 50% of the lesions occurred in patients between the ages of 5 and 25 years, with a peak incidence at 13 years. In addition, he reported that the female was more often affected than the male and that 80% of the lesions occurred anterior to the molar areas.

The lesion is usually asymptomatic and, although frequently discovered by the patient himself, comes to professional attention during a routine examination. In our experience it is often associated with irritation (e.g., overextended margins of faulty restorations, deposits of calculus), which indicates that it most likely represents an inflammatory hyperplastic-type lesion such as a pyogenic granuloma or a hormonal tumor involving a segment of the periodontal ligament. Certainly it appears to pass through the same clinical stages as the inflammatory hyperplasias: the early lesions are soft, quite vascular, and red and bleed readily; the more mature lesions are firm, fibrous, and pale pink.

DIFFERENTIAL DIAGNOSIS

The following lesions should be included in the differential diagnosis for the peripheral fibroma with calcification: other inflammatory hyperplastic lesions of the gingiva, osteogenic sarcoma, and chondrosarcoma.

The *chondrosarcoma* and *osteogenic sarcoma*, considered together, are less frequent gingival lesions than the peripheral fibroma with calcification. Although a slight bony resorption may occur beneath the peripheral fibroma with calcification, severe bony changes would classically be seen if the lesion were malignant. Also a band-like asymmetric widening of the periodontal ligaments of involved teeth is an expected finding with chondrosarcoma and osteogenic sarcoma but is not a feature of the peripheral fibroma with calcification (Fig. 20-11).

The common varieties of *gingival inflammatory hyperplastic lesions* (hormonal tumor, pyogenic granuloma) occur much more often than does the peripheral fibroma with calcification, but they share many identical clinical features with it. In contrast, the peripheral fibroma with calcification may cause a separation of the adjacent teeth, not frequently seen with the other inflammatory hyperplasias. Also, if calcified foci are present within the soft tissue overgrowth, the clinician should exclude the other inflammatory hyperplasias since these foci suggest rather the peripheral odontogenic fibroma, the osteogenic sarcoma, and the chondrosarcoma.

MANAGEMENT

The peripheral fibroma with calcification should be excised, with special care to remove the lesion's attachment in the periodontal ligament. As a rule the adjacent teeth do not have to be extracted. These lesions occasionally recur, but their management is not a problem. All excised tissue should be examined microscopically.

MUCOCELE AND RANULA

The mucocele and ranula are retention phenomena of the minor salivary glands and the sublingual major salivary glands, respectively. Although they are discussed in detail in Chapter 9 as bluish lesions, it is noteworthy to mention that in a review of 63 oral mucoceles, Cohen (1965) observed 52 (82%) on the lower lip and 8%, 2%, and 1% on the cheek, in the retromolar area, and on the palate, respectively.

DIFFERENTIAL DIAGNOSIS

When the mucosal covering is thicker than usual, the lesion will appear pink, be soft to rubbery in consistency, and be fluctuant but not emptiable.

In such instances it must be differentiated from a *superficial cyst, lipoma, plexiform neurofibroma, relatively deep cavernous hemangioma, lymphangioma,* and *mucus-producing salivary gland tumor.*

If aspiration of the lesion produces a sticky, viscous, clear, mucuslike fluid, all the foregoing lesions can be eliminated except the mucus-producing salivary gland tumors; and these are uncommon lesions.

Although retention phenomena should be initially considered as a possible mucus-producing malignant salivary gland tumor (e.g., mucoepidermoid tumor, mucous adenocarcinoma), these occur most often on the posterior hard palate, retromolar area, and posterolateral aspect of the floor of the mouth. An induration at the base of a retention phenomenon may be just fibrous tissue, but it should alert the clinician to the possibility of a malignant tumor.

MANAGEMENT

If the conservative approach of marsupialization is followed, the base of the lesion must be examined carefully for pathosis and a cautious periodic follow-up must be maintained. If the lesion is treated by complete excision, the specimen must be examined microscopically.

HEMANGIOMA, LYMPHANGIOMA, AND VARICOSITY

Hemangiomas, lymphangiomas, and varicosities are discussed as bluish lesions in Chapter 9.

If a hemangioma, lymphangioma, or varicosity is covered with a thicker than usual layer of oral mucosa, however, its bluish color will be masked and it will be seen as a pink, smooth nodular or dome-shaped lesion.

The differential diagnosis of such lesions is similar to that described for the mucocele and ranula, in which significant information can be obtained by sampling the material within the lesion by aspiration.

CENTRAL EXOPHYTIC LESIONS

Central lesions of the jawbones frequently produce exophytic masses as the result of expansion, erosion, or invasion. Thus, for the differential diagnosis of oral lesions, the possibility that an exophytic mass could be central in origin must always be considered. Usually a complete examination, including a history and clinical and radiographic surveys, will indicate whether the lesion is central in origin. Since lesions of bone are discussed in detail in Part III of this text, only a list of the more common pathoses that may pro-

Fig. 7-19. Exophytic lesions that are central in origin. **A,** Eruption cyst. **B,** Follicular cyst. **C,** Palatal space abscess from a maxillary molar. (**A** courtesy D. Bonomo, D.D.S., Flossmoor, Ill. **B** courtesy R. Nolan, D.D.S., Waukegan, Ill.)

duce these exophytic growths will be reiterated here (Fig. 7-19):

Benign tumors

Cysts

Infections

Malignant tumors

Odontogenic tumors

Soft tissue abscesses such as the foregoing, resulting from odontogenic infection, are central in origin; but because their peripheral manifestations are usually exophytic dome-shaped masses (Fig. 7-19), they must often be considered in the differential diagnosis of peripheral lesions. Actually such abscesses will be readily recognized by their location, by the fact that they are rubbery, fluctuant, painful, and hot, and by the fact that they yield pus on aspiration.

PAPILLOMA AND VERRUCA VULGARIS

The papilloma and verruca vulgaris are benign exophytic growths of the surface epithelium, as their rough surfaces would indicate. Because their surfaces often retain a significant amount of keratin, these lesions are discussed with the white lesions in Chapter 5. Nevertheless, occasionally keratinization will not be a feature and the lesions will appear pink. Papillomas and verrucae vulgari seldom measure more than 1 cm in diameter (Fig. 7-20).

Fig. 7-20. Pink papilloma. **A,** Midline of the palate. **B,** Maxillary lingual alveolus. Both lesions were pedunculated.

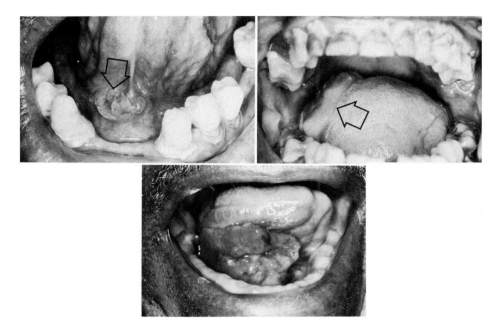

Fig. 7-21. Exophytic types of squamous cell carcinoma.

DIFFERENTIAL DIAGNOSIS

Solitary examples of a lightly keratinized papilloma and verruca must be differentiated from a pyogenic granuloma, papillary squamous cell carcinoma, condyloma acuminata, condyloma lata, and lesions such as peripheral ameloblastomas that may show extensive pseudoepitheliomatous hyperplasia. With the exception of the pyogenic granuloma the differentiating features of the other lesions are covered in Chapter 5 (p. 80).

The rounded smooth contours of the *pyogenic granuloma,* except for a possible area of ulceration, would permit the differentiation between the pyogenic granuloma and the papilloma and verruca, as would the tendency for the pyogenic granuloma to readily bleed (in contrast to the papilloma and verruca).

If several lesions are present, the examiner should consult the list of rare multiple lesions at the end of this chapter for additional entities that may be included in his list of possibilities. A detailed discussion of all these lesions is beyond the scope of the text.

EXOPHYTIC SQUAMOUS CELL CARCINOMA

Squamous cell carcinoma is discussed in Chapter 5 as a white lesion, in Chapter 6 as an ulcerative lesion, and in Chapter 10 as a red lesion. In this chapter the exophytic variety of squamous cell carcinoma will be described.

Verrucous carcinoma is not included in the discussion because, although an exophytic lesion, it has markedly different characteristics.

FEATURES

Exophytic carcinoma in our experience occurs most often on the lateral borders of the tongue, the floor of the mouth, and the soft palate. Approximately 55% of all the squamous cell carcinomas of the tongue in a series reported by Whitaker and co-workers (1972) were exophytic-type lesions.

The lesions are very firm to palpation, and their bases may be indurated because of infiltration of the underlying tissue. They may be nodular or polypoid in shape, are usually somewhat pink to red, and invariably have at least one ulcerated patch on their surfaces (Figs. 7-21 and 7-22). In some cases the surfaces may be entirely necrotic and have a whitish-gray ragged appearance. Pain or a tendency to bleed are not early characteristics.

It is generally believed that the majority of exophytic carcinomas are less aggressive than the ulcerative varieties; but all lesions must be evaluated on an individual basis. Cervical lymph node involvement is the usual route of metastatic spread.

Fig. 7-22. Exophytic squamous cell carcinoma. **A,** Ulcerated exophytic lesion in a 54-year-old woman. **B,** Large exophytic lesion of the floor of the mouth, ridge, and lateral border of the tongue. (**B** courtesy J. Lehnert, D.D.S., Minneapolis.)

Occasionally an exophytic squamous cell carcinoma will have a polypoid shape and a papillated surface (Fig. 7-23). Such lesions are sometimes referred to as papillary squamous cell carcinomas. They represent a variation of exophytic carcinoma and need to be differentiated from papillomas, verrucae, condyloma acuminatum, condyloma latum, pseudoepitheliomatous hyperplasia, and verrucous carcinoma.

DIFFERENTIAL DIAGNOSIS

The following lesions must be distinguished from the exophytic carcinoma: pyogenic granuloma, verrucous carcinoma, malignant salivary gland tumors, peripheral malignant mesenchymal tumors, peripheral metastatic tumors, and amelanotic melanoma.

Amelanotic melanoma is a rare oral tumor which, when it becomes ulcerated, is clinically indistinguishable from an exophytic carcinoma. Because of its low frequency of occurrence, however, it would have a low rank in the differential diagnosis.

Peripheral metastatic tumors in their early stages may be rather innocent appearing, firm, and nodular, dome shaped, or polypoid with smoothly contoured surfaces and covered with normal-appearing mucosa. Later, when their surfaces become ulcerated, they may be indistinguishable from squamous cell carcinomas. Again, because this pathosis has such a low incidence, it would be assigned a low rank in the list of possible entities unless there is evidence from the history or examination suggesting the presence of a parent tumor.

Peripheral malignant mesenchymal tumors (e.g., fibrosarcoma, myosarcoma, neurosarcoma,

Fig. 7-23. Papillary squamous cell carcinoma. Early invasion of the underlying tissue was observed microscopically. The obvious swelling under the lesion was produced by a recent injection of local anesthetic solution, not by gross invasion.

liposarcoma) are also rare oral lesions. In their early stages, like most metastatic lesions, they are often firm, smooth surfaced, and nodular, dome shaped, or polypoid. The fact that their surfaces are smooth and covered with normal-appearing mucosa permits the differentiation between these early lesions and the rough-surfaced ulcerated squamous cell carcinomas. Later, though, when these malignant mesenchymal tumors become ulcerated, they may appear very similar to an exophytic squamous cell carcinoma. Evidence of metastatic involvement of cervical lymph nodes would be very unusual in most mesenchymal tumors and would strongly support a diagnosis of squamous cell carcinoma. On the basis of its low incidence, a clinician would have to conclude that an ulcerated exophytic lesion was more likely a squamous cell carcinoma than a peripheral malignant mesenchymal tumor.

Malignant salivary gland tumors are second to squamous cell carcinoma as the most common oral malignancy. The firm types are under consideration here. The fluctuant mucus-producing varieties (e.g., low-grade mucoepidermoid tumors, mucous adenocarcinomas) have necessarily been grouped in the differential diagnosis with the retention phenomena. Like the early secondary tumors and early peripheral malignant mesenchymal tumors, the malignant salivary gland tumors originate in tissue situated deep to and separate from the surface epithelium. Thus in their early stages they are nodular or dome shaped, have a smooth contour, and are covered with normal-appearing epithelium. Later, when their surfaces become ulcerated because of the trauma of mastication or biopsy, or perhaps as a result of the rupturing of retained fluid, they may appear to be malignant (i.e., have ulcerated, necrotic, friable surfaces). At this stage the malignant salivary gland tumors may not be readily differentiated from exophytic squamous cell carcinomas. The following clues, however, are helpful:

1. Squamous cell carcinoma is not so common on the posterior hard palate as are malignant salivary gland tumors.
2. Salivary gland tumors occur more frequently in women, and squamous cell carcinoma occurs two to four times as frequently in men. The significance of this difference between the two tumors must be modified, however, because approximately 95% of the oral malignancies are squamous cell carcinomas whereas only about 4% are malignant minor salivary gland tumors.
3. Malignant minor salivary gland tumors frequently maintain their dome shape even after their surfaces become ulcerated.

The *verrucous carcinoma* is a much slower growing lesion than the exophytic squamous cell carcinoma and is most often associated with the prolonged use of chewing tobacco or snuff. The sites frequently affected are the vestibule and buccal mucosa. The surface of the lesion is usually papillomatous and frequently white because of the retention of keratin. Exophytic squamous cell carcinoma, on the other hand, is most often observed on the lateral border of the tongue or floor of the mouth and frequently has a partly ulcerated surface that is not papillomatous or keratotic. The verrucous carcinoma seldom metastasizes; in contrast, the exophytic squamous

Fig. 7-24. Verrucous carcinoma. Note the pebbly white surface of this slow-growing lesion, which has a relatively sessile base. (From Claydon, R. J., and Jordan, J. E.: J. Oral Surg. **36:**564-567, 1978. Copyright by the American Dental Association. Reprinted by permission.)

cell carcinoma commonly spreads to the cervical lymph nodes.

The large *pyogenic granuloma* with an ulcerated surface may be a suspicious-appearing lesion. It is usually moderately soft to palpation and bleeds easily, however, whereas the exophytic carcinoma is very firm and usually does not bleed when manipulated.

In addition, a great many rare exophytic lesions such as the following may be confused with exophytic squamous cell carcinoma; but an in-depth discussion of all these possibilities is beyond the scope of this text:

Condyloma acuminatum
Granulomatous fungal diseases
Gumma
Keratoacanthoma
Lethal midline granuloma
Sarcoidosis
Tuberculosis

MANAGEMENT

The management of intraoral squamous cell carcinomas is discussed in detail in Chapter 6.

VERRUCOUS CARCINOMA

Verrucous carcinoma is a specific kind of low-grade* squamous cell carcinoma that occurs as a verrucous type of exophytic lesion (Fig. 7-24). It seldom metastasizes, is usually cured by ade-

---

*Low-grade carcinomas are slow growing, do not metastasize early, tend to develop into bulky tumors, may often be successfully treated by simple local excision, and have a favorable prognosis.

quate local excision, and carries a better prognosis than does regular squamous cell carcinoma. The lesion frequently has a white keratotic surface and is discussed with the white lesions in Chapter 5.

On occasion, the surface of the verrucous carcinoma will not be heavily keratinized and will appear pink. The differential diagnosis in such cases is discussed under the differential diagnosis section of exophytic squamous cell carcinoma (p. 141).

MINOR SALIVARY GLAND TUMORS

Most of the minor salivary gland tumors are exophytic lesions, which explains their inclusion in this chapter. The intraoral minor salivary glands are predominantly of the mucous type and are normally distributed throughout the oral mucosa except for the anterior hard palate, attached gingivae, and anterior two thirds of the dorsal surface of the tongue. Unusual cases of salivary gland tumors occurring in these locations have been reported and are considered to have arisen in ectopic minor salivary glands.

The mucous glands are not attached to the surface mucosa except by the common ducts that drain a cluster of glands. These clusters of mucous glands are situated deep to the surface mucosa and usually lie just superficial to the loose connective tissue layer if such a layer is present. Thus as a tumor originates in these glands and enlarges, it becomes a nodular or dome-shaped exophytic mass with a smooth surface (Chapter 3).

Because of the great variety of neoplasms that occur in the salivary glands, the establishment and adoption of a uniform classification and nomenclature for these tumors have not yet been achieved. (With only one or two exceptions, all the tumors occurring in the major salivary glands are also found in the minor salivary glands.)

To establish some common order that will contribute to a universal comprehension of descriptions and discussions of this homogeneous group of lesions, the World Health Organization has introduced the following classification (Thackray and Sabin, 1972).

1. Epithelial tumors
   a. Adenomas
      (1) Pleomorphic adenoma (mixed tumor)
      (2) Monomorphic adenomas
         (a) Adenolymphoma [Warthin's tumor, papillary cystadenoma lymphomatosum]*
         (b) Oxyphilic adenoma [oncocytoma]*

      b. Mucoepidermoid tumor
      c. Acinic cell tumor
      d. Carcinomas
         (1) Adenoid cystic carcinoma [cylindroma]*
         (2) Adenocarcinoma
         (3) Epidermoid carcinoma
         (4) Undifferentiated carcinoma
         (5) Carcinoma in pleomorphic adenoma (malignant mixed tumor)
2. Nonepithelial tumors
3. Unclassified tumors

Most North American oral pathologists would recommend some modification of the WHO classification as illustrated by the minutes of an ESTOP† meeting at London, Ontario, on October 17, 1976. This group suggested the following modifications: (1) the term "adenolymphoma" for papillary cystadenoma lymphomatosum was unsatisfactory; (2) papillary cystadenoma lymphomatosum should not be included under monomorphic adenoma and possibly the same for oxyphilic adenoma; (3) a considerable number of oral pathologists felt that the term mucoepidermoid "tumor" was unacceptable because they believed that all of these lesions are carcinomas; (4) most favored the term acinic cell "carcinoma" over acinic cell "tumor" for similar reasons.

As with other groups of lesions, the diagnostician would be aided considerably if there were certain clinical features of salivary gland tumors that would enable him to conclude whether the tumors were malignant or benign. In our opinion, though, nothing distinctive can be found about the clinical features of either malignant or benign minor salivary gland tumors that will signal their identity. The clinical appearance of both are so similar that in most cases a tumor cannot be ranked in the working diagnosis according to its malignancy or lack of malignancy.

One exception to this circumstance would be the highly malignant tumor recognizable by its rapid growth.

Early minor salivary gland tumors, whether benign or not, are usually nodular or dome-shaped elevations with smooth contours; and the overlying mucosa either is normal or appears smoother and glossier because of the tension created by the underlying expanding tumor (Figs. 7-25 and 7-26). As the overlying mucosa becomes thinned by the expanding tumor and

---

*Contents of brackets are ours.

*Contents of brackets are ours.
†Eastern Society of Teachers of Oral Pathology.

Fig. 7-25. Minor salivary gland tumors. **A** and **B**, Pleomorphic adenomas. **C**, Adenoid cystic carcinoma that became ulcerated after an incisional biopsy. (**B** and **C** courtesy E. Kasper, D.D.S., Maywood, Ill.)

traumatized during mastication or as the pooled mucus ruptures or a biopsy of the growth is made, an ulcer appears that is persistent and usually becomes necrotic. We have been impressed by several benign tumors that have taken on the appearance of angry malignant-looking lesions as the result of an incisional biopsy or other traumatic episode. Consequently, although the more rapidly growing malignant varieties of minor salivary gland tumor may tend to ulcerate earlier, the number of benign tumors ulcerating is sufficiently high to keep this feature from being clinically useful in distinguishing between the types.

Likewise the firmness (induration) of a lesion is no better a prognostic sign than is surface ulceration for clinically distinguishing between the malignant and the benign salivary tumors, because the majority of both malignant and benign tumors are firm. The fact that some malignant salivary tumors as well as some benign ones are moderately soft and fluctuant, or have soft and firm areas, further emphasizes this point.

Although it is not possible to establish clinical guidelines that will enable the examiner to determine whether a particular minor salivary gland tumor is malignant or benign, salivary tumors can be categorized into two clinical classes: (1) those that are firm to palpation and (2) those that are moderately soft and fluctuant.

The following tumors are almost categorically firm to palpation. They are ranked, as much as possible, in order of frequency of occurrence:

Pleomorphic adenoma (benign mixed tumor)
Adenoid cystic carcinoma
Mucoepidermoid tumor of high-grade malignancy
Carcinoma in pleomorphic adenoma (malignant mixed tumor)
Acinic cell carcinoma
Oncocytoma

The firmness in these tumors results from the presence of dense aggregates, nests, and cords of closely packed tumor cells, fibrous tissue, and hyaline areas as well as cartilagelike and bonelike tissue (pleomorphic adenoma).

The following tumors, on the other hand, are moderately soft and are frequently fluctuant. Again, an attempt has been made to arrange them in descending order of incidence:

Well-differentiated mucoepidermoid tumor
Papillary cyst adenoma
Mucus-producing adenocarcinoma
Warthin's tumor or papillary cystadenoma lymphomatosum

The softness of these tumors results from the

Fig. 7-26. Palatal masses. **A,** Palatal space abscess from infected lateral incisor tooth. **B,** Naso-palatine cyst. **C,** Fibroma. **D,** Palatal space abscess from periapical abscess of first premolar tooth. **E,** Pleomorphic adenoma. **F,** Small midline fissural cyst of palate. **G,** Large benign salivary tumor. **H,** Large squamous cell carcinoma of the soft palate. (**B** and **E** courtesy W. Heaton, D.D.S., Chicago. **H** courtesy J. Lehnert, D.D.S., Minneapolis.)

fluid produced and the consequent retention phenomena; in other words, mucus is produced in well-differentiated mucoepidermoid tumors and in mucous adenocarcinomas whereas cyst fluid is produced in the papillary cyst adenoma and in Warthin's tumor. The tumors in this group are fluctuant because of the enclosed fluid.

FEATURES

Most of the intraoral minor salivary gland tumors occur on the posterior aspect of the hard palate (Figs. 7-25 and 7-26). In a series studied by Soskolne and co-workers (1973), 66% of the tumors were found in this site, and in a review by Chaudhry and co-workers (1961), 57.7% of the tumors occurred on the palate. The next most frequent sites, in approximate descending order of frequency, are the upper lip, buccal mucosa, retromolar region, tongue, and floor of the mouth. In the Canadian series reported by Main and co-workers (1976) approximate percentage by location was as follows: palate, 53%; buccal mucosa, 17%; tongue, 8%; upper lip, 5%; gingiva, 4%; bone, 2.6%; unspecified, 7%. Concerning incidence of mixed tumors of the lips it is interesting that in the AFIP series the ratio of occurrence in the upper lip to lower lip was 75:13 (Krolls and Hicks, 1973). The vast majority of malignant intraoral salivary gland tumors are mucoepidermoid carcinomas and adenoid cystic carcinomas.

The incidence according to sex varies from series to series and from type to type, but most reports indicate a higher frequency in women. The peak age for the benign tumors lies between 30 and 39 years, whereas for the malignant tumors it is between 40 and 49 years (Soskolne et al., 1973).

The ratio of benign to malignant lesions among minor salivary gland tumors slightly favors the benign variety—as illustrated in the series examined by Soskolne and co-authors (1973), in which 67% were benign, and by the series of Chaudhry and his group (1961), in which 60% were benign. Interestingly Main and co-workers (1976) reported that 62.2% from their Scottish series were benign whereas only 34.7% of their Canadian series were benign. The pleomorphic adenoma accounted for 60.9% of all tumors described by Soskolne's group and 55.7% of the tumors reviewed by Chaudhry's.

These tumors may be present and tolerated for several months or even years because they are characteristically asymptomatic; consequently they usually come to professional attention only during routine examination. The adenoid cystic carcinoma, however, may be painful, especially if it has extended into a perineural space.

Benign salivary gland tumors may produce a well-defined saucerlike depression in the underlying bone. In contrast, malignant tumors may invade the bone and produce a ragged radiolucent defect with poorly defined borders (Fig. 20-9). Such tumors positioned on the lateral aspect of the posterior hard palate may destroy the alveolar bone and invade the maxillary sinus.

The malignant types may spread via lymphatic vessels to the cervical lymph nodes. The lungs are the most common site of distant metastasis. The adenoid cystic carcinoma frequently spreads along the perineural spaces, and other types also occasionally do this.

Comprehension of the histopathology of the minor salivary gland tumors is difficult because of the many varieties of tumors. The following have clear-cut histologic features, which makes their identification relatively easy:

Acinic cell carcinoma
Adenoid cystic carcinoma
Canalicular adenoma
Mucoepidermoid tumor
Papillary cyst adenoma
Pleomorphic adenoma
Oncocytoma
Warthin's tumor

Some of the unclassified adenocarcinomas are difficult to identify; and in the case of the low-grade lesions, it is frequently difficult to determine whether the tumors are malignant or benign. Occasionally this also happens when a carcinoma occurs within a pleomorphic adenoma. Often many slides must be prepared from different areas of the specimen before a malignant change can be detected, and even then the changes may not be pronounced. A detailed discussion of the histopathology of the minor salivary gland tumors is beyond the scope of this text.

DIFFERENTIAL DIAGNOSIS

Since the following tumors account for from 82% (Soskolne et al., 1973) to 94% (Chaudhry et al., 1961) of all minor salivary gland tumors the clinician is likely to encounter, he should initially include them in his differential diagnosis when it seems probable that the lesion is a minor salivary tumor: pleomorphic adenoma, adenoid cystic carcinoma, unclassified or undifferentiated adenocarcinomas, mucoepidermoid tumor, and carcinoma in pleomorphic adenoma.

To facilitate the consideration of the differential diagnosis, the discussion has been divided into two sections: the first includes the firm tumors; the second includes the softer fluctuant ones. As previously noted, we do not believe that there are enough clinical differences between the lesions within each group to attempt a differentiation between the individual minor salivary tumors. Nevertheless, the following facts may be useful prognostic aids:

1. The pleomorphic adenomas make up about 60% of all minor salivary gland tumors.
2. The majority of intraoral adenoid cystic carcinomas and mucoepidermoid tumors occur on the posterolateral aspect of the hard palate.
3. An ulcerated minor salivary tumor, in the absence of a history of incisional biopsy or other traumatic incident, is more likely to be malignant.

Firm minor salivary tumors. Several lesions must be included in the differential diagnosis for a firm minor salivary tumor: mature lesions of inflammatory hyperplasia (fibromas), benign and malignant mesenchymal tumors, necrotizing sialometaplasia, focal hyperplasia of minor salivary glands, and the rare granulomatous lesions of tuberculosis, syphilis (gumma), and fungal infections.

The very low incidence of the last-mentioned *rare lesions of tuberculosis, syphilis,* and *fungal infections* would prompt a low ranking for these tumors.

Likewise, the relatively low incidence of oral *benign* and *malignant mesenchymal tumors* would prompt the clinician to rank the minor salivary tumors above this group in the differential diagnosis, except in special cases (e.g., von Recklinghausen's disease) (Fig. 7-28).

The *mature lesions of inflammatory hyperplasia (fibromas)* are much more common than the minor salivary tumors; but unlike the minor salivary tumors, they are seldom dome shaped. The fibromas are usually slightly polypoid or sessile. Also the agent causing the chronic irritation usually can be identified. In addition, the posterolateral aspect of the hard palate is not a common site for a solitary inflammatory hyperplastic lesion but is the most frequent site for a minor salivary tumor.

Soft minor salivary gland tumors. Several lesions must be considered in the differential diagnosis for a soft fluctuant minor salivary gland tumor: mucoceles, superficial cavernous hemangiomas, submerged lipomas, and plexiform neurofibromas.

The *plexiform neurofibroma* is uncommon

except in patients with von Recklinghausen's disease. It and the *submerged lipoma* cannot be differentiated from the minor salivary tumors in this group through palpation or visual examination. Aspiration, however, will be productive in the case of soft and fluctuant minor salivary gland tumors although not with plexiform neurofibromas or lipomas. The yellow color of the superficial lipoma will prompt the clinician to identify this lesion.

Superficial cavernous hemangiomas will be bluish, whereas deeper ones will be pink. Both are emptiable by carefully applied digital pressure, and this fact differentiates hemangiomas from both mucoceles and soft salivary gland tumors.

Mucoceles are encountered much more often than are minor salivary gland tumors; but approximately 82% of them occur on the lower lip, which is not a common site for a minor salivary gland tumor (Cohen, 1965). In practical terms, mucoceles cannot be differentiated from some of the early malignant tumors containing mucus (e.g., mucoepidermoid tumor, mucus-producing adenocarcinoma). Thus it is important to do a biopsy of all mucoceles. The relative incidences of mucoceles and minor salivary gland tumors would prompt the diagnostician to conclude that a small superficial retention-phenomenon type of lesion is much more likely to be a mucocele than a salivary gland tumor.

Ulcerated minor salivary tumors. The possible causes of a large ulcerated lesion or ulcerated exophytic lesion of the posterior hard palate include the following: tumors of the minor glands, squamous cell carcinomas (usually commence on the soft palate), antral malignancies, major aphthous ulcers, gummas, necrotizing sialometaplasia, lethal midline granulomas, Wegener's granulomatosis, lymphomas, actinomycosis, blastomycosis, tuberculosis, rhinoscleroma, mucormycosis, and noma.

Fig. 7-26 illustrates a variety of lesions that may occur as palatal swellings.

MANAGEMENT

The recurrence rates for the minor salivary gland tumors vary greatly from series to series but are relatively high even in the case of benign tumors. This is probably because the original tumor was incompletely excised. Although many of these benign tumors appear encapsulated, a few tumor cells frequently penetrate the pseudocapsule and escape excision (Clairmont et al., 1977; Krolls and Boyers, 1972). Thus it is expedient to include a wide margin of normal tissue in the removal of benign or malignant lesions. Frozen sections completed at surgery will help to indicate whether or not the margins are free of tumor and whether a wider excision should be undertaken. Malignant tumors are treated by surgery or a combination of surgery and radiation.

Close posttreatment surveillance should be maintained to detect early recurrences. In malignant cases, chest radiographs every 6 months are imperative to detect the earliest stage of possible pulmonary metastasis.

PERIPHERAL BENIGN MESENCHYMAL TUMORS

Individual types of oral peripheral mesenchymal tumors are uncommon lesions; but when considered as a group, they demonstrate a more impressive incidence. Such a group would include the following:

Lipomas

Myomas (rhabdomyoma and leiomyoma)

Peripheral nerve tumors (neurofibroma, plexiform type of neurofibroma, schwannoma, traumatic neuroma)

FEATURES

All the peripheral benign mesenchymal tumors are nodular, polypoid, or dome shaped with smooth contours and are characteristically covered with normal mucosa unless chronically traumatized. They may be located on the tongue, buccal mucosa, lips, hard and soft palates, floor of the mouth, and vestibule. They usually are asymptomatic, grow slowly, and can be moved over the deeper tissue. When situated within loose connective tissue, they are often exceptionally movable.

The lipoma, although the most frequently occurring true peripheral mesenchymal tumor, is an uncommon oral lesion. It is soft, spongy, fluctuant, sessile, and usually nodular or dome shaped and asymptomatic. The superficial lesion will have a definite yellow color, and in the thinned mucosa over its surface there are often small red blood vessels that blanch on pressure (Fig. 7-28). The lipoma that is deeper in the tissue will have a normal pink mucosal color, however, and its margin may be so diffuse as to be difficult to define by palpation.

Greer and Richardson (1973) reviewed a large series of oral lipomas and reported that most of the lesions were discovered in patients between ages 27 and 70 years, with an average age of 51. The female-to-male ratio in the patients they studied was 7:1. Fifty percent of the lesions were located on the buccal mucosa; the next most frequent site was the mandibular retromolar area. These authors found that whether a particular lesion was yellow or not depended on its depth in the tissue and the amount of fibrosis present.

In contrast, MacGregor and Dyson (1966) reported that males and females were equally involved in their series; but they also found that the most frequent site was the buccal mucosa, followed by the buccal sulcus, tongue, lower lip, and floor of the mouth.

Hatziotis (1971) reviewed a large series of oral lipomas and reported that there was a higher incidence in men. Vindenes (1978) reported that in his series the lesions were distributed equally in men and women. The buccal mucosa was the most frequent site in his study, followed by the lips.

The remainder of the benign mesenchymal tumors (i.e., myomas, schwannomas, firm neurofibromas, traumatic neuromas) are so different from the lipoma that they must be discussed separately. With the exception of the fibromas, most of which are actually mature inflammatory hyperplastic lesions, these other lesions seldom occur in the oral cavity—although some have been reported on the tongue, lip, buccal mucosa, floor of the mouth, and posterior palate (Figs. 7-27 and 7-28). They are invariably firm with discrete borders; and if situated in the loose connective tissue layer, they will be freely movable.

DIFFERENTIAL DIAGNOSIS

Since the lipoma is so different from the other benign mesenchymal tumors, its differential diagnosis is best discussed separately. Lesions that should be included in the differential diagnosis are dense focal aggregates of Fordyce's granules, the buccal fat pads, the superficial cavernous hemangioma, lymphangioma, myxomas, and varicosity, the superficial retention phenomena (e.g., mucoceles, ranulas, mucus-producing salivary gland tumors) as well as deeper vascular lesions, and the plexiform neurofibroma.

The *plexiform neurofibroma* may be difficult to distinguish from a nonyellow lipoma, because both lesions are soft, fluctuant, and nonproductive on aspiration. Because of their rarer occurrence, however, the plexiform neurofibromas should follow the lipoma in the differential diagnosis, except in patients with von Recklinghausen's disease (Fig. 7-28, C and D).

Superficial retention phenomena (mucoceles,

Fig. 7-27. Mesenchymal tumors. **A,** Leiomyoma of the tip of the tongue. **B,** Amputation neuroma on the ventral surface of the tongue. (From Kelly, D. E., and Harrigan, W. F.: J. Oral Surg. **35:** 316-318, 1977. Copyright by the American Dental Association. Reprinted by permission.)

Fig. 7-28. Benign mesenchymal tumors. **A** and **B,** Lipomas. **C,** Neurofibroma on the palate. **D,** Multiple neurofibromatosis. (**C** courtesy R. Nolan, D.D.S., Waukegan, Ill. **D** courtesy P. D. Toto, D.D.S., Maywood, Ill.)

ranulas, mucus-producing minor salivary gland tumors) will be bluish in color whereas the *deeper lesions* will be pink. Aspiration of a clear sticky viscous fluid (mucus) will distinguish the retention phenomena from the lipoma.

The *superficial cavernous hemangioma, lymphangioma,* and *varicosity* will also be blue in color, so the clinician should be able to distinguish them from the yellow lipoma. When they are deeper and covered with normal pink mucosa, they may be differentiated from the lipoma by the fact that they are emptiable by pressure. Also aspiration of hemangiomas and varicosities will produce venous blood and of lymphangiomas a frothy lymph fluid whereas aspiration of a lipoma will be nonproductive.

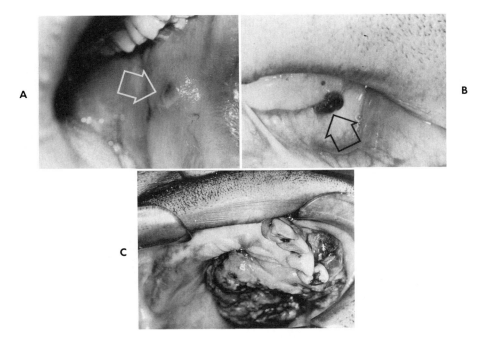

Fig. 7-29. Nevus and melanoma. **A,** Intramucosal nevus. **B,** Melanoma. **C,** Large melanoma. (**A** courtesy E. Kasper, D.D.S., Maywood, Ill. **B** courtesy D. Skuble, D.D.S., Hinsdale, Ill. **C** courtesy R. Oglesby, D.D.S., Chicago.)

The *buccal fat pads* in some individuals may become so hypertrophied as to be mistaken for a lipoma by the inexperienced clinician. They should be recognized, however, by their characteristic bilateral position in the posterior cheek. They are usually symmetric in size, except when one has herniated after trauma or a surgical procedure.

If the lipoma is superficial, its yellow color will distinguish it from all the foregoing entities except the *dense focal aggregates of Fordyce's granules*. These should not pose a problem, though, since the accumulations of spots are seldom larger than a few millimeters in diameter, and the presence of individual granules scattered in the surrounding mucosa will aid the clinician in recognizing them.

Since the myoma, schwannoma, firm neurofibroma, and traumatic neuroma have so many similar features and few if any distinguishing characteristics, they are difficult to discern from each other clinically and attempts to make a differential diagnosis are not of any potential value.

Lesions that must be considered with this group include the *fibroma,* the *firm minor salivary gland tumors,* and the *granular cell myoblastoma.*

When a firm smoothly contoured lesion covered with normal pink mucosa is encountered on the oral mucosa, the examiner would normally conclude (on the basis of incidence) that it is a fibroma. If it is on the posterolateral aspect of the palate, he would likely consider it a minor salivary gland tumor. Finally, if it is on the dorsal surface or lateral border of the tongue, it could be a granular cell myoblastoma. In addition, Cherrick and co-workers (1973) found that the tongue is the most frequent intraoral site for a leiomyoma.

MANAGEMENT

The recommended treatment for the peripheral benign mesenchymal tumors is excision, microscopic examination of the tumor tissue, and postoperative surveillance to prevent an undetected recurrence.

NEVUS AND MELANOMA

Nevus and melanoma are uncommon intraoral tumors that are discussed in detail in Chapter 9 as macular and exophytic brownish, bluish, or black lesions. If individual lesions are typical in appearance (i.e., pigmented and firm), the list of possibilities is quite restricted (Fig. 7-29).

Fig. 7-30. Exophytic metastatic tumors. **A,** Metastatic melanoma. **B,** Metastatic adenocarcinoma from the lung. **C,** Three metastatic lesions from a carcinoma of the esophagus in a 46-year-old man. (**A** from Mosby, E. L., et al.: Oral Surg. **36:**6-10, 1973. **B** courtesy R. Kallal, D.D.S., Chicago. **C** courtesy E. Robinson, D.D.S., Toledo, Ohio.)

If a lesion is amelanotic and is discovered in its early stage of development, however, it will appear as a firm, smoothly contoured, nodular or somewhat polypoid mass covered with normal-appearing mucosa (Fig. 7-30, *A*). The list of possible lesions then must include fibromas and benign mesenchymal tumors; and if its surface is ulcerated as the result of trauma, it may mimic a pyogenic granuloma.

As the intraoral amelanotic melanoma grows and is traumatized, its surface will ulcerate and become necrotic. At this stage it will have the clinical appearance of a malignant tumor. Then, based on the incidence of similar-appearing lesions, the possible diagnoses would be ranked as follows: squamous cell carcinoma, malignant salivary gland tumor, peripheral metastatic tumor, malignant primary mesenchymal tumor, and amelanotic melanoma.

PERIPHERAL METASTATIC TUMORS

Intrabony metastatic tumors are much more common than peripheral metastatic tumors of the oral cavity (Hatziotis et al., 1973) and are discussed in detail in Chapter 20.

Much of what has been described for the central tumors is true for the peripheral variety, so this material will not be repeated here. In addition, peripheral metastatic tumors are discussed in Chapter 10 under solitary red lesions. The most common tumors to metastasize to the oral cavity originate in the kidney, lung, gastrointestinal tract, breast, and prostate gland.

FEATURES

There may be a history of a primary tumor, or the symptoms of such a tumor may indicate its probable existence.

Bhaskar (1971) stated, however, that 33% of

the oral secondary tumors he examined were the first recognized indication of the presence of the primary tumor.

The secondary lesion may be asymptomatic and thus be detected on routine examination; or the patient may describe any or all of the following as the chief complaint: intraoral swelling that may or may not relate to an ill-fitting denture, pain, or paresthesia. Although the secondary malignancy may occur anywhere on the oral mucosa, it is more frequently seen on the tongue and gingivae (Hatziotis et al., 1973).

Because the nests of tumor cells are expanding beneath the surface epithelium, the early lesions are usually nodules or dome-shaped masses— smooth surfaced and covered with normal-appearing mucosa. At this stage the lesions will frequently appear deceptively benign (Fig. 7-30). Later, as a result of trauma, their surfaces may ulcerate and become necrotic. When this occurs, they will appear clinically to be malignant.

As the tumor invades the deeper tissue, it will become fixed. In some cases underlying bone is destroyed, and this circumstance causes the appearance of an ill-defined, ragged, saucerlike radiolucency on the periphery of the bone.

DIFFERENTIAL DIAGNOSIS

The advanced ulcerated lesion of a peripheral metastatic tumor may appear very similar to an *exophytic squamous cell carcinoma, malignant salivary tumors, malignant mesenchymal tumors,* and an *amelanotic melanoma.*

If the patient has a history of a tumor elsewhere, this would prompt the clinician to consider the possibility that the oral lesion is a metastatic tumor. If there is no history of a primary tumor or suggestive symptoms, however, the incidence of these tumors would prompt the clinician to pursue the possibility of the entities in foregoing groups in the indicated order. If the patient is less than 20 years old, the probability that the lesion is a squamous cell carcinoma or a malignant salivary gland tumor is considerably lessened.

MANAGEMENT

The rationale of the management of metastatic tumors is considered in Chapter 19.

PERIPHERAL MALIGNANT MESENCHYMAL TUMORS

Since reports of intraoral peripheral malignant mesenchymal tumors (e.g., neurosarcomas, malignant schwannomas, fibrosarcomas, rhabdo-

Fig. 7-31. Rhabdomyosarcoma of the dorsal surface of the tongue. (Courtesy N. Choukas, D.D.S., Maywood, Ill.)

myosarcomas, hemangiosarcomas, liposarcomas) are found only occasionally in the lierature, it must be concluded that this group of lesions is quite uncommon. The intraoral osteogenic sarcoma and chondrosarcoma occur relatively more frequently, but these usually are central in origin and consequently are discussed in Part III of the text.

There is very little that is distinctive about the mesenchymal tumors that would differentiate them from any of the clinically benign or malignant-appearing lesions, except possibly the age factor (Fig. 7-31). These tumors usually affect a considerably younger age group than does squamous cell carcinoma.

RARITIES
Solitary lesions

The rare solitary exophytic lesions represent a formidable number of entities (Figs. 7-32 and 7-33). In spite of the fact that these lesions are rare, the clinician must at least be aware of the possibilities they represent when he is examining a specific lesion.

The circumstances and special characteristics may prompt him to include one or more of these lesions in the differential list.

Actinomycosis
Ameloblastoma (peripheral)
Antral neoplasms
Blastomycosis
Bohn's nodule (Epstein's pearl)
Chondroma of soft tissue
Choristoma
Condyloma acuminatum

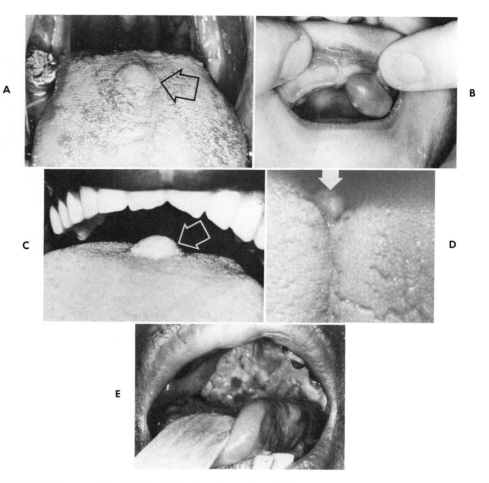

Fig. 7-32. Rare exophytic lesions. **A,** Granular cell myoblastoma. **B,** Epulis of the newborn. **C,** Lingual thyroid gland. **D,** Persistent tuberculum impar. **E,** Lymphosarcoma in the pharynx. (**A** courtesy R. Kallal, D.D.S., Chicago. **C** and **D** courtesy E. Kaspar, D.D.S., Maywood, Ill. **E** courtesy E. Evans, D.D.S., St. Cloud, Minn.)

Fig. 7-33. Rare exophytic lesions. **A,** Sialolith in Wharton's duct. **B,** Two dome-shaped masses on lower lip are focal hyperplasias of minor salivary glands. Each aggregation of minor glands drained through one duct opening in the middle of each mass.

Condyloma lata
Congenital epulis of the newborn
Early chancre
Early gumma
Eruption cyst
Extraosseous odontogenic tumor
Focal hyperplasia of the minor salivary glands
Giant cell fibroma
Gingival cyst
Granular cell myoblastoma
Granulomatous fungal disease
Hamartoma
Histiocytosis X
Juvenile nasopharyngeal angiofibroma
Juvenile xanthogranuloma
Keratoacanthoma
Lead poisoning
Lethal midline granuloma
Leukemic enlargement
Lingual thyroid gland
Lymphoma
Median nodule of the upper lip
Median rhomboid glossitis (nodular variety)

Molluscum contagiosum
Myxoma of soft tissue or oral focal mucinosis
Necrotizing sialometaplasia
Neuroectodermal tumor of infancy
Nodular leukoplakia
Plasmacytoma of soft tissue
Pseudosarcomatous fasciitis
Sarcoidosis
Sialolith
Squamous acanthoma
Sturge-Weber syndrome
Teratoma
Tuberculosis
Verruciform xanthoma

Multiple lesions

As are the solitary rarities, the rare exophytic pathoses that occur as multiple lesions are almost impossible to rank according to frequency; they are listed therefore in alphabetical order (Figs. 7-34 and 7-35).

Acanthosis nigricans
Acrokeratosis verruciformis of Hope

Fig. 7-34. Multiple gingival masses. **A,** Mouth-breathing gingivitis. **B,** Phenytoin (Dilantin) hyperplasia. **C,** Familial gingival fibromatosis. (**C** courtesy W. Heaton, D.D.S., Chicago.)

Fig. 7-35. Multiple exophytic masses. **A,** Amyloidosis in multiple myeloma. **B,** Multiple blood clots in heroin-induced thrombocytopenic purpura. **C,** Multiple condyloma lata of the lower lip. **D,** Multiple papules of palate in a patient with Darier's disease. (**A** from Kraut, R. A., Buhler, J. E., LaRue, J. R., and Acevedo, A.: Oral Surg. **43:**63-68, 1977. **B** from Kraut, R. A., and Buhler, J. E.: Oral Surg. **46:**637-640, 1978. **C** courtesy S. Smith, D.D.S., Chicago. **D** courtesy M. Bernstein, D.D.S., Louisville.)

Amyloidosis (Fig. 7-35, *A*)
Bohn's nodules
Chronic granulomatous disease
Condyloma acuminata
Condyloma lata (Fig. 7-35, *C*)
Cowden's disease
Crohn's disease
Cysticercosis
Darier's disease (Fig. 7-35, *D*)
Eruption cysts
Focal dermal hypoplasia (Goltz's syndrome)
Focal epithelial hyperplasia (Fig. 7-36)
Gardner's syndrome
Giant cell fibromas
Hereditary telangiectasia
Histiocytosis X
Idiopathic gingival fibromatosis
Kaposi's sarcoma
Lichenoides chronica
Lymphangiomas of neonates

Lymphomas
Lymphomatoid papulosis
Lymphoproliferating disease of the palate
Molluscum contagiosum
Multiple exostoses
Multiple expansile metastatic carcinomas
Multiple fibroepithelial hyperplasias (Fig. 7-37)
Multiple gingival cysts
Multiple hamartoma neoplasia syndrome
Multiple lipomas
Multiple melanomas
Multiple mucoceles
Multiple myeloma
Multiple papillomas
Multiple peripheral brown giant cell lesions (hyperparathyroidism)
Multiple verrucae
Noonan's syndrome
Orodigitofacial syndrome (multiple hamartomas of the tongue)

Fig. 7-36. Focal epithelial hyperplasia in an Israeli patient. (From Buchner, A.: Oral Surg. **46:** 64-69, 1978.)

Fig. 7-37. Multiple fibroepithelial hyperplasia seen on the tongue, buccal mucosa, and lips of a patient. (From Buchner, A., and Sandbank, M.: Oral Surg. **46:**34-39, 1978.)

Oral florid papillomatosis
Phenytoin hyperplasia
Pyostomatitis vegetans
Sarcoidosis
Syndrome of multiple mucosal neuromas, pheochromocytoma, and carcinoma of the thyroid
Syphilitic papules
Thrombocytopenic purpura
Urticaria pigmentosa
von Recklinghausen's disease
Xanthoma disseminatum

SPECIFIC REFERENCES

Adkins, K. F.: Lymphoid hyperplasia in the oral mucosa, Aust. Dent. J. **18:**38-40, 1973.

Angelopoulos, A. P.: Pyogenic granuloma of the oral cavity: statistical analysis of its clinical features, J. Oral Surg. **29:** 840-847, 1971.

Bhaskar, S. N.: Oral manifestations of metastatic tumors, Postgrad. Med. **49:**155-158, 1971.

Bhaskar, S. N., and Cutright, D. E.: Giant cell reparative granuloma (peripheral): report of 50 cases, J. Oral Surg. **29:**110-115, 1971.

Chaudhry, A. P., Vickers, R. A., and Gorlin, R. J.: Intraoral minor salivary gland tumors, Oral Surg. **14:**1194-1226, 1961.

Cherrick, H. M., Dunlap, C. L., and King, O. H.: Leiomyomas of the oral cavity, Oral Surg. **35:**54-66, 1973.

Clairmont, A. A., Richardson, G. S., and Hanna, D. C.: The pseudocapsule of pleomorphic adenomas (benign mixed tumors), Am. J. Surg. **134:**242-243, 1977.

Cohen, L.: Mucoceles of the oral cavity, Oral Surg. **19:**365-372, 1965.

Cundiff, E. J.: Peripheral ossifying fibroma. A review of 365 cases, M.S.D. thesis, Indiana University, 1972. Cited in Shafer, W. G., Hine, M. K., and Levy, B. M.: A textbook of oral pathology, ed. 3, Philadelphia, 1974, W. B. Saunders Co.

Cutright, D. E.: The histopathologic findings in 583 cases of epulis fissuratum, Oral Surg. **37:**401-411, 1974.

Eversole, L. R., and Rovin, S.: Reactive lesions of the gingiva, J. Oral Pathol. **1:**30-38, 1972.

Giansanti, J. S., and Waldron, C. A.: Peripheral giant cell granuloma: review of 720 cases, J. Oral Surg. **27:**787-791, 1969.

Greer, R. O., and Richardson, J. F.: The nature of lipomas and their significance in the oral cavity: a review and report of cases, Oral Surg. **36:**551-557, 1973.

Hatziotis, J.: Lipoma of the oral cavity, Oral Surg. **31:**511-524, 1971.

Hatziotis, J., Constantinidou, H., and Papanayotou, P. H.: Metastatic tumors of the oral soft tissues, Oral Surg. **36:** 544-550, 1973.

King, D. R., and Moore, G. E.: An analysis of torus palatinus in a transatlantic study, J. Oral Med. **31:**44-46, 1976.

King, R. E., Altini, M., and Shear, M.: Basal extensions in human mucosa, J. Oral Pathol. **8:**140-146, 1979.

Knapp, M. J.: Oral tonsils: location, distribution, and histology, Oral Surg. **29:**155-161, 1970a.

Knapp, M. J.: Pathology of oral tonsils, Oral Surg. **29:**295-304, 1970b.

Krolls, S. O., and Boyers, R. C.: Mixed tumors of salivary glands: long-term follow-up, Cancer **30:**276-281, 1972.

Krolls, S. O., and Hicks, J. L.: Mixed tumors of the lower lip, Oral Surg. **35:**212-217, 1973.

MacGregor, A. J., and Dyson, D. P.: Oral lipoma. A review of the literature and report of twelve new cases, Oral Surg. **21:**770-777, 1966.

Main, J. H. P., McGurk, F. M., McComb, R. J., and Mock, D.: Salivary gland tumors: review of 643 cases, J. Oral Pathol. **5:**88-102, 1976.

Miller, E. L.: Clinical management of denture-induced inflammations, J. Prosthet. Dent. **38:**362-365, 1977.

Soskolne, A., Ben-Amar, A., and Ulmansky, M.: Minor salivary gland tumors: a survey of 64 cases, J. Oral Surg. **31:**528-531, 1973.

Thackray, A. C., and Sabin, L. H.: International histological classification of tumors. No. 7. Histological typing of salivary gland tumors, Geneva, 1972, World Health Organization.

Tomich, C. E.: Oral focal mucinosis: a clinicopathologic and histochemical study of eight cases, Oral Surg. **38:**714-724, 1974.

Uohara, G. I., and Federbusch, M. D.: Removal of papillary hyperplasia, J. Oral Surg. **26:**463-466, 1968.

Vindenes, H.: Lipomas of the oral cavity, Int. J. Oral Surg. **7:**162-166, 1978.

Weathers, D. R., and Callihan, M. D.: Giant-cell fibroma, Oral Surg. **37:**374-384, 1974.

Whitaker, L. A., Lehr, H. B., and Askovitz, S. I.: Cancer of the tongue, Plast. Reconstr. Surg. **30:**363-370, 1972.

GENERAL REFERENCES

Abbey, L. M., Sawyer, D. R., and Syrop, H. M.: Oral squamous acanthoma, Oral Surg. **45:**255-260, 1978.

Acevedo, A., and Buhler, J. E.: Plasma-cell granuloma of the gingiva, Oral Surg. **43:**196-200, 1977.

Ackerman, L. V.: Verrucous carcinoma of the oral cavity, Surgery **23:**670-678, 1948.

Akin, R. K., Kreller, A. J., and Walters, P. J.: Papillary cystadenoma of the lower lip: report of case, J. Oral Surg. **31:**858-860, 1973.

Baden, E., Moskow, B. S., and Moskow, R.: Odontogenic gingival epithelial hamartoma, J. Oral Surg. **26:**702-714, 1968.

Baden, E., and Newman, R.: Liposarcoma of the oropharyngeal region, Oral Surg. **44:**889-902, 1977.

Ballard, B. R., Suess, G. R., Pickren, J. W., et al.: Squamous-cell carcinoma of the floor of the mouth, Oral Surg. **45:**568-579, 1978.

Batsakis, J. G., Wozniak, K. J., and Regezi, J. A.: Acinous cell carcinoma: histogenetic hypothesis, J. Oral Surg. **35:**904-906, 1977.

Baughman, R. A.: Lingual thyroid and lingual thyroglossal tract remnants, Oral Surg. **34:**781-799, 1972.

Berg, R., Eisenbud, L., Sciubba, J., and Stern, M.: Adenoid cystic carcinoma of the palate: twenty-five years of active disease, J. Oral Med. **34:**81-84, 1979.

Bhaskar, S. N.: Lymphoepithelial cysts of the oral cavity: report of twenty-four cases, Oral Surg. **21:**120-128, 1966.

Bhaskar, S. N., and Jacoway, J. R.: Peripheral fibroma and peripheral fibroma with calcification: report of 376 cases, J. Am. Dent. Assoc. **73:**1312-1320, 1966.

Bhaskar, S. N., and Jacoway, J. R.: Pyogenic granuloma—clinical features, incidence, histology, and result of treatment: report of 242 cases, J. Oral Surg. **24:**391-398, 1966.

Birkholz, H., Sills, A. H., and Reid, R. A.: Peripheral ameloblastoma, J. Am. Dent. Assoc. **97:**685-660, 1978.

Blair, A. E., and Edwards, D. M.: Congenital epulis of the newborn, Oral Surg. **43:**687-691, 1977.

Blok, P., van Delden, L., and van der Waal, I.: Non-Hodgkin's lymphoma of the hard palate, J. Oral Surg. **47:**445-452, 1979.

Brandjord, R. M., Reaume, C. E., and Wesley, R. K.: Leiomyosarcoma of the floor of the mouth: review of the literature and report of case, J. Oral Surg. **35**:590-594, 1977.

Brown, C. R., Merrill, S. S., and Lambson, G. O.: Microbiologic aspects of papillary hyperplasia, Oral Surg. **28**:545-551, 1969.

Buchner, A., and Mass, E.: Focal epithelial hyperplasia in an Israeli family, Oral Surg. **36**:507-511, 1973.

Buchner, A., and Sandbank, M.: Multiple fibroepithelial hyperplasia of the oral mucosa, Oral Surg. **46**(1):34-39, 1978.

Cardo, V. A., and Stratigos, G. T.: Verrucous carcinoma of the palate: report of case, J. Oral Surg. **31**:61-63, 1973.

Chen, S.: Adenoid cystic carcinoma of minor salivary gland, Oral Surg. **42**:606-619, 1976.

Chen, S., and Miller, A. S.: Neurofibroma and schwannoma of the oral cavity, Oral Surg. **47**:522-528, 1979.

Cherrick, H. M.: Benign neural sheath neoplasm of the oral cavity, Oral Surg. **32**:900-909, 1971.

Choukas, N. C.: Lymphosarcoma of the maxilla, Oral Surg. **23**:567-572, 1967.

Christensen, R. E., Jr., Hertz, R. S., and Cherrick, H. M.: Intraoral juvenile xanthogranuloma, Oral Surg. **45**:586-590, 1978.

Christensen, R. E., Jr., Sanders, B., and Mudd, B.: Local recurrence of solitary plasmacytoma of the mandible, J. Oral Surg. **36**:311-313, 1978.

Clairmont, A. A., and Conley, J. J.: Malignant schwannoma of the parapharyngeal space, J. Otolaryngol. **6**:28-30, 1977.

Clairmont, A. A., and Conley, J. J.: Malignant mixed tumor of the soft palate, J. Oral Surg. **36**:394-395, 1978.

Cohen, N., Plaschkes, Y., Peuzner, S., and Loewenthal, M.: Review of 57 cases of keratoacanthoma, Plast. Reconstr. Surg. **49**:138-144, 1972.

Crocker, D. J., Cavalaris, C. J., and Finch, R.: Intraoral minor salivary gland tumors, Oral Surg. **29**:60-68, 1970.

Doyle, J. L.: Benign lymphoid lesions of the oral mucosa, Oral Surg. **29**:31-37, 1970.

Dreyer, W. P., and Thomas, C. J.: Diphenylhydantoinate-induced hyperplasia of the masticatory mucosa in an edentulous epileptic patient, Oral Surg. **45**:701-706, 1978.

Drummond, J. F., Giansanti, J. S., Sabes, W. R., and Smith, C. R.: Sialadenoma papilliferum of the oral cavity, Oral Surg. **45**:72-75, 1978.

Dunlap, C. L., and Barker, B. F.: Necrotizing sialometaplasia, Oral Surg. **37**:722-727, 1974.

Dunley, R. E., and Jacoway, J. R.: Necrotizing sialometaplasia, Oral Surg. **47**:169-172, 1979.

Eisenbud, L., Katzka, I., and Platt, N.: Oral manifestations in Crohn's disease: report of case, Oral Surg. **34**:770-773, 1972.

Elzay, R. P., and Dutz, W.: Myxomas of the paraoral-oral soft tissue, Oral Surg. **45**:246-254, 1978.

Epker, B. N., and Henny, F. A.: Clinical, histopathologic, and surgical aspects of intraoral minor salivary gland tumors, J. Oral Surg. **27**:792-804, 1969.

Eversole, L. R.: Mucoepidermoid carcinoma: review of 815 reported cases, J. Oral Surg. **28**:490-494, 1970.

Eversole, L. R., Rovin, S., and Sabes, W. R.: Mucoepidermal carcinoma of minor salivary glands: report of 12 cases with follow-up, J. Oral Surg. **30**:107-112, 1972.

Eversole, L. R., and Sabes, W. R.: Granular cell sheath lesions: report of cases, J. Oral Surg. **29**:867-871, 1971.

Eversole, L. R., Schwartz, W. D., and Sabes, W. R.: Central and peripheral fibrogenic and neurogenic sarcoma of the oral regions, Oral Surg. **36**:49-62, 1973.

Eversole, L. R., and Sorenson, H. W.: Oral florid papillomatosis in Down's syndrome, Oral Surg. **37**:202-207, 1974.

Farman, A. G., and Kay, S.: Oral leiomyosarcoma: report of a case and review of the literature pertaining to smooth-muscle tumors of the oral cavity, Oral Surg. **43**:402-409, 1977.

Fejerskov, O., and Nybroe, L.: Primary malignant melanoma of the hard palate: report of case, J. Oral Surg. **31**:53-55, 1973.

Fendell, L. D., and Smith, J. R.: Betel-nut–associated cancer: report of case, J. Oral Surg. **28**:455-456, 1970.

Fin, P.: Rare oral viral disorders (molluscum contagiosum, localized keratoacanthoma, verrucae, condyloma acuminatum, and focal epithelial hyperplasia), Oral Surg. **34**:604-618, 1972.

Firfer, H., Sohn, D., Heurlin, R., and Stuteville, O. H.: Neurilemmoma of the tongue, Oral Surg. **21**:139-142, 1966.

Fitzpatrick, B. N.: Parathyroid adenoma, Oral Surg. **27**:653-658, 1969.

Forney, S. K., Foley, J. M., Sugg, W. E., Jr., and Oatis, G. W., Jr.: Necrotizing sialometaplasia of the mandible, Oral Surg. **43**:720-726, 1977.

Freedman, G. L., Hooley, J. R., and Gordon, R. C.: Congenital epulis in the newborn: report of 2 cases, J. Oral Surg. **26**:61-64, 1968.

Freedman, P. D., and Lumerman, H.: Sialadenoma papilliferum, Oral Surg. **45**:88-94, 1978.

Friedman, J. M., Gormley, M. B., Kupfer, S., and Jarrett, W.: Cavernous hemangioma of the oral cavity: review of the literature and report of case, J. Oral Surg. **31**:617-619, 1973.

Frim, S. P., and Giunta, J.: Monomorphic adenoma (basal cell adenoma): report of case, J. Oral Surg. **37**:426-427, 1979.

Gallo, W. J., Moss, M. Shapiro, D. N., and Gaul, J. V.: Neurilemmoma: review of the literature and report of five cases, J. Oral Surg. **35**:235-236, 1977.

Gardner, G. D.: Peripheral ameloblastoma: a study of 21 cases, including 5 reported as basal cell carcinoma of the gingiva, Cancer **39**:1625-1633, 1977.

Giansanti, J. S., Baker, G. O., and Waldron, C. A.: Intraoral mucinous, minor salivary gland lesions, presenting clinically as tumors, Oral Surg. **32**:918-922, 1971.

Giunta, J., and Cataldo, E.: Lymphoepithelial cysts of the oral mucosa, Oral Surg. **35**:77-84, 1973.

Godby, A. F., Sonntag, R. W., and Cosentino, B. J.: Hypernephroma with metastasis to the mandibular gingiva, Oral Surg. **23**:696-700, 1967.

Gold, B. D., Sheinkopf, D. E., and Levy, B.: Dermoid epidermoid, and teratomatous cysts of the tongue and the floor of the mouth, J. Oral Surg. **32**:107-111, 1974.

Goldberg, M. H., Nemarich, A. N., and Danielson, P.: Lymphangioma of the tongue: medical and surgical therapy, J. Oral Surg. **35**:841-844, 1977.

Greer, J. L., Crine, J. D., and Tilson, H. B.: Malignant lymphomas of the oral soft tissues, J. Oral Surg. **36**:971-974, 1978.

Greer, R. O., and Goldman, H. M.: Oral papillomas, Oral Surg. **38**:435-440, 1974.

Greer, R. O., and Hammond, W. S.: Extraosseous ameloblastoma: light microscopic and ultrastructural observations, J. Oral Surg. **36**:553-556, 1978.

Greer, R. O., and Sanger, R. G.: Primary intraoral sarcoidosis, J. Oral Surg. **35**:507-509, 1977.

Hanks, C. T., Fischman, S. L., and Guzman, M. N.: Focal epithelial hyperplasia, Oral Surg. **33**:934-943, 1973.

Hatziotis, J. C.: Lipoma of the oral cavity, Oral Surg. **31**:511-524, 1971.

Hicks, J. L., and Nelson, J. F.: Juvenile nasopharyngeal angiofibroma, Oral Surg. **35**:807-817, 1973.

Howland, W. J., Armbrecht, E. C., and Miller, J. A.: Oral manifestations of multiple idiopathic hemorrhagic sarcoma of Kaposi: report of two cases, J. Oral Surg. **24**:445-449, 1966.

Jacobson, S., and Shear, M.: Verrucous carcinoma of the mouth, J. Oral Pathol. **1**:66-75, 1972.

Jelso, D. J.: A light microscope study of mixed tumors of human salivary glands, J. Oral Surg. **32**:353-362, 1974.

Kahn, L. B.: Adenoid cystic carcinoma of the salivary gland and its histologic variants, Oral Surg. **44**:394-404, 1977.

Kapstad, B., and Bang, G.: Verrucous carcinoma of the oral cavity treated with Bleomycin, Oral Surg. **42**:588-590, 1976.

Kerpel, S. M., Freedman, P. D., and Lumerman, H.: The papillary cystadenoma of minor salivary gland origin, Oral Surg. **46**:820-826, 1978.

Kessel, L. J., and Stewart, J. B.: Malignant lymphoma of the tongue: a case report, Br. J. Oral Surg. **14**:31-35, 1976.

King, O. H., Jr. Blankenship, J. P., King, W. A., and Coleman, S. A.: The frequency of pigmented nevi in the oral cavity: report of 5 cases, Oral Surg. **23**:82-90, 1967.

Kraut, R. A., and Buhler, J. E.: Heroin-induced thrombocytopenic purpura, Oral Surg. **46**:637-640, 1978.

Kraut, R. A., Buhler, J. E., LaRue, J. R., and Acevedo, A.: Amyloidosis associated with multiple myeloma, Oral Surg. **43**:63-68, 1977.

Krolls, S. O., and Hicks, J. L.: Mixed tumors of the lower lip, Oral Surg. **35**:212-217, 1973.

Kuepper, R. C., and Harrigan, W. F.: Actinomycosis of the tongue: report of case, J. Oral Surg. **37**:123-125, 1979.

LaForgia, P., and Mangini, F.: Nodular isolated actinomycosis of the tongue—a case report, Dent. Survey **55**:48-51, 1979.

Lekkas, C., and van Hoof, R.: Lipoma of the tongue, Oral Surg. **48**:214-215, 1979.

Lumerman, H., Bodner, B., and Zambito, R.: Intraoral (submucosal) pseudosarcomatous nodular fasciitis, Oral Surg. **34**:239-244, 1972.

Mader, C., and Gay, W.: Intraoral adenoid cystic carcinoma, J. Am. Dent. Assoc. **99**:212-214, 1979.

Mandel, L.: Bilateral ranulas: report of case, J. Oral Surg. **28**:621-622, 1970.

Matsumura, T., and Kawakatsu, K.: Verrucous carcinoma of oral mucosa: histochemical patterns and clinical behaviors, J. Oral Surg. **30**:349-356, 1972.

McDaniel, R. K., Luna, M. A., and Stimson, P. G.: Lingual thyroid: report of case, J. Am. Dent. Assoc. **81**:1156-1158, 1970.

Melrose, R. J., Abrams, A. M., and Howell, F. V.: Mucoepidermoid tumors of the intraoral minor salivary glands: a clinicopathologic study of 54 cases, J. Oral Pathol. **2**:314-324, 1973.

Miller, A. S., Leifer, C., Chen, S., and Harwick, R. D.: Oral granular-cell tumors: report of twenty-five cases with electron microscopy, Oral Surg. **44**:227-237, 1977.

Miller, A. S., and Pullon, P. A.: Enlarging lump on posterior dorsum of the tongue, Dent. Survey **55**:56, 1979.

Mittelman, D., and Kaban, L. B.: Recurrent "non-Hodgkin's lymphoma" presenting with gingival enlargement: report of a case, Oral Surg. **42**:792-800, 1976.

Mosby, E. L., Sugg, W. E., and Hiatt, W. R.: Gingival and pharyngeal metastasis from a malignant melanoma, Oral Surg. **36**:6-10, 1973.

Nelson, J. F., Tsaknis, P. J., and Konzelman, J. L.: Noonan's syndrome: report of a case with oral findings, J. Oral Med. **33**:94-96, 1978.

Page, L. R., Drummond, J. F., Daniels, H. T., et al.: Blastomycosis with oral lesions: report of two cases, Oral Surg. **47**:157-160, 1979.

Papanayotou, P. H., and Kayavis, J. G.: Epidermoid implantation cyst of the lower lip: report of case, J. Oral Surg. **35**:585-586, 1977.

Parks, C. R., and Bottomley, W. K.: Lymphoblastic lymphosarcoma, Oral Surg. **33**:297-301, 1972.

Peterson, L. J.: Granular-cell tumor: review of the literature and report of a case, Oral Surg. **37**:728-735, 1974.

Pisanty, S.: Keratoacanthoma of the face, Oral Surg. **21**:506-510, 1966.

Pisanty, S.: Bilateral lipomas of the tongue, Oral Surg. **42**:451-453, 1976.

Praetorius-Clausen, F.: Rare oral viral disorders (molluscum contagiosum, localized keratoacanthoma, verrucae, condyloma acuminatum, and focal epithelial hyperplasia), Oral Surg. **34**:604-618, 1972.

Pryse, J. C., Kuftinec, M. M., and Burzynski, N. J.: A dentocranio-facial study of the multiple endocrine neoplasia (men) type 3 syndrome, J. Oral Med. **34**:85-88, 1979.

Prystowsky, S. D., and Rogers, J. G.: A median nodule of the upper lip as a familial trait, Oral Surg. **42**:653-655, 1976.

Pullon, P. A., and Cohen, D. M.: Oral metastasis of retinoblastoma, Oral Surg. **37**:583-588, 1974.

Quinn, J. H., McDonnell, H. A., and Leonard, G. L.: Multifocal angiosarcoma of the gingiva: report of case, J. Oral Surg. **28**:215-217, 1970.

Reaume, C. E., and Sofie, V. L.: Lingual thyroid, Oral Surg. **45**:841-845, 1978.

Regezi, J. A., Batsakis, J. G., and Courtney, R. M.: Granular cell tumors of the head and neck, J. Oral Surg. **37**:402-406, 1979.

Robinson, E. R., and Stuteville, O. H.: Metastatic tumors to the tongue: review of the literature and report of a case, Oral Surg. **15**:980-985, 1962.

Russel, E. A., and Nelson, J. F.: Adenocarcinoma of the palate—diagnosis and management, Oral Surg. **45**:528-531, 1978.

Samit, A. M., Mashberg, A., and Greene, G. W.: Necrotizing sialometaplasia, J. Oral Surg. **37**:353-356, 1979.

Schneider, L. C.: Cellular hemangiomas of the oral mucosa, J. Oral Med. **33**:9-11, 1978.

Schuler, S., McDonald, J. S., Strull, N. J., and Alpert, B.: Soft-tissue reticulum-cell sarcoma of the oral cavity, Oral Surg. **45**:984-991, 1978.

Scofield, H. H., Werning, J. T., and Shukes, R. C.: Solitary intraoral keratoacanthoma, review of the literature and report of case, Oral Surg. **37**:889-898, 1974.

Sela, J., and Ulmansky, M.: Mucous retention cysts of salivary glands, J. Oral Surg. **27**:619-623, 1969.

Seldin, H. M., Seldin, S. D., Rakowes, W., and Jarrett, W. J.: Lipomas of the oral cavity: report of 26 cases, J. Oral Surg. **25**:270-274, 1967.

Setia, A. P.: Severe bleeding from a pregnancy tumor, Oral Surg. **36**:192-194, 1973.

Seward, M. H.: Eruption cyst: an analysis of its clinical features, J. Oral Surg. **31**:31-35, 1973.

Shapiro, D. N.: Lipoma of the oral cavity, Oral Surg. **27**:571-576, 1969.

Smith, J. F.: Salivary gland lesions—variations and predictability, Oral Surg. **27**:499-521, 1969.

Solomon, M. P., Rosen, Y., and Delman, A.: Intraoral submucosal pseudosarcomatous fibromatosis, Oral Surg. **38**:264-269, 1974.

Strader, R. J.: Review of a technique in the treatment of mucoceles, Oral Surg. **37**:695-698, 1974.

Suckiel, J. M., Davis, W. H., Patakas, B. M., and Kaminishi, R. M.: Early and late manifestations of necrotizing sialometaplasia, J. Oral Surg. **36**:902-905, 1978.

Sugimura, M., Sakamoto, T., Tsubakimoto, M., et al.: Analysis of 102 lesions diagnosed as "palatal tumor" in a spot diagnosis, Int. J. Oral Surg. **4**:143-150, 1975.

Summers, C. J.: Prevalence of tori, J. Oral Surg. **26**:718-720, 1968.

Summers, L., and Booth, D. R.: Intraoral condyloma acuminatum, Oral Surg. **38**:273-278, 1974.

Svirsky, J. A., Freeman, P. D., and Lumerman, H.: Solitary

intraoral keratoacanthoma, Oral Surg. **43:**116-122, 1977.

Swart, J. G. N., van der Kwast, W. A. M., Snow, G. B., and van der Waal, I.: Possible myxoma of the floor of the mouth: report of case, J. Oral Surg. **35:**501-503, 1977.

van der Waal, I., Bruggenkate, T. M., and van der Kwast, W. A. M.: Focal epithelial hyperplasia in a child from Surinam, Int. J. Oral Surg. **4:**168-171, 1975.

van Wyk, C. W., Staz, J., and Farman, A. G.: Focal epithelial hyperplasia in a group of South Africans: its clinical and microscopic features, J. Oral Pathol. **6:**1-13, 1977.

Weitzner, S., and Hentel, W.: Metastatic carcinoma in tongue, Oral Surg. **25:**278-281, 1968.

Weitzner, S., Lockey, M. W., and Lockard, V. G.: Adult rhabdomyoma of soft palate, Oral Surg. **47:**70-73, 1979.

Wertheimer, F. W., and Georgen, G. J.: Abbreviated case report: intraoral acinic cell adenocarcinoma, Oral Surg. **32:**923-926, 1971.

Wesley, R. K., and Zielinski, R. J.: Osteocartilaginous choristoma of the tongue: clinical and histopathologic considerations, J. Oral Surg. **36:**59-61, 1978.

Wiener, A. P.: Monomorphic adenoma, canalicular variant: report of case, J. Oral Surg. **35:**414-415, 1977.

Wilson, D. F., and MacEntee, M. I.: Papillary cystadenoma of ectopic minor salivary gland origin, Oral Surg. **37:**915-918, 1974.

Wysocki, G. P., and Brooke, R. I.: Oral manifestations of chronic granulomatous disease, Oral Surg. **46:**815-819, 1978.

Wysocki, G. P., and Hardie, J.: Ultrastructural studies of intraoral verruca vulgaris, Oral Surg. **47:**58-62, 1979.

Yoshimura, Y.: Two cases of plasmacytoma in the oral cavity, Int. J. Oral Surg. **5:**82, 1976.

Young, W. G., and Claman, S. M.: A lymphoepithelial cyst of the oral cavity: report of case, Oral Surg. **23:**62-70, 1967.

Yurosko, J. J., Wall, T. M., Vopal, J. J., and Gossman, J. R.: Clinical-pathological Conference Case 20. Part 1. Idiopathic gingival fibromatosis, J. Oral Surg. **35:**820-821, 1977.

Zegarelli, D. J.: Chondroma of the tongue, Oral Surg. **43:**738-745, 1977.

8

Pits, fistulas, and draining lesions

Henry M. Cherrick

Pits, fistulas, and draining lesions of the oral cavity include the following:

Pits
Fovea palatinae
Commissural lip pit
Postsurgical pit
Postinfection pit
Rarities
  Congenital lip pits

Intraoral fistulas and sinuses
Chronic draining alveolar abscess
Suppurative infection of the parotid and submandibular glands
Draining mucocele and ranula
Oroantral fistula
Oronasal fistula
Draining chronic osteomyelitis
Draining cyst
Patent nasopalatine duct

Cutaneous fistulas and sinuses
Pustule
Sinus draining a chronic dentoalveolar abscess or chronic osteomyelitis
Extraoral draining cyst
Specific sinuses
  Thyroglossal duct
  Second branchial sinus
  Congenital aural sinuses
Salivary gland fistula or sinus
Auriculotemporal syndrome
Orocutaneous fistula
Rarities
  First branchial arch sinus and fistula

Pits, fistulas, and draining lesions of the cervicofacial complex may present perplexing diagnostic problems partially because of the numerous types that may occur in the oral cavity as well as in the skin of the face and neck. The process of differential diagnosis may be facilitated, however, by dividing these lesions into three categories: (1) pits, (2) intraoral fistulas and sinuses, and (3) cutaneous fistulas and sinuses.

The terms "fistula" and "sinus" will be used in the present discussion as prescribed by their traditional definitions. A *fistula* (Latin, reed instrument or pipe) is an abnormal pathway between two anatomic cavities; it has two openings. A *sinus* (Latin, hollow, bay, or curve) represents the tract of a lesion; it has but one opening. The fistula and the sinus are designated according to the surfaces or surface on which they open (e.g., oroantral fistula, cutaneous sinus). The clinician is undoubtedly aware that most writers in the relevant literature do not strictly adhere to these definitions. There is, furthermore, an increasing tendency to use the terms interchangeably.

Pits

A "pit" is defined as a hollow fovea or indentation. Pits, generally being blind tracts lined with epithelium, are normal anatomic landmarks or else are congenital, postsurgical, or inflammatory defects.

FOVEA PALATINAE

The foveae palatinae are two indentations formed by a coalescence of several mucous gland ducts near the midline of the palate. These round to oval-shaped depressions are always located in soft tissue on the anterior part of the soft palate. They can usually be accentuated by the patient's holding his nose while attempting to blow it. They may be probed to a depth of 0.5 to 2 mm and, when manipulated, may secrete a clear mucinous fluid. On rare occasion the foveae palatinae are abnormally large and may be confused with fistulas or sinuses (Fig. 8-1).

COMMISSURAL LIP PIT

The commissural lip pit is a relatively common developmental disorder, although there is no

Fig. 8-1. Fovea palatinae located on the anterior aspect of the soft palate.

Fig. 8-2. Bilateral commissural lip pits. (Courtesy D. Bonomo, D.D.S., Flossmoor, Ill.)

Fig. 8-3. Postsurgical pit after incision and drainage.

agreement concerning its incidence. Everett and Wescott (1961) reported that approximately 0.2% of the population showed this anomaly; however, Baker (1966) found that 12% of whites and 20% of blacks in his series demonstrated it.

The commissural lip may be bilateral or unilateral. Unilateral examples occur equally on the right and on the left sides of the mouth. The pits are located at the angles of the mouth, with the tracts diverging dorsolaterally into the cheek (Fig. 8-2). They range in length from a shallow dimple to a tract measuring up to 4 mm in length, and the tissue is slightly raised about the opening.

Microscopically the tract is lined with stratified squamous epithelium that continues into the vermilion tissue of the lip. Mucous gland ducts may empty into the sinus, and as a result mucus frequently can be milked from the tract.

DIFFERENTIAL DIAGNOSIS

The differential diagnosis of the commissural lip pit is discussed in the differential diagnosis section at the end of the chapter (p. 176). The commissural lip pit especially must be differentiated from the *congenital lip pit*, which is seen on the vermilion border of the lower lip but not at the commissures. The congenital lip pit, however, is extremely rare—occurring in about one of 2 billion births (Gorlin and Pindborg, 1964, p. 117).

MANAGEMENT

The commissural lip pit is asymptomatic and requires no treatment.

POSTSURGICAL PIT

The postsurgical pit is the result of wound breakdown secondary to infection or of failure to

obliterate dead space in wound closure (i.e., improper layer closure and inadequate eversion of the wound). The postsurgical pit clinically appears as a dimple or puckering of a portion or the entire surface of a wound with a comparatively shallow depression that can be easily probed (Fig. 8-3).

DIFFERENTIAL DIAGNOSIS

The differential diagnosis of the postsurgical pit is discussed in the differential diagnosis section under "Postinfection Pit."

MANAGEMENT

The management of the postsurgical pit is discussed in the management section under "Postinfection Pit."

POSTINFECTION PIT

The postinfection pit usually results from loss of tissue often due to necrosis. After the infection

Fig. 8-4. Postinfection pit after successful treatment of actinomycosis with antibiotic therapy.

has been resolved, there is a subsequent inversion of the surface tissue into the resultant defect, forming a postinfection pit. The clinical appearance is similar to that of the postsurgical pit (Fig. 8-4). Accurate diagnosis may be determined from facts obtained through the patient interview.

DIFFERENTIAL DIAGNOSIS

The postsurgical pit and the postinfection pit may have similar appearances to a *stitch abscess, sinus, fistula,* or *congenital pit;* however, they may be distinguished from the latter entities by a careful history and physical examination, including depth exploration (with lacrimal probes), and by radiographic examination (i.e., with lacrimal probes or gutta-percha points inserted into the pits).

MANAGEMENT

Shallow postsurgical and postinfection pits within the oral cavity do not usually require treatment. If food debris tends to become deposited in them, however, they should be surgically eliminated. Esthetic consideration would prompt the same excision and layer closure as for extraoral pits.

RARITIES

The congenital lip pit represents one of the rarest defects in the human body, occurring in about one out of every 2 billion births (Gorlin and Pindborg, 1964, p. 117). Thus it will not be discussed further here.

Intraoral fistulas and sinuses

CHRONIC DRAINING ALVEOLAR ABSCESS

The dentoalveolar abscess is one of the most common lesions observed by the dental profession and frequently occurs as a draining lesion. The pathogenesis and radiologic appearance of this lesion are discussed in Chapter 16.

The vast majority of dentoalveolar abscesses result from a direct extension of an acute pulpitis or an acute nonsuppurative periodontitis or from an acute exacerbation of a periapical granuloma, cyst, or chronic abscess. Less commonly the dentoalveolar abscess is of the postoperative type, arising from an infection of the alveolar socket after surgical removal of a tooth. The pulp tissue of the extracted tooth may or may not have been infected before removal, or the infection may have been implanted during the extraction. In either case the process remains essentially the same: a pyogenic infection of the periodontal ligament and bone (Eisenbud and Klatell, 1951).

The surrounding tissue attempts to localize the pyogenic infection by forming an enclosure of granulation tissue, which in turn is surrounded by fibrous connective tissue. This results in a well-circumscribed lesion containing necrotic tissue, disintegrated and viable polymorphonuclear leukocytes, and other inflammatory cells in the periapical region of the tooth or alveolus.

This well-circumscribed periapical abscess may penetrate the surrounding fibrotic capsule and form a sinus that opens on the mucosa or the skin of the face or neck—usually as a result of one or more of the following circumstances:

1. Inability of the body to completely contain or localize the causative organisms
2. Increase in the number of the causative organisms, or introduction of a more virulent organism through the carious tooth or by surgical intervention
3. Lowering of the patient's general resistance during the course of formation of the periapical abscess
4. Trauma or surgical intervention, mechanically producing an opening in the fibrous capsule

The enlarging dentoalveolar abscess contains purulent material that is under pressure. Because of this pressure, the pus proceeds through the bone along the path of least resistance until it reaches the surface, where because of the limiting fibrous periosteal layer, it temporarily forms

Fig. 8-5. Intraoral sinus from a chronic alveolar abscess of the central incisor. Note the parulis on the labial aspect.

Fig. 8-6. Palatal sinus openings draining chronically infected pulpless teeth. **A,** Lateral incisor. **B,** Maxillary first molar.

a subperiosteal abscess. Eventually it will erode through the periosteum and penetrate the soft tissue, again following the path of least resistance.

The path of least resistance is determined by the location of the breakthrough in the bone and the anatomy of the muscles and fascial planes in the area. In the majority of cases, the expanding abscess points and discharges onto the nearest external surface in the oral cavity; however, there are other more complicated paths of infection, but their discussion is beyond the scope of this text.

FEATURES

In the majority of cases, the intraoral sinuses open on the labial and buccal aspects of the alveolus (Fig. 8-5) because usually the apices of both the maxillary and the mandibular teeth are located nearer to the buccal than to the lingual cortical plate. Thus this route offers the shorter distance for the burrowing pus.

In the maxilla, however, the roots of the lateral incisors and the palatal roots of the molars frequently lie closer to the palatal cortical plate than to the buccal plate; therefore an infection in these roots often produces a palatal abscess and perhaps a sinus (Fig. 8-6). Also the mandibular molar roots, particularly of the third molars, are located closer to the lingual plate. In addition, since most of the root tips of these teeth lie below the mylohyoid muscle, the pus drains into the submandibular space and the deeper planes of the neck instead of through an intraoral sinus.

Clinically the sinus opening has the appearance of a small ulcer. This opening is most commonly found on the buccal alveolus adjacent to the infected tooth. The palatal sinus, on the other

hand, may burrow for a variable distance on the palate before it points and erodes through the palatal mucosa. The mucosal sinus opening may be red and will bleed easily. It may be level with the mucosa or raised (a parulis). Occasionally, after temporary emptying of an abscess, the sinus will heal and form a slightly raised pale papule. After a period of time, pus will accumulate and another sinus opening will develop. Therefore the clinician may find multiple sinus scars and/or patent sinuses in some cases. Palpation of the surrounding mucosa may cause the expression of pus from the sinus(es).

The patient will frequently give a history of pain that started as a dull ache and progressed to an increasingly severe throbbing. A sudden decrease in the pain usually signals the formation of a sinus; and the pain may disappear completely at this stage. Although the offending tooth will often be tender to percussion, vitality tests will be negative since the pulp is nonvital.

Radiographically dentoalveolar abscesses and sinuses usually appear as radiolucent areas of bone resorption around a root apex. The radiolucent area is frequently ragged in outline and generally lacks a sclerotic margin, although such a margin may develop. This aspect is discussed in detail in Chapter 16.

DIFFERENTIAL DIAGNOSIS

The differential diagnosis of a chronic draining alveolar abscess is discussed in the differential diagnosis section at the end of the chapter (p. 176).

MANAGEMENT

The management of pulpoperiapical sequelae is discussed at length in Chapter 16.

SUPPURATIVE INFECTION OF THE PAROTID AND SUBMANDIBULAR GLANDS

Purulent discharge from Stensen's papillae and the sublingual caruncles indicates the presence of a suppurative infection of the parotid and/or submandibular salivary glands, respectively (Fig. 8-7). Thus pus-forming infections of these two major salivary glands are included in this discussion of intraoral draining lesions.

Suppurative infection of the parotid or submandibular salivary glands characteristically occurs in the very ill or debilitated patient. Most often these patients are over 65 years or within the first 4 weeks after birth (Gustafson, 1951; Krippachne et al., 1962; Shulman, 1950). In the delicate or debilitated newborn infant of low birth weight, inflammation of the glands usually develops from complicating diseases that produce dehydration (Gustafson, 1951). In the older individual there are many predisposing factors, among which are dehydration, malnutrition, and oral cancer. Surgery, especially abdominal and orthopedic procedures, is one of the most common predisposing factors for suppurative infection of the salivary glands (Krippachne et al., 1962).

The route taken by the microbes is thought to

be either (1) retrograde, from the oral cavity to the affected gland via the secretory duct, or (2) antegrade, from the bloodstream to the gland (Shulman, 1950). *Staphylococcus aureus* is the most frequent infectious agent found, but infections of *Streptococcus viridans* and *Escherichia coli* are also common; in addition, many bacteria of the oral flora may induce this infection.

For an infection to be introduced via the secretory duct, a change in the person's well-being must have occurred, usually in one of four ways:

1. Increase in the number of microorganisms in the oral cavity, or introduction of a more virulent type than is normally present at the duct opening
2. Lowering of the individual's general resistance
3. Decrease in salivary secretion
4. Decrease in the bactericidal effect of the saliva (Gustafson, 1951)

The infection commences in the epithelial cells of the large secretory duct and spreads progressively to the smaller ducts and finally to the gland parenchyma. Once infection of the parenchyma has occurred, multiple abscesses may form and then coalesce. If the infection is not eradicated, pus may penetrate the gland capsule and spread into the surrounding tissue, usually along one of three pathways: (1) downward into the deep fascial planes of the neck, (2) backward into the external auditory canal, or (3) outward onto the skin of the face (Gustafson, 1951; Krippachne et al., 1962).

FEATURES

Often the first manifestation of a parotid infection is pain in the temporomandibular joint region; this is followed by swelling of the gland, which usually becomes hot, indurated, and tender to palpation. Redness may be found around the orifices of the infected gland's duct, and pus may be expressed by pressure on the gland (Fig. 8-7).

The patient may be febrile and quite ill, often out of proportion to what would be expected from such a localized infection. In the majority of cases, there is a concomitant rise in the number of leukocytes, especially in the neutrophil fraction.

DIFFERENTIAL DIAGNOSIS

The differential diagnosis of suppurative infection of the parotid and/or submaxillary glands is discussed in the differential diagnosis section at the end of the chapter (p. 176).

Fig. 8-7. Purulent discharge from Wharton's duct during an acute infection of the submandibular gland.

MANAGEMENT

Treatment of choice is the immediate institution of antibiotic therapy. Since many of the infections are resistant to the most frequently used antibiotics, the most effective treatment is with type-specific antibiotics—indicated by typing the causative organism from pus expressed from the duct. If there is no improvement within 3 to 4 days, incision and drainage should be undertaken.

DRAINING MUCOCELE AND RANULA

The mucocele and ranula are retention phenomena of the minor salivary glands and the sublingual salivary gland, respectively. These lesions are included in Chapter 7 as exophytic lesions and are discussed in Chapter 9 with the bluish lesions. They are included in this chapter because occasionally they occur as chronic draining lesions.

As a mucocele or a ranula increases in size, the overlying epithelium and mucous membrane become stretched. As it grows progressively larger, it may cause the mucous membrane to become extremely thin and undergo spontaneous rupture. Often a traumatic incident in the oral cavity will promote rupture. The exudate is usually clear, viscous, and sticky. When drainage occurs, the mucocele or ranula decreases in size; however, healing of the rupture occurs rapidly and the lesion gradually fills and expands again. Continual repetition of these events can produce a chronic sinus (Fig. 8-8).

DIFFERENTIAL DIAGNOSIS

The differential diagnosis of mucocele and ranula is discussed in Chapters 7 and 9 and at the end of this chapter (p. 176).

MANAGEMENT

Treatment consists of either total enucleation or marsupialization. During the surgical correction other salivary ducts or glands may be injured, so recurrences are not uncommon.

OROANTRAL FISTULA

The oroantral fistula is a pathologic pathway connecting the oral cavity and the maxillary sinus (Fig. 8-9). In the majority of cases, it is caused by the extraction of a tooth; but it may also be caused by other trauma, tuberculosis (Juniper, 1973), syphilis (Shafer et al., 1974, p. 376), or leprosy (Lighterman et al., 1962). Occasionally it results from tooth-associated pathoses, such as periapical infection or cyst formation. The oroantral fistula is discussed also in Chapter 30.

Most oroantral fistulas are initiated by the extraction of a maxillary tooth—the primary reason being the proximity of the sinus floor to the apex of the tooth. Usually the apices of the posterior teeth are within 3 mm of the cortical floor of the maxillary sinus, or they may project into the maxillary sinus with only a small amount of bony covering. The roots of the second molar are closest to the maxillary sinus, followed by those of the first molar, third molar, second premolar, first premolar, and canine.

The palatal root apices of the molars are most frequently involved in the formation of a fistula. Extraction of the maxillary first molar accounts for 50% of the oroantral fistulas with the other 50% almost evenly accounted for by extraction of the second and third molars (Killey and Kay, 1967; Mustian, 1933; Wowern, 1971).

An oroantral fistula generally forms as a result of inadequate blood clot formation in the alveolus

Fig. 8-8. Sinus opening from a chronically draining mucocele.

Fig. 8-9. Oroantral fistula in an edentulous patient. (Courtesy P. Akers, D.D.S., Chicago.)

after violation of the maxillary sinus. This may be consequential to a sinusitis or secondary infection or the introduction of packs or other hemostatic agents in the socket.

FEATURES

Clinically an oroantral fistula will frequently be seen immediately after extraction of a tooth, especially if the root has been fractured and displaced into the antrum; however, it may not always be apparent or suspected, especially if the extraction was atraumatic.

A patient with a chronic oroantral fistula may experience one or more symptoms. The most frequent complaint is the passage of fluids from the oral cavity into the nose, or the patient may have a foul or salty taste in his mouth. Facial pain or an associated frontal headache may develop from an acute maxillary sinusitis. The headache is generally of a throbbing nature and is exacerbated by any movement of the head. A unilateral nasal discharge accompanied by a sensation of nasal obstruction or nocturnal coughing due to the draining of exudate into the pharynx may also occur. The swallowed exudate may produce a morning anorexia. The patient may also experience an epistaxis on the affected side.

Other less common symptoms are the eversion of an antral polyp through the fistula, resulting in the sudden appearance of an exophytic mass on the alveolar crest, the aspiration of air into the mouth through the tooth socket, and the inability to blow out the cheeks or draw on a cigarette (Killey and Kay, 1967).

A patient with an oroantral fistula will have a pathologic pathway by which microorganisms of the oral flora may enter the maxillary sinus and cause a sinusitis. The severity of the sinusitis will depend on several factors, varying usually inversely with the diameter of the fistula. If the opening is large, pressure will not increase because the exudate will escape freely into the oral cavity; hence the patient will complain of little if any pain. On the other hand, if the diameter of the fistula is quite small, an acute sinusitis will be more likely to develop.

A patient with an acute maxillary sinusitis may experience swelling and redness overlying the sinus and the molar eminence as well as pain beneath the eye. Palpation over the maxilla will increase the pain, and the teeth with roots adjacent to the sinus will often be painful or sensitive to percussion. The pain may also be referred to other teeth in the arch and to the ear.

In a chronic sinusitis from an oroantral fistula, nasal and postnasal discharges are ordinarily present along with a fetid breath and a vague pain or stuffiness in the affected side of the face (Burket, 1971, p. 233; Shafer et al., 1974, p. 470).

Radiologically the maxillary sinus may appear cloudy because of an accumulation of blood, mucus, or purulent exudate. In some cases there may be a distinct fluid level evident (Worth, 1963, p. 706).

DIFFERENTIAL DIAGNOSIS

When the fistula is large and a definite communication between the oral cavity and the maxillary sinus can be demonstrated, the diagnosis is obvious. In other cases, when the inflammation of the sinus mucosa has sealed the fistula, the diagnosis may be more difficult because the clinician is unable to clinically identify the tract. A radiograph, however, may reveal a break in the continuity of the sinus floor, which identifies the site of the previously patent defect.

MANAGEMENT

An oroantral fistula should be repaired as soon as possible after it has occurred. When there is a sinusitis or an infection, however, the surgical repair of the fistula must wait until the infection has been eliminated. An intensive course of antibiotic therapy should be instituted for a minimum of 1 week, the duration depending on the extent of the infection. A decongestant should also be employed to encourage free drainage of the pus and mucus. Antral lavage is needed in some cases and may be accomplished through the fistulous opening. Occasionally an antrostomy may be needed to help in draining the sinus (Anderson, 1969; Killey and Kay, 1967).

Many elaborate surgical methods have been developed for closing oroantral fistulas. In all the methods the fistula is excised and the surrounding necrotic tissue is curetted. The various methods include utilization of bone grafts, gold foil grids, and buccal and palatal flap techniques (Goldman et al., 1969; Ziemba, 1972). Once the antral infection has been eliminated, closure of the defect will usually be successful regardless of the surgical technique employed; however, some surgeons prefer to augment the closure by packing the maxillary sinus with gauze and subsequently removing the gauze through a nasal antrostomy. This procedure helps to ensure that a sinusitis does not develop during the critical stage of fistula closure.

ORONASAL FISTULA

The oronasal fistula is a pathologic epithelium-lined defect connecting the oral and nasal cav-

Fig. 8-10. Oronasal fistulas in a patient with congenital cleft palate. (Courtesy P. Akers, D.D.S., Chicago.)

Fig. 8-11. Oronasal fistula as a result of a healed syphilitic gumma.

ities. The most frequent causes of this type of fistula are congenital cleft palate, trauma, infection, neoplasm, or an unsuccessful surgical procedure. The most common traumatic injuries are automobile accidents and gunshot wounds (Clarkson et al., 1946).

Although a complete midline cleft of the palate is not a diagnostic problem, occasionally a partial cleft, an unsuccessful repair of a complete cleft, or some cases of anterior clefts will resemble an oronasal fistula from some other cause (Fig. 8-10).

Occasionally an acute dentoalveolar abscess of a maxillary central incisor will burrow through the maxilla into the floor of the nasal cavity. Infrequently the abscess may exit high on the nasolabial aspect of the maxilla and tunnel up beneath the periosteum into the floor of the nose, where it usually forms an opening in the anterior portion of the nasal cavity (Gorlin and Goldman, 1970). Other less frequent infectious causes are leprosy, syphilitic gumma, and mycotic infections (Gorlin and Goldman, 1970, p. 346; Lighterman et al., 1962) (Fig. 8-11). The fistula may also be produced during the surgical removal of buried roots, teeth, odontomas, tori, cysts, or benign and malignant neoplasms.

FEATURES

When there is an obvious defect in the maxilla, the patient will complain of food passing into his nose and will often demonstrate nasal speech. Probing of the defect, in conjunction with radiographic examination, will usually establish a definitive diagnosis of an oronasal fistula.

MANAGEMENT

The indicated treatment is usually the surgical removal of the fistula with subsequent flap ad-

vancement. When the fistula is considered too large to close surgically, a prosthetic appliance can be utilized to cover the defect.

DRAINING CHRONIC OSTEOMYELITIS

Chronic osteomyelitis is discussed in Chapter 16 as a periapical radiolucency, in Chapter 20 as an ill-defined radiolucency, in Chapter 24 as a mixed radiolucent-radiopaque lesion, and in Chapter 27 as a radiopacity. In the present chapter its draining aspect will be featured.

FEATURES

Clinically a sinus will be present extending from the medullary bone through the cortical plate to the mucous membrane or skin (Figs. 8-12 and 8-13). Should the infection exit the bone above a muscle attachment, the sinus opening may be a considerable distance from the offending infection. The mandible is much more frequently involved than the maxilla (Chapter 20). Chronic draining cases are ordinarily painless unless there is an acute or subacute exacerbation. Radiographically the involved bone may be radiolucent, mixed radiolucent-radiopaque, or completely radiopaque, depending on the course of the infection. Sequestra and involucra formation are often noted.

DIFFERENTIAL DIAGNOSIS

The differential diagnosis of a draining chronic osteomyelitis is discussed in the differential diagnosis section at the end of the chapter (pp. 176 and 177).

MANAGEMENT

The management of a draining chronic osteomyelitis is discussed in detail in Chapter 20.

Fig. 8-12. Cutaneous sinus secondary to chronic osteo-myelitis at a fracture site.

Fig. 8-13. Cutaneous sinus secondary to osteoradio-necrosis.

DRAINING CYST

Odontogenic and nonodontogenic cysts of intraosseous origin may perforate and produce sinuses that drain onto the oral mucosa. Secondary infections, or direct extensions by expansion of the cysts, generally produce these lesions. Cysts caused by inflammation and cysts that frequently become large (e.g., periapical cysts, dentigerous keratocysts, odontogenic keratocysts) are the greatest offenders.

FEATURES

Prior to sinus formation, there is usually pain or swelling of the involved area. When the periosteum and mucosa are perforated, the pain ceases and a purulent discharge ensues. If the sinus is small, the drainage may continue as a chronic case. If the sinus is large, however, the infection will regress because of the excellent drainage established and the cyst may disappear completely because of its decompression. Clinically, when the cyst is large, there is expansion of the cortical plate. Palpation of the area will commonly elicit pain, crepitus, and a purulent or cheesy discharge. Radiologically a well-delineated radiolucency is noted.

DIFFERENTIAL DIAGNOSIS

The differential diagnosis of a draining cyst is covered in the differential diagnosis section at the end of the chapter (p. 176).

MANAGEMENT

After the infection has been eliminated, the cyst must be treated by enucleation, marsupialization, or decompression. Associated teeth may require extraction or root canal therapy.

PATENT NASOPALATINE DUCT

A completely patent nasopalatine duct or canal is an extremely rare condition, especially in the adult. It arises when the embryologic nasopalatine ducts fail to become obliterated. In embryonic life the nasopalatine ducts are paired epithelium-lined tubes extending from the nasal cavity to the oral cavity within the incisive canal. The nasal orifices of the ducts lie on each side of the nasal septum in the anterior nasal floor.

The nasopalatine duct is funnel shaped and continuous with the nasal epithelium. It extends downward in an anterior direction more or less parallel with the facial contour of the premaxilla to exit as two slits—one on each side of the palatine papilla, which overlies the incisive foramen (Hill and Darlow, 1945; Rosenberger, 1944).

The nasopalatine duct is lined with ciliated pseudostratified columnar epithelium to within 3 or 4 mm of the palatal opening. At this level there is a transition to cuboidal epithelium and then to stratified squamous epithelium (Abrams et al., 1963; Burket, 1937; MacGregor, 1964).

Under normal circumstances the nasopalatine ducts disintegrate during fetal life and this oronasal communication is eliminated. In unusual cases all or part of the duct persists and remains patent in postnatal life. The completely patent nasopalatine duct is rare; however, circumstances in which only sections of the duct are

Fig. 8-14. Bilateral patent nasopalatine ducts with gutta-percha cones inserted into the defects. (Courtesy W. Goebel, D.D.S., Edwardsville, Ill.)

Fig. 8-15. Cutaneous sinus secondary to a periapical infection. This cutaneous lesion resembles a pustule.

patent at the nasal or oral end are more frequent. These sections exist as variable-length cul-de-sacs, with the nasal variety being more common. The oral variety of the patent nasopalatine duct may be identified by exposing a radiograph of the region with an orthodontic wire or gutta-percha point inserted into the defect (Fig. 8-14).

FEATURES

The patent nasopalatine duct is usually asymptomatic except when small particles of food or liquid are aspirated into the nose via the duct. This happens most often after the patient has begun wearing dentures, which may force liquid up the canal and into the nose.

DIFFERENTIAL DIAGNOSIS

The differential diagnosis of a patent nasopalatine duct is discussed in the differential diagnosis section at the end of the chapter (p. 175).

MANAGEMENT

Since the nasopalatine duct is usually asymptomatic, it generally does not require treatment.

Cutaneous fistulas and sinuses

PUSTULE

A pustule is a small superficial elevation of the skin or mucous membrane filled with pus. Pustules are included in this chapter primarily because they become draining lesions for a short time after they rupture; and they are included

secondarily because a solitary pustule on the skin overlying the jaws may easily be mistaken for a draining sinus from a chronic alveolar abscess or a chronic osteomyelitis (Fig. 8-15).

Pustules in the skin are common lesions and generally are the result of psoriasis, impetigo, acrodermatitis continua, or superficial bacterial diseases. Intraoral pustules are less common and are the result of superficial foreign bodies or specific diseases such as pustular psoriasis or subcorneal pustular stomatitis. Pustules are classified as primary or secondary (i.e., preceded by a vesicle or papule).

FEATURES

Clinically the pustule appears as a small superficial elevation filled with pus and possibly surrounded by a small area of erythema. These lesions are generally asymptomatic but may be tender or painful.

DIFFERENTIAL DIAGNOSIS

The differential diagnosis of a pustule is discussed in the differential diagnosis section at the end of the chapter (p. 177).

MANAGEMENT

A pustule seldom requires definitive treatment.

SINUS DRAINING A CHRONIC DENTOALVEOLAR ABSCESS OR CHRONIC OSTEOMYELITIS

As discussed previously under the intraoral draining lesions, pus from an enlarged dentoalveolar abscess or chronic osteomyelitic lesion burrows along the path of least resistance in both

Fig. 8-16. Cutaneous sinuses. **A,** Secondary to a draining dentoalveolar abscess. **B,** Caused by a submandibular space infection. **C,** Secondary to a canine space infection. (**A** courtesy S. Rosen, D.D.S., Los Angeles.)

hard and soft tissues. This burrowing usually results in the formation of a sinus that empties into the vestibule adjacent to the offending tooth. In some instances, however, the path of least resistance leads to the skin and thus to the formation of cutaneous sinuses (Figs. 8-15 and 8-16).

If the pus exits from bone deep within soft tissue, its spread will be governed by structures such as muscles and fascial sheets. Usually the infection will spread via fascial planes to the most available potential fascial space. A fascial space is a potential space that exists between two or more fascial investing layers or planes and is occupied by loose areolar tissue.

The infections of the head and neck are usually classified by their anatomic location. *Maxillary* dentoalveolar infections generally spread to the canine fossa, the buccal space, and the infratemporal space, whereas *mandibular* infections

spread to the mandibular, submandibular (submaxillary), submental, pterygomandibular, masseteric, parapharyngeal, parotid, and carotid spaces. The infection may spread by direct continuation from the dentoalveolar abscess along the fascial planes or by the lymphatic and blood systems. A detailed discussion of the individual space abscesses is beyond the scope of this chapter; the space abscesses of the neck are discussed in Chapter 14.

EXTRAORAL DRAINING CYST

The phenomenon of intraoral draining cysts was discussed earlier in the chapter (p. 168). This same situation can occur on the skin of the face and neck (Fig. 8-17). The more common cysts to occur in these cutaneous regions are sebaceous, epidermoid, dermoid, thyroglossal, preauricular, and branchial—which are dis-

Fig. 8-17. Chronic draining sebaceous cyst.

cussed more completely in Chapter 14 with masses in the neck.

SPECIFIC SINUSES
Thyroglossal duct

The thyroglossal duct is a hollow tube of epithelial cells marking the embryonic descent of the thyroid anlage from the tongue to the normal position of the thyroid gland in the neck. It normally becomes a solid stalk and usually undergoes degeneration and disappears. The original opening of the thyroglossal duct persists as a vestigial pit, the foramen cecum of the tongue. Occasionally this communcation fails to become obliterated and persists as a thyroglossal duct.

FEATURES

The thyroglossal duct is most commonly seen within the first two decades of life although a duct may begin to drain later in life because of local irritation, with resultant proliferation of the duct tissue. The sexes are approximately equally affected (Marshal, 1949; Stahl and Lyall, 1954; Ward, 1949).

The sinus opening from the thyroglossal duct may be at any level in the midline of the neck from the foramen cecum to the suprasternal notch. Most frequently it is located in the area adjacent to the hyoid bone, being more often noted just below the hyoid than just above (Fig. 14-13).

Only rarely is the duct seen in the suprasternal area or in the foramen cecum region. Although mainly a midline phenomenon, it is found on either side of the midline in a small percentage

of cases; and only rarely is it far enough from the midline to be confused with a branchial cleft sinus (Pollock and Stevenson, 1966). The epithelial lining of the duct is generally squamous epithelium or ciliated pseudostratified columnar epithelium. Ducts that have had recurrent bouts of inflammation may show little or no epithelial lining. Chronic inflammation is generally present in the surrounding connective tissue. On rare occasion, thyroid tissue is entrapped in the duct lining and neoplastic transformation into papillary thyroid carcinoma occurs (Jacques, 1970).

The literature suggests that the duct opening is usually secondary to infection of a thyroglossal duct cyst or to incomplete removal in previous operations. The cutaneous openings are 1 to 3 mm in diameter with a reddish, inflamed margin. Mucoid (clear) or purulent exudate may be expressed from the opening. The tract may be palpable back to the cyst. Rarely there are patent thyroglossal ducts emptying into the oral cavity via the foramen cecum. The patient will then usually complain of a bad taste in his mouth. A purulent exudate may be seen emanating from the foramen cecum and results from an infection with oral microorganisms.

DIFFERENTIAL DIAGNOSIS

The differential diagnosis of a thyroglossal duct is discussed in the differential diagnosis section at the end of the chapter (pp. 172 and 177).

MANAGEMENT

The indicated treatment is complete surgical excision of all thyroglossal duct epithelium. Because such excision is frequently difficult to complete, however, the recurrence rate is quite high (Brown, 1961).

Second branchial sinus (lateral cervical sinus)

A sinus or fistula of the second branchial cleft or pouch is fairly common, making up the vast majority of sinuses and fistulas of the lateral neck. This anomaly is thought to occur when the second branchial cleft or the second pharyngeal pouch or both fail to obliterate in the embryologic development of the fetus. The second branchial cleft separates the second and third branchial arches and, continuous with the second pharyngeal pouch internally, forms the second branchial membrane. The second branchial cleft and membrane usually become obliterated and disappear whereas the endoderm of the pouch gives rise to the palatine tonsil and tonsillar fossa. The line of obliteration of the second branchial cleft extends from the lower anterior border of the sternocleidomastoid muscle, through the fork of the carotid artery bifurcation, and upward toward the tonsillar fossa (Gore and Masson, 1959). Thus there can be three distinct types of branchial tracts (Bailey, 1933):

1. A cutaneous sinus that results from failure of obliteration of the second branchial cleft
2. A mucosal sinus that results from failure of obliteration of the second pharyngeal pouch
3. A fistula with both external and internal openings that results from failure of obliteration of both the cleft and the pouch

FEATURES

A second branchial sinus occurs equally in males and females; and although there appears to be a strong familial tendency at times, the majority of sinuses lack any known hereditary influence (Carp and Stout, 1928; Hyndman and Light, 1929). The sinus or fistula may be unilateral, bilateral, or rarely near the midline. The majority of anomalies are either external sinuses (50%) or complete fistulas (39%); and only occasionally an internal sinus is observed (Neel and Pemberton, 1945). The sinus or fistula is usually found at birth or within the first year. Adults with this anomaly will generally give a history of intermittent drainage since childhood or of a spontaneous discharge due to infection and rupture of a cervical cyst.

These branchial sinuses or fistulas appear as small dimples or small openings in the lateral region of the neck. The openings are usually close to the anterior border of the sternocleidomastoid muscle, the majority being in the lower neck just above the sternoclavicular joint. They sometimes occur in the middle or upper third of the neck along the anterior border of the sternocleidomastoid, however, but in these cases there is the possibility that the sinus was acquired through the formation of a sinus tract after infection of a branchial cyst.

DIFFERENTIAL DIAGNOSIS

A second branchial sinus may be differentiated from any other fistulas or sinuses of the neck by its position.

A *thyroglossal duct sinus* or *fistula* is found high in the midline, and the *first branchial sinus* may be found high in the neck posterior and inferior to the angle of the mandible. Rarely is a second branchial sinus ever seen near the midline or high in the neck.

The only other common draining lateral sinus in the neck is *suppurative lymphadenitis,* most commonly *tuberculous adenitis.* This entity can usually be differentiated by the history or by appropriate clinical diagnostic tests. Sometimes radiographs taken after the injection of radiopaque dye into the sinus or fistula are of diagnostic help.

MANAGEMENT

Once the diagnosis is made, the sinus or fistula must be excised in its entirety or there will be recurrence.

Congenital aural sinuses (auricular fistulas, preauricular fistulas, preauricular pits)

Congenital aural sinuses occur in approximately 1% of the population (Ewing, 1946). They are more common in blacks and Orientals than in whites (Selkirk, 1935) and are present equally in males and females, occurring bilaterally in approximately 25% of the cases. They are believed to be a non-sex-linked mendelian dominant trait with variable expressivity (Cowley and Calman, 1971). Occasionally they will be associated with other ear and facial anomalies, but as a rule they occur alone.

Current opinion on the cause of aural sinuses maintains that they evolved during the embryologic development of the external ear from the six ectoderm-covered mesenchymal nodules (the auditory tubercles) of the first two branchial arches. By the third fetal month these six nodules have proliferated and merge around the primitive external auditory meatus to form the external ear. Abnormal development may have resulted in the formation of congenital sinuses between the auditory tubercles.

FEATURES

There are seven possible sites about the ear for these pits to occur (Fig. 8-18). By far the most common is the marginal helix (90%). Sinuses are rarely seen at the other possible sites. The majority of congenital aural sinuses open at the anterior margin of the ascending limbs of the helices where the skin of the face joins the skin of the external ear.

The openings of the aural sinuses vary in size from pinpoint to 2 mm in diameter and, unless infected, are level with the surrounding skin.

The aural sinuses usually range in size from a slight fossa to a depression 1 cm deep, running internally in an inferoposterior direction anterior to the cartilaginous external auditory meatus (Fig. 8-19). They may be attached to the meatus by a ribbon of fibrous tissue, but they never pierce or open into the meatus (Sykes, 1972).

The majority of aural sinuses are asymptomatic, but sometimes occlusion of the orifices will result in formation of a cyst. Once the sinuses have been infected, they seldom become completely asymptomatic but usually undergo a chronic low-grade inflammation with occasionally recurring acute inflammatory exacerbations.

Fig. 8-18. Congenital aural sinus and cyst.

Fig. 8-19. Note the auricular tags and the instrument in a congenital aural sinus.

DIFFERENTIAL DIAGNOSIS

Most commonly these sinuses are confused with *first branchial cleft anomalies.* The two can be differentiated by remembering that the aural sinuses never open into the external auditory canal and are generally located on the anterosuperior aspect of the external ear whereas the first branchial cleft anomalies commonly open into the external auditory canal and produce a purulent discharge with no evidence of middle ear infection. Also the first branchial anomalies usually have another opening on the inferoposterior side of the angle of the mandible, forming a fistula.

MANAGEMENT

Treatment is rendered only when the aural sinuses become cystic or infected, which circumstance necessitates complete removal of the tract or recurrence of symptoms will result.

SALIVARY GLAND FISTULA OR SINUS

Parotid and submandibular gland fistulas are relatively rare lesions and are caused primarily by accidental trauma, surgery, or infection. For a fistula to be produced, there must usually be damage to the parotid or submandibular duct or one of its large branches. The saliva that escapes from the damaged duct either forms a pool within the soft tissue or drains through a fistula in the skin (Figs. 8-20 and 8-21).

The parotid duct lies in the middle third of a line drawn across the face from the tragus of the ear to a point midway between the vermilion border of the lip and the ala of the nose. It arises from the merger of numerous smaller branches at the anterior border of the gland. Occasionally there is an accessory parotid duct that joins the main duct somewhat distal to this border.

Fig. 8-20. Posttraumatic parotid fistula caused by laceration of the parotid duct.

Fig. 8-21. Multiple fistulas from a chronic parotitis.

The main parotid duct then crosses superficially to the masseter muscle and turns inward at the anterior border of the muscle, passing through the fat pad of the cheek and forward in an oblique direction to open into the oral cavity opposite the maxillary second molar. When it crosses the outer surface of the masseter muscle, it lies close to the skin and is vulnerable to injury at this site (Baron, 1960).

Parotid gland fistula has been reported to occur from infection due to actinomycosis, tuberculosis, syphilis, cancrum oris, salivary calculi, and malignancies.

A fistula of the submandibular salivary gland complex is rare and will not be discussed.

DIFFERENTIAL DIAGNOSIS

Differential diagnosis of salivary gland fistula includes the consideration of *fistulas and sinuses from specific and nonspecific infections and foreign bodies* in the area of the salivary glands. Definitive diagnosis is accomplished by the history, probing the involved duct, and the use of sialography.

MANAGEMENT

Once diagnosed, there are various surgical modes of treating salivary gland fistula:
1. The most common method is apposition of the severed duct ends if the fistula is the result of trauma.
2. Another method is creation of a second mucosal opening by suturing the proximal intact portion of the duct to the buccal mucosa.
3. Yet another method is formation of an artificial internal fistula, using various materials.

4. If a chronic fistula will not respond to these conservative operations, the gland may be removed.

AURICULOTEMPORAL SYNDROME (FREY'S SYNDROME)

The auriculotemporal syndrome is included in the present chapter because patients with this disorder experience profuse sweating from a small cutaneous area in the temporal region. Perspiration exuding from such a small area could be confused with an exudate from a draining lesion.

This disorder is caused by damage to the auriculotemporal nerve and subsequent reinnervation of the sweat glands by parasympathetic salivary fibers. Surgical procedures involving the partoid gland, ramus, or condyle of the mandible are the most common cause of the nerve injury. In other cases accidental trauma and infections have been implicated.

FEATURES

Clinically the auriculotemporal syndrome becomes evident approximately 5 weeks after damage to the auriculotemporal nerve. The first signs are sweating on the involved side of the face during and after gustatory stimuli. Eventually a feeling of warmth may precede flushing and sweating (Laage-Hellman, 1957).

DIFFERENTIAL DIAGNOSIS

The definitive diagnosis of auriculotemporal syndrome is made by eliciting a history of trauma or infection in the involved area. The simplest method of identifying the fluid as sweat is by utilization of the Minor starch-iodine test (Laage-Hellman, 1957). Other aspects of the differential diagnosis are discussed in the differential diagnosis section at the end of the chapter (p. 177).

MANAGEMENT

The auriculotemporal syndrome is usually considered to be permanent, although an estimated 5% of these patients experience regression or disappearance of the disorder.

OROCUTANEOUS FISTULA

Orocutaneous fistula is a troublesome defect because it permits the continual leaking of saliva onto the lower face or neck. It is a common sequela of trauma to the head and neck regions. The lesion is also seen with oral malignancies and inflammatory conditions. Cancrum oris, a lesion rarely seen in the United States, may produce an orocutaneous fistula.

FEATURES

Clinically there is an abnormal communication of the oral cavity with the skin surface. A traumatic fistula primarily involves soft tissue, but in many neoplastic and infectious conditions the fistula may involve the osseous structures of the jaws.

Traumatic fistula is generally an epithelial lined communication resulting from either an accident or an attempt at surgical repair. It usually does not exhibit the signs of inflammation commonly seen in neoplastic or inflammatory-induced fistulas.

Neoplastic fistula may be the result of disease that has progressed through soft tissue and/or bone, beginning either in the oral cavity or on the skin surface (Fig. 8-22). Often the fistula will be the result of surgical intervention for the neoplastic disease.

Inflammatory fistula is generally not lined with epithelium unless it is of long duration. The fistula may originate in either soft tissue or bone (e.g., actinomycosis).

DIFFERENTIAL DIAGNOSIS

Establishing a diagnosis of orocutaneous fistula is usually readily accomplished, and the cause plainly evident.

MANAGEMENT

Surgical repair may be successful in most cases of traumatic fistula; but a fistula caused by malignancy is usually hopeless because of the advanced stage of the tumor.

Small infectious-type fistulas may heal spontaneously after elimination of the infection.

RARITIES

Rare defects such as the first branchial arch sinus and fistula would be included in this category.

DIFFERENTIAL DIAGNOSIS OF PITS, FISTULAS, AND SINUSES

Pits, fistulas, and sinuses may readily be misdiagnosed if the clinician fails to employ a systematic diagnostic approach. When he encounters these lesions, he should be certain to establish the following facts from the patient interview:

1. Was the defect present at birth? If not, when did it become apparent?
2. Is there fluid draining from it?
3. Does the patient complain of a bad taste in his mouth?

Fig. 8-22. Orocutaneous fistula resulting from a squamous cell carcinoma.

During the clinical examination pressure should be exerted on the surrounding or associated tissue to determine whether fluid can be expressed from the pit. If fluid is obtained, it should be carefully scrutinized to determine its nature—saliva, pus, blood, or cyst fluid.

In addition, the clinician should attempt to probe the depression to determine whether it is just a shallow diverticulum or indeed a tract. If the instrument or gutta-percha cone can be inserted to a considerable depth, a radiograph of the area should be obtained to aid in determining the depth, direction, and termination of the tract.

Routine radiographs of the adjacent bone will aid in identifying lesions of bone as origins of such tracts.

In some cases shallow pits represent all that remains of quiescent or eradicated tracts.

Intraoral pits, fistulas, and sinuses

The following entities must be considered, in this approximate order of frequency:

Fovea palatinae
Chronic draining dentoalveolar abscess
Commissural lip pits
Postsurgical and postinfection pit or depression
Oroantral fistula
Oronasal fistula
Draining cyst
Draining chronic osteomyelitis
Draining mucocele or ranula
Suppurative infection of the parotid and submaxillary salivary glands
Patent nasopalatine duct

The *patent nasopalatine duct* is a very rare entity. When it is present, the patient may complain of a bad taste. The diagnosis is established by its course through the incisive canal, which can be illustrated by exposing a radiograph after a gutta-percha cone has been inserted into the tract.

Suppurative infection of the parotid and submaxillary salivary glands is also quite uncommon. It should be suspected especially when there is a predisposing dehydration. Expressing pus from the respective duct openings by application of pressure on the glands establishes the diagnosis and differentiates this disorder from infections involving other tissues.

Draining mucocele or ranula is slightly more common. The mucocele is most often located on the lower lip, and the ranula occurs in the floor of the oral cavity. A history of repeated episodes of swelling and draining with regression in these locations prompts the clinician to assign a high rank to mucocele and ranula, especially when the fluid is clear, viscous, and sticky.

A *chronic osteomyelitis* more frequently drains through an extraoral sinus opening than through an intraoral opening. Suggestive changes in the basal bone plus the finding that pus can be expressed by exerting pressure on a tender or painful expansion of the mandible would suggest the assignment of a high rank to osteomyelitis. The probability that chronic osteomyelitis is the likely diagnosis is enhanced if any of the following are true:

1. The patient has an uncontrolled systemic disease, such as diabetes.
2. The jawbone has been previously irradiated.
3. The patient has Paget's disease.

Drainage from a cyst is almost always caused by infection. If the cyst is in bone, a radiograph will reveal the defect but may not help differentiate between an abscess and a cyst. Such a distinction is academic anyway because an infected cyst may be considered an abscess. Soft tissue cysts within the oral cavity are uncommon.

A large *oronasal fistula* is easily recognized, so a discussion of its differential features is not necessary. Small fistulas in the anterior midline could be confused with a patent nasopalatine duct, but these two entities can be distinguished by noting the position on an occlusal radiograph of an inserted gutta-percha point.

Since the majority of *oroantral fistulas* occur on the ridge in the premolar-molar area, a defect in this region that permits passage of food or drink into the nose is almost certainly an oroantral fistula. Small tracts from *infected cysts* or *abscesses* in this region could be confused with purulent drainage of an infected sinus through an oroantral fistula; however, a radiograph taken after the insertion of a gutta-percha cone would reveal the image of the cone terminating inferior to the antrum if the case were an infected cyst or abscess.

A *postsurgical or postinfection defect* is seen most often on the alveolus and is diagnosed by learning of the causative experience.

Commissural lip pits always occur in the characteristic location, so the probability that other pits or sinus openings could occur in this location is quite remote.

Chronic draining dentoalveolar abscesses comprise the majority of intraoral draining lesions. If pus can be expressed from the opening by pressing on a tender tooth, then the diagnosis is almost certainly chronic abscess. This impression is confirmed if a radiograph exposed after the insertion of a gutta-percha cone shows the image of the cone leading to the tooth.

The *foveae palatinae* are normal anatomic landmarks; however, in some patients these depressions are so prominent that they could resemble fistulas or sinus openings. Their characteristic location on each side of the midline of the anterior soft palate and the fact that mucus can be expressed from them by pressing on the surrounding soft tissue should permit proper identification.

Fistulas and sinuses of the face and neck

The following entities must be considered in the differential diagnosis when a draining lesion is encountered on the skin of the face and neck:

Pustule
Draining cyst
Chronic alveolar abscess or osteomyelitis
Salivary gland fistula
Orocutaneous fistula
Congenital aural sinus
Auriculotemporal syndrome
Thyroglossal sinus
Lateral cervical sinus

Determination of the location, depth, and course of tracts in the neck and face often permits the differentiation of these lesions. Thus injecting radiopaque dye into the defects, along with the use of radiographs, is frequently beneficial as a diagnostic indicator.

Identifying the fluid draining from these lesions may provide a valuable clue for diagnosis. In various cases the fluid may prove to be sweat, pus, cyst fluid, or saliva.

Saliva will be found emanating from orocutaneous and salivary gland fistulas and through the second branchial arch sinus.

1. The *second branchial arch sinus* can be differentiated from the orocutaneous fistula by the fact that the former is a developmental lesion and so is usually observed early in life. Also in most cases the former defect is more posterior, extending inferiorly to the hyoid bone through to the lateral tonsillar fossa.

2. The *orocutaneous fistula* may be differentiated from the salivary fistula by the fact that the defect is not through and through in the latter. Also the characteristic location of the salivary gland fistula will aid in the differentiation.

When the drainage is *clear, thin cyst fluid*, a tract from a *branchial* or *thyroglossal cyst* must be suspected. If the sinus is in the lateral neck, it is most likely draining a branchial cyst. If it is in or near the midline in the region of the hyoid bone, however, and if it is stressed when the tongue protrudes, then the lesion is most likely thyroglossal in origin.

If *purulent material* is emanating from a cutaneous sinus, the following entities must be considered: pustule, infected cyst, chronic alveolar abscess or chronic osteomyelitis, and infected congenital aural sinus.

1. If the lesion is an infected *aural sinus*, swelling and tenderness will be present as well as a small sinus opening in or just anterior to the external ear. This entity may be confused with a *first branchial arch sinus*, but the latter is very rare (only 24 cases have been reported in the literature).

2. A *draining alveolar abscess* or *chronic osteomyelitis* of the mandible may empty onto the skin of the lower face or upper neck. Radiographically bony changes will be evident with both entities. If the cause is *Actinomyces*, there will frequently be fine yellow granules present in the purulent material (which usually emanates from multiple sinuses).

3. *Infected draining cysts* most often encountered in these regions are the thyroglossal, branchial, sebaceous, and dermoid.
   a. The *sebaceous* and *dermoid* varieties can usually be differentiated from the other two by their more superficial location. The dermoid cyst occurs most often in the midline and is firm whereas the sebaceous variety may occur anywhere and is not so firm.
   b. The deeper *thyroglossal* and *branchial* types usually can be differentiated by the fact that the former are near or in the midline whereas the latter are situated more laterally.

4. *Purulent infections in lymph nodes* and *draining space infections* must also be considered.

A *pustule* is the most common of all purulent draining lesions and is readily recognized by its short course and superficial location as well as by the presence of multiple skin lesions.

The *auriculotemporal syndrome* need not be confused with any of the other entities included in this chapter. A history of trauma to the parotid region followed by sweating on gustatory stimulation is practically pathognomonic.

SPECIFIC REFERENCES

Abrams, A. M., Howell, F. V., and Bullock, W. K.: Nasopalatine cysts, Oral Surg. **16**:306-332, 1963.

Anderson, M. F.: Surgical closure of oroantral fistula: report of a series, J. Oral Surg. **27**:862-863, 1969.

Bailey, H.: The clinical aspects of branchial fistulas, Br. J. Surg. **21**:12-21, 1933.

Baker, B. R.: Pits of the lip commissures in Caucasoid males, Oral Surg. **21**:56-60, 1966.

Baron, H. D.: Surgical correction of salivary fistula, Gen Pract. **21**:89-98, 1960.

Brown, P. M., and Judd, E. S.: Thyroglossal duct cysts and sinuses, Am. J. Surg. **102**:494-501, 1961.

Burket, L. W.: Nasopalatine duct structures and a peculiar bony pattern observed in the anterior maxillary region, Arch. Pathol. **23**:793-800, 1937.

Burket, L. W.: Oral medicine: diagnosis and treatment, ed. 6, Philadelphia, 1971, J. B. Lippincott Co.

Carp, L., and Stout, A. P.: Branchial anomalies and neoplasms: a report of thirty-two cases with follow-up results, Ann. Surg. **87**:186-209, 1928.

Clarkson, P., Wilson, T. H. H., and Lawrie, R. S.: Treatment of 1,000 jaw fractures, Br. Dent. J. **80**:69-75, 1946.

Cowley, D. J., and Calman, J. S.: Pre-auricular fistulae in four generations: a study in heredity, Br. J. Plast. Surg. **24**:388-390, 1971.

Eisenbud, L., and Klatell, J.: Acute alveolar abscess, Oral Surg. **4**:208-224, 1951.

Everett, F. G., and Wescott, W. B.: Commissural lip pits, Oral Surg. **14**:202-209, 1961.

Ewing, M. R.: Congenital sinuses of the external ear, J. Laryngol. Otolaryngol. **61**:18-23, 1946.

Goldman, E. H., Stratigos, G. T., and Arthur, A. L.: Treatment of oroantral fistula by gold foil closure: report of a case, J. Oral Surg. **27**:875-877, 1969.

Gore, D., and Masson, A.: Anomaly of the first branchial cleft, Ann. Surg. **150**:309-312, 1959.

Gorlin, R. J., and Goldman, H. M.: Thoma's oral pathology, ed. 6, St. Louis, 1970, The C. V. Mosby Co.

Gorlin, R. J., and Pindborg, J. J.: Syndromes of the head and neck, New York, 1964, McGraw-Hill Book Co.

Gustafson, J. R.: Acute parotitis, Surgery **29**:786-801, 1951.

Hill, W. C., and Darlow, H. M.: Bilateral perforate nasopalatine communication in the human adult, J. Laryngol. Otolaryngol. **60**:160-165, 1945.

Hyndman, O. R., and Light, A.: The branchial apparatus; its embryologic origin and the pathologic changes to which it gives rise, with presentation of a familial group of fistulas, Arch. Surg. **19:**410-452, 1929.

Jacques, D. A., Chambers, R. G., and Oertel, J. E.: Thyroglossal tract carcinoma: a review of the literature and additions of eighteen cases, Am. J. Surg. **120:**439-446, 1970.

Juniper, R. P.: Tuberculosis causing bilateral oroantral fistulae, Br. J. Oral Surg. **10:**352-356, 1973.

Killey, H. C., and Kay, L. W.: An analysis of 250 cases of oro-antral fistula treated by the buccal flap operation, Oral Surg. **24:**726-739, 1967.

Krippachne, W., Hunt, T. K., and Dunphy, J.: Acute sup-purative parotitis: study of 161 cases, Ann. Surg. **156:**251-257, 1962.

Laage-Hellman, J. E.: Gustatory sweating and flushing after conservative parotidectomy, Acta Otolaryngol. **48:**234-252, 1957.

Lighterman, I., Watanabe, Y., and Hidaku, T.: Leprosy of the oral cavity and adnexa, Oral Surg. **15:**1178-1194, 1962.

MacGregor, A. J.: Patent nasopalatine canal, Oral Surg. **18:**285-292, 1964.

Marshall, S. F.: Thyroglossal cysts and sinuses, Ann. Surg. **129:**642-651, 1949.

Mustian, W. F.: The floor of the maxillary sinus and its dental, oral and nasal relations, J. Am. Dent. Assoc. **20:**2175-2187, 1933.

Neel, H. B., and Pemberton, J.: Lateral cervical (branchial) cysts and fistulas, Surgery **18:**267-286, 1945.

Pollock, W. F., and Stevenson, E. O.: Cysts and sinuses of the thyroglossal duct, Am. J. Surg. **112:**225-232, 1966.

Rosenberger, H. C.: Fissural cysts, Arch. Otolaryngol. **40:**288-290, 1944.

Selkirk, T. K.: Fistula auris congenita, Am. J. Dis. Child. **49:**431-447, 1935.

Shafer, W. A., Hine, M. K., and Levy, B. M.: A textbook of oral pathology, ed. 3, Philadelphia, 1974, W. B. Saunders Co.

Shulman, B. H.: Acute suppurative infections of the salivary glands in the newborn, Am. J. Dis. Child **80:**413-416, 1950.

Stahl, W. M., and Lyall, D.: Cervical cysts and fistulae of thyro-glossal tract origin, Ann. Surg. **139:**123-128, 1954.

Sykes, P. J.: Pre-auricular sinus: clinical features and the prob-lems of recurrence, Br. J. Plast. Surg. **25:**175-179, 1972.

Ward, G. E.: Thyroglossal tract abnormalities: cysts and fis-tulas, Surg. Gynecol. Obstet. **89:**727-734, 1949.

Worth, H. M.: Principles and practice of oral radiologic inter-pretation, Chicago, 1963, Year Book Medical Publishers.

Wowern, N. V.: Oroantral communications and displacements of roots into the maxillary sinus: a follow-up of 231 cases, J. Oral Surg. **29:**622-627, 1971.

Ziemba, R. B.: Combined buccal and reverse palatal flap for closure of oral-antral fistula, J. Oral Surg. **30:**727-729, 1972.

GENERAL REFERENCE

Azaz, B., and Taicher, S.: Facial sinus tracts in children, J. Dent. Child. **43:**167, 1976.

9

Intraoral brownish, bluish, or black conditions

Norman K. Wood
Paul W. Goaz

The intraoral conditions classified as brownish, bluish, or black may be categorized according to whether they produce distinct and discretely circumscribed lesions or a generalized and diffuse discoloration of the patient. (Refer to the list below and also to Tables 9-1 and 9-2.)

Distinct circumscribed types
Melanoplakia
Varicosity
Amalgam tattoo
Petechia and ecchymosis
Early hematoma
Late hematoma
Hemangioma
Oral melanotic macule
Mucocele
Ranula
Superficial cyst
Giant cell granuloma
Black hairy tongue
Lymphangioma
Pigmented fibroma
Melanoma
Nevus
Mucus-producing salivary gland tumors
von Recklinghausen's disease
Albright's syndrome
Heavy metal lines
Rarities
    Acanthosis nigricans
    Acromegaly
    Addison's disease (distinct circumscribed lesions)
    Chlorpromazine therapy
    Cushing's syndrome
    Fabry's disease
    Gaucher's disease
    Hereditary hemorrhagic telangiectasia
    Kaposi's sarcoma
    Lentigo
    Lichen planus
    Lupus erythematosus

    Lymphangiomas of neonates
    Lymphoma (superficial)
    Melanotic neuroectodermal tumor of infancy
    Pernicious anemia
    Peutz-Jeghers syndrome
    Pheochromocytoma
    Rheumatic fever
    Scleroderma
    Submucous fibrosis
    Superficial cartilaginous tumor in patient with ochronosis
       or alkaptonuria
    Superficial *Pseudomonas aeruginosa* infection
    Thyrotoxicosis
    Uremia (petechiae)
    Xeroderma pigmentosa

Generalized brownish, bluish, or black conditions
Cyanosis
Chloasma gravidarum
Addison's disease
Hemochromatosis
Argyria
Rarities
    Aniline intoxication
    Arsenic poisoning
    Carotenemia
    Chloroquine therapy
    Dermatomyositis
    Idiopathic familial juvenile hypoparathyroidism, Addison's disease, superficial candidiasis
    Pellagra
    Porphyria
    Sprue
    Wilson's disease

    The brownish, bluish, or black color that serves as the basis for this category of disorders originates from one of two sources: (1) the accumulation of colored material in abnormal amounts or locations in the superficial tissues or (2) a pooled clear fluid just beneath the epithelium. The amassed material that effects these color changes may be either exogenous or endogenous in origin.

The exogenous substances producing the brownish, bluish, or black conditions usually include heavy metals not normally found in the body, commercial dyes, vegetable pigments, and various other stains that have been either ingested or introduced directly into the tissues. The point of introduction may be at the site of or remote from the lesion in question.

The endogenous chromatic materials producing the brownish, bluish, or black conditions usually result from increased melanin states or are derived from blood pigments or abnormal aggregations of metals normally found in the body. It is interesting that the color imparted by such exogenous or endogenous materials is a function of not only the amount of pigment but also the depths at which the pigments have been deposited in the tissues. For example, the more superficial melanin deposits appear browner whereas the deeper melanin deposits seem more bluish.

Refraction phenomena cause abnormal coloration in superficial fluid-filled cavities such as some cysts and retention phenomena in the minor salivary glands. Although in these pathoses the distinctive bluish color might appear to be due to pigment in the area, it is actually the result of altered reflection and absorption of light in the area.

Distinct circumscribed types

MELANOPLAKIA (BLACK PIGMENTATION)

All people, except albinos,* have a discernible degree of melanin pigmentation distributed throughout the epidermis of the skin.

Melanin is thought to be produced by the dendritic melanocytes in the basal layer of the epidermis (Fig. 9-1). It is formed by the oxidation of tyrosine—a reaction that is catalyzed by the copper-containing enzyme tyrosinase and mediated by the melanocyte-stimulating hormone (MSH), from the anterior pituitary. The melanin is secreted by the melanocytes and then picked up by the adjacent basal cells of the epithelium.

FEATURES

The clinical appearance of melanin varies from light brown through blue to black, depending

on the amount present and its depth in the tissues. The deeper and heavier the deposit of melanin in the skin or mucosa, the darker it appears. There is great variation in the degree of pigmentation of the skin between the races and between individuals of the same race. Although much of this variation is genetically controlled, the remainder is due to various degrees of tanning from exposure to sunlight.

Light-skinned individuals normally have a relatively even coloration throughout the oral cavity; however, dark-complexioned people, especially those of the black race, frequently have macules of pigmentation (melanoplakia) of various configurations and sizes on their oral mucosae (Fig. 9-2). The gingivae are frequent sites of this patchy pigmentation, but variation in physiologic pigmentation is not limited to the gingivae. Such areas of melanoplakia on the oral mucous membranes in blacks are not usually a cause for concern; but if they are known to be of recent origin, they may complicate the formulation of a differential diagnosis and prompt and biopsy procedure.

DIFFERENTIAL DIAGNOSIS

A solitary, small, circumscribed, darkly pigmented lesion in a black cannot be clinically distinguished from an *amalgam tattoo, junctional nevus, melanoma,* or local area of *hemosiderin deposition* after trauma. Should such an area be observed in a white, it is unlikely to be melanoplakia but more likely an oral melanotic macule or one of the entities just mentioned.

Microscopically the increased pigmentation present in the basal layer is the only significant observation in melanoplakia.

MANAGEMENT

The diagnosis of melanoplakial patches in blacks is seldom a problem and after correct identification this entity requires no further attention. However, it is not always possible to differentiate between a patch of melanoplakia and a superficial spreading melanoma on a clinical basis. Hence if one or more of the following characteristics exist then the pigmented patch should be excised along with an adequate border of normal-appearing tissue and submitted for microscopic study: if the pigmented patch has (1) appeared recently rather than being present since birth or childhood, (2) decreased or increased in size, (3) become elevated in part or whole, (4) undergone color changes of any type, or (5) undergone surface ulceration or fissuring.

---

*Melanin formation is impaired by a congenital decrease in tyrosinase in albinism.

Fig. 9-1. The clear cells in the basal cell layer of the epithelium are melanocytes. The arrow indicates three melanocytes.

Fig. 9-2. Melanoplakia. **A,** Arrows indicate three areas of involvement. **B,** Unusual ribbonlike appearance of melanoplakia.

VARICOSITY

A varicosity is a distended vein and is a common occurrence in the oral cavity, especially in older individuals. It may also result from partial blockage of the vein proximal to the distension either by a structure causing external pressure or from a plaque that has formed on the lumen side of the wall as a result of an injury.

FEATURES

The varicosities most frequently observed by the clinician are superficial, painless, and bluish; they appear somewhat congested and accentuate the shape and distribution of the vessel. The most frequent site is the ventral surface of the tongue (Fig. 9-3 and Plate 1, A).

When many of the sublingual veins are involved, this condition is called "caviar tongue" (or phlebectasia linguae) (Fig. 9-3). The clinician should be cognizant of the fact that varicosities in the oral cavity, although occurring for the most part in normal patients, may on rare occasions be caused by a tumor pressing on the superior vena cava at a proximal site such as in the mediastinum. Congested veins in the head and neck region are also seen in apprehensive individuals and in children who are holding their breath.

DIFFERENTIAL DIAGNOSIS

The clinical identification of a lesion as a varicosity usually does not present a problem, but occasionally one will be found having a bulbous shape (Fig. 9-3, C and Plate 1) and then must be differentiated from all the other fluid-filled bluish lesions of the oral cavity: hemangioma, aneurysm, mucocele, ranula, and superficial nonkeratotic cyst (Plate 1, A).

Contrasting with the *superficial nonkeratotic cyst, ranula,* and *mucocele,* which are fluctuant and cannot be emptied by digital pressure because they contain fluid in a closed chamber, the varicosity, the hemangioma (especially the cavernous variety), and the aneurysm do not demonstrate fluctuance and usually can be emptied by digital pressure.

An *aneurysm* is exceedingly rare in the oral cavity and will demonstrate a pulse, as will also an *arteriovenous shunt.* An angiogram may be an additional aid in the identification of an arteriovenous lesion.

Although the *cavernous hemangioma* can be readily emptied into the afferent and efferent vessels by digital pressure, the *capillary hemangioma* cannot be as readily emptied because the vascular spaces and the afferent and efferent

Fig. 9-3. A, Caviar tongue (phlebectasia linguae). **B,** Small varicosity. **C,** Large bulbous varicosity that resembled a ranula.

Plate 1. A, Dome-shaped varicosity that resembles a ranula. **B,** Four dome-shaped bluish eruption cysts in a neonate. **C,** Follicular cyst that has destroyed the buccal bony plate and appears as a bluish mass (arrow). **D,** Bluish peripheral giant cell granuloma of the gingiva. **E,** Addison's disease. Note the diffuse tanning on the neck and the discrete brownish macules on the face. **F,** Addison's disease. Brownish macules are scattered over a mucosa that is tanner than normal in this white patient. **G,** Argyria. This patient developed argyria from the self-administration of nose drops containing silver. Note how the skin of the face (which is exposed to sunlight) shows more color change than does the skin of the palm (not exposed to sunlight). **H,** Palate of a patient with argyria. (**D** courtesy J. Ireland, D.D.S., Maywood, Ill. **F** and **H** courtesy S. Svalina, D.D.S., Maywood, Ill.)

Plate 2. A, Denture stomatitis. Exfoliative cytology of the reddened mucosa was positive for *Candida albicans*. The stomatitis disappeared after 1 week of therapy with nystatic troches. **B,** Candidosis. Multiple erythematous palatal lesions proved to be acute atrophic candidosis (same lesion as in Fig. 10-16). **C,** Erosive lichen planus involving the lateral border of the tongue. **D,** Erosive lichen planus of the buccal mucosa. **E,** Erythroplakia of the floor of the mouth. This lesion proved on biopsy to be squamous cell carcinoma. **F,** Large erythroplakic lesion of the lateral soft palate proved on biopsy to be squamous cell carcinoma. **G,** Erythema multiforme. Lesions were confined to the oral mucosa. **H,** Allergic mucositis due to cold tablets. (All illustrations except **E** courtesy G. G. Blozis, D.D.S., Columbus, Ohio.)

Plate 3. A, Plasma cell gingivitis. Note the restriction of the erythematous reaction to the gingiva.
B, Benign mucous membrane pemphigoid. There is focal involvement of the gingiva by red patches,
and some areas of superficial necrosis are present. The palate was also involved. **C,** Benign mucous
membrane pemphigoid. There is diffuse involvement of the labial gingiva. Note the gingival bleb
produced by a stream of air. **D,** Radiation mucositis. Note the whitish patches of fibrinous exudate
scattered over the erythematous mucosa. This patient had received 2,600 R for treatment of a
squamous cell carcinoma of the floor of the mouth. **E,** Chemotherapy mucositis. This patient was
receiving methotrexate. Erythematous areas appeared as the surface cells were exfoliated.
F, Fordyce's granules. **G,** Odontogenic abscess on the buccal aspect of the alveolus. **H,** Lipoma
of the lower lip. (**A** courtesy P. D. Toto, D.D.S., Maywood, Ill. **B** to **E** courtesy G. G. Blozis, Columbus, Ohio. **G** courtesy G. MacDonald, D.D.S., Belleville, Ill.)

Plate 4. A, Recurrent aphthous stomatitis. **B,** Atrophic candidosis. **C** and **D,** Pemphigus. **E,** Reaction to periodontal dressing. **F,** Reiter's syndrome. **G,** Primary herpetic gingivostomatitis. **H,** Erosive lichen planus with both an erosive and a ketatotic component. (**B** courtesy S. Raibley, D.D.S., Maywood, Ill. **C** and **D** courtesy S. Fischman, Buffalo, N.Y. **F** courtesy J. Lehnert, D.D.S., Minneapolis. **G** courtesy S. Smith, D.D.S., Chicago. **H** courtesy S. Raibley, D.D.S., Maywood, Ill.)

vessels are so small that they may be immediately sealed when pressure is applied to the lesion. Also the capillary hemangioma is seldom a bluish domed mass like its cavernous counterpart but is more reddish.

The varicosity, on the other hand, will collapse if the vein distal to it is occluded by digital pressure (provided the proximal end is not totally blocked by a process that may have caused the varicosity). A hemangioma, however, usually will not collapse when manipulated in this manner because the blood tends to pool in the many vascular spaces.

A more dependable test to identify a varicosity is to completely occlude the vessel proximally by digital pressure and try to evacuate the lesion by massaging in a distal direction. If the lesion is a varicosity, it cannot be easily evacuated in a distal direction because the valves in the normal segment of the vein distal to the varicosity will not readily permit the retrograde passage of blood.

MANAGEMENT

Usually all that is required is to positively diagnose the lesion as a varicosity. Except for the large bulbous types, which may be regularly irritated, oral varicosities seldom require treatment. It is extremely important, however, that they be differentiated from other pathoses. The clinician must develop a thorough differential diagnosis and a positive working diagnosis of varicosity, and he must completely rule out other vascular lesions.

If the lesion relates to a general cardiovascular condition, contemplated dental work should be deferred until the patient's physician indicates that it is safe to proceed.

AMALGAM TATTOO

The amalgam tattoo is a frequently occurring asymptomatic dark bluish lesion usually seen on the gingiva in mouths in which teeth have been restored with silver amalgam (Fig. 9-4). It usually is produced when the gingiva is abraded at the time a tooth is prepared for restoration. Subsequently, when the amalgam is placed, some of the silver or mercury contacts the abraded tissue and precipitates the protein of the immature collagen fibers, thus fixing them.

The amalgam tattoo is a permanent stain and can also be seen in histologic sections of the tissue (Fig. 9-4). Radiographs of the region are normal except when actual fragments of amalgam have been introduced into the tissue; the fragments are then detectable as dense radiopacities.

Fig. 9-4. Amalgam tattoo. **A,** Dark macule on the crest of the ridge in the mandibular molar area. **B,** The black granules forming the wavy lines are particles of silver that have stained reticulin fibers.

DIFFERENTIAL DIAGNOSIS

On visual examination, an amalgam tattoo often cannot be differentiated from a junctional nevus, an oral melanotic macule, a macular type of melanoma, or a hemangioma (Figs. 9-11 and 9-17).

A *superficial hemangioma* will blanch on pressure, and a *nevus* or *melanoma* seldom occurs in the oral cavity.

Furthermore, an increase in size or a change in color would be expected with a melanoma; and if there is an amalgam restoration adjacent to such a quiescent lesion, this is almost conclusive evidence that the suspected area is an amalgam tattoo.

MANAGEMENT

Amalgam tattoos do not require treatment; but if there is a suspicion that the lesion could be a nevus or a melanoma, it should be excised and microscopically examined. A similar course should be followed if the patient is unduly worried about the nature of the lesion.

PETECHIA AND ECCHYMOSIS (PURPURA)

Petechiae and ecchymoses are purpuric submucous or subcutaneous hemorrhages. They have the same basic mechanism: both appear as bluish macules differing only in size; petechiae are minute pinpoint hemorrhages, whereas ecchymoses are larger than 2 cm in diameter (Figs. 9-5 to 9-7). If these lesions are observed soon after their inception they will be red. Within a few hours they will have changed to a bluish-brown color.

FEATURES

The hemorrhaging is quite slow in this spectrum of lesions; hence there is not sufficient blood to pool and develop the fluctuant swellings characteristic of the early hematomas. Trauma and perhaps more frequently disorders of the hemostatic mechanisms or other systemic disease may be the causative factors involved. It is important to obtain a complete history from a patient who is discovered to have these lesions. If the person has experienced several such episodes, he almost certainly has a systemic problem and must be examined for hemostatic defects such as thrombocytopenia, leukemia, and hemophilia or other diseases such as subacute bacterial endocarditis, Waterhouse-Friderichsen syn-

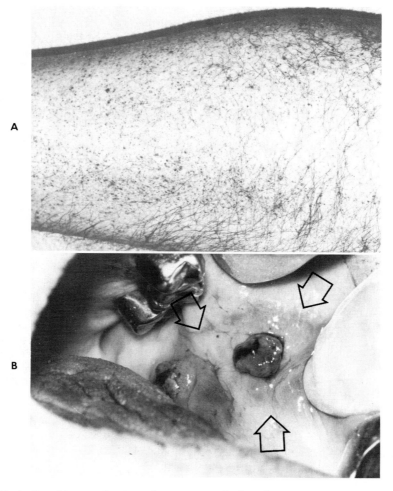

Fig. 9-5. A, Petechiae on the arm of a patient with thrombocytopenic purpura. **B,** Ecchymosis (arrows) surrounding an exophytic blood clot in the same patient. (Courtesy S. Svalina, D.D.S., Maywood, Ill.)

Fig. 9-6. Large purpuric lesion in the buccal and palatal mucosa after a mandibular fracture. (Courtesy D. Bonomo, D.D.S., Flossmoor, Ill.)

Fig. 9-7. Purpuric macules in hemostatic disease. **A,** Petechial purpuric macules that occurred during a sickle cell crisis. **B,** Petechiae and gingival bleeding occurring in a patient with acute myelogenous leukemia. **C,** Purpuric macules and blood clots in a patient with heroin-induced thrombocytopenic purpura. **D,** Purpuric macules in a patient with leukemia. (**A** courtesy S. Smith, D.D.S., Chicago. **B** courtesy J. Canzona, D.D.S., Chicago. **C** from Kraut, R. A., and Buhler, J. E.: Oral Surg. **46:**637-640, 1978. **D** courtesy J. Lehnert, D.D.S., Minneapolis.)

drome, infectious mononucleosis, sickle cell anemia, polycythemia, disseminated fat emboli, or
vitamin C deficiency.

DIFFERENTIAL DIAGNOSIS

Clinically petechiae and ecchymoses begin as
reddish macules of varying shape and outline. On
palpation their consistency is similar to that of
normal mucosa. They do not blanch on pressure;
but within a few days their color changes from
red to blue to green-blue to yellow-green to yellow
and then disappears as the hemoglobin is de-
graded to hemosiderin and removed.

A single petechial macule resulting from local trauma will take on a bluish brownish appearance in a day or two and must be differentiated
from an *amalgam tattoo,* an *oral melanotic
macule,* a *junctional nevus,* and a *melanoma.* A
history of recent trauma, accompanied by the
change in color to green to yellow and then finally
disappearing within 4 or 5 days, will indicate its
true identity.

Early petechial lesions must be differentiated
from *telangiectasias* in patients with Rendu-
Osler-Weber syndrome (hereditary hemorrhagic
telangiectasia). This syndrome manifests itself as
small reddish macule-papule lesions that are dilated capillaries situated just under the epithelium that will blanch on pressure. They can
thus be differentiated from petechiae.

Palatal petechiae and ecchymotic patches deserve special attention when they occur as a solitary lesion at or near the junction of the hard and
soft palate. The following diagnoses need to be
considered: (1) trauma from fellatio, (2) trauma
from severe coughing, (3) trauma from severe
vomiting, (4) prodromal sign of infectious mononucleosis, and (5) prodromal sign of hemostatic
disease.

There seems little doubt that *oral sexual practices* are on the increase. Thus the dentist must
consider this possibility first when a reddish or
bluish macule is detected on the posterior palate
and has been produced by extravasated blood
(Fig. 10-4). If the lesion is indeed due to fellatio
the bruise will disappear in a few days after passing through the various color changes: blue,
green, and yellow. Frequently it will reappear
in another week or so. A careful history taken in
confidential surroundings will reveal the cause
in almost all cases.

Bruising of the palate from severe attacks of
vomiting and *coughing* will appear as a broad
linear red or bluish bruise that follows the junction of the hard and soft palate. Again the history
would be diagnostic in these cases.

Prodromal signs of *infectious mononucleosis*
may occur as 6 to 20 petechiae in the soft palate
a few days before the patient becomes ill. These
petechiae may also occur between the fifth and
twentieth days of illness. This feature along with
malaise, enlarged nodes in the neck, and a positive Monospot test followed by a positive Paul-
Bunnell heterophil test establishes the diagnosis
of the disease.

Because the soft palate sustains a considerable
degree of stimulation and mild trauma during
swallowing of food this location is frequently the
first to show the petechiae that may herald the
onset of *hemostatic disease.* A complete blood
workup will usually identify the specific diagnosis. However, the clinician must remember that
some individuals bruise easily and so a few scattered petechiae may be present from time to time
on the palates of these normal individuals.

MANAGEMENT

The associated hemostatic disorders may be
conveniently divided into three groups according
to the basic defect: disorders of the vessels, disorders of the platelets, and disorders affecting
coagulation. A suitable study of the patient, including a good history, clinical examination, and
the appropriate laboratory tests, will identify the
specific underlying systemic defect. Surgery
should not be undertaken until the defect has
been identified and corrected, or at least the
surgical procedure modified on the basis of the
defect's recognition and nature.

EARLY HEMATOMA

The hematoma is a pool of effused blood confined within the tissues. If it is superficial, it will
appear as an elevated bluish swelling in the mucosa (Fig. 9-8). The early hematoma is fluctuant,
rubbery, and somewhat discrete in outline; and
the overlying mucosa is readily movable. The
temperature of the overlying mucosa may be elevated slightly. Digital pressure on the surface
may produce a stinging sensation as a further dissection of the tissues is effected by this procedure.

DIFFERENTIAL DIAGNOSIS

A history of a traumatic incident (e.g., accident, surgery, administration of a local anesthetic) can almost always be elicited from the patient and is useful in establishing the diagnosis of
early hematoma. Not to be overlooked is the possibility of spontaneous hemorrhage with the development of a hematoma in patients who have a
blood dyscrasia or other bleeding diathesis; and
this may be the first indication of their systemic

Fig. 9-8. Hematoma. **A,** A small lesion on the buccal mucosa. **B,** Large dome-shaped hematoma in the right sublingual region caused by damage to the lingual artery during a surgical procedure.

disease. Generally, however, petechia and ecchymosis are more often seen in these patients than is a hematoma; however, a hematoma may be encountered after a surgical procedure in such patients who have not been properly prepared for surgery.

Early hematoma must be differentiated from all the soft and rubbery bluish lesions that occur in the oral cavity: *mucocele, ranula, varicosity, hemangioma, lymphangioma,* and *superficial cyst.* The history of a sudden onset after a recent traumatic incident strongly favors a diagnosis of early hematoma. The lesion is tender and fluctuant and cannot be evacuated by digital pressure. Although an early hematoma is usually not painful, palpation will generally induce a stinging sensation as the pressure on the contained pool of blood causes further separation of the tissues. There is no thrill or crepitus. It is almost always a solitary lesion that will yield dark blue blood on aspiration.

MANAGEMENT

The hematoma will generally be self-limiting in size, because the increasing pressure of the blood in the tissue will equalize with the hydrostatic pressure in the injured vessel and thus terminate the extravasation. If a large arteriole is damaged, however, a pressure bandage may be placed over accessible areas to control the hemorrhage and the expansion of the hematoma.

Occasionally evacuation with an aspirating syringe may be feasible in an expanding or painful hematoma and then a pressure bandage placed to prevent its re-formation. If indicated, the patient may be hospitalized for observation and the offending vessel located surgically and ligated.

An enlarging hematoma in the neck or sublingual area may encroach on the airway, and its management must be evaluated in the light of this possibility.

Since the hematoma presents an excellent medium for the growth of opportunistic bacteria, the clinician must be aware that the probability of infection is high if the patient is not immediately protected with a suitable antibiotic for several days.

LATE HEMATOMA

A hematoma is usually completely clotted within 24 hours and then becomes a hard, black, painless mass. It often requires this prolonged period to completely clot because blood continues to leak into the clotting pool from the injured vessels. If the hematoma is superficially located, color changes may be observed from black to blue to green to yellow during the days following. It disappears finally when all the hemosiderin from the extravasated blood has been removed from the tissues.

If a hematoma becomes infected, it will be painful. Although the clot will initially be firm, if the infection is a pyogenic type, the firm clot will soften and become fluctuant as pus accumulates.

DIFFERENTIAL DIAGNOSIS

Clinicians frequently see postextraction patients with a hematoma that has formed inferior to the extraction site. The submaxillary space is a frequent site for the development of such post-extraction hematomas, which must be differentiated from an *early space infection.*

The late hematoma will be very firm and painless, whereas the infection will also be firm but acutely painful to palpation. In addition, the tissue over the infection will have an increased temperature and may be inflamed. Later the infection may become fluctuant and yield pus on aspiration.

MANAGEMENT

If the patient with a hematoma of considerable proportions has not been protected with antibiotics, such prophylactic treatment should be initiated immediately and the patient observed carefully for the next few days. If the patient has or appears to be developing a problem with respiration, he should be hospitalized and appropriate measures instituted to establish and maintain a patent airway.

HEMANGIOMA

The hemangioma is a benign tumor of patent blood vessels that may be congenital or traumatic in origin. It may appear similar to a telangiec-

tasia, which is a dilatation of a previously existing vessel, in contast to the hemangioma, which is a new formation of blood vessels. Seventy-three percent occur within the first year of life (Watson and McCarthy, 1940).

Only those hemangiomas that occur superficially will be considered in this section. The deeper hemangiomas are rarely detected and do not appear blue since the deeper tissue covering obscures the color imparted by the vascular mass; also the capillary hemangiomas will not be included in this discussion since they are usually a reddish lesion.

The cavernous hemangioma is a soft, nonfluctuant, domelike, bluish nodule that may vary in size from a millimeter or less to several centimeters in diameter (Fig. 9-9). It frequently appears on the lips, buccal mucosa, palate, and other sites in the oral cavity.

DIFFERENTIAL DIAGNOSIS

The hemangioma blanches and may be emptied by the application of digital pressure, which forces the blood from the vascular spaces. This feature accounts for the finding that the lesion is not fluctuant and, in turn, helps to differentiate

Fig. 9-9. Cavernous hemangioma. **A,** Of the lip. **B,** Of the anterolateral border of the tongue. **C,** Of the floor of the mouth mimicking a ranula. (Courtesy G. MacDonald, D.D.S., Belleville, Ill.)

the cavernous hemangioma from the *mucocele, ranula,* and *superficial cysts,* which though soft are, in contrast, fluctuant and nonemptiable. (Refer to Chapter 3 for a broader discussion of these differences.) A varicosity usually is seen as an elongated enlargement of a superficial vein rather than as a nodule or dome-shaped mass.

Furthermore, a pulse is not detectable within the cavernous hemangioma. This feature serves to distinguish the hemangioma from an *arteriovenous shunt* or an *aneurysm*—both of which may occur as rubbery, nonfluctuant, domelike, bluish nodules with a usually discernible throbbing.

In addition to the foregoing characteristics, the aspiration of bluish blood with a fine-gauge needle contributes convincing evidence for a working diagnosis of cavernous hemangioma.

MANAGEMENT

Surgery or sclerosing techniques or both are used for treatment of a hemangioma. Sclerosing solutions, such as sodium psylliate or sodium morrhuate, are injected into the lesion for the purpose of inducing the formation of fibrous tissue, which scleroses and shrinks the vascular spaces (Fig. 9-10). This technique is often used before surgery to reduce the amount of surgery needed and to reduce the hemorrhage that attends the removal of these conditions.

Minkow and co-workers (1979) reported on treating a series of 24 hemangiomas of the oral cavity and lips with sodium tetradecyl sulfate (Sotradecol). The smaller lesions disappeared after injection, while the larger lesions required up to ten treatments with 2 weeks between treatment. These investigators reported that all lesions disappeared without scarring and no side effects were experienced.

The injection of a sclerosing agent is frequently all that is required. A lesion treated thus will become firm and lose much of its bluish color. The exact size and extent of the tumor must be determined prior to any treatment, however, since the visible portion may represent just the "tip of the iceberg." Angiograms are used to advantage for this purpose. The excision of a moderate or large hemangioma should not be attempted in the dental office; rather the patient should be hospitalized and the procedure done in an operating room, where there is blood ready for transfusions and where extraoral ligation of cervical arteries may be accomplished more readily.

In recent years cryotherapy has gained some acceptance in the treatment of hemangiomas (Leopard, 1975; Murphy, 1978).

ORAL MELANOTIC MACULE

The oral melanotic macule is a pigmented entity of the oral mucosa and lips that has just recently achieved recognition (Buchner and Hansen, 1979a; Page et al., 1977; Weathers et al., 1976). Apparently this lesion is the most common pigmentation to occur in the oral cavity of light-skinned individuals. Concerning incidence Buchner and Hansen (1979) studied 105 cases and reported that the oral melanotic macule accounted for 0.5% of cases accessioned in their laboratory. The cause of the oral melanotic macule is uncertain in the majority of cases but may represent posttraumatic (inflammatory) pigmentation in some cases. Buchner and Hansen suggested the possibility that it is an atypical manifestation of physiologic pigmentation since the

Fig. 9-10. A, Photomicrograph of a cavernous hemangioma showing the many vascular spaces separated by thin connective tissue septa. **B,** Photomicrograph of a cavernous hemangioma that has been sclerosed by an injected agent. Note the decreased number of vascular spaces and the increased fibrous tissue component.

Fig. 9-11. Oral melanotic macule of the lower lip.

histologic appearance is identical to that of melanoplakia.

FEATURES

The oral melanotic macule is usually a solitary lesion that occurs mostly in light-skinned individuals. The lesion is usually well circumscribed and gray, brownish, black, or bluish (Fig. 9-11). The majority measured less than 1 cm across. The largest reported lesion was 2.0 cm across (Page et al., 1977). In Buchner and Hansen's study the most frequent site was the lower lip (28.7%) followed by the gingiva (22.8%), the buccal mucosa (16.2%), and the hard palate (6.7%). The Page study and the Weathers study, although separating the lip lesions as a separate entity from the oral lesions, reported the same site predilections.

The mean age was 41.0 years, 45.4 years, and 31.5 years, respectively, for the Buchner, Page, and Weathers (labial melanotic macule) studies. Buchner and Hansen reported that the female-male ratio was 2.2:1. Page and co-workers reported an approximately equal sex spread. The majority of the lesions remain constant in size and do not tend to become malignant. The only significant histologic observation is the increased pigment contained in the basal cell layer. Lesions also may show melanin in the lamina propria some of which is contained in melanophages. In some instances an increase in the number of clear cells is seen. The microscopic picture is identical to that seen in melanoplakia.

DIFFERENTIAL DIAGNOSIS

The following entities need to be included in the differential discussion of oral melanotic macule: melanoplakia, amalgam tattoo, ecchymotic patch, superficial spreading melanoma, nevi, lentigo, and focal melanosis.

Melanoplakia will not always be distinguishable from the oral melanotic macule but usually the latter entity is smaller and has a different configuration than the melanoplakic patches that are present in the rest of the mucosa of the black patient in question.

The *amalgam tattoo* in most cases will be in a location where it could be associated with a juxtaposed amalgam filling. However, that is not always the case, amalgam tattoos being seen on mucosa that is quite far removed from the alveolar processes.

The *ecchymotic patch* can be easily differentiated from all the melanin-containing macules. The former entity usually has a browner color and disappears within a few days.

Superficial spreading melanoma is much less common, is seen in patients who are on the average 8 years older than those with an oral melanotic macule, and slowly grows by circumferential growth. Oral melanoma occurs twice as frequently in males as does the oral melanotic macule, and the palate is the most common site affected.

Flat *nevi* and *lentigo* are rare lesions in the oral cavity but may look identical clinically to the oral melanotic macule.

Focal melanosis as described by Buchner and Hansen (1979a) shows a similar increase in pigmentation of the basal cell layer. However, focal melanosis, unlike the oral melanotic macule, is not seen as a pigmented lesion clinically. Hence focal melanosis must be considered in the *histologic* differential diagnosis process.

If multiple melanotic patches are present in the oral cavity of a patient the following conditions should be considered: melanoplakia, multiple oral melanotic macules, melanoma, Addison's disease, Albright's syndrome, Peutz-Jeghers syndrome, and postinflammatory pigmentation.

MANAGEMENT

The oral melanotic macule should be excised as soon as possible along with an adequate border of normal tissue and submitted for microscopic study. This is necessary because these lesions cannot be differentiated from small superficial spreading melanomas on a clinical basis. Only one exception is permitted: if a melanin patch has been known to be present for at least 5 years and *no* changes have occurred then it is sufficient to observe the lesion every 6 months. If the patient is known to be unreliable such a

Fig. 9-12. Mucocele. (**B** courtesy G. MacDonald, D.D.S., Belleville, Ill.)

lesion should be excised without further surveillance.

MUCOCELE

The superficial mucocele is one of the most frequent bluish lesions to occur on the lower lip, but it can occur anywhere on the oral mucosa. It is unlikely to be found on the attached gingiva or the anterior hard palate, however, because of the usual absence of minor salivary glands in these regions. The upper lip is also an uncommon location for a mucocele.

The mucocele is thought to occur when a duct of a minor salivary gland is severed by trauma and the secretion is spilled and pooled in the superficial tissues. It seldom possesses an epithelial lining and thus is classified as a false cyst.

A superficial mucocele appears as a bluish mass (Fig. 9-12) because the thin overlying mucosa permits the pool of mucous fluid to absorb most of the visible wavelengths of light except the blue, which is reflected. A deep mucocele, on the other hand, may be normal mucosal pink due to the thickness of the covering mucosa. If it is subjected to chronic irritation, its mucosal covering will be inflamed.

DIFFERENTIAL DIAGNOSIS

A mucocele is usually a fluctuant, bluish, soft, nodular or dome-shaped elevation that is freely movable on the underlying tissue but cannot be moved independently of the mucosal layer. It cannot be emptied by digital pressure, and on aspiration it yields a sticky, viscous, clear fluid. This result helps to rule out the *vascular lesions* and also a *superficial nonkeratotic cyst,* which usually contains a thin straw-colored fluid.

The patient may report that the swelling is somewhat paroxysmal—suddenly recurring, rupturing, and draining periodically. In spite of these rather characteristic features, the differential diagnosis developed for a mucocele must include *early mucoepidermoid tumor* and *mucinous adenocarcinoma*. Both these neoplastic entities may mimic a mucocele inasmuch as superficial pools of mucus may be apparent in all three. Hence the clinician must inspect and palpate the tissue at the base and periphery of the mucocele for induration, which might indicate the presence of such tumors. A salivary tumor is rare in the lower lip but occurs with a higher frequency in the palate, buccal mucosa, and upper lip (Krolls and Hicks, 1973).

MANAGEMENT

Any mucocele should be completely removed and the excised tissue examined microscopically. This is particularly important because some mucin-producing salivary tumors will mimic a mucocele clinically. The lesion should be excised in such a way as to sever a minimum of the ducts of adjacent acini. A good practice is to remove all the glandular units that protrude into the incision because their ducts will likely have been severed. This practice will help to avoid the embarrassing occurrence of numerous iatrogenic satellite mucoceles.

Recently investigators (Wilcox and Hickory, 1978) have suggested steroid injection as an alternative to surgery in the treatment of mucoceles. Abrams (1978) pointed out the danger of missing early mucin-producing tumors using such a treatment approach.

RANULA

A ranula is, in effect, a mucocele that occurs in the floor of the mouth—a retention cyst in the sublingual salivary gland (Fig. 9-13). It derives its name from the diminutive form of the Latin word for frog, *rana;* it is said to resemble a frog's belly.

FEATURES

A pertinent feature to be noted in the history of a ranula is fluctuation in size. The lesion is gen-

Fig. 9-13. Ranula. **A,** Small unilateral dome-shaped bluish lesion. **B,** Large bluish ranula occupying the floor of the mouth.

erally smallest early in the morning before rising and largest just before meals, which reflects the increased secretory activity during periods of gustatory stimulation and water absorption from the pooled mucus during inactive periods of sleep.

When superficially located, a ranula is quite bluish (Fig. 9-13); but a deep ranula will appear pinker, reflecting the thicker mucosal covering. It usually occurs unilaterally, is dome shaped, and may vary greatly in size. It is soft and fluctuant and cannot be emptied by digital pressure. It does not pulsate, and on aspiration it yields the sticky clear fluid characteristic of salivary retention phenomena.

DIFFERENTIAL DIAGNOSIS

The differential diagnosis for a ranula would be identical with that described for a mucocele (p. 191). It is interesting how closely the vascular lesions depicted in Figs. 9-3, *C,* and 9-9, *C,* resemble a ranula both in location and appearance.

MANAGEMENT

Initially, conservative treatment by marsupialization is recommended—excising the entire roof of the ranula and permitting the area to heal

without a dressing. Such an approach necessitates the very careful examination of the lesion's base in case the mucin-producing entity is really a salivary tumor. For the same reason close postoperative surveillance is necessary. Recurrence of the lesion treated in this manner may be expected in a low percentage of the cases. When the lesion does recur, it is an indication that ducts from neighboring sublingual gland units have been severed during operation or occluded by scarring.

Recurrences of the condition may well signal the necessity to adopt a more radical form of treatment, such as the removal of sections of the involved gland or at times the entire gland. If the ranula is very large and a considerable degree of postoperative swelling is anticipated, the patient must be hospitalized to care for airway problems that may develop.

SUPERFICIAL CYST

The odontogenic as well as some of the "fissural" cysts that occur just under the epithelial surface and contain straw-colored fluid appear clinically as bluish, nodular swellings. Although they do occur in patients with a mixed dentition, the most common example of the condition is the eruption type of follicular cyst seen in infants (Plate 1).

Actually several types of odontogenic cysts (radicular, follicular, or residual, or eruption) will appear as nodular, bluish, fluctuant swellings if they are not confined in bone and are located near enough to the surface that the intervening soft tissues can transmit some light to the cyst's mass (Plate 1 and Fig. 9-14).

Epidermoid cysts, however, are filled with keratin so they appear white and are called "Epstein's pearls" when they are small and situated superficially. Also superficial keratocysts will appear white for the same reason.

DIFFERENTIAL DIAGNOSIS

The superficial cyst must be differentiated from all the other soft bluish lesions.

A *cavernous hemangioma* can be evacuated by digital pressure whereas a superficial cyst cannot.

A radiograph will help differentiate a superficial cyst from a *mucocele* since the bony superficial cyst will cause demonstrable bone destruction whereas the mucocele will not be radiographically apparent.

A *gingival cyst* generally will not involve bone, so a radiograph will not be helpful in differentiating it from a mucocele. In addition, a muco-

Fig. 9-14. Bluish cysts. **A,** Bluish translucent shallow dome-shaped mass (arrow), which proved to be a gingival cyst. **B,** Bluish eruption cyst involving the left central incisor tooth. The eruption hematoma would look like this too. (**A** courtesy E. Seklecki, D.D.S., Tucson, Ariz. **B** courtesy A. C. W. Hutchinson collection, Northwestern University Dental School Library, Chicago.)

cele, unlike a gingival cyst, rarely if ever occurs on the gingiva or the alveolar ridges since minor salivary glands are not normally present in these locations.

Provided the cyst is not infected, a thin straw-colored fluid will be obtained on aspiration whereas a clear, viscous, sticky fluid will be found in the mucocele.

MANAGEMENT

The treatment of intrabony cysts is discussed in detail in Chapters 17 and 18.

GIANT CELL GRANULOMA

The giant cell granuloma may be either central or peripheral. The central variety is discussed in detail in Chapter 18, whereas the peripheral type is described in Chapter 7 as an exophytic lesion. The exophytic giant cell granuloma, as well as some of the other inflammatory hyperplastic lesions, may be bluish, so it is also included in this chapter.

Apparently the exophytic giant cell granuloma tends to undergo intermittent episodes of internal hemorrhage, for there is often a considerable amount of hemosiderin observed in the tissue. If the hemosiderin is located near the surface, it often imparts a bluish-brown appearance to the superficial (peripheral) lesion (Plate 1). The numerous vascular spaces filled with bluish blood also account for the bluish color.

DIFFERENTIAL DIAGNOSIS

The following lesions should be considered in the differential diagnosis of the peripheral giant cell granuloma (PGCG): other inflammatory hy-perplastic lesions, hemangioma, lymphangioma, metastatic tumors of the gingiva, nevi, and nodular melanomas.

Other *inflammatory hyperplastic* lesions need not really be differentiated because they represent the same basic pathosis as the peripheral giant cell granuloma.

The majority of *hemangiomas* have been present from birth. In contradistinction the PGCG is of relatively recent onset. Also congenital hemangiomas seldom occur on the gingiva yet the gingiva and alveolar mucosa are the only locations of the PGCG.

Oral *lymphangiomas* are much less common than the PGCG and rarely occur on the gingiva. In addition, the lymphangioma will have a much paler color.

Metastatic carcinoma to the gingiva must be considered also. However, in the absence of a history of a primary tumor elsewhere this entity would deserve a low ranking. Evidence of bone destruction under the exophytic lesions would prompt the clinician to consider metastatic tumor as more likely.

Oral nevi and nodular melanomas occur much less frequently than does the PGCG and will in almost all cases be firmer to palpation, also they are usually darker in color except for the amelanotic varieties. Finally, a nodular melanoma will produce a history of rapid growth.

MANAGEMENT

The cardinal rule is that radiographic examination is a necessary adjunct in the clinical evaluation of all exophytic lesions. Therefore adequate radiographs of the area in question must be available to determine whether underlying bone is involved. Also the giant cell lesion of hyperparathyroidism must be ruled out by examining the serum for the biochemical signs of this disease. Surgical excision is the treatment of choice.

Although less than 10% of these lesions recur after excision, patients who have had them removed should receive two or three yearly examinations so that any recurrence will not go undetected.

BLACK HAIRY TONGUE

Hairy tongue is a harmless entity occurring on the dorsum of the tongue; it occurs in approximately 0.15% of the general population (Farman, 1977). This condition is the result of an elongation of the filiform papillae, in some cases to such

an extent that they resemble hair (Fig. 9-15). This alteration in the papillae results from an increased retention and accumulation of keratin (hyperkeratosis) (Fig. 9-15). The condition has been thought to be provoked by irritation from one or a combination of the following local factors:

1. Food debris remaining on the tongue and becoming impacted between the papillae in people not practicing good oral hygiene
2. Habitual use of oxidizing or astringent agents in oral preparations
3. Local use of some antibiotics
4. Use of tobacco
5. *Candida albicans* infection

Systemic influences such as systemic antibiotic therapy, anemia, and general debilitation have been suspected to play an etiologic role (Farman,

Fig. 9-15. Black hairy tongue. **A** and **B,** Clinical views of patients. **C,** High-magnification photomicrograph shows elongated filiform papillae with increased keratin retention. (**C** courtesy A. C. W. Hutchinson collection, Northwestern University Dental School Library, Chicago.)

1977). It is interesting that Mann and co-workers (1974) showed that zinc deficiency in sheep was associated with hairy tongue.

The hyperplastic, hyperkeratotic papillae are essentially light colored, but the color they assume is a consequence of local factors in and about them. Chromogenic bacteria, mineral and vitamin preparations, drugs, and dark-colored food materials may be responsible for changing a white hairy tongue to tan, to brown, and then to black. Pain is usually not a feature, but gagging may be a problem.

Farman (1977) in a large study of hairy tongue reported that patients with malignant neoplasia are much more prone to develop this condition (22.06% of his patients with a malignant neoplasm had hairy tongue). This investigator found a slightly increased incidence in elderly patients also (0.72%). Additional findings indicated that hairy tongue is generally associated with candidal organisms and that the pH of saliva on hairy tongues was 6 or less. The majority of Farman's patients with hairy tongue were not smoking at the time of the study but most had smoked previously in their lives.

MANAGEMENT

Improved tongue-brushing techniques after shearing the elongated papillae with scissors are generally all that is necessary.

LYMPHANGIOMA
FEATURES

A lymphangioma is very similar to a cavernous hemangioma. Like the hemangioma it is congenital; but it is much less common. Its most frequent intraoral sites are the dorsal surface and lateral borders of the tongue (Fig. 9-16). Its color is less blue than that of a hemangioma, ranging from normal mucosal pink to bluish, and may be quite translucent. Aspiration yields lymph fluid that is high in lipid content.

The dilated lymphatic channels of a lymphangioma characteristically reach high into the lamina propria and often contact epithelial basement membranes. This feature is often pronounced enough to impart a pebbly appearance to the surface of the lesion. In addition, this feature may hinder the evacuation of the lesion by digital pressure.

DIFFERENTIAL DIAGNOSIS

The differential diagnosis of a lymphangioma would be identical to that for a cavernous hemangioma. Aspiration with a fine-gauge needle may be used to differentiate these two lesions.

Fig. 9-16. Lymphangioma. **A,** Pebbly surfaced lesion on the dorsum of the tongue. **B,** Note the numerous lymphatic spaces, some of which appear to be in intimate contact with the surface epithelium. (**A** courtesy D. Bonomo, D.D.S., Flossmoor, Ill.)

MANAGEMENT

Even small lesions on the dorsal surface and lateral borders of the tongue are often continually irritated and become a worry to the patient. It follows that surgical excision is the treatment of choice; but a hemangioma must be ruled out before the excisional procedure is undertaken. Excision of a lymphangioma is not as hazardous a procedure as is excision of a hemangioma; still, if the lesion is larger than 2 cm and is located on the tongue, the patient should be hospitalized because of the possibility of extensive postoperative edema and a related airway problem.

PIGMENTED FIBROMA (PIGMENTED EPULIS)

The pigmented fibroma occurs occasionally in the oral cavity. It is a small, moderately firm, nodular or polypoid mass light bluish or brownish in appearance. It is frequently mistaken for a nevus, and its true identity is dependent on microscopic examination—which demonstrates it to be a fibroma or a myxofibroma with increased melanin deposition in the basal layer of the epithelium (fibroma in melanoplakic patch). The entity, then, must be included in the differential diagnosis of "nevoidlike" lesions.

MELANOMA

Melanoma is a moderately uncommon malignant tumor of melanocytes; 9000 new cases for all body sites are diagnosed each year: oral melanomas are rare, accounting for approximately 1% of all melanomas (Weathers et al., 1976).

In the past melanomas of the skin have been lumped more or less as a single entity with a uniformly poor prognosis. During the last decade or two new information has changed this concept dramatically (Clark et al., 1969; McGovern, 1976). Most primary melanomas of the skin may now be classified into three separate lesions on a clinical, histologic, and behavioral basis: (1) lentigo maligna melanoma, (2) superficial spreading melanoma, and (3) nodular melanoma (Regezi et al., 1978). These have been listed in ascending order of malignant behavior.

Lentigo maligna melanoma has a predilection for the exposed surfaces of older patients. Clinically it is seen as a pigmented macule with an ill-defined margin. During phase one it grows slowly in a radial (developing uniformly around a central axis) and a superficial manner. This slow growth phase usually continues for many years, and then behavior becomes more aggressive as phase two takes over. In this second stage invasion becomes advanced and metastasis frequent (Regezi et al., 1978). Prognosis for the lentigo maligna melanoma is considered to be good particularly if it is completely excised during the radial growth phase.

Superficial spreading melanoma is the most common form of melanoma and shows some behavioral characteristics similar to lentigo maligna melanoma. It begins as a pigmented macule that enlarges slowly over several years in a superficial radial growth pattern (Fig. 9-17). As the name implies, the malignant melanocytes are very superficial, being restricted mostly to the epithelium and the junction. If the lesion is left untreated it will shift into the more aggressive vertical growth phase and show as a pigmented nodule or nodules within the larger pigmented patch. Metastasis usually does not occur while the lesion is in the superficial spreading (radial)

growth phase. Thus if the lesion is completely excised during the superficial phase the prognosis is much better than for nodular melanoma.

Nodular melanoma arising by itself without a superficial spreading component grows rapidly, may metastasize early, and carries the poorest prognosis of all.

Clark and co-workers (1969) reported the following mortality rate for the three types of skin melanomas: lentigo maligna melanoma, 10.3%; superficial spreading melanoma, 31.5%; and nodular melanoma, 56.1%.

Oral melanomas and melanomas of the lips are rare tumors. Like their skin counterparts, over the years the oral tumors have been grouped as one entity with a uniformly grave prognosis (Bina, 1979; Chaudry et al., 1960; Eneroth, 1975). Recently it has been recognized that there are behavioral differences among oral melanomas (Jackson and Simpson, 1975; Liversedge, 1975). Also a few superficial spreading melanomas of the oral cavity have been reported (Bennett et al., 1976; Regezi et al., 1978; Robertson et al., 1979). In addition to these developments there has been a history of a previously existing pigmented patch (melanosis) in a significant number of large nodular melanomas that have been reported (Regezi et al., 1978). Thus it seems likely that a significant number of oral melanomas are of the superficial spreading type that have been present for some years but have not been diagnosed until the lesion has changed to the more aggressive vertical growth phase.

FEATURES

The oral melanoma may be encountered as one of four enlarging clinical lesions: a pigmented macule, a pigmented nodule, a large pigmented exophytic lesion, or an amelanotic (unpigmented) variety of any of these three forms (Figs. 9-17 and 9-18). It may vary in color from a mucosal pink through brown and blue to black. It is usually quite firm to palpation but not as firm as a squamous cell carcinoma. The oral variety ulcerates with some frequency but does not possess a rolled raised border. There is often an erythematous border in the mucosa surrounding the tumor, which represents an inflammatory reaction of the surrounding tissue to the tumor.

The oral melanoma occurs most frequently in the maxillary alveolar mucosa and on the hard and soft palates (Figs. 9-17 and 9-18). The rate of growth in superficial spreading melanoma is very slow until the vertical phase is reached. The growth rate for the nodular melanoma,

Fig. 9-17. Superficial spreading melanomas. **A** and **B,** Two views of a superficial spreading melanoma on the maxillary ridge of a 45-year-old white man. The patient had watched it slowly grow for several months. **B,** Mirror shot showing spread of tumor from the labial gingiva through the interproximal area to involve the lingual gingiva. **C,** Superficial spreading melanoma of the lower lip in a 59-year-old white man had been present for 8 years, spreading from two small pigmented patches. Nodules were now present on the mucosal surface. (**A** and **B** from Robertson, G. R., Defiebre, B. K., and Firtell, D. N.: J. Oral Surg. **37:**349-352, 1979. Copyright by the American Dental Association. Reprinted by permission. **C** from Regezi, J. A., Hayward, J. R., and Pickens, T. N.: Oral Surg. **45:**730-740, 1978.)

Fig. 9-18. Advanced melanomas of the maxillary ridge and palate. **A,** Nodular melanoma appeared to have a superficial spreading component at the periphery. **B,** Large advanced nodular melanoma in a 56-year-old woman. (**A** courtesy S. Smith, D.D.S., Chicago.)

though usually very rapid, may be variable. The tumor is usually painless unless ulcerated or infected or both. Rapid infiltration of the adjacent deep tissues frequently occurs in the nodular type and fixes the superficial tissues to the deeper layers.

DIFFERENTIAL DIAGNOSIS

The early melanoma, which appears clinically as a small brownish-blue macule, may be readily confused with an *amalgam tattoo*, an *oral melanotic macule*, a *focal hemosiderin deposit* after trauma, or a localized area of *melanoplakia*.

The clinician will have difficulty arriving at a working diagnosis when he must choose between these entities with only the information available from the patient examination.

The early nodular melanoma is difficult or impossible to differentiate clinically from an *intramucosal, compound,* or *blue nevus,* a *pigmented fibroma,* or a small pigmented *peripheral giant cell granuloma* that contains a large amount of hemosiderin. Occasionally the nodular melanoma will have an irregular, fissured, or ulcerated and bleeding surface—features that strongly suggest malignancy. Rapid growth would point to melanoma.

Although the rapidly enlarging pigmented exophytic variety is not easily confused with other entities, the clinician may be confronted with a lesion in a patient he is seeing for the first time and the patient may not be able to tell how long the lesion has been present or whether it is enlarging.

If the melanin is deposited near the surface, the *melanotic neuroectodermal tumor of infancy* may be quite similar in appearance to the pigmented melanoma. A good number of these appear clinically with a nonpigmented pink surface, however, because the melanin is deposited in the deeper tissue. The anterior maxilla is a common site for either of these tumors; but the average age of occurrence of an oral melanoma is in the 50s (the youngest occurrence reported was in a child 5 years old) whereas the melanotic tumor of infancy occurs in children under 1 year of age.

The amelanotic melanoma is sometimes mistaken clinically for a *pyogenic granuloma* or it may resemble many of the *benign* or *malignant tumors* that have nodular, polypoid, or exophytic shapes.

The macular bluish, brownish, or black lesions such as melanoplakia, the oral melanotic macule, and ecchymotic patch need to be considered in the differential diagnosis of superficial spreading

melanoma. All are macules with similar coloring.

The *ecchymotic patch* will disappear within a few days, passing through the various characteristic color changes. Frequently these may be related to a traumatic episode.

Melanoplakia, the physiologic pigmentation found in the oral cavities of blacks, will have been present since infancy or puberty without change. Most designs are similar throughout the mouth and so if a patch of unusual design were present the clinician would be more likely to suspect a superficial spreading type of melanoma. If the patch had appeared 2 or 3 years ago in an adult between 40 and 70 years of age and had increased in size then the working diagnosis would be superficial spreading melanoma.

The *oral melanotic macule* cannot be differentiated from an early lesion of superficial spreading melanoma. If the pigmented patch is over 2 cm in size and has shown evidence of enlargement it must be considered a superficial spreading melanoma until proven otherwise by microscopic study.

MANAGEMENT

If the suspicion index is very low, a melanoma may be ruled out by just observing the small pigmented area for a time. An example could be the amalgam tattoo; if the working diagnosis is amalgam tattoo, then the lesion should be watched for a period to see whether it changes.

If the suspicion index is higher and the lesion is small, however, it should be excised early with a wide margin of normal tissue and microscopically examined. Radical resection with removal of regional lymph nodes may be necessary for larger lesions.

The prognosis for oral melanomas is poor because characteristically they are discovered in advanced stages and they metastasize early to the regional nodes and via vascular routes to the lungs, liver, skin, brain, and bones. However, the prognosis is much improved if the tumor is of the superficial spreading type and is excised in the radial growth phase when the lesion is small. The possibility that the oral lesion is a secondary (metastatic) lesion should always be considered (Fig. 7-29).

NEVUS

A nevus is a congenital or acquired benign tumor of the melanocytes or nevus cells that occurs on the skin but seldom intraorally. It is usually but not always pigmented, ranging in color from gray to light brown to blue to black. There are four types of oral nevi: intramucosal, junctional, compound, and blue.

The intramucosal (intradermal*) nevus is composed of a bulk of nevus cells in the lamina propria, which do not contact the basement membrane. Because this bulk of cells is packed within the usually dense collagenous connective tissue stroma, the nevus is firm to palpation and is generally raised in the form of a smooth nodule but sometimes it appears as a polypoid mass (Fig. 9-19). The intramucosal nevus must be differentiated from a *pigmented fibroma* and a *nodular melanoma*.

The junctional nevus derives its name from the fact that the nevus cells are in the basal layer just above the junction of the epidermis and dermis. It is usually not raised because there are just a few nevus cells present (Fig. 9-19). This lesion must be differentiated from *melanoplakia*, an *amalgam tattoo*, a *melanotic macule*, and a *melanoma*.

The compound nevus cells are in both locations—lamina propria and basal layer of the epithelium. This lesion therefore is a firm, raised nodule or polypoid mass having a clinical appearance identical with that of the intramucosal nevus.

The blue nevus is also a raised nodule generally dark blue in color with stellate and fusiform cells usually containing melanin. These cells are usually located deep in the lamina propria, which is why the lesion may appear more darkly pigmented than the other nevi. It can be moved over the submucosal structures but cannot be moved independently of the mucosa. It must be differentiated from a melanoma, but this cannot be done clinically.

Buchner and Hansen (1979b) reported on 32 new cases of intraoral nevi: 66% were intramucosal type, 25% were common blue nevi, 6% were compound, and 3% were the junctional type. The locations of the lesions were as follows: 37.5% on the hard palate, 16% on the buccal mucosa, and 12.5% each on the labial mucosa, the vermilion border, and the gingiva. Ninety-one percent of the nevi exhibited pigmentation clinically. The mean age of the patients was 29.6 years and the female-male ratio was 3.6:1.

DIFFERENTIAL DIAGNOSIS

The firmness of a nevus to palpation distinguishes this lesion from a *cyst,* a *retention phenomenon* of the minor salivary glands, and a

---

*The intradermal nevus or common mole is one of the most frequently occurring pigmented lesions of the skin.

Fig. 9-19. Nevus. **A** and **B,** Junctional nevi. **C,** Histopathology of a junctional nevus. **D,** This exophytic lesion proved to be an intramucosal nevus. (**D** courtesy N. Herrod, D.D.S., Provo, Utah.)

hemangioma. An exception might be a *sclerosing hemangioma;* but even it will have some vascular spaces that are reddish and will blanch on digital pressure, a characteristic not shared by the nevi.

The occurrence of a dark bluish lesion in proximity to an amalgam restoration, or the probability of such a previous relationship in an edentulous area, lends support to identifying the condition as an *amalgam tattoo.*

Small areas of hemorrhage may resemble a junctional nevus but will change color and disappear within a week or so.

A nevus cannot be definitely differentiated from an early *melanoma* except by microscopic study; but a change in degree of pigmentation, bleeding, or surface appearance is an ominous sign.

The *oral melanotic macule* looks identical to a nonraised nevus or early superficial spreading melanoma. The two latter lesions are much less common, however, and so would be ranked much lower in the differential process.

MANAGEMENT

A nevus should be excised with a wide border of normal tissue and carefully studied microscopically. The opinion still persists today that some melanomas may arise from nevi.

MUCUS-PRODUCING SALIVARY GLAND TUMORS

The mucoepidermoid tumor is a malignancy of the salivary glands that originates with some frequency in the oral cavity. Three cell types are seen:

1. A mucous cell
2. An epidermoid cell
3. An intermediate-type cell

The greater the percentage of mucous cells, the less malignant the tumor is thought to be. This low-grade variety is included with the blue lesions because pools of mucus are frequently present (Fig. 9-20). Thus the tumor may resemble a mucocele clinically.

The mucous cell adenocarcinoma is another tumor of salivary glands that produces a moderate quantity of mucus and can likewise mimic a mucocele in its early stages.

An advanced tumor of these two types might have an overall firm consistency with discrete, soft, fluctuant areas intermixed.

DIFFERENTIAL DIAGNOSIS

The lower lip is a very uncommon site for a salivary gland tumor but a frequent site for a mucocele. Hence a bluish, fluctuant, dome-shaped, nonemptiable swelling on the lower lip is most likely a *mucocele.*

A lesion resembling a mucocele on the palate or even the buccal mucosa or upper lip, however, should be viewed with suspicion since mucoceles are less common in these areas.

MANAGEMENT

The base of any clinical mucocele should be examined carefully for induration, which might

Fig. 9-20. Low-grade mucoepidermoid tumor showing pools of mucus *(m),* which may cause this lesion to clinically mimic a mucocele.

indicate an infiltrating tumor. Of course, all excised tissue from a lesion of this type must be microscopically examined to establish the true nature of the lesion. Wide resection is the treatment of choice for a mucoepidermoid tumor.

VON RECKLINGHAUSEN'S DISEASE (MULTIPLE NEUROFIBROMATOSIS)

Multiple neurofibromatosis is a hereditary disease that is thought to be transmitted as an autosomal dominant trait. The two most common features of this disorder are the multiple neurofibromas and the café-au-lait spots (Fig. 9-21). The tumors are frequently of the plexiform variety and thus are soft, smooth, fluctuant, usually flesh colored, and nodular or pedunculated; however, they will occasionally assume large pendulous flabby proportions.

Multiple cutaneous neurofibromas are a characteristic sign. Axillary freckling, when present, is also characteristic. These spots, as their color suggests, are the result of increased pigment in the basal layer and, like the neurofibromas, are sometimes encountered in the oral cavity.

The café-au-lait spots are brownish macules that occur at any cutaneous site, including the genitalia, soles, and palms. They are present in more than 90% of the cases and are diagnostic when more than five are present and they are larger than 1.5 cm in diameter.

DIFFERENTIAL DIAGNOSIS

The multiple cutaneous neurofibromas identify von Recklinghausen's disease.

Although the *multiple basal cell nevus syndrome* has cutaneous tumors and is accompanied by cysts in the jaws, unlike the neurofibromas of von Recklinghausen's disease, the tumors of the basal cell nevus syndrome are restricted to the skin of the face, neck, and chest. Furthermore, pigmentation is not a feature of this syndrome.

Multiple mucosal plexiform neurofibromas are also seen as part of a syndrome with *nodular carcinoma of the thyroid gland* and *pheochromocytoma,* but cutaneous neurofibromas and pigmentation are not features.

Multiple desmoid tumors, fibromas, and epidermoid cysts occur on the skin of patients who have *Gardner's syndrome,* but there are no pigmented macules present. In addition, patients with Gardner's syndrome have multiple osteomas of the cranial and facial bones, including the jaws, and multiple polyposis of the colon.

The differential diagnosis of diseases with café-au-lait spots is presented under Albright's syndrome, discussed next.

MANAGEMENT

The café-au-lait component does not require treatment, but surgical excision of individual neurofibromas may be necessary for various reasons. Approximately 7% of these patients develop a neurogenic sarcoma.

ALBRIGHT'S SYNDROME

Albright's syndrome is a developmental defect of unknown cause in which the following three features are present:
1. Café-au-lait macules
2. Single or multiple involvement of bones with fibrous dysplasia leading to deformity and fractures
3. Precocious puberty in girls

This entity is uncommon in its complete form and more frequently occurs with features 1 and 2 only, which combination is known as Jaffe's type. The café-au-lait spots are irregularly shaped, brownish-tan macules seen in the skin and sometimes in the oral mucosa. They represent melanin deposition.

DIFFERENTIAL DIAGNOSIS

When pigmented macules are found on the skin and oral mucosa, the following syndromes and diseases must be considered: Albright's syndrome, von Recklinghausen's disease, Peutz-Jeghers syndrome, and Addison's disease.

Patients with *Addison's disease* in some instances will have discrete macules instead of the diffuse tanning (Fig. 9-22). The classic symptoms

Fig. 9-21. Café-au-lait spots on a patient with von Recklinghausen's disease. Note the small nodular multiple neurofibromas. (Courtesy P. D. Toto, D.D.S., Maywood, Ill.)

Fig. 9-22. Perioral macular pigmentation in patient with Addison's disease. (Courtesy S. Smith, D.D.S., Chicago.)

A

B

C

D

Fig. 9-23. Peutz-Jeghers syndrome. **A** and **B,** Perioral pigmentation. **C,** Radiograph showing intestinal polyposis. **D,** Specimen of intestine showing numerous polyps on the luminal surface. (Courtesy D. Cooksey, D.D.S., Los Angeles.)

of adrenal insufficiency will differentiate this disease from the others.

Peutz-Jeghers syndrome also can be excluded since the pigmented macules on the skin in this disorder are restricted to the area surrounding body orifices and/or the fingers (Fig. 9-23). Then too the symptoms that result from the accompanying intestinal polyposis will preclude confusing Peutz-Jeghers syndrome with Albright's syndrome and von Recklinghausen's disease.

The café-au-lait spots occurring in *Albright's syndrome* are seen in young patients with fibrous dysplasia and precocious puberty. In contrast, the café-au-lait spots occurring in *von Recklinghausen's disease* are associated with concomitant cutaneous and mucosal multiple neurofibromas.

MANAGEMENT

The café-au-lait feature of Albright's syndrome does not require treatment. The jaws, however, may be affected with the lesions of fibrous dysplasia and thus may require recontouring for esthetic considerations.

HEAVY METAL LINES

Chronic poisoning with heavy metals (e.g., mercury, lead, bismuth) may result in a dark brownish to blue-black discoloration in the oral cavity. Most frequently the heavy metals are deposited as a line or band on inflamed marginal gingiva.

This particular pattern of deposition is the result of increased capillary permeability in the free gingivae caused by inflammation, permitting perivascular infiltration of the tissues by the metal. The pigmentation will not disappear when the irritation is removed and the accompanying inflammation resolved. Information obtained from the history will be the most useful in establishing a positive identification of the offending metal.

More stringent regulations on working conditions in factories that use heavy metals, more careful inspection and elimination of chipping lead paint in the interior of old houses, and also elimination of these metals from medicines have greatly reduced the incidence of this type of lesion.

RARITIES

Although the disease conditions mentioned as rarities do have distinctly circumscribed brownish, bluish, or black oral lesions, either they occur very rarely or, if found more frequently, oral lesions are seldom a feature. No ranking according to frequency of occurrence has been attempted:

Acanthosis nigricans
Acromegaly
Addison's disease (distinct circumscribed lesions)
Chlorpromazine therapy
Cushing's syndrome
Fabry's disease
Gaucher's disease
Hereditary hemorrhagic telangiectasia
Kaposi's sarcoma
Lentigo
Lichen planus
Lupus erythematosus
Lymphangiomas of neonates
Lymphoma (superficial)
Melanotic neuroectodermal tumor of infancy
Pernicious anemia
Peutz-Jeghers syndrome
Pheochromocytoma
Rheumatic fever
Scleroderma
Submucous fibrosis
Superficial cartilaginous tumor in patient with ochronosis or alkaptonuria
Superficial *Pseudomonas aeruginosa* infection
Thyrotoxicosis
Uremia (petechiae)
Xeroderma pigmentosa

Generalized brownish, bluish, or black conditions

CYANOSIS

Cyanosis is caused by a substantial rise in the proportion of reduced hemoglobin to oxygenated hemoglobin in the blood. It may be local or generalized according to the cause. For instance, a tourniquet that has been applied to a patient's arm for a considerable length of time will produce a local cyanosis of the arm whereas a hysterical crying child who is hypoventilating will have a generalized cyanosis.

A rule of thumb holds that cyanosis will become clinically apparent when the reduced hemoglobin reaches 5 g/dl. The generalized bluish cast to the skin is readily seen in whites but is easier to overlook in dark-skinned individuals. It can be detected quite readily in the oral mucous membranes of individuals of all races and complexions.

Coldness may cause a peripheral cyanosis on

the lips and extremities, but the cause of this condition is readily apparent.

Basically there are three causes of generalized cyanosis:

1. Respiratory deficiency
2. Cardiovascular pathology
3. Abnormal hemoglobin metabolism

Examples of respiratory disease causing generalized cyanosis are advanced tuberculosis, emphysema, and pneumonia. Common cardiovascular diseases that cause generalized cyanosis are congenital heart defects, right ventricular failure, and ventricular fibrillation. Clubbing of the fingers will often accompany cyanosis if it has persisted as a chronic condition.

DIFFERENTIAL DIAGNOSIS

The diagnosis of the general medical problem should be placed in the hands of a competent physician.

MANAGEMENT

Before the clinician composes a treatment plan or initiates any dental treatment for the cyanotic patient, he must be aware of the serious implications and potential problems that may be encountered. Thus it is imperative that the physician's advice be sought, obtained, and followed. Of course, if the patient is having an acute attack, the dental clinician must initiate emergency measures supporting circulation and respiration until the patient is in the hands of a competent medical team.

CHLOASMA GRAVIDARUM

Chloasma gravidarum is the tanned mask seen on the cheeks, nose, and infraorbital areas of pregnant light-skinned women during the latter half of pregnancy. It is occasionally accompanied by a diffuse browning of the oral mucosa. The pigmentation slowly disappears after delivery. The increased ACTH level during pregnancy is thought to account for the increased melanocyte activity.

ADDISON'S DISEASE

Addison's disease occurs in approximately one in 100,000 of the population and is extremely rare in children. Bilateral adrenocortical destruction after tuberculous or fungal infection and an idiopathic atrophy are the most frequent causes. Occasionally bilateral tumor metastasis, leukemic infiltration, and amyloidosis of the adrenal cortex have been found to be responsible. Whatever the cause, the loss of adrenal cortex results in a deficiency in both glucocorticoids and mineralocorticoids.

It has been shown that ACTH and MSH are similar in structure, and ACTH is believed to have some degree of melanocyte-stimulating activity. Normally the pituitary gland produces ACTH, which in turn causes the adrenal cortex to produce glucocorticoids (e.g., hydrocortisone), which are secreted into the circulation. When the glucocorticoids reach a certain blood level, they cause the anterior pituitary to cease production of ACTH. In Addison's disease, however, the defective cortex is unable to produce much glucocorticoid, so this feedback mechanism is not activated and the pituitary continues to produce ACTH. As a result the increased production of melanin changes the color of the skin to a smoky tan or a chestnut brown (Plate 1).

Pigmentation usually appears early and is one of the most prominent signs of the disease. It may take one of two forms, the more usual being a deep tanning of the skin and mucous membranes with heavier deposits of melanin over pressure points. The cheek is the most common site for this pigmentation in the oral mucosa. More infrequently the increased melanocytic activity is expressed by the development of distinct brownish macules on the oral mucosa and skin (Plate 1 and Fig. 9-22).

Other clinical features that attend the disease are hypotension, lymphocytosis, hyperkalemia, hypoglycemia, hyponatremia, and a reduced basal metabolic rate.

DIFFERENTIAL DIAGNOSIS

A good history coupled with an alert clinical appraisal should guide the practitioner to the correct working diagnosis. The type that produces an overall deep tanning of the skin as well as of the mucous membranes must be differentiated from hemochromatosis, argyria, and several rarer entities (e.g., hyperpituitarism).

Addison's disease may be distinguished from *hyperpituitarism* by the fact that urine levels of 17-ketosteroids are decreased in the former but elevated in the latter condition. Although *chronic adrenal insufficiency* is rare in children, it does occur to complete the occasional and little understood genetic syndrome characterized by superficial candidiasis, idiopathic familial juvenile hypoparathyroidism, and Addison's disease.

A history of silver ingestion identifies *argyria*.

An accompanying hepatic fibrosis, diabetes, other endocrinopathies, and iron deposition in the affected organs and the skin differentiate *hemochromatosis* from Addison's disease.

The macular type of discoloration that occasionally develops in place of the more generalized tanning might be mistaken for *Peutz-Jeghers syndrome, Albright's syndrome,* or *von Recklinghausen's disease;* however, the attending features of these individual syndromes should preclude any such confusion.

MANAGEMENT

The dentist should not begin treatment without first consulting the patient's physician. If the disease is well controlled, the patient will be able to withstand dental procedures. Supplementation of their corticosteroid medication is always required prior to dental work.

HEMOCHROMATOSIS (BRONZE DIABETES)

Bronze diabetes is a disorder in which excess iron is deposited in the body and results in eventual sclerosis and dysfunction of the tissues and organs so involved. The iron is stored in the form of hemosiderin and ferritin. Three circumstances are generally believed to be contributing influences—idiopathy, diet, and excessive blood transfusions—and all three relate to increasing iron levels in the body.

No agreement has yet been reached as to the exact pathogenesis of the three types of hemochromatosis (or even whether they are different). The most frequent organs involved are the liver, the skin, and the endocrine glands, especially the pancreas and the adrenal glands.

In the idiopathic type there appears to be a defect in the iron-absorption mechanism permitting increased intestinal absorption. The gradual surplus of iron accumulates until enough is present to produce the symptoms, usually in the fourth and fifth decades.

The cause of the tanning in hemochromatosis, like that in Addison's disease, is an increased melanin production and not the deposition of hemosiderin in the skin. This, as in Addison's disease, results from the high levels of ACTH that accompany the destruction of the adrenal cortex by the heavy iron deposits. The effect is a blue-gray color of the skin, especially over the genitalia, face, and arms.

The disease is primarily manifested in males, with over 80% of the cases occurring in men. This difference is attributed to the greater intake of dietary iron in men, which they are unable to excrete. On the other hand, women apparently lose enough iron during menses and pregnancy to preclude the tissue deposits of iron from reaching toxic levels. In addition, the genetic defect in the iron absorption mechanism that has been proposed may have greater penetrance in males.

DIFFERENTIAL DIAGNOSIS

Similar skin and oral pigmentation is seen in *Addison's disease, argyria,* and some of the rare diseases (e.g., *Wilson's disease* [hepatolenticular degeneration] and *porphyria*). A careful history and clinical examination will rule out the other states. When the triad of hemochromatosis (i.e., skin pigmentation, liver disease, diabetes) is present in a male patient, the diagnosis is not difficult.

Although a skin biopsy showing iron deposits is of value in confirming the diagnosis, determination of the iron content and iron-binding capacity of the serum and biopsies of the bone marrow and liver are considered more reliable than the skin biopsy.

MANAGEMENT

The dental clinician must work closely with the patient's physician when oral treatment is planned. The patient will be more susceptible to infection, to cardiovascular collapse, and to hypoglycemic episodes—tendencies that are characteristic of adrenal insufficiency and diabetes.

ARGYRIA (SILVER PIGMENTATION)

Whites who have silver pigmentation develop a striking bluish-gray (slate-colored) skin, especially in the exposed areas (Plate 1). They invariably give a history of having used some type of self-medication, such as nose drops, which contains silver salts, over a long period. Silver deposition often causes accompanying neurologic and hearing damage, which in turn affects the equilibrium. It also stimulates melanocyte activity in the skin, hence the more intense color in exposed areas. The bluish-gray discoloration has been reported to also occur in the oral mucosa (Plate 1).

DIFFERENTIAL DIAGNOSIS

The bluish-gray color is usually easily distinguished from the more brownish *Addisonian color. Hemochromatosis* also will produce a browner color. The fact that exposed areas of the skin are not more discolored than the covered areas differentiates *cyanotic states* from argyria. Histologic identification of silver particles fixed

Table 9-1. Distinct circumscribed types of brownish, bluish, or black conditions

MACULES

Condition	Appearance	Usual history	Usual age of occurrence (years)	Frequency
Melanoplakia	Macules of varying size, shape, and location on oral mucosa	No symptoms	Under 1	Very common in dark-skinned races
Amalgam tattoo	Macule on gingiva or edentulous ridge	No symptoms Amalgam fillings	5 and over	Common
Petechia Ecchymosis	Macule anywhere in oral cavity or skin	Recent trauma and/or bleeding diathesis	Young children Older adults	Occasional
Melanotic macule	Small macule (under 2 mm) on lower lip, gingiva, or buccal mucosa	No symptoms	Mean age = 41-42	Occasional Male-female ratio = 1:2.2
Superficial spreading melanoma	Enlarging macule on palate or maxillary gingiva	Present for several years Slowly enlarging	Mean age = 50.5	Rare Male-female ratio = 2:1
Junctional nevus	Macule anywhere on oral mucosa (palate, lips)	No symptoms	Mean age = 38	Rare in oral cavity Equal frequency for males and females
Heavy metal lines	Macular ribbon following free gingivae	Malaise Anemia	Working age	Rare
Peutz-Jeghers syndrome	Macules around lips, buccal mucosa, fingers, and other body orifices	Melena Intestinal colic	More distinct at puberty	Rare
Albright's syndrome	Macules (café-au-lait spots) anywhere on skin or mucous membranes	Skeletal problems Precocious puberty in girls	6-10	Rare

EXOPHYTIC LESIONS OF SOFT CONSISTENCY

Condition	Appearance	Fluctuance	May be emptied	Usual history	Usual age of occurrence (years)	Frequency
Black hairy tongue	Patch of hairy growth, varying in length, on dorsal surface of tongue	No	No	Feels like hairs on tongue Gagging sensation	Over 30	Occasional
Mucocele	Nodular swelling	Yes	No	Variation in size Occasional rupture and drainage	Over 40	Occasional Significantly more common in males
Ranula	Nodular swelling on floor of mouth	Yes	No	Slowly enlarging Smaller in early morning		Occasional Significantly more common in females
Cavernous hemangioma	Nodular swelling	Usually not	Yes	Present from birth or after trauma Occasional bleeding		Occasional
Early hematoma	Nodular swelling	Yes	No	Recent trauma and/or bleeding diatheses		Occasional
Superficial cyst	Nodular swelling	Yes	No	Displaced teeth Slowly enlarging swelling		Occasional

Table 9-1. Distinct circumscribed types of brownish, bluish, or black conditions—cont'd

Condition	Appearance	Fluctu-ance	May be emptied	Usual history	Usual age of occurrence (years)	Frequency
Lymphangioma	Nodular swelling Surface frequently has pebbly appearance	Usually not	Partially	Present from birth or after trauma		Rare
Mucoepidermoid tumor	Mucocelelike nodule	Some areas	No	Slowly expanding mass	40	Rare Mucocelelike epidermoid tumor is rare
Multiple neurofibromatosis	Macules (café-au-lait) present on skin and occasionally oral mucosa	Macules —no Tumors —yes		Multiple skin tumors present from birth		Rare
Hereditary hemorrhagic telangiectasia (Rendu-Osler-Weber)	Purple papules on skin and mucous membranes, which blanch on pressure	No	Yes	Bleeding from lesions and body orifices	12	Rare

FIRM LESIONS

Condition	Appearance	Usual history	Usual age of occurrence (years)	Frequency
Amalgam fragment	Macule on gingiva or edentulous alveolus	Present for some years Firm mass in tissue	5 and over	Common
Late hematoma	Mass or swelling	Previous trauma and/or bleeding diatheses with repeated bleeding episodes		Occasional
Giant cell granuloma	Moderately firm macule, nodule, or polypoid mass on gingiva or alveolus	Slowly expanding mass	30 and over	Occasional
Pigmented fibroma	Papule, nodule, or polypoid mass Usually on buccal mucosa	Present for some time		Occasional
Intramucosal nevus	Papule Nodule Polypoid mass	Present from birth		Rare
Compound nevus	Papule Nodule Polypoid mass	Present from birth		Rare
Melanoma	Pigmented or amelanotic Nodule Polypoid mass on palate or maxillary gingiva	Rapidly enlarging mass	Mean age = 50.5	Rare Twice as common in males
Neuroectodermal tumor	Expansion of labial alveolus Pigmented or pink	Slowly expanding mass in anterior maxilla	Under 1	Rare

Table 9-2. Generalized brownish, bluish, or black discolorations*

Condition	Distribution	Usual history	Usual age of occurrence (years)	Accompanying conditions	Special tests
Cyanosis	Total skin surface Oral mucosa (if systemic type)	Increased severity of symptoms on exertion	Infant 60s, 70s, 80s	Malaise Dyspnea Orthopnea	Color decreases when circulation and oxygenation of blood is increased
Chloasma gravidarum	Skin of face, most frequently over nose and cheek Oral mucosa	Increased brownish color of skin as pregnancy progresses	Over 13	Pregnancy	
Addison's disease	Skin, especially exposed areas Oral mucosa	Hypoglycemia Weakness Decreased resistance to stress	Adult	Symptoms and signs of adrenocortical insufficiency	Negative ACTH test Improvement with cortisone and aldosterone administration
Hemochromatosis†	Skin, especially exposed areas Oral mucosa	Slowly increasing pigmentation, recent increased iron intake, or multiple blood transfusions	Over 35	Liver disease Diabetes Adrenocortical insufficiency	Skin, liver, and bone marrow positive for iron Serum iron-binding capacity
Argyria	Skin, especially exposed areas Oral mucosa	Chronic self-administration of silver-containing medication	Adult	Equilibrium and hearing problems Headaches	Skin biopsy positive for silver

*With the exception of argyria, which is rare, all these entities are of occasional frequency. Chloasma gravidarum, of course, is not seen in males.
†Eighty percent of the patients are male.

to protein complexes in the corium is diagnostic for the disease.

MANAGEMENT

There are no special precautions to take during oral treatment except to consider the patient's disturbance in equilibrium. Hence the clinician should avoid rapid changes in the position of the patient while he is seated in the dental chair.

RARITIES

Although the disease conditions included in this section may show generalized brownish, bluish, or black conditions, they either occur very rarely or else seldom show this feature. No ranking according to frequency of occurrence has been attempted:

Aniline intoxication
Arsenic poisoning
Carotenemia
Chloroquine therapy
Dermatomyositis

Idiopathic familial juvenile hypoparathyroidism, Addison's disease, superficial candidiasis
Pellagra
Porphyria
Sprue
Wilson's disease

SPECIFIC REFERENCES

Abrams, A. M.: Danger of treating mucoceles by steroid injection, J. Oral Surg. **36**:583, 1978.

Bennett, A. J., Solomon, M. P., and Jarrett, W.: Superficial spreading melanoma of the buccal mucosa: report of case, J. Oral Surg. **34**:1109-1111, 1976.

Bina, S.: Primary malignant melanoma of the oral cavity in Iranians (review of 18 cases), J. Oral Med. **34**:51-52, 1979.

Buchner, A., and Hansen, L. S.: Melanotic macule of the oral mucosa. A clinicopathologic study of 105 cases, Oral Surg. **48**:244-249, 1979a.

Buchner, A., and Hansen, L. S.: Pigmented nevi of the oral mucosa: a clinicopathologic study of 32 new cases and review of 75 cases from the literature. I. A clinicopathologic study of 32 new cases, Oral Surg. **48**:131-142, 1979b.

Chaudry, A. P., Burke, R. J., and Gorlin, R. J.: Malignant melanoma of the oral cavity, Oral Surg. **13**:584-588, 1960.

Clark, W., From, L., Bernardina, E., and Mihm, M.: The histogenesis and biologic behavior of primary human malignant melanomas of the skin, Cancer Res. **29**:705-726, 1969.

Eneroth, C. M.: Malignant melanoma of the oral cavity, Int. J. Oral Surg. **4**:191-197, 1975.

Farman, A. G.: Hairy tongue (lingua villosa), J. Oral Med. **32**:85-91, 1977.

Krolls, S. O., and Hicks, J. L.: Mixed tumors of the lower lip, Oral Surg. **35**:212-217, 1973.

Jackson, D., and Simpson, H. E.: Primary malignant melanoma of the oral cavity, Oral Surg. **39**:553-559, 1975.

Leopard, P. J.: Cryosurgery and its application to oral surgery, Br. J. Oral Surg. **13**:128-152, 1975.

Liversedge, R. L.: Oral malignant melanoma, Br. J. Oral Surg. **13**(1):40-55, 1975.

Mann, S. O., Fell, B. F., and Dalgarno, A. C.: Observations on the bacterial flora and pathology of the tongue of sheep deficient in zinc, Rev. Vet. Sci. **17**:91-101, 1974.

McGovern, V. J.: Malignant melanoma: clinical and histological diagnosis, New York, 1976, John Wiley & Sons, pp. 55-84.

Minkow, B., Laufer, D., and Gutman, D.: Treatment of oral hemangiomas with local sclerosing agents, Int. J. Oral Surg. **8**:18-21, 1979.

Murphy, J. B.: The management of a large hemangioma of the oral cavity with cryotherapy, J. Oral Med. **33**:104-106, 1978.

Page, L. R., Corio, R. L., Crawford, B. E., et al.: The oral melanotic macule, Oral Surg. **44**:219-226, 1977.

Regezi, J. A., Hayward, J. R., and Pickens, T. N.: Superficial melanomas of oral mucous membrane, Oral Surg. **45**:730-740, 1978.

Robertson, G. R., Defiebre, B. K., and Firtell, D. N.: Primary malignant melanoma of the mouth, J. Oral Surg. **37**:349-352, 1979.

Watson, W. L., and McCarthy, W. D.: Blood and lymph vessel tumors: a report of 1,056 cases, Surg. Gynecol. Obstet. **71**:569-588, 1940.

Weathers, D. R., Corio, R. L., Crawford, B. E., et al.: The labial melanotic macule, Oral Surg. **42**:196-205, 1976.

Wilcox, J. W., and Hickory, J. E.: Nonsurgical resolution of mucoceles, J. Oral Surg. **36**:478, 1978.

GENERAL REFERENCES

Ashur, H., Mizarhi, S., Ben-Hur, N., and Dolberg, L.: Metastatic malignant melanoma to the palatine tonsils: report of case, J. Oral Surg. **37**:110-112, 1979.

Batsakis, J. G., Bauer, R., Regezi, J. A., and Campbell, T.: Desmoplastic melanoma of the maxillary alveolus, J. Oral Surg. **37**:107-109, 1979.

Batsakis, J. C., and Rice, D. H.: Melanomas (cutaneous and mucosal) of the head and neck, Univ. Mich. Med. Cent. J. **37**:87-98, 1971.

Bhaskar, S. N., Cutright, D. E., Beasley, J. D., and Perez, B.: Giant cell reparative granuloma (peripheral): report of 50 cases, J. Oral Surg. **29**:110-115, 1971.

Bhaskar, S. N., and Jacoway, J. R.: Blue nevus of the oral mucosa, Oral Surg. **19**:678-683, 1965.

Brekke, J. H., Minn, V., and Gorlin, R. J.: Melanotic neuroectodermal tumor of infancy, J. Oral Surg. **33**:858-865, 1975.

Brener, M. D., and Harrison, B. D.: Intraoral blue nevus, report of a case, Oral Surg. **28**:326-330, 1969.

Browne, W. G.: Oral pigmentation and root resorption in Gaucher's disease, J. Oral Surg. **35**:153-155, 1977.

Cataldo, E., and Mosadomi, A.: Mucoceles of the oral mucous membrane, Arch. Otolaryngol. **91**:360-365, 1970.

Darnis, F.: Hémochromatosis (à propos de 100 observations), Ann. Biol. Clin. **30**:349-378, 1972.

DeLeon, E. L.: Treatment of hemangioma with sclerosing solution, Dent. Survey **47**:29-33, 1971.

Eversole, L. R., Rovin, S., and Sabes, W. R.: Mucoepidermoid carcinoma of minor salivary glands: report of 17 cases with follow up, J. Oral Surg. **30**:107-112, 1972.

Fejerskou, O., and Nybrae, L.: Primary malignant melanoma of the hard palate: report of case, J. Oral Surg. **31**:53-55, 1973.

Frantzis, T. F., Sheridan, P. J., Reever, C. M., and Young, L. L.: Oral manifestations of hemochromatosis, Oral Surg. **33**:186-190, 1972.

Giansanti, J. S., Drummond, J. F., and Sabies, W. R.: Intraoral melanocytic cellular nevi, Oral Surg. **44**:267-270, 1977.

Giansanti, J. S., Tillery, D. E., and Olanksy, S.: Oral mucosal pigmentation resulting from antimalarial therapy, Oral Surg. **31**:66-69, 1971.

Giansanti, J. S., and Waldron, C. A.: Peripheral giant cell granuloma: review of 720 cases, J. Oral Surg. **27**:787-791, 1969.

Gordon, N. C., Brown, S., Khosle, U. M., and Hansen, L. S.: Lead poisoning, Oral Surg. **47**(6):500-512, 1979.

Gormley, M. B., Jarrett, W., and Seldin, R.: Ranulas: a series of eighteen cases of extravasation cysts, J. Acad. Gen. Dent. **21**:29-32, 1973.

Grace, N. D.: Hepatic iron overload, Postgrad. Med. **53**(1):125-129, 1973.

Gutmann, J., Cifuentes, C., Gandulfo, P., and Guesalaga, F.: Intradermal nevus associated with epidermoid cyst in the mucous membrane of the cheek, Oral Surg. **45**:76-82, 1978.

Hansen, L. S., Silverman, S., and Beumer, J.: Primary malignant melanoma of the oral cavity, Oral Surg. **26**:352-359, 1968.

Harper, J. C., and Waldron, C. A.: Blue nevus of the palate, Oral Surg. **20**:145-149, 1965.

Hasse, C. D., Zoutendam, G. L., and Gombas, O. F.: Intraoral blue (Jadasson-Tieche) nevus, Oral Surg. **45**:755-761, 1978.

Hatziotis, J. C., and Mylona-Hatziotis, A. J.: Blue nevi of the oral cavity: review of the literature and report of two cases, J. Oral Surg. **31**:773-775, 1973.

Kraut, R. A., and Buhler, J. E.: Heroin-induced thrombocytopenic purpura, Oral Surg. **46**:637-640, 1978.

Lopez, J., Jr.: Melanotic neuroectodermal tumor of infancy: review of the literature and report of case, J. Am. Dent. Assoc. **93**:1159-1164, 1976.

Mack, L. M., and Woodward, H. W.: Blue nevus of oral mucosa membrane: report of case, Oral Surg. **25**:929-932, 1968.

Mandel, L., and Baurmash, H.: Bilateral ranulas: report of a case, J. Oral Surg. **28**:621-622, 1970.

Mark, H. I., and Kaplan, S. I.: Blue nevus of the oral cavity: review of the literature, Oral Surg. **24**:151-157, 1967.

McCrae, M. W., Miller, A. S., and Rosenthal, S. L.: Intraoral blue nevus: report of two additional cases, Oral Surg. **25**:590-593, 1968.

Miller, A. S., and Pullon, P. A.: Case of the month: translucent lesion on ventral tip of tongue, Dent. Survey **55**:34, 1979.

Murti, P. R., Bhonsle, R. B., Daftary, D. K., and Mehta, F. S.: Oral lichen planus associated with pigmentation, J. Oral Med. **34**:23-24, 1979.

Nagel, N. J.: Oral nevi: report of case and review of literature, J. Oral Surg. **30**:835-838, 1972.

Ogbusawa, O., Trowell, J., Williams, J. T., et al.: Hyperpigmentation of pernicious anemia in blacks, Arch. Intern. Med. **138**:388-389, 1978.

Powell, L. W.: Changing concepts in hemochromatosis, Postgrad. Med. J. **46**:200-209, 1970.

Rask, K. R., Topp, C. W., and Tilson, H. B.: Intraoral blue nevus: review of the literature and report of case, J. Oral Surg. **30**:212-214, 1972.

Robbins, A. H.: Hemochromatosis, melanosis and hypovitaminosis C, Arch. Dermatol. **106:**768, 1972.

Seward, M. H.: Eruption cyst: an analysis of its clinical features, J. Oral Surg. **31:**31-35, 1973.

Shapiro, L., and Zegarelli, D. J.: The solitary lentigo, Oral Surg. **31:**87-92, 1971.

Shira, R.: Simplified technique for the management of mucoceles and ranulas, J. Oral Surg. **20:**374-379, 1962.

Smirne, J. M.: Melanoameloblastoma: report of case, J. Oral Surg. **27:**279-280, 1969.

Sohn, D. M., Hasler, J. F., and Levy, S.: Pigmented nevus of the oral mucosa: report of a case, J. Am. Dent. Assoc. **72:**895-898, 1966.

Svejda, J., Skach, M., and Plackova, A.: Hairlike variations of filiform papillae in the human tongue, Oral Surg. **43:**97-105, 1977.

Trodahl, J. N., Schwartz, S., and Gorlin, R. J.: The pigmentation of dental tissues in erythropoietic (congenital) porphyria, J. Oral Pathol. **1:**159-171, 1972.

Weitzner, S.: Blue nevus of the hard palate, J. Oral Surg. **34:**934-936, 1976.

Wesley, R. K., Delaney, J. R., and Pensler, L.: Mucocutaneous melanosis and gastrointestinal polyposis (Peutz-Jegher's syndrome): clinical considerations and report of case, J. Dent. Child. **44:**131-134, 1977.

10

Solitary red lesions

Norman K. Wood
George G. Blozis
Paul W. Goaz

This chapter deals primarily with pathologic conditions that appear as single red lesions or else diffuse lesions that affect only one mucosal surface. These are as follows:

Traumatic erythematous macule
Purpuric macule (early stage)
Inflammatory hyperplastic lesion (early stage)
Reddish ulcers or ulcers with red halos
Nonpyogenic soft tissue odontogenic infection (cellulitis)
Chemical or thermal erythematous macule
Nicotinic stomatitis
Erythroplakia, carcinoma in situ, and red macular squamous cell carcinoma
Exophytic, red squamous cell carcinoma
Atrophic candidosis (denture stomatitis, angular cheilitis, acute atrophic candidosis)
Macular hemangioma and telangiectasia
Allergic manifestations
Herald lesion of generalized stomatitis or vesiculobullous disease
Metastatic tumors
Rarities
    Actinomycosis
    Amyloidosis
    Blastomycosis
    Coccidioidomycosis
    Erysipelas
    Exfoliative cheilitis
    Herpangina
    Histoplasmosis
    Hyperemic oral tonsils
    Plasma cell gingivitis
    Ludwig's angina
    Secondary syphilis
    Tuberculosis

NORMAL VARIATION IN ORAL MUCOSA
Masticatory and lining mucosa

As discussed in Chapter 5, the normal oral mucosa demonstrates a wide spectrum of pink colors.

The healthy masticatory mucosa (over the hard palate, the gingiva, and dorsal surface of the tongue) is light pink in color (Fig. 10-1). These surfaces are exposed to heavy mechanical forces of friction and pressure during mastication and have adapted to meet these stresses by producing (1) a protective layer of keratin and (2) a subepithelial connective tissue that is densely fibrous, relatively avascular, and firmly attached to bone or muscle.

In contrast, the lining mucosa (the oral mucosa over the vestibule, cheeks, lips, floor of the mouth, and ventral surface of the tongue) is not subjected to such intense mechanical and chemical stimulations as the masticatory mucosa and so similar tissue modification does not occur in these areas. As a consequence of this different morphology the color from the underlying vasculature is transmitted through the more transparent overlying tissue and imparts a more reddish color to the surface in comparison to the pinkish hue of the masticatory mucosa.

Palatoglossal arch region

Occasionally in a significant number of apparently normal individuals, areas of their mucosa covering the palatoglossal arch region are a deep dusky red in contast to the lighter red color of the surrounding tissues (Fig. 10-2).

These red macular bands are usually present bilaterally, are entirely painless, and although the size and shape of the areas in the same individual may not be uniform, they persist unchanged. In some cases they are also found on the mucosa lining the tonsillar fossa, particularly in individuals who have had tonsillectomies some years before. It would seem to us

Fig. 10-1. Clinical view showing the paler pink of the attached gingiva (masticatory mucosa) in contrast to the deeper pink of the vestibular mucosa (lining mucosa).

Fig. 10-2. Note the red appearance of the palatoglossal arch (arrows) in this healthy asymptomatic patient.

that these regions have a richer blood supply than the surrounding tissues and may be associated with Waldeyer's ring. Although this entity must be considered to be a normal variation in the individuals in which it occurs, it is important that the clinician be familiar with the condition because it is often misdiagnosed as "sore throat."

Pathologic red lesions

The red color of a lesion is, to some extent, usually the result of increased vascularity in the underlying tissues. The loss of part or all of the covering epithelium also contributes to the measures of color developed; a thick membrane will obscure the underlying red color whereas more color will be transmitted through a thin one. The degree of redness is also, in part, a function of the amount of the pigment hemoglobin present in the area, as well as the extent of its oxygenation. Red lesions frequently have a thin mucosa that covers numerous dilated and engorged vessels and as a consequence will frequently hemorrhage after minimal trauma.

A red color can also be imparted to the tissues by another pigment, melanin. This color may vary from light brown to a reddish brown to a bluish black. The reddish-brown color is seen infrequently in melanin-producing lesions.

When the surface of a red lesion is smooth it is presumptive evidence that the epithelium is uniformly atrophic and somewhat edematous. When some irregularities are present on the surface, the epithelium will often show variable degrees of hyperplasia or surface keratinization or both, and these changes are responsible for a

granular or papillary appearance. Sloughing white patches, representing necrotic tissue and fibrinous exudate, may also appear in areas where the mucosa is erythematous.

In summary the basic tissue changes or causes that produce abnormal red conditions are as follows:

1. Marked increase in hemoglobin concentration of circulating blood (polycythemia)
2. Vascular dilatation from:
   a. Inflammation (erythema)
      (1) Mechanical trauma (e.g., cheek biting, ill-fitting denture)
      (2) Thermal trauma (e.g., hot food)
      (3) Chemical trauma (strong mouthwashes, iatrogenic spills)
      (4) Infection (cellulitis, Ludwig's angina)
      (5) Allergy or autoimmune disease (e.g., Sjögren's syndrome)
      (6) Ulcer with inflamed rim (e.g., recurrent herpetic lesion)
   b. Congenital defects (e.g., hemangioma)
3. Extravasation of blood (e.g., trauma or hemostatic disease or both)
4. Atrophy or thinning of mucosa (e.g., atrophic candidiasis) (inflammatory component usually present too)

TRAUMATIC ERYTHEMATOUS MACULES AND EROSIONS

Mechanical trauma to the oral mucosa can produce a variety of clinical lesions depending on the nature and circumstances of the insult. The following are some of the clinical lesions that may be produced: (1) a keratotic lesion (increased retention of keratin), (2) a necrotic white lesion (necrosis of the epithelium and possibly the sub-

Fig. 10-3. Traumatic erythematous macules. These red patches all blanched on digital pressure. **A,** Palatal lesion caused by ill-fitting palatal connector of a partial denture. **B,** Red lesion at antero-lateral border of tongue caused by a carious tooth with a sharp edge. **C,** Red and white traumatic lesion of the tongue caused by the patient chewing his tongue while it was anesthetized. The darker areas (red) are erythematous, and the white areas are necrotic. **C,** Small red macule on lip of middle-aged woman who repeatedly touched this spot with the incisal edge of her maxillary incisor.

epithelial tissue to some extent), (3) a reddish erythematous macule (an area of inflammation), (4) a purpuric macule (subepithelial hemorrhage within the tissue spaces), (5) a bleb (a pooling of tissue fluid in the tissue), (6) an erosion, (7) an ulcer, and (8) an exophytic lesion (inflammatory hyperplasia). Three of these, the erythematous macule and erosion, the purpuric macule, and the granulomatous stage of the inflammatory hyperplastic lesion, are essentially red and are discussed in this chapter.

Traumatic erythematous macules are produced by a low-grade usually chronic physical insult. A more intense degree of brief trauma would be expected to produce a purpuric macule, an erosion, or a frank ulcer in order of increasing severity. Common causes include sharp margins of teeth or restorations and ill-fitting prostheses. Self-inflicted trauma such as cheek biting or other habits also may produce traumatic erythematous macules.

FEATURES

The usual sites for erythematous macules are on the anterior and lateral borders of the tongue, the floor of the mouth, the posterior palate, buccal mucosa, and mucosal surfaces of the lips. The macule may show considerable variation in the intensity of its red color. The size of the red zone corresponds closely to the size of the traumatic agent. Consequently size and shape may vary considerably. The margins of macular lesions are not usually sharply defined but may be in some instances (Fig. 10-3). Symptoms may vary from mild tenderness to considerable pain. The causative agent is usually easily identified either through the history or the clinical examination. The lesion generally regresses quickly after the cause is removed; however, if the lesion is located on the tongue it may persist for several weeks and heal as a bald pink area devoid of papillae.

Microscopic changes include an inflamed

lamina propria covered with perhaps a slightly thinned or eroded stratified squamous epithelium that is completely nonkeratinized. Because this lesion is basically inflammatory in nature it may blanch when digital pressure is applied.

DIFFERENTIAL DIAGNOSIS

For a discussion of the differential diagnosis of traumatic erythematous macules and erosions refer to the differential diagnosis section under purpuric macules.

MANAGEMENT

The mechanical irritant should be identified and eliminated and the lesion kept under surveillance until it disappears. Healing will usually take place in 3 or 4 days. If it does not disappear soon then additional workup should be done. If the suspicion index is high a biopsy should be done in order to rule out more serious conditions such as erythroplakia, squamous cell carcinoma, and fungal diseases such as candida and histoplasmosis.

PURPURIC MACULES (EARLY STAGE)

The purpuric macule is produced by a blunt traumatic insult to the mucosa or skin of sufficient force to cause the superficial extravasation of blood. If the patient is examined soon after the traumatic incident has occurred, petechial (small pinpoint) or ecchymotic (larger) areas will be observed, which are quite red in color. If sufficient time has lapsed to permit some breakdown of the hemoglobin pigment then the "bruise" will be bluish, undergoing the color changes described in Chapter 9, "Intraoral Brownish, Bluish, or Black Conditions."

FEATURES

The size of the purpuric macule will vary according to the size and force of the physical agent inflicting the damage. Usually the borders are poorly demarcated, blending almost imperceptibly with the surrounding normal tissue (Fig. 10-4). The lesion does not usually blanch on pressure because the red blood cells are within

Fig. 10-4. Red purpuric macules. These lesions either blanched minimally or did not blanch at all to digital pressure. **A,** Palatal ecchymosis caused by fellatio. **B,** Palatal petechiae apparently caused by violent coughing although a history of fellatio was not satisfactorily ruled out. **C,** Palatal petechiae in a patient with hemophilia. **D,** Reddish ecchymotic patch of the buccal mucosa following an oral surgical procedure.

the tissues rather than in vessels. Nevertheless, purpuric macules may also have an accompanying inflammatory component and in such cases the clinician may observe some blanching on palpation. Virtually any of the oral surfaces may be involved but in our experience the palate, buccal mucosa, and floor of the mouth are the most common sites.

Frequently reddish elliptic purpuric macules occurring on the palatal mucosa near the junction of the hard and soft palate may be due to oral sexual practices and are caused by the repeated bumping of the male organ on the soft tissue in this region (Fig. 10-4). In such a case the lesion disappears within 2 or 3 days only to return again when the act is repeated (Giansanti et al., 1975). A judicious history taken in a confidential setting will frequently reveal the true identity of such a lesion.

DIFFERENTIAL DIAGNOSIS

When transient reddish macules are observed near the junction of the hard and soft palate, the following entities need to be considered: traumatic erythematous macule, purpuric macule of oral sex, palatal bruising due to severe coughing or severe vomiting, macular hemangioma, atrophic candidasis, mononucleosis, and herpangina. The first four lesions are usually painless, and a careful history will establish the occurrence of a traumatic incident. Hemangiomas seldom occur on the posterior palate, and both the erythematous macule and the hemangioma will blanch somewhat on pressure. In contradistinction to the purpuric macule and the erythematous macule the hemangioma would not be transient in nature.

MANAGEMENT

Once the diagnosis of purpuric macule has been established the patient should be advised of its nature. He should be seen at a later date to ensure that the diagnosis was correct and that the lesion has disappeared.

If several purpuric areas are present the patient should be asked if he has always bruised excessively and how extensive the trauma was. If the correlation is unsatisfactory the patient should be tested for the presence of a bleeding diathesis.

INFLAMMATORY HYPERPLASTIC LESIONS (GRANULOMATOUS STAGE)

Inflammatory hyperplastic lesions are discussed in considerable detail in Chapter 7, "Pe-

ripheral Oral Exophytic Lesions." They are similar in etiology to the traumatic erythematous macule and the purpuric macule except that the precipitating insults are invariably chronic irritants such as calculus, ragged margins of cavities, overhanging restorations, overextended denture flanges, sharp spicules of bone, or chronic biting of the cheek or lip. Such prolonged chronic insults stimulate the production of granulation tissue. A list of inflammatory hyperplastic lesions includes the following: pyogenic granuloma, hormonal tumor, traumatic hemangioma, fibroma, epulis fissuratum, epulis granulomatosum, papillary hyperplasia, peripheral giant cell granuloma, parulis, and the peripheral fibroma with calcification.

In the life cycle of one of these lesions the entity initially develops as a mass of inflamed granulation tissue and so clinically appears quite soft and very red. Later when fibrous tissue is laid down the lesion becomes firmer and less red. If the irritant is eliminated at this stage the remainder of the inflammation disappears, the lesion shrinks noticeably, becomes very firm, and takes on a pale hue. This end-point lesion is a "garden-variety" fibroma.

FEATURES

Features of inflammatory hyperplastic lesions are covered in detail in Chapter 7. In the stage being considered here, the lesions are quite red, moderately soft, polypoid or nodular masses (Fig. 10-5).

Microscopy of the early hyperplastic lesion reveals granulomatous tissue covered with an intact layer of stratified squamous epithelium that is nonkeratinized. If the surface becomes traumatized the lesion will usually develop a white necrotic area in the region of the injury and will have become a pyogenic granuloma.

DIFFERENTIAL DIAGNOSIS

The early inflammatory hyperplastic lesion must be differentiated from hemangioma, a metastatic tumor, a primary malignant tumor, a papilloma, condylomas, and verrucae. In the case of most inflammatory hyperplastic lesions in their early stages of development, a precipitating irritant is usually identifiable. This strengthens the impression and supports a working diagnosis.

However, if such an irritant is not apparent the possibility that the lesion is either a primary or secondary malignant tumor beginning below a normal epithelium is given more consideration in the differential diagnosis. A history of treat-

Fig. 10-5. Reddish inflammatory hyperplastic lesions. All these lesions contained a large inflammatory component. **A,** Red pyogenic granuloma of the lingual gingiva caused by the sharp edges of a large carious lesion on the lateral incisor. **B,** Large red epulis fissuratum. **C,** Red papillary hyperplasia in its earliest stages, caused by an ill-fitting upper denture. **D,** Red parulis on the labial mucosa in an early stage of development. The lesion occurred at the opening of a sinus that was draining the infected periapical region of the maxillary right central incisor. (**A** courtesy E. Seklecki, D.D.S., Tucson, Ariz.)

ment or symptoms of a primary tumor elsewhere would in turn prompt the ordering of these possibilities in favor of a metastatic tumor (Fig. 10-21). Primary malignant tumors of the oral soft tissue are rare. Likewise, it is rare for a squamous cell carcinoma to appear as a small exophytic red lesion with a smooth unulcerated surface.

In the case of gingival lesions juxtaposed with unrelated alveolar bony changes it is most important to differentiate the inflammatory hyperplastic lesions from malignant tumors.

A congenital *hemangioma* would be present from birth while a traumatic (acquired) hemangioma is really a type of inflammatory hyperplastic lesion.

Papillomas, condylomas, and verrucae are included for the sake of completeness. However, since the inflammatory hyperplastic lesions are red and have a basically smooth, evenly contoured surface they should be readily differentiated from these epithelial growths that are frequently white with a cauliflowerlike surface. The pyogenic granuloma may have an area on its otherwise smooth surface that is white but this is necrotic material and can be easily removed, leaving a raw bleeding surface.

MANAGEMENT

Excisional biopsy in combination with elimination of the irritant is the treatment of choice for lesions of substantial size. Small red lesions may shrink to a size that precludes treatment when the irritant is eliminated.

ULCERS WITH RED HALOS

Solitary ulcers are discussed at length in Chapter 6. They are included here for completeness because ulcerative conditions frequently are first manifested as erythematous macules, for example, the recurrent herpetic lesion and the recurrent aphthous ulcer. Furthermore, in these conditions when the reddish area ultimately ulcerates the defect will frequently have a reddish border (Fig. 10-6). Such an observation might prompt the clinician to classify such an entity as a red lesion; however, experience has demon-

Fig. 10-6. Reddened mucosa surrounding three recurrent aphthous ulcers in the floor of the mouth.

Fig. 10-7. Cellulitis of the mucosa of the cheek and surrounding pterygomandibular region originating from a pericoronitis involving the erupting third molar tooth. The white necrotic material represents a localized ANUG. (Courtesy G. Blozis, D.D.S., Columbus, Ohio.)

strated that it is more beneficial from a differential diagnosis aspect to classify such lesions as ulcers.

DIFFERENTIAL DIAGNOSIS

The differential diagnosis of the various oral ulcers is covered in Chapter 6, "Oral Ulcers and Fissures."

NONPYOGENIC SOFT TISSUE ODONTOGENIC INFECTION (CELLULITIS)

This section includes a discussion of soft tissue odontogenic infections that either are caused by nonpyogenic bacteria or else represent prepyogenic or postpyogenic infections. That is, the causative bacteria may be either nonpyogenic or else the infection has not reached the pus-forming or pus-pooling stage. Odontogenic infection may originate in three sites: (1) the canals and the periapex of pulpless teeth, (2) the gingiva in periodontal disease, (3) the gingival operculum over an erupting tooth.

FEATURES

In most of these cases a suitable historical, clinical, and radiographic examination coupled with pulp testing will usually clearly indicate the diagnosis of dental infection (Fig. 10-7).

The alveolar mucosa and gingiva are the most frequent sites of dental infection, but if the infection is permitted to spread, a number of the oral mucosal surfaces, as well as the overlying skin, may become involved. Various degrees of swelling will be present, showing a hot, red, tender to painful surface. However, if sufficient pus has formed and pooled near the surface of the swollen

tissue it would impart a yellowish-white color to the central region of the swelling. Also the swelling would feel rubbery and demonstrate fluctuance (see Chapter 3).

Ludwig's angina is an unusual example of a reddish soft tissue infection that is produced by a mixed infection of nonspecific microorganisms but a nonpyogenic strain of streptococcus is almost invariably present. This condition causes a sudden swelling of the floor of the mouth and also of the submental and submaxillary spaces, often of such a magnitude that obstruction of the airway is threatened. In most cases a very red, moderately firm, painful swelling of the floor of the mouth produces an elevation of the tongue. The skin of the neck overlying the swollen submental and submaxillary spaces is usually also red and feels hot on palpation (Fig. 10-8).

Cervical or intraoral actinomycosis is a specific infection that frequently occurs as a tender very reddish swelling (Fig. 10-8).

DIFFERENTIAL DIAGNOSIS

When a patient has a reddish painful swelling of the oral soft tissues with an accompanying tender cervical lymphadenitis the diagnosis of infection is reasonably certain. An extremely high percentage of these infections will be odontogenic in origin and hence bacterial in etiology. However, the clinician should also at least consider actinomycosis, tuberculosis, and various fungal infections such as histoplasmosis, coccidioidomycosis, and blastomycosis as unlikely possibilities.

Fig. 10-8. Red infectious lesions. **A,** Ludwig's angina. Note the swelling of the submental and submandibular spaces. Unfortunately the redness of the overlying skin does not show in this black-and-white photo. The patient also had a red painful sublingual swelling. **B** and **C,** A case of actinomycosis in the submandibular space of a 56-year-old man. **C** shows the redness of the lesion. (**B** and **C** courtesy E. Seklecki, D.D.S., Tucson, Ariz.)

MANAGEMENT

When a diagnosis of odontogenic infection has been established, the associated dental problem should be eliminated by root canal therapy, extraction, curettage, excision, or incision and drainage. In addition, we recommend concomitant coverage with an adequate dose of an appropriate antibiotic.

Patients with infections that are or may become a threat to their airway should be hospitalized so that any respiratory complication can be managed properly.

CHEMICAL OR THERMAL ERYTHEMATOUS MACULE

The cause of a chemical or thermal erythematous macule is usually a caustic drug or hot foods or beverages. Obviously the severity of the tissue damage varies with the intensity and duration of the insult and so several different clinical appearances may be produced. Very caustic or very hot agents may produce a coagulation necrosis of the superficial tissue that will appear whitish and can be scraped off. Fig. 5-43 illustrates such a change precipitated by aspirin. Still more intense or prolonged insults may result in frank ulceration or stripping of the mucosa. Milder agents or briefer applications of strong agents will produce the mildest clinically detectable reaction, an *erythema* of the superficial tissues, thus explaining why this condition is included in this chapter (Fig. 10-9). Sometimes a mixed reaction is produced and so the clinical lesion may appear as necrotic white dots or patches on an erythematous base (Fig. 10-9).

FEATURES

The red area is tender to painful, may blanch somewhat on pressure, and will generally bleed on the slightest manipulation. The size and shape corresponds to the area of contact with the caustic agent. The buccal and palatal mucosa are the sites most commonly affected. Mild aspirin burns are good examples as are mild palatal burns from hot food stuffs (Fig. 10-9). A careful history will elicit the facts concerning the causative agent in almost all cases.

DIFFERENTIAL DIAGNOSIS

Many of the lesions discussed in this chapter should be considered in the differential diagnosis: e.g., erythema from mechanical trauma, purpuric macule, cellulitis (nonpyogenic odontogenic infection), allergic manifestations, erythroplakia, atrophic candidosis, herald spot of disseminated red conditions, and fungal infections. A recent history of chemical or thermal injury along with uncomplicated resolution of the lesion in question would eliminate these possibilities and establish the correct diagnosis.

MANAGEMENT

The majority of these cases are quite mild and relatively painless. If pain is a problem systemic analgesics and topical applications of hydrocortisone in an emollient base (Kenalog in Orbase) can be used. If any doubt persists as to the correct diagnosis or if the injury appears to be superimposed on a serious lesion then surveillance is required and a biopsy should be done if the lesion in question does not resolve.

Fig. 10-9. Reddish lesions caused by chemical burns. **A,** Red and white acetaminophen (Tylenol) burn. **B,** Reddish area on mucosa of lower lip represents a stage in healing of lesion caused by the overzealous use of Listerine mouthwash. (**B** from Bernstein, M.: Oral Surg. **46:**781-789, 1978.)

NICOTINIC STOMATITIS

Nicotinic stomatitis is discussed at length as a white lesion of the palate in Chapter 5. This lesion is included in the present chapter because it is a red lesion in its earliest stage before keratosis has been produced (Shafer et al., 1974). Also, in the later keratotic stage the inflamed minor salivary duct openings appear as small red dots in the center of low flat nodules of hyperplastic tissue. Nicotonic stomatitis is seen primarily on the palate of pipe smokers.

DIFFERENTIAL DIAGNOSIS

The following conditions particularly have to be considered as somewhat similar clinical pictures when nicotinic stomatitis is suspected: multiple papillomatosis, denture stomatitis, and atrophic candidiasis. Generally multiple papillomatosis and denture stomatitis can be quickly excluded if the condition is on the hard palate because nicotinic stomatitis does not occur under a denture as the former two entities do. A smear would quickly identify atrophic candidiasis. A history of pipe smoking as well as the relatively greater prevalence of nicotinic stomatitis would cause it to be a more likely possibility in the differential diagnosis than atrophic candidiasis.

ERYTHROPLAKIA, CARCINOMA IN SITU, AND RED, MACULAR SQUAMOUS CELL CARCINOMA

The term "erythroplakia" is used in this book as a clinical term for a specific red lesion much as "leukoplakia" is used for white lesions of a specific spectrum. Thus an "erythroplakic" lesion can be defined as a persistent velvety red patch that cannot be identified as any other specific red lesion such as inflammatory erythemas or those produced by blood vessel anomalies. Mashberg and Morrisey (1973) and Mashberg (1978) identified erythroplasia (erythroplakia) as the earliest sign of asymptomatic cancer and reported that invasion may occur in small lesions of less than 1 cm in diameter. Indeed the term "erythroplakia" carries a more serious implication than its white counterpart "leukoplakia" because almost all erythroplakias show malignant changes. In a study of 58 cases by Shafer and Waldron (1975) 51% were invasive carcinoma and 41% were carcinoma in situ or severe epithelial dysplasia.

On a microscopic basis these authors reported that the lesion's reddish color is due to the absence of a surface keratin layer and also to the fact that the connective tissue papillae, containing enlarged capillaries, project very close to the surface. They also described a general failure of the epithelial cells to achieve significant maturation (keratinization). Interestingly their work showed that when actual invasion occurs, cellular maturation may commence.

FEATURES

Erythroplakia usually appears as a velvety red or granular red macule (patch) that may be slightly raised (Fig. 10-10). The lesion is painless and varies greatly in size; the borders may be either well circumscribed or may blend imperceptibly with the surrounding normal mucosa. Small lesions are easily overlooked, but the chances for their detection are greatly enhanced by first drying the mucosa with a gauze since this intensifies the red color.

Three different clinical appearances have been described by Shear (1972): (1) the *homogenous form*, which is completely red in appearance (Fig. 10-10); (2) *patches* of erythroplakia and leukoplakia occurring together (Fig. 10-11); and (3) *speckled* erythroplakia in which small leukoplakic specks are scattered over an area of erythroplakia (Fig. 10-12). The term "speckled leukoplakia" used in Chapter 5 is synonymous with the term "speckled erythroplakia" used here.

Shafer and Waldron (1975) found no difference in the sexual distribution of erythroplakia. They reported that the peak age of occurrence fell in the 50s and 60s. Interestingly these authors found that there is a difference in the frequency of occurrence between males and females when anatomic location is considered. The floor of the mouth proved to be the most common site affected in males, while the mandibular gingival and alveolar mucosa and mandibular sulcus make up the most common site in females. The retromolar region was the second most common site in both sexes.

DIFFERENTIAL DIAGNOSIS

Although all the red macular lesions listed in this chapter should be considered in a differential diagnosis of an erythroplakic lesion the lesions that are obviously macular hemangiomas and telangiectasias can be readily eliminated by their characteristic features. In a similar way the traumatic lesions, odontogenic infections, and allergies can be given a low ranking on the basis of their transient nature, their pain, and often obvious events in the history. The traumatic erythematous macules of the tongue are often

Fig. 10-10. Homogeneous erythroplakia. **A,** Very small red lesion on ventral surface of tongue, which showed invasion microscopically. This 52-year-old woman had had two previous oral squamous cell carcinomas removed from other locations. **B,** Small red lesion on the soft palate at upper extent of pterygomandibular raphe. Lesion was barely discernible until the tissue was dried with a gauze. **C,** Red macule involving the sublingual papilla on the right side. Excisional biopsy revealed early invasion in some sections and carcinoma in situ in others. (**B** courtesy R. Lee, D.D.S., Findlay, Ohio.)

Fig. 10-11. Erythroplakic patches and leukoplakic patches in the same lesion. **A,** Lateral border of the tongue in a 64-year-old man. The red patch showed carcinoma in situ. **B,** Facial gingiva in a 57-year-old man. Some of the red areas showed invasive squamous cell carcinoma. (**A** courtesy R. Crum, D.D.S., Hines, Ill. **B** courtesy E. Seklecki, D.D.S., Tucson, Ariz.)

Fig. 10-12. Speckled erythroplakia of the oral floor. All lesions proved to be invasive squamous cell carcinoma on biopsy. (**A** courtesy J. Lehnert, D.D.S., Minneapolis. **B** courtesy R. Lee, D.D.S., Findlay, Ohio.)

more difficult to differentiate because these may persist for weeks after the irritant has been eliminated. Also red lesions of atrophic candidiasis may be indistinguishable clinically. In cases of candidiasis features in the history are often suggestive of susceptibility and a smear would be diagnostic. Tuberculosis and fungal lesion such as histoplasmosis should be considered (Shear, 1972), but their probability would be low on the basis of incidence alone.

MANAGEMENT

We concur with Mashberg and Morrissey's recommendation (1973) that if a red lesion persists for more than 14 days after all local trauma and infectious foci have been eliminated then a biopsy is mandatory. Obviously if the suspicion index is high, arrangements should be made for immediate biopsy and further care.

EXOPHYTIC, RED SQUAMOUS CELL CARCINOMA

Exophytic squamous cell carcinoma is discussed in Chapter 7 without emphasis on color. Macular, red squamous cell carcinomas have

been discussed under erythroplakia earlier in this chapter. To further develop the differential picture it is necessary to include and describe an additional clinical lesion: the exophytic, red squamous cell carcinoma. Fig. 10-13 illustrates two examples of this entity.

FEATURES

The lesions of exophytic squamous cell carcinoma nicely illustrate the rule of thumb (Chapter 7) which holds that a mass that arises in the covering epithelial surface will have a rough surface and contour. These exophytic, red squamous cell carcinomas usually have a broad base and are usually domelike or nodular in shape. The surface may vary considerably in roughness from lesion to lesion and also from area to area on the same lesion (Fig. 10-13). The surface may range from granular to pebbly to deeply creviced. The lesion may be completely red or the red surface may be sprinkled with white necrotic or white keratotic foci. The lesion itself is firm to palpation and the base will usually show induration and fixation to the deeper structures such as the periosteum. Pain is seldom a complaint.

Fig. 10-13. Red exophytic squamous cell carcinoma. **A,** Small lesion on the lower lip. **B,** Large red lesion in the retromolar region. (**A** courtesy James Love, D.D.S., Raleigh, N.C.)

DIFFERENTIAL DIAGNOSIS

All red exophytic lesions such as inflammatory hyperplasias (granulomatous stage), hemangiomas, minor salivary tumors, primary mesenchymal tumors, metastatic tumors, amelanotic melanoma, and rare proliferating lesions such as tuberculosis, gummas, actinomycosis, and histoplasmosis must be considered.

Red inflammatory hyperplastic lesions are more common than exophytic squamous cell carcinoma, and they will be considerably softer to palpation and in almost all cases the mechanical irritant will be evident.

Many of the *hemangiomas* will empty or partialy empty on digital pressure, which will be accompanied by a similar degree of blanching. Consequently these lesions will usually be readily identified.

Because approximately 90% of all oral malignancies are primary squamous cell carcinomas, the chance of the red lesion being either a *metastatic tumor* or a *primary mesenchymal tumor* is unlikely but it must be considered. However, in contrast to the exophytic squamous cell carcinoma the majority of primary mesenchymal tumors have a smooth nonulcerated surface in the early stages of development; this is also true of minor salivary gland tumors.

MANAGEMENT

A good working recommendation to follow is to promptly do a biopsy of any red exophytic lesion of the oral cavity that does not appear to be an infection, an inflammatory hyperplastic lesion, or a hemangioma. If it is not one of these lesions then it is likely malignant or else a rare proliferative infectious disorder.

ATROPHIC CANDIDOSIS

Atrophic candidosis is an interesting clinical variant of the candidal infection that produces a red appearance rather than the better known white pseudomembranous lesion that is discussed in Chapter 5. The red color is produced by a thinning or even a complete erosion of the surface epithelium with an accompanying inflammation of the underlying connective tissue.

Denture stomatitis

The diffuse redness of the palate seen under dentures has posed a diagnostic dilemma for many years. The tissue reaction has often been attributed to an allergic response to the denture base material, but that particular association has seldom been substantiated. Current studies offer strong evidence that the lesion is the result of a chronic infection by *Candida albicans*. The redness is not the typical change described in candidosis (candidiasis), however, but represents a tissue response that has been labeled "chronic atrophic candidosis." *Candida* organisms are almost always found in smears from the red lesions of these patients.

Of specific interest is the observation that the *Candida* organisms can be identified in larger quantities on the denture base material than on the palatal mucosa. This observation has prompted the suggestion that *Candida* organisms are residents on or in the denture base and the clinical lesion is a result of extremely irritating toxins produced by the fungus (Davenport, 1970).

FEATURES

Denture stomatitis occurs under either complete or partial dentures and is found more frequently in women. The lesions are almost always confined to the palate and seldom if ever involve the mandibular ridge. In approximately 50% of the patients, there is an associated angular cheilitis with or without an inflammatory papillary hyperplasia of the palate. A significantly high correlation has also been established between the occurrence of this condition and the wearing of dentures at night. There is some question as to what role trauma by ill-fitting dentures plays in the pathogenesis of the lesions. Chronic injury may predispose the tissue to infection by *Candida* organisms, which are considered to be normal inhabitants of the oral cavity. At times there is an underlying chronic debilitating disease that predisposes patients to infection by *Candida* organisms.

The lesions may be totally asymptomatic, or the patient may complain of a soreness and dryness of the mouth. This soreness may also be described as a burning sensation. The palatal tissue is bright red, somewhat edematous, and granular. Only the tissue covered by the denture is involved. The redness usually involves the entire area covered by the denture but may be focal in its distribution (Fig. 10-14 and Plate 2).

When seen microscopically, the lesion is rather nonspecific. The epithelium is atrophic and may be ulcerated in areas. An intense chronic inflammatory infiltrate is present in the lamina propria and also involves the epithelium. Usually the *Candida albicans* organism is not found in tissue specimens. The most accurate diagnostic test is a smear from the area of the lesion stained with periodic acid–Schiff reagent. This will show the yeast and hyphal forms of *Candida*. Cultures are not as useful, however, since they will also be positive in patients who are carriers but do not have lesions.

DIFFERENTIAL DIAGNOSIS

The clinical picture of denture stomatitis is rather specific; few if any other diseases appear the same. Infections by other organisms, however, could be responsible for a similar diffuse redness.

MANAGEMENT

Currently the most useful antifungal agent is nystatin (Ritchie et al., 1969). Since it is not absorbed, nystatin is beneficial only when in contact with the *Candida* organisms; therefore the vaginal tablets used as oral troches are more beneficial than the oral suspension because they provide longer contact with the organism. The tablets should be dissolved in the mouth four times a

Fig. 10-14. Denture stomatitis. **A,** Only the palatal tissue contacted by an acrylic transitional partial denture is inflamed. Smears containing *Candida* were obtained from both the palatal tissue and the denture. **B,** Patchy redness covers the entire palate in a patient who wears a full denture. An exfoliative cytologic smear was positive for *Candida*. **C,** Same patient after therapy with nystatin for 1 week.

day after meals and at bedtime. Dentures should be placed in a nystatin solution during the night and covered by a nystatin ointment while being worn during the day. Usually new dentures are necessary because the effort to eliminate the fungus from the denture base is frequently met with failure.

Angular cheilitis

Angular cheilitis is usually a reddish ulcerative or proliferative condition marked by one or a number of deep fissures spreading from the cor-

Fig. 10-15. Red lesions of angular cheilosis. *Candida albicans* had secondarily infected this condition, which was primarily caused by wearing dentures with decreased vertical dimension.

Fig. 10-16. Candidosis. **A,** Palatal lesion of acute pseudomembranous candidosis. **B,** Same area after the white plaque was removed by means of a tongue blade. **C,** Same area 1 week after the plaque was removed. An exfoliative cytologic smear of the palatal tissue was positive for *Candida*. The lesions are typical of acute atrophic candidosis. **D,** Same area after therapy with nystatin for 1 week.

ners of the mouth. The lesions are bilateral, usually do not bleed, and are restricted to the skin surface (Fig. 10-15). Although such factors as decreased vertical dimension of dentures, anemia, and vitamin B deficiencies may be predisposing factors or at least be associated with the development of this lesion, infection with *Candida albicans* and in some cases with a mixture of other microorganisms seems to represent a major cause. Thus the lesions usually persist even though the predisposing factors have been eliminated, unless they are treated with an antifungal ointment such as nystatin.

Acute atrophic candidosis (Candidiasis)

The lesion of acute atrophic candidosis represents another though less common form of a *Candida* infection. It usually is the sequela of the typical lesion of *Candida*, the acute pseudomembranous candidosis. When the white plaque of pseudomembranous candidosis is shed or removed, a red, atrophic, and sore mucosa is often left (Fig. 10-16 and Plate 2). At times the lesion may be asymptomatic. It may resolve spontaneously or require treatment with nystatin (Lehner, 1964, 1967).

FEATURES

The lesions will be seen in essentially the same types of patients—persons who are prone to develop acute pseudomembranous candidosis. Included are individuals who are taking broad-spectrum antibiotics, steroids, or immunosuppressive agents. In addition, the lesions occur during pregnancy and may accompany diabetes, hypothyroidism, and other debilitating diseases. They are also found in apparently normal healthy individuals.

Tissue sections show an atrophic epithelium that may contain a few hyphae in the superficial layers. The lamina propria usually has a mild acute inflammatory infiltrate and increased vascularity. An exfoliative cytologic smear of the lesion is most useful in establishing a diagnosis.

DIFFERENTIAL DIAGNOSIS

Frequently the red lesions of acute atrophic candidosis are seen in association with those of the pseudomembranous type and do not pose a diagnostic problem. When discovered as isolated red lesions, they are rather nonspecific in appearance. Lesions produced by chemical burns, drug reactions, and other organisms have a similar clinical appearance but can usually be excluded or included on the basis of the history.

MANAGEMENT

The lesions of acute atrophic candidiasis respond well to either an oral suspension of nystatin or nystatin vaginal tablets used as oral troches.

MACULAR HEMANGIOMAS AND TELANGIECTASIAS

The majority of the oral hemangiomas of soft tissue are exophytic and bluish and so have been discussed in Chapters 7 and 9. However, red macular hemangiomas and exophytic red hemangiomas occur both as nonsyndrome entities and also as syndrome manifestations (Figs. 10-17 and 10-18). Red hemangiomas are usually of the capillary variety rather than cavernous, which are usually more bluish in color. These reddish macular hemangiomas are also known as port-wine stains or nevus flammeus on the skin. Sturge-Weber syndrome usually has both facial and intraoral macular hemangiomas (Fig. 10-18) although the intraoral hemangiomas may also be of the exophytic variety. An additional characteristic is the "tramline" calcifications seen in lateral skull roentgenograms.

The macular hemangiomas are readily differ-

Fig. 10-17. Red macular hemangioma on the buccal mucosa, which had been present since birth.

entiated from erythemas by their history of long duration, by their nontenderness, and by the fact that an inflammatory component is not present. They can be differentiated from red purpuric macules by the absence in the history of a recent traumatic episode as well as the transience of the latter condition.

Telangiectasias represent permanently enlarged end-capillaries that are located superficially just under the skin or mucosa. They are red, are seldom over 5 mm in diameter, and blanch readily on digital pressure, which easily and rapidly differentiates them from red petechiae. They may occur as solitary red macular or multiple lesions where they are usually a manifestation of the Rendu-Osler-Weber syndrome, also known as hereditary telangiectasia.

MANAGEMENT

Woods and Tulumello (1977) listed the following methods of treatment for the oral hemangioma: conscientious observation, use of radiation, steroids, embolization, antimetabolites, sclerosing solutions, surgical removal, or a combination of sclerosing agents and surgery.

ALLERGIC MACULES

Allergic manifestations in the oral cavity usually occur as a generalized eruption. Occasionally solitary lesions occur, generally as the result of a contact allergy and hence have to be differentiated from the other solitary red lesions (Fig. 10-19). When appearing as a red lesion they may be either an erythema or an ulcer. Usually the offending allergen can be identified by taking a careful history.

Fig. 10-18. Red macular hemangiomas associated with Sturge-Weber syndrome. **A** and **B,** Macular hemangiomas on the lip and alveolar mucosa in a 17-year-old patient who also had a port-wine stain on the left side of the face. The intraoral lesions blanched readily on digital pressure. **C** and **D,** Another patient with Sturge-Weber syndrome. **C,** Full-face view showing large superficial hemangioma (port-wine stain) on the left side of the face and upper lip terminating at the midline. **D,** Intraoral view of same patient showing the large red macular hemangioma that has involved the maxillary alveolar and gingival mucosa on the left side of the midline. The lip involvement on the left side can also be seen. (Courtesy S. Raibley, D.D.S., Maywood, Ill.)

Fig. 10-19. Red allergic manifestations. **A,** Petechiae in red patch (arrows), which was allergic reaction to topical anesthetic (unfortunately the red patch is not clearly visible in this black-and-white picture). **B,** Allergic reaction to agents in periodontal dressing. Note the deep mostly uniform color of all the mucosa in this picture. (**A** courtesy E. Ranieri, D.D.S., Maywood, Ill.)

HERALD LESION OF GENERALIZED STOMATITIS OR VESICULOBULLOUS DISEASE

Vesiculobullous disease and other conditions that may cause a generalized stomatitis are discussed in Chapter 11. Occasionally such conditions will occur first as a solitary lesion (erythema, bleb, or ulcer) perhaps one or several months before a full-blown attack occurs. Examples of this are patients who have had occasional, single, recurrent aphthous ulcers and then suddenly experience a widespread involvement of their oral mucosal membranes, that is, a recurrent aphthous stomatitis.

Fig. 10-20, A, illustrates the case of a woman who originally was seen with two small blebs on the buccal mucosa. These soon disappeared, but several months later the woman developed a full-blown attack of pemphigus.

The solitary lesion illustrated in Fig. 10-20, B, illustrates a herald lesion of erosive lichen planus. When the 45-year-old woman first presented for diagnosis and treatment only the one lesion was found. Several months later she experienced a severe attack of erosive lichen planus.

METASTATIC TUMORS

Exophytic metastatic tumors are discussed in Chapter 7. It will be helpful to reiterate that this group of lesions includes those that arise in bone and extend into the soft tissue, as well as those that begin in the soft tissue. On the basis of a number of reports it appears that the following represent the more common locations of the primary tumors that metastasize to the jaws (listed in descending order of frequency): breast, lung, kidney, gastrointestinal tract, thyroid, and prostate.

Metastatic tumors in the oral cavity are uncommon lesions, representing about 1% of all oral malignancies (Clausen and Poulsen, 1963; Meyer and Shklar, 1965). The vast majority are located in bone although some of these central lesions involve the oral soft tissue by extension (Hatziotis et al., 1973). In Meyer and Shklar's series (1965) 92% arose in jawbone, compared to 8% in the oral soft tissue; 85% of these secondary bone tumors occurred in the mandible. It is interesting that 70% of their cases were adenocarcinomas. Metastatic carcinoma of the gingiva is even more rare as evidenced by the sparsity of reports (Ellis et al., 1977; Sanner et al., 1979, Sato et al., 1978).

FEATURES

Exophytic metastatic tumors are usually rapidly growing nodular or polypoid masses. The surfaces may be smooth and covered with intact mucosa, which will vary from light pink to normal mucosal pink to red, depending on the integrity of the covering epithelium, the vascularity, and the amount of inflammation present (Fig. 10-21). When the lesions become larger they frequently develop an ulcerated surface as a result of chronic trauma from mastication. As a result the appearance will vary from one of red and white patches to part or complete ulceration of the entire surface, which will have a tendency to bleed easily.

The location of metastatic lesions varies considerably but most occur in the lower half of the oral

Fig. 10-20. Herald lesion of generalized stomatitis. **A,** Two vesicles with red rims on the buccal mucosa of a patient. These soon disappeared but the patient developed a full-blown case of pemphigus several months later. **B,** Solitary reddish lesion with a keratotic white component that was observed in a 45-year-old woman. Several months later the patient experienced a severe disseminated attack of erosive lichen planus.

cavity. The premolar/molar region of the mandible is the most commonly involved site. Other areas in the oral soft tissue and bone are the alveolus, body of the jawbone, ramus, lip, tongue, and gingiva.

Although the diagnostic features of metastatic tumors may vary the following should add to the suspicion index: paresthesia, rapid swelling or expansion of the jaws, pain, loose or extruded teeth without apparent cause, or failure of an extraction site to heal (Birkholz and Reed, 1979).

Osseous involvement will usually be quite evident in radiographs and may present a wide spectrum of possible appearances: (1) solitary, ragged, poorly marginated radiolucency, (2) cystlike radiolucency, (3) multilocular radiolucency, (4) multiple separate radiolucencies, (5) mixed radiolucency/radiopacity, and (6) complete radiopacity.

DIFFERENTIAL DIAGNOSIS

The following lesions should be included in the differential diagnosis: inflammatory hyperplasia, primary mesenchymal malignant tumors, traumatized minor salivary tumors, and amelanotic melanoma.

Inflammatory hyperplastic lesions are the most common by far. They can usually be tentatively identified by the identification of a chronic irritant.

Minor salivary tumors are almost never red but if the red exophytic tumor in question is located in the posterolateral hard palate then the possibility of a tumor of the minor salivary glands would have to be considered.

As *primary malignant mesenchymal tumors* represent less than 1% of all oral malignancies

they are less common than the metastatic variety. Nevertheless, some of these primary tumors will be red, especially the vascular variety, and must be considered though they will be assigned a low ranking in the differential diagnosis.

Amelanotic melanoma of the oral cavity is a very rare tumor but can be indicated by a pink or reddish exophytic lesion (Fig. 7-30, *A*) so it cannot be completely dismissed.

The suspicion of *metastatic tumor* is enhanced by symptoms of a primary tumor elsewhere or a history of previous treatment of such a tumor. However, it is important to consider that the metastatic oral lesion may be the first indication of the presence of a primary tumor.

MANAGEMENT

Treatment of individual cases of metastatic carcinoma in the oral cavity may be careful observation, palliative measures, or aggressive measures, depending on the general condition of the patient. If the patient is dying as a result of disseminated tumor then observation or palliative measures will be the management of choice. On the other hand, if the oral lesion appears to be the only metastatic lesion existing then attempts should be made to eradicate it.

RARITIES

The following intraoral conditions are rare but nevertheless must be considered when a red lesion is detected: actinomycosis, amyloidosis, blastomycosis, coccidioidomycosis, erysipelas, herpangina, histoplasmosis, plasma cell gingivitis, Ludwig's angina, secondary syphilis, and tuberculosis (Plate 3).

Fig. 10-21. Red metastatic tumors. **A,** Mass of 3 cm on the right maxillary gingiva of a 58-year-old white man, which proved to be a metastatic adenocarcinoma from the lung. **B,** Reddish granulomalike mass on the anterior gingiva of a 27-year-old white man, which proved to be metastatic synovial sarcoma. (**A** and **B** from Ellis, G. L., Jensen, J., Reingold, I. M., and Barr, R. J.: Oral Surg. **44:**238-245, 1977.)

SPECIFIC REFERENCES

Birkholz, H., and Reed, J. H.: Bronchogenic carcinoma metastatic to the lip and the mandible, J. Am. Dent. Assoc. **98:**414-416, 1979.

Clausen, F., and Poulsen, H.: Metastatic carcinoma to the jaws, Acta Pathol. Microbiol. Scand. **57:**361-374, 1963.

Davenport, J. C.: The oral distribution of *Candida* in denture stomatitis, Br. Dent. J. **129:**150-156, 1970.

Ellis, G. L., Jensen, J. L., and Barr, R. J.: Malignant neoplasms metastatic to gingivae, Oral Surg. **44**(2):238-245, 1977.

Giansanti, J. S., Craner, J. R., and Weathers, D. R.: Palatal erythema: another etiologic factor, Oral Surg. **40:**379-381, 1975.

Hatziotis, J. C., Constantinido, H., and Papanayotto, P. H.: Metastatic tumors of the oral soft tissues, Oral Surg. **36**(4): 544-550, 1973.

Lehner, T.: Oral thrush, or acute pseudomembranous candidiasis, Oral Surg. **18:**27-37, 1964.

Lehner, T.: Oral candidosis, Dent. Pract. **17:**209-216, 1967.

Mashberg, A.: Erythroplasia: the earliest sign of asymptomatic oral cancer, J. Am. Dent. Assoc. **96:**615-620, 1978.

Mashberg, A., and Meyers, H.: Anatomical site and size of 222 early asymptomatic oral squamous cell carcinomas, Cancer **37:**2149-2157, 1976.

Mashberg, A., and Morrissey, J. B.: A study of the appearance of early asymptomatic oral squamous cell carcinoma, Cancer **32:**1436-1445, 1973.

Meyer, I., and Shklar, G.: Malignant tumors metastatic to mouth and jaws, Oral Surg. **20**(3):350-362, 1965.

Ritchie, G. M., Fletcher, A. M., Main, D. M. G., and Prophet, A. S.: The etiology, exfoliative cytology, and treatment of denture stomatitis, J. Prosthet. Dent. **22:**185-200, 1969.

Sanner, J. R., Ramin, J. E., and Yang, C.: Carcinoma of the lung metastatic to the gingiva: review of the literature and report of case, J. Oral Surg. **37:**103-106, 1979.

Sato, M., Nishio, J., Yoshida, H., et al.: Metastatic choriocarcinoma involving the gingiva, Int. J. Oral Surg. **7:**182-196, 1978.

Shafer, W. G., Hine, M. K., and Levy, B. M.: A textbook of oral pathology, ed. 3, Philadelphia, 1974, W. B. Saunders Co.

Shafer, W. G., and Waldron, C. A.: Erythroplakia of the oral cavity, Cancer **36:**1021-1028, 1975.

Shear, M.: Erythroplakia of the mouth, Int. Dent. J. **22:**460-473, 1972.

Woods, W. R., and Tulumello, T. N.: Management of oral hemangioma, Oral Surg. **44:**39-44, 1977.

GENERAL REFERENCES

Briggs, P. C.: Submandibular duct stenosis as a complication of Ludwig's angina, Oral Surg. **47:**14-15, 1979.

Brooke, R. I.: Exfoliative cheilitis, Oral Surg. **45:**52-55, 1978.

Ciola, B., and Yesner, R.: Radiographic manifestations of a lung carcinoma with metastases to the anterior maxilla, Oral Surg. **44**(5):811-816, 1977.

Fiumara, N. J., Grande, D. J., and Giunta, J. L.: Papular secondary syphilis of the tongue, Oral Surg. **45:**540-542, 1978.

Friedlander, A. H., and Singer, R.: Renal adenocarcinoma of the kidney with metastasis to the tongue, J. Am. Dent. Assoc. **97:**989-991, 1978.

Hayward, J. R., and Regezi, J. A.: Oral dysplasia and in situ carcinoma: clinicopathologic correlations of eight patients, J. Oral Surg. **35:**756-762, 1977.

Holland, C. S.: The management of Ludwig's angina, Br. J. Oral Surg. **13:**153-159, 1975.

Knapp, M. J.: Pathology of oral tonsils, Oral Surg. **29:**295-304, 1970.

Kotilainen, R.: Denture stomatitis: a clinical, mycological and histologic investigation of maxillary denture wearers after a prolonged use of the denture. Thesis. University of Kuopio, 1977, pp. 9-72.

Murphy, N. C., and Bissada, N. F.: Iron deficiency: an overlooked predisposing factor in angular cheilitis, J. Am. Dent. Assoc. **99:**640-641, 1979.

Pindborg, J. J., Daftary, D. K., and Mehta, F. S.: A follow-up study of sixty-one oral dysplastic precancerous lesions in Indian villagers, Oral Surg. **43:**383-390, 1977.

Robinson, H. B. G.: Look out for those red spots: erythroplakia. Editor's chair, Dent. Survey **54:**4, Nov. 1978.

Sciubba, J. J., and Brown, A. M.: Oral-facial manifestations of Klippel-Trenaunay-Weber syndrome, Oral Surg. **43:**227-232, 1977.

Shafer, W. G.: Oral carcinoma in situ, Oral Surg. **39:**227-238, 1975.

Slade, E., Danielson, O., and Goldberg, M.: Erysipelas: facial lymphadenitis, J. Oral Surg. **35:**416-417, 1977.

Zegarelli, D. J.: Red and white intraoral lesions, Dent. Survey **55:**34-42, March 1979.

11

Generalized red conditions

Stuart L. Fischman
Russell J. Nisengard
George G. Blozis

This chapter deals primarily with the diffuse red conditions that occur in the oral cavity and affect several oral surfaces simultaneously. The majority of these will occur as multiple ulcerations distributed over erythematous mucosal surfaces. They include:

Recurrent aphthous stomatitis and Behçet's syndrome
Primary herpetic gingivostomatitis
Erosive lichen planus
Erythema multiforme
Acute atrophic candidosis
Benign mucous membrane pemphigoid
Pemphigus
Desquamative gingivitis
Radiation and chemotherapy mucositides
Xerostomia
Plasma cell gingivitis
Stomatitis areata migrans
Allergies
Polycythemia
Lupus erythematosus
Rarities
    Actinomycosis
    Acute gangrenous stomatitis
    Agranulocytosis
    Amyloidosis
    Bullous pemphigoid
    Cheilitis granulomatosa (Melkersson-Rosenthal
        syndrome)
    Diabetic ulcerations
    Epidermolysis bullosa
    Gonococcal stomatitis
    Granulomatous disease of the newborn
    Hand-foot-and-mouth disease
    Heavy metal poisoning
    Hereditary mucoepithelial dysplasia
    Hereditary telangiectasia
    Herpangina
    Histoplasmosis
    Impetigo
    Kaposi's sarcoma (multiple)
    Leukemia
    Major aphthous ulcerations

Measles
Metastatic hemangiosarcomas
Mycosis fungoides
Psoriasis
Psoriasis variants
    Pustular psoriasis
    Acrodermatitis continua
    Impetigo herpetiformis
Reiter's syndrome
Scurvy
Streptococcal stomatitis
Thermal and chemical burns (mild, recent)
Ulcerative colitis
Uremic stomatitis
Varicella zoster (primary and secondary)
Vincent's angina
Vitamin B deficiencies (severe)

Chapter 10 is devoted to the solitary reddish lesions. In contrast, this chapter discusses those diseases that produce reddish changes on several different mucous membranes simultaneously. They may also appear on other body surfaces (mucous membranes and skin). Also included are those vesicular lesions that appear red both prior to the eruption of the vesicles and after rupture.

These conditions represent the most difficult challenge to clinical diagnosis. There are several reasons for this. (1) In many instances the specific cause is unknown. (2) Frequently, laboratory and biopsy results are nonspecific or overlap. (3) Many of these conditions are relatively uncommon so that even the specialist seldom has the opportunity to study a sufficient quantity of cases in order to gain expertise. (4) The degree of severity of individual cases varies widely. (5) The initial clinical appearance varies, but they appear similar in their later stages. For example, the vesiculobullous group is quite distinctive in

231

the early stages, but after the "blisters" rupture and disappear, the resultant ulcerative stomatitis is quite nonspecific in appearance.

The vesicular diseases are a particular enigma because the "blisters" may form and rupture within 24 hours; hence the clinician and patient may be unaware that vesicles ever were present in a given case. (6) Presentation, remission, and recurrence make up the frequent course of many of these diseases. (7) Treatment is palliative for the vast majority of these conditions.

An overview of the various conditions reveals a considerable divergence: for instance, polycythemia manifests itself as a painless deep dusty red color of the mucosa usually without inflammation, blisters, or ulcerations. The stomatitis accompanying xerostomia does not produce bullae but is otherwise nondistinctive except for the decrease in salivary pooling. The bullous diseases are similar in that vesicles or blebs are the first lesions to appear; however, these soon rupture to form ulcers on inflamed mucosal surfaces. Diseases such as lichen planus, lichenoid drug reaction, lupus erythematosus, stomatitis areata migrans, and psoriasis may form a fifth group frequently demonstrating both white (keratotic) and red lesions.

These conditions have in common the generalized reddened appearance of the oral mucosa. Pain is usually a symptom.

ETIOLOGY

The spectrum of causes of generalized red conditions is especially broad and varied. It includes the following (unfortunately the specific cause is unknown in a considerable number of conditions):

Hereditary conditions
Allergic conditions
Autoimmune conditions
Infections (bacterial, fungal, viral)
Altered host state (e.g., diabetes, uremia)
Altered local resistance (e.g., xerostomia)
Trauma
Iatrogenic conditions
Neoplasia
Secondary to gastrointestinal conditions
Deficiency states (vitamins, etc.)
Idiopathic conditions

RECURRENT APHTHOUS STOMATITIS

Solitary recurrent aphthous *ulcers* are discussed in detail in Chapter 6, "Oral Ulcers and Fissures." Their characteristic history and clin-

Fig. 11-1. Recurrent aphthous stomatitis. This middle-aged woman had many ulcers scattered throughout the oral mucosa. Note the characteristic reddened (darker) mucosa surrounding these ulcers in the sublingual region.

ical picture permit ready recognition. However, a patient will occasionally be seen with what will prove to be multiple aphthous ulcers distributed over several inflamed mucosal surfaces (Fig 11-1 and Plate 4). This condition is known as recurrent aphthous *stomatitis* and when the clinician initially sees such a case it is more convenient for differential purposes to think of it as a generalized reddish ulcerated condition.

The cause of this condition is presently unknown. There are excellent data suggesting that immunologic factors (humoral immune response, cell-mediated immune responses, and immune complexes) may play an important role in recurrent aphthous ulceration.

FEATURES

The ulcers of recurrent aphthous stomatitis are basically round or ovoid, have yellowish necrotic bases, and are surrounded by a region of inflamed mucosa. When the lesions are less than 1 cm they are referred to as "minor" ulcers; if larger than 1 cm they are referred to as "major." The lesions are multiple, invariably painful, and most frequently occur on the labial or buccal mucosa, floor of the mouth, and soft palate (Fig. 11-1 and Plate 4). The attacks are recurrent. Each attack lasts for about 10 days although if major aphthous ulcers are present they may persist for months. The patient then enjoys a disease-free period of anywhere from a few weeks to several months before suffering a recurrence of aphthous stomatitis. As with all of the other stomatitides a painful lymphadenitis accompanies each ulcerative episode.

If extraoral problems accompany recurrent aphthous stomatitis the diagnosis of Behçet's syndrome may be made. Behçet's syndrome is characterized by oral and genital ulcers and ocular inflammation. At least two of these symptoms are required to establish the diagnosis. Behçet's syndrome is currently classified as mucocutaneous (oral, genital, or skin lesions, or all three), arthritic (arthritis in addition to mucocutaneous lesions), and neuroocular (neurologic or ocular symptoms or both in addition to symptoms from the first two types).

DIFFERENTIAL DIAGNOSIS

All the ulcerative mucositides listed at the beginning of the chapter need to be considered. The absence of vesicles and blebs would rule out *benign mucous membrane pemphigoid* and *pemphigus* and partially eliminate *erythema multiforme*. The fact that the ulcers in recurrent aphthous stomatitis are quite uniform in appearance and also somewhat similar in size would differentiate this condition from erythema multiforme, which will appear as lesions that vary greatly from one another in appearance: erythematous macules, blebs, ulcers, and crusted lesions on the lip. If crusted lesions are present on the vermilion border this would not be compatible with a diagnosis of recurrent aphthous ulceration.

The fact that a white (keratotic) component is not present would tend to rule out *lichen planus, lichenoid drug reaction, lupus erythematosus*, and *psoriasis*.

Considering the possibility of *atrophic candidiasis* one would expect to discover predisposing conditions in the patient workup. Also most cases of candidiasis, even the atrophic type, will pass through a white necrotic phase or perhaps will have a minor keratotic component. A negative cytology test for *Candida albicans* would rule out the possibility.

Ulcerative mucositis due to *xerostomic* conditions should be deemphasized if a decrease in the salivary pool is not a feature. Actually in recurrent aphthous stomatitis increased salivation is a usual feature.

Primary herpetic gingivostomatitis can be differentiated from recurrent aphthous stomatitis by the fact that the former condition is usually accompanied by a fever, small vesicles precede ulceration, the vesicles and ulcers are pinpoint size, and the attached gingivae are almost invariably involved. In recurrent aphthous stomatitis the gingivae are seldom ever involved. Also frequently a history of contact with an active lesion on another person can be established in primary herpetic infection.

Herpetiform ulcers are characterized by recurrent crops of as many as 100 small (1 to 2 mm) painful ulcers that may involve any part of the oral mucosa.

MANAGEMENT

Because the cause of the lesions is currently obscure, there is no specific treatment. Patients are generally given supportive therapy, including the use of systemic analgesics and topical anesthetic agents. In especially severe cases the use of topical or systemic steroids should be considered. Tetracycline mouth rinse has been reported to be effective in reducing the severity of lesions of recurrent aphthous ulcerations (Graykowski and Hooks, 1978).

PRIMARY HERPETIC GINGIVOSTOMATITIS

Primary infections with herpes simplex virus (herpesvirus hominis) are a relatively common cause of multiple oral ulcerations.

FEATURES

Approximately 30% of Americans have been infected with type 1 herpesvirus (Rowe, 1977). The initial infection with the herpesvirus is usually subclinical or else heralded by the appearance of a vesicular lesion on the vermilion border. Occasionally the primary infection is characterized by the acute onset of a systemic illness. Following an incubation period of 5 to 10 days, the patient complains of malaise, irritability, headache, and fever, and within a few days the mouth becomes very uncomfortable. Oral examination at this time reveals a widespread inflammation of the marginal and attached gingivae. Numerous small vesicles are seen throughout the oral mucosa and on the lips (Fig. 11-2 and Plate 4). These vesicles soon rupture and become pinpoint ulcers, and secondary infection generally occurs. Ulcers on the lips may become bloody and crusted, and saliva may "drool" from the oral cavity. Cervical lymphadenopathy is also a frequent finding. In young children, the diagnosis of the infection may be missed and the symptoms may be assumed to result from teething.

Dental personnel should be aware of the possibility of implantation of the virus on the hands. Herpetic whitlow is a primary infection of the finger with this virus (Brightman and Guggen-

Fig. 11-2. Primary herpetic gingivostomatitis. **A** and **B,** Example in a woman. Note the inflamed gingivae and the ragged appearance with a faint whitish pattern. Close inspection revealed that the ragged white appearance was produced by the rupture and ulceration of the many pinpoint vesicles. **C,** Example in a 9-year-old boy; the primary infection was mostly confined to the gingivae. **D,** Case in a 13-year-old girl in which the prominent manifestations involved the mucosa of the lip and the anterior portion of the tongue. **E,** Gingival inflammation and swelling in leukemia. The ragged appearance along with the multiple pinpoint ulcerations is not present in this disease. (**A** and **B** courtesy E. Ranieri, D.D.S., Maywood, Ill. **E** courtesy P. Akers, D.D.S., Evanston, Ill.)

heimer, 1970). It may be seen in dental personnel who examine mouths of patients with primary herpetic gingivostomatitis or in patients who have a habit of biting the cuticle.

Approximately one third of those patients who have had a primary infection will develop recurrent herpetic infections. Herpes labialis is the most frequent type of recurrent infection. It usu-

ally is seen as a cluster of vesicles appearing around the lips following a systemic illness or other stressful situation. Ultraviolet light and mechanical stimuli may also produce recurrences.

DIFFERENTIAL DIAGNOSIS

The differential diagnosis of primary herpetic gingivostomatitis has been covered in the differential diagnosis section of recurrent aphthous stomatitis. In addition, *hand-foot-and-mouth disease* (viral etiology) needs to be considered because multiple pinpoint oral vesicles and ulcers as well as fever are common to both. The absence of these lesions on the palms and soles would eliminate hand-foot-and-mouth disease. *Herpangina* (coxsackievirus) can generally be identified by the fact that the small vesicles and ulcers are usually limited to the soft palate and oropharynx.

Occasionally a very large intraoral manifestation of *recurrent herpes* occurs (e.g., small pinpoint vesicles and ulcers covering the whole palate). It is important to note that only one surface is involved in the recurrence whereas multiple surfaces are involved in primary herpetic gingivostomatitis.

Establishment of diagnosis. The diagnosis of primary herpetic gingivostomatitis is usually made on a clinical basis. The patient has a number of vesicles or small painful ulcers throughout the oral cavity. A history of systemic signs and symptoms of a viral illness is helpful in establishing the diagnosis.

Confirmation of the viral infection by laboratory methods is available but not utilized routinely. The virus may be isolated in tissue culture if fluid can be obtained from an intact vesicle. Primary infections are associated with an increase in antibody titer, and acute and convalescent sera may be studied. Histologic and cytologic examination of tissue may be done, but it will not permit identification of the specific virus.

There are two types of herpes simplex virus that cause disease in humans. The type I virus is primarily associated with infections of the skin and mucous membrane and type II with infections of the genitalia (although the converse can and does occur). Epidemiologic studies have suggested a relationship between carcinoma of the uterine cervix and herpes simplex virus type II; however, a relationship between oral infection with the type I virus and oral carcinoma has not been demonstrated. The frequency of oral herpesvirus infection is so high that these relationships are statistically difficult to demonstrate (Shillitoe and Silverman, 1979).

MANAGEMENT

There is no specific treatment of primary herpetic gingivostomatitis although vidarabine has recently been highly successful in reducing the mortality rates of herpetic meningitis (F.D.A., 1978-79). The usual supportive measures for an acute viral infection should be instituted. These include maintenance of proper oral hygiene, adequate fluid intake to prevent dehydration, and the use of systemic analgesics for control of pain. Antipyretic agents are also prescribed when fever is a symptom. In severe cases, it may be necessary to use a topical anesthetic mouth rinse such as viscous lidocaine or elixir of diphenhydramine (Benadryl). The patient is often able to tolerate cold liquids, and they may aid in preventing dehydration. If secondary infection becomes a major problem, appropriate antibiotics should be instituted.

EROSIVE LICHEN PLANUS

The lesions of lichen planus may take several different forms and have been classified into the following types: keratotic vesiculobullous, atrophic, and erosive (Shklar, 1972). Although the lesions of the atrophic and erosive forms are somewhat distinct, they are usually combined and discussed under the heading of erosive lichen planus. The cause of the disease is obscure, but some studies have implicated emotional stress.

FEATURES

The keratotic form of lichen planus (discussed in Chapter 5 as a white lesion) has been considered to be the most common, but a recent report suggests that the erosive form may be seen more often (Silverman and Griffith, 1974). The disease occurs about twice as often in women as in men, with the average age being about 50 years. The initial lesion usually does not occur until after 40 years of age.

Lichen planus is a disease primarily of whites and seldom involves blacks or Orientals. The most common site of involvement is the buccal mucosa. The following sites are also involved (in decreasing order of frequency): tongue, gingiva, palate, lip, and floor of the mouth. Reports of concurrent skin involvement are quite variable, placing this phenomenon in the range of 20%. A spontaneous remission has been reported in many cases. The oral lesions are especially prone to recurrence and remission.

Although the keratotic form of lichen planus is usually asymptomatic the patient with the atrophic or erosive variety will almost always complain of a burning sensation or pain. The atrophic lesions appear smooth and erythematous and may have a feathery white keratotic border. In the erosive form the surface is usually granular and bright red and tends to bleed when traumatized. A pseudomembrane composed of necrotic cells and fibrin covers more severe areas of erosion.

The patterns of involvement change from week to week. However, almost invariably there is a clinically apparent white keratotic component present either in a reticular, feathery, or plaque pattern (Fig. 11-3 and Plates 3 and 4).

Cases have been reported in which lichen planus was associated with a squamous cell carcinoma; and as a consequence, lichen planus has been speculated to be a premalignant lesion (Fulling, 1973; Silverman and Griffith, 1974).

In recent follow-up studies, however, the number of patients with lichen planus who developed squamous cell carcinoma ranged from less than 1% to 2.5%. These results do not confirm the previous reports and leave the question unresolved. As a matter of precaution, such patients should be observed carefully so that any changes can be detected early and investigated.

The histopathology of the atrophic form shows a thinned epithelium with hydropic degenera-

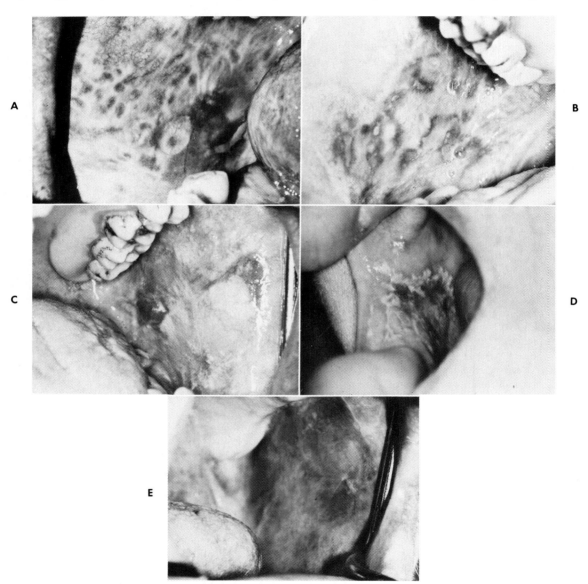

Fig. 11-3. Erosive lichen planus. **A** to **D,** Four cases of erosive lichen planus. Note the various proportions of keratotic and erythematous involvement in each. **E,** Case of erosive lichen planus in which almost no keratotic component was present. Two weeks later a considerable keratotic component was observed in this same case.

tion in the basal cell layer. A dense bandlike infiltrate of lymphocytes is confined to the area immediately beneath the epithelium. In the erosive form either the epithelium is completely missing or only remnants of epithelial tissue are seen. The underlying inflammatory infiltrate becomes mixed with polymorphonuclear leukocytes and loses its distinctive bandlike pattern. The diagnosis of lichen planus can be confirmed only by a biopsy.

In the atrophic lesions where the epithelium still is intact, the changes are usually characteristic. Unfortunately an intact epithelium does not exist in erosive lesions, and the diagnosis may be difficult if not impossible. A biopsy from the edge of an erosive lesion is usually more helpful in diagnosis. When more typical lesions are present on other areas of the mucosa or skin, it may be assumed that the red lesions represent lichen planus (Fig. 11-3 and Plate 4). However, if the lesions are clinically suggestive of squamous cell carcinoma, biopsy is imperative.

DIFFERENTIAL DIAGNOSIS

Other diseases that contain a clinically apparent keratotic component in combination with a mucositis and so present lesions similar to those of lichen planus are squamous cell carcinoma, lichenoid drug reaction, psoriasis, stomatitis areata migrans, atrophic candidiasis with a keratotic border, and discoid lupus erythematosus.

When red lesions are confined only to the gingiva, it is virtually impossible to clinically and histologically distinguish atrophic or erosive lichen planus from benign mucous membrane pemphigoid and desquamative gingivitis. Immunofluorescent findings in gingival biopsies, however, are diagnostic of benign mucous membrane pemphigoid and some forms of desquamative gingivitis. Characteristic, but not diagnostic, immunofluorescent findings occur in lichen planus.

Special diagnostic procedures. In lichen planus, immunofluorescent studies of biopsies reveal characteristic but not diagnostic findings (Table 11-1). Globular deposits, sometimes called cytoid bodies or Civatte bodies, that contain immunoglobulins, fibrin, or complement are observed in the papillary dermis along the dermoepidermal junction (Fig. 11-4). Cytoid bodies are more often seen in active stages of the disease and are more common in lesions than in normal tissue. While cytoid bodies are not disease specific or diagnostic, their identification can be helpful when routine histopathologic studies are inconclusive. Cytoid bodies are seen in biopsy

Table 11-1. Immunofluorescent findings important in the diagnosis of red conditions

Disease	Serum		Tissue		
	Types of antibodies	Findings	Pattern of staining	Findings	Significance
Benign mucous membrane pemphigoid or cicatricial pemphigoid	Basement membrane antibodies	– or + (<25%)	Basement membrane	+	Diagnostic
Bullous pemphigoid	Basement membrane antibodies	+(80%)	Basement membrane zone	+(100%)	Diagnostic
Lichen planus	Negative		Globular deposits or cytoid bodies in dermis and epidermis; fibrin deposits along dermoepidermal junctions	+(97%)	Characteristic
Pemphigus, all forms	Intercellular antibodies of epithelium	+(>95%)	Intercellular epithelial deposits	+(100%)	Diagnostic
Discoid lupus erythematosus	Negative or low titer of antinuclear antibodies		Dermoepidermal deposits of immunoglobulins and complement: lesion only	+(80%)	Highly characteristic
Systemic lupus erythematosus	High titer of antinuclear antibodies	+(90-100%)	Dermoepidermal deposits of immunoglobulins and complement: lesion and normal tissue	+(>90%)	Diagnostic

specimens in 97% of lichen planus, 41% of systemic lupus erythematosus, 70% of discoid lupus erythematosus, 75% of dermatomyositis, 50% of erythema multiforme, 50% of pemphigoid, 40% of pemphigus, and 40% of normal specimens. The findings in lichen planus can partially be differentiated from the other diseases and the normal specimens on the basis of size and number of cytoid bodies and other immunologic findings. In lupus erythematosus, pemphigus, and pemphigoid, diagnostic immunofluorescent findings can also be seen in biopsy specimens (Table

Fig. 11-4. A, Direct immunofluorescence test on oral biopsy from patient with lichen planus demonstrating IgG deposits in cytoid or globular pattern in the dermis. Similar deposits of IgA, IgM, fibrin, and complement can also be seen. Such findings are characteristic. **B,** Direct immunofluorescence test on oral biopsy from patient with lichen planus demonstrating fibrin deposits in a granular pattern along the dermoepidermoid junction.

11-1). In normal biopsy specimens smaller and fewer cytoid bodies are observed.

MANAGEMENT

A specific and uniformly successful treatment for symptomatic lichen planus is not available. Symptomatic relief and at times complete remission can be obtained by using a topical steroid such as betamethasone or triamcinalone. Intralesional injections of steroids have also been beneficial in some instances. Triamcinalone diacetate suspension can be injected into the lesions. The usual regimen is 40 mg/wk. Systemic cortisone taken in tablet form will effect a rapid regression of symptoms and induce a remission for varying periods. In attempts to partly eliminate the side effects of administering cortisone systemically the following method has been successfully used: an elixir of cortisone taken at the same dosage as is prescribed for systemic administration is held in the mouth for 15 minutes four times per day. The mouth is then rinsed gently with the elixir and the elixir is expectorated.

ERYTHEMA MULTIFORME

Erythema multiforme is a disease of unknown cause that has many different manifestations; however, when seen in its classic form, it is easily recognized. It is a vesiculobullous disease, but vesicles and bullae usually are present for only a limited time.

Although an attack of erythema multiforme usually occurs without apparent reason, certain agents have been identified as precipitating the disease. The most common is a herpes simplex infection, but other infections and drugs have also been implicated.

FEATURES

The disease occurs primarily in young adults, usually males. It has a sudden onset and runs a course of 2 to 6 weeks. Recurrences are common. In many cases lesions are limited to the oral mucosa and involve the following sites, listed in descending order of frequency: buccal mucosa, lips, palate, tongue, and fauces (Fig. 11-5 and Plates 3 and 4). The gingivae are rarely involved.

A sloughing mucosa and diffuse redness are

A

B

C

Fig. 11-5. Erythema multiforme. **A,** 26-year-old black man with extensive lesions of the lips and oral mucous membranes. **B,** A milder case with erythematous patches, blebs, erosions, and ulcers restricted to the mucosa of the cheeks. **C,** Target lesion on the skin of another patient with erythema multiforme. (**A** courtesy W. Heaton, D.D.S., Chicago.)

the most frequent clinical features. The initial lesions are small red macules that may enlarge and develop a whitish center. The macules progress to form bullae that rupture, leaving a sloughing mucosal surface. A bright red raw surface is seen when the tissue is lost. In time the denuded surface becomes covered with a pseudomembrane of fibrin and cells and assumes a grayish appearance (Brandtzaeg, 1964). Involvement of the oral tissues may be limited to merely a diffuse redness (Wooten et al., 1967).

Skin lesions may accompany the oral condition, or there may be cutaneous manifestation without oral involvement. Skin lesions often have a characteristic bull's-eye or target appearance (Fig. 11-5). Although the palms of the hands are a classic location these lesions may occur anywhere on the skin.

A microscopic examination of vesicles and bullae reveals a subepithelial cleft. The underlying connective tissue contains a mixed inflammatory infiltrate with numerous eosinophils. The light microscopic changes and immunologic findings seen in immunofluorescent examination of biopsy specimens are not diagnostic but can be used to rule out other diseases. There are no specific laboratory studies that are useful.

The diagnosis is made on the basis of clinical information. Obviously this can pose a problem if the lesions are limited to the oral cavity. A history of previous attacks that involved other mucous membranes or the skin is most useful in making the diagnosis.

DIFFERENTIAL DIAGNOSIS

Similar oral lesions may be seen in pemphigus vulgaris, benign mucous membrane pemphigoid, allergic reactions, erosive lichen planus, primary herpetic gingivostomatitis, and xerostomia. All of these diseases must be considered in a differential diagnosis. Oral lesions that occur because of drug reactions may appear similar to those of erythema multiforme and may vary from focal or diffuse areas of erythema to areas of erosion and ulceration that began as vesicles or bullae. It then becomes a question of whether the drug precipitated an attack of erythema multiforme or whether the lesions actually resulted from drug allergy.

MANAGEMENT

Since erythema multiforme is a self-limiting disease, usually only supportive care is necessary. When areas other than the oral cavity are involved, the patient is best managed through a cooperative effort of physician and dentist. If the oral cavity is severely involved, systemic steroids or a steroid oral suspension used as a mouthwash may provide symptomatic relief.

ACUTE ATROPHIC CANDIDOSIS (CANDIDIASIS)

The lesion of acute atrophic candidosis represents a less common form of a *Candida* infection. It usually is the sequel of the typical lesions of *Candida,* or acute pseudomembranous candidosis. When the white plaque of pseudomembranous candidiasis is shed or removed, often a red, atrophic, and sore mucosa is left (Fig. 11-6 and Plate 4). At times the lesion may be asymptomatic. It may resolve spontaneously or require treatment with nystatin (Lehner, 1964, 1967).

FEATURES

The lesions will be seen in the same types of patients who are prone to develop acute pseudomembranous candidosis, for example, those taking broad-spectrum antibiotics, steroids, or immunosuppressive agents. In addition, the lesions

Fig. 11-6. Erythematous papules of candidosis that were an incidental finding and resolved without treatment. An exfoliative cytologic smear was positive for *Candida.*

occur with diabetes, hypothyroidism, other debilitating diseases, and pregnancy. They are sometimes found in apparently normal healthy individuals.

Tissue sections show an atrophic epithelium that may contain a few hyphae in the superficial layers. The lamina propria usually has a mild, acute, inflammatory infiltrate and increased vascularity. An exfoliative cytologic smear of the lesions is most useful in establishing a diagnosis.

DIFFERENTIAL DIAGNOSIS

Frequently the red lesions of acute atrophic candidosis are seen in association with those of the pseudomembranous type and do not pose a diagnostic problem. When present as multiple red lesions, they are rather nonspecific in appearance. Lesions produced by chemical burns, drug reactions, and other organisms have a similar clinical appearance as may predominantly red lesions of erosive lichen planus, mild cases of erythema multiforme, and discoid lupus lesions.

MANAGEMENT

The lesions of acute atrophic candidosis respond well to either a nystatin oral suspension or vaginal tablets used as oral troches. A typical therapeutic regimen would include the use of nystatin oral suspension four times daily. The preparation is dispensed with a measured dropper and the patient should be instructed to use 4 ml (400,000 units) in each side of the mouth. The medication should be retained in the mouth as long as possible before swallowing. Treatment should be continued for at least 2 days after the patient is asymptomatic and cultures are normal.

Nystatin vaginal tablets can be used as troches and dissolved in the mouth. The patient should be advised to use one tablet four times per day. Obviously, the patient should be advised to ignore any prepackaged instructions that accompany the tablets.

BENIGN MUCOUS MEMBRANE PEMPHIGOID

The cause of benign mucous membrane pemphigoid or cicatricial pemphigoid is still unknown; however, immunopathologic changes are associated with the lesions. Immunoglobulins or complement or both can be found deposited in the basement membrane zone. Occasionally the serum also contains antibodies to the basement membrane zone.

FEATURES

Benign mucous membrane pemphigoid is seen in women twice as frequently as in men. The disease affects older individuals, with the highest incidence occurring in the late 50s. It has rarely been reported in other than whites. Lesions are found primarily on the mucous membranes, with infrequent involvement of the skin. Of the mucous membranes, the oral cavity and eyes are involved most often. Lesions occur on the gingiva, buccal mucosa, and palate.

The gingiva becomes edematous and bright red—a rather striking feature of the disease (Plate 3). This involvement may be patchy or diffuse. Subsequent to bullae formation or trauma the surface epithelium may be lost, leaving a raw, red bleeding surface. The vesiculobullous lesions in other areas of the oral cavity do not appear as red, nor do they bleed as much. The ulcers that result from the collapse of bullae are surrounded by a zone of erythema (Fig. 11-7) and surprisingly are relatively asymptomatic. Unless treated, the disease follows a chronic course of partial remission and exacerbation.

The histologic changes are not diagnostic since the vesicles and bullae are subepithelial. Frequently, the epithelial roof of the bulla is lost and the histologic changes become nonspecific, characterized by a chronic inflammatory infiltrate of the connective tissue. If the surface is intact, direct immunofluorescent study of the biopsy is particularly important since the immunofluorescent findings are diagnostic: basement membrane zone deposition of immunoglobulins and complement (Fig. 11-8). In contrast to routine histology, the immunofluorescent findings can be observed in the adjacent clinically normal mucosa. The biopsy site of choice is actually the perilesional or clinically normal mucosa since these areas have the dermal/epidermal relationships necessary for immunofluorescent evaluation (Table 11-1). In approximately 25% of the cases, low titers of serum antibodies to the basement membrane are also observed. When these occur, they are also diagnostic of pemphigoid.

Immunofluorescence is an important and useful diagnostic technique because it can help separate the gingival lesions of benign mucous membrane pemphigoid from those of erosive lichen planus and desquamative gingivitis (Skhlar and McCarthy, 1971). A clinical feature common to these three diseases is the production of a gingival bleb by a strong jet of air (Plate 3). This occurs because of the defect in the basement membrane region.

Fig. 11-7. Benign mucous membrane pemphigoid. This illustration shows whitish areas of intact and collapsed bullae as well as some erythematous and ulcerated areas.

DIFFERENTIAL DIAGNOSIS

Other diseases that should be considered in a differential diagnosis of benign mucous membrane pemphigoid are pemphigus vulgaris, bullous pemphigoid, bullous lichen planus, and early cases of erythema multiforme.

MANAGEMENT

The patient with benign mucous membrane pemphigoid may be extremely difficult to treat. Steroids have been the only useful form of therapy; but unfortunately their side effects may be quite severe. Using steroids on alternate days has been somewhat successful in avoiding these complications.

PEMPHIGUS

Pemphigus is a vesiculobullous disease of unknown cause that may affect mucous membranes and skin. The four major forms of pemphigus are pemphigus vulgaris, pemphigus vegetans, pemphigus foliaceus, and pemphigus erythematosus. They have similar immunologic findings, which are diagnostic (Table 11-1).

FEATURES

Pemphigus affects the sexes approximately equally, and the vast majority of patients are white. In a report by Rosenberg and co-workers (1976) 74% of the cases with the vulgaris or vegetans type were in Jewish people; approximately 98% of the cases were over 31 years of age at the time of onset; and 80% of the vulgaris variety (by far the most common type) first occurred intraorally. In this 20-year follow-up study, mortality was 32% with more than half of these deaths occurring within the first 12 months of the disease.

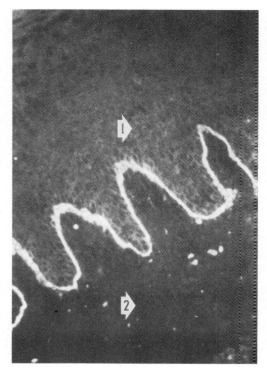

Fig. 11-8. Direct immunofluorescence on oral biopsy from patient with benign mucous membrane pemphigoid revealing complement deposits along the basement membrane zone in a linear pattern (1, epithelium; 2, lamina propria). Similar deposits of IgG and other immunoglobulins also occur. These findings are diagnostic.

The lesions of pemphigus vulgaris may appear as areas of erosion but more often they are seen as ulcers, bullae, or areas of sloughing mucosa or skin (Fig. 11-9 and Plate 4). Diffuse erythematous involvement of the gingiva has been reported but is not the typical manifestation of the disease.

The microscopic study of intact vesicles or bullae reveals that the basic defect is intraepithelial where the individual cells separate from one another and a pooling of fluid occurs. The basal layer of epithelial cells remains in position on the basement membrane.

DIFFERENTIAL DIAGNOSIS

All the vesiculobullous conditions listed at the beginning of this chapter should be considered in the differential diagnosis. As a general rule the size of the bullae in pemphigus is smaller than those that occur in benign mucous membrane

Fig. 11-9. Pemphigus. **A** and **B,** Clinical views of the same case. The mucosa of the lower lip is much more severely involved than the buccal mucosa. **C,** Direct immunofluorescence on oral biopsy from patient with pemphigus revealing IgG deposits intercellularly in the epithelium. Epithelial intercellular antibodies are also seen in the serum. Both are diagnostic. (**A** and **B** courtesy M. Lehnert, D.D.S., Minneapolis.)

pemphigoid and considerably larger than those that occur in the viral diseases such as herpes and hand-foot-and-mouth disease.

Special diagnostic procedures. Immunofluorescent studies of sera and biopsy specimens reveal a diagnostic finding of antibodies limited to the intercellular substance of epithelium and intercellular deposits of IgG (Fig. 11-9).

The sera from over 95% of pemphigus patients with active disease contain intercellular epithelial antibodies. During early stages of the disease or remission the antibody titers may be low or negative. The significance of the antibody titer must be considered together with the clinical and histologic findings. Low titers (10 to 20) are significant when there are typical clinical and histologic findings. Low titers of intercellular antibodies with atypical clinical and histologic findings may be termed "pemphiguslike" antibodies rather than true pemphigus antibodies. Pemphiguslike antibodies that occur as a result of extensive burns and some drug eruptions do not bind in vivo as in true pemphigus.

The intercellular antibody titer frequently relates to disease activity by rising and falling with exacerbations and remissions. In many cases, the titer changes of two or more doubling dilutions precede the clinical changes and provide a prognostic test for control of drug therapy. Sera should be tested every 2 to 4 weeks until the patient is in remission and then every 1 to 6 months.

Almost all patients with active pemphigus have intercellular deposits of IgG and sometimes IgA, IgM, and complement in biopsy specimens. These findings are diagnostic. Biopsies of oral lesions should be taken from the periphery of the lesion where the epithelium is still intact.

MANAGEMENT

Corticosteroid therapy is the preferred treatment for severe pemphigus. Other modes of treatment currently being evaluated include alternate-day steroid and gold therapy and immunosuppressive treatment with methotrexate or azathioprine (Imuran) (Rosenberg et al., 1976).

DESQUAMATIVE GINGIVITIS

There is some question as to whether desquamative gingivitis is a specific disease entity or a clinical manifestation of several different diseases. In a study of 40 patients with clinical desquamative gingivitis, McCarthy and Shklar (1964) histologically identified 17 cases of benign mucous membrane pemphigoid, two cases of pemphigus, and four cases of lichen planus. The remainder were considered hormonal, idiopathic, or abnormal responses to local factors. In an immunofluorescent study of 50 patients with clinical desquamative gingivitis, 14 were identified as benign mucous membrane pemphigoid, two were identified as pemphigus, and one case was identified as psoriasis. Of the remaining 33, 16 had findings consistent with lichen planus (Nisengard and Neiders, 1979). While the cause of desquamative lesions of the gingivae is not always known, it is generally considered to represent a degenerative pathosis of the gingivae. Because it occurs more frequently in postmenopausal women, there may also be an underlying hormonal factor.

FEATURES

Desquamative gingivitis is seen in both sexes but is far more prevalent in women (Glickman and Smulow, 1964). Generally it occurs after the

Fig. 11-10. Desquamative gingivitis. Note areas of erosion on the gingiva (arrows). (Courtesy E. Ranieri, D.D.S., Maywood, Ill.)

age of 40, but it may occur at any age after puberty. The changes are usually confined to the gingivae, most often the labial surface. Usually the palatal and lingual surfaces are not involved. The gingivae become bright red and edematous. Changes may be limited to a few small areas (Fig. 11-10) of the palate or they may be diffuse and extend throughout the gingivae. The epithelium is quite friable and can be removed from the underlying connective tissue easily, leaving a red surface that bleeds readily after minimal trauma. Patients may complain of a burning sensation but often are asymptomatic.

Microscopically the epithelium is thin and atrophic. The rete ridges are blunted, and there may be clefting below the basement membrane. Edema and a mild chronic inflammatory infiltrate are seen in the underlying connective tissue. The microscopic findings are not diagnostic and serve only to exclude other diseases. Immunofluorescent studies of gingival biopsies are of particular importance where the underlying cause is benign mucous membrane pemphigoid, pemphigus, or lichen planus. A diagnosis is made on the basis of a good history and physical examination.

DIFFERENTIAL DIAGNOSIS

As previously mentioned, the other diseases that produce similar lesions are erosive lichen planus, benign mucous membrane pemphigoid, bullous pemphigoid, and rarely pemphigus vulgaris.

MANAGEMENT

Treatment is directed at providing symptomatic relief. Initially it is important that the possible local irritating factors be removed. Different drugs such as estrogens and steroids have been

Fig. 11-11. Radiation mucositis. **A,** Squamous cell carcinoma appearing clinically as a large area of erythroplakia in the retromolar and soft palate region. **B,** Same patient about midway through radiation therapy. Note the areas of erythema and the fibrinous exudate.

applied topically and do provide variable degrees of improvement. Systemic steroids have been used with limited success.

RADIATION AND CHEMOTHERAPY MUCOSITIDES

The diagnosis of the mucositis that occurs as a result of radiation or chemotherapy should be easily established from the information contained in the patient history.

Radiation mucositis
FEATURES

Radiation therapy produces rather characteristic and dramatic changes. During the course of therapy, which usually continues for 6 weeks, the patient develops a diffuse inflammatory change in the mucosa. The amount of tissue involved will be determined by the portal used for the radiation therapy.

Tissue change does not become apparent until the last part of the first week or the beginning of the second week. Distinct blebs may be produced or else the change starts as a whitish area resulting from decreased cellular division and retention

of squamous cells. In subsequent weeks, the surface layers are lost and a thin erythematous mucosa is seen. Focal areas break down and ulcerate. These ulcerations then become covered with a tan-yellow fibrous exudate (Fig. 11-11 and Plate 3). The tissue response varies considerably among patients. Profound changes resolve a few weeks after therapy is completed, but there is some residual redness for variable periods of time (Blozis and Robinson, 1968).

MANAGEMENT

Symptomatic relief is necessary for these patients because the pain can be quite severe, especially when eating. Topical anesthetics such as elixir of diphenhydramine or lidocaine can be combined with either milk of magnesia, Maalox, or Kaopectate and used as mouthwash. Analgesics may be necessary.

Chemotherapy mucositis
FEATURES

Oral lesions resulting from chemotherapy are relatively infrequent and occur only during the course of therapy. Initially patients may complain of a burning sensation. Lesions may or may not be associated with this burning sensation. The lesions begin as focal areas of redness that may persist and that ultimately ulcerate (Plate 3). Infrequently the ulcerations become rather numerous and large.

MANAGEMENT

Treatment is directed toward providing symptomatic relief. If the lesions become debilitating, it may be necessary to briefly interrupt chemotherapy. Usually they become secondarily infected and respond well to an oral suspension of tetracycline used as a mouthwash and then swallowed.

XEROSTOMIA

Dryness of the mouth is not a disease but a sign of impaired function of the salivary glands, which may be reversible or irreversible. Infectious and inflammatory lesions of the salivary glands such as mumps will produce a transient xerostomia. When the primary disease resolves, the flow of saliva will return to normal. Diseases such as Mikulicz's disease or Sjögren's syndrome produce irreversible changes that result in a progressive decrease in the production of saliva. Radiation to the head neck area causes atrophy of the glands and a decrease in the amount of saliva secreted.

Fig. 11-12. Reiter's syndrome. **A,** Erythema involving the sclera. **B,** Anterior intraoral view. Note small erythematous patches (arrows). **C,** View showing reddish macules on tongue. **D,** View of palate showing reddish patches. (Courtesy M. Lehnert, D.D.S., Minneapolis.)

Dehydration and senile atrophy of the glands will reduce the amount of saliva produced by the glands (Bertram, 1967). Many medications currently in wide use decrease salivary gland activity. Ganglionic blocking agents used to control hypertension, many psychotherapeutic agents (tranquilizers and antidepressants), and antihistamines have this side effect. Eisenberg (1978) discussed the causes of xerostomia in considerable detail.

FEATURES

In mild short-term cases of xerostomia the patient may be asymptomatic and the mucosa appear normal. In moderately severe cases the patient may complain of a dry mouth or a burning sensation. When these symptoms are intense, there will be difficulty with speech, mastication, and the retention of artificial appliances. Patches of mucosa will appear very atrophic and take on a dark dusky red appearance (Fig. 11-12 and Plate 4). In severe xerostomia, erosion and ulceration of the inflamed mucosa will occur.

The combined features of decreased salivary and lacrimal production indicate a diagnosis of Mikulicz's disease. In Sjögren's syndrome decreased salivary production, decreased lacrimal production, and arthritis are seen.

DIFFERENTIAL DIAGNOSIS

A lack of saliva enables the clinician to differentiate the mucositis of xerostomia from the other types listed in this chapter.

Historical evidence is very useful in establishing the type of xerostomia. A history of radiation treatment, antisialagogue medication, and combinations of features suggesting one of the syndromes associated with xerostomia are clues that direct the clinician to the correct diagnosis.

PLASMA CELL GINGIVITIS

Plasma cell gingivitis is a disease that was recognized as a distinct entity several years ago. It has also been reported under the name of atypical gingivostomatitis. Studies indicate that the lesions may be caused by some ingredient in chewing gum; and the disease has been suggested as a type of allergic response (Kerr et al., 1971; Perry et al., 1973). It is interesting that although this condition was frequently seen in the 1960s and early 1970s, it is seen much less frequently now (Silverman and Lazada, 1977).

FEATURES

Plasma cell gingivitis occurs much more frequently in women and is seen predominantly in young adults. The patient complains of a sore or burning mouth. The most striking and characteristic feature of the disease is the involvement of the gingiva. The entire free and attached gingivae are edematous and bright red (Fig. 11-13 and Plate 3). Frequently there are associated lesions of the lips, tongue, and buccal mucosa, a scaling of the lips, and an angular cheilitis. The tongue is erythematous and devoid of filiform papillae. The patient may state that the problem has been present for as long as 3 years.

The most spectacular microscopic changes are seen in the lamina propria, which is densely infiltrated by plasma cells. The other changes are rather nonspecific. A diagnosis is made primarily on the basis of the clinical appearance of the lesions and is supported by a biopsy.

DIFFERENTIAL DIAGNOSIS

The clinical features of plasma cell gingivitis are rather distinctive and are not simulated by other diseases. An early leukemic infiltrate of the gingiva may appear somewhat similar.

MANAGEMENT

The patient usually shows a marked improvement shortly after he stops chewing gum. Other patients show marked improvement after changing brands of toothpaste. Complete remission of the disease takes place in approximately 4 weeks.

STOMATITIS AREATA MIGRANS

Stomatitis areata migrans is a recently recognized disorder that is also known as migratory mucositis or ectopic geographic tongue.

FEATURES

Most frequently the lesions of geographic tongue are confined to the dorsal surface and lateral borders of the tongue. Occasionally lesions similar to those seen on the tongue have been reported on other mucosal surfaces of the oral cavity (Weathers et al., 1974). These lesions are considered to be a more extensive involvement of the same process and have been referred to as stomatitis areata migrans or ectopic geographic tongue. The basic appearance is that of red patches of various sizes and shapes that are surrounded by white (keratotic) raised rims (Fig.

Fig. 11-13. Diffuse and rather striking erythematous changes of plasma cell gingivitis are confined to the gingiva.

Fig. 11-14. Stomatitis areata migrans on the buccal mucosa.

11-14). The white rims may show a radiating, feathery appearance as they fade into the surrounding normal mucosa. The patterns change continuously and finally fade out completely as the condition enters a remission. Stomatitis areata migrans is usually asymptomatic and found on routine oral examination.

The histopathology of stomatitis areata migrans shows a thinning of the surface epithelium in some areas and an epithelial hyperplasia in others. The epithelium may show spongiosis and infiltration by acute and chronic inflammatory cells, often in a focal arrangement (Munro's abscesses).

DIFFERENTIAL DIAGNOSIS

The following lesions need to be differentiated from stomatitis areata migrans: lichen planus, psoriasis, lupus erythematosus, Reiter's syndrome, and electrogalvanically induced lesions (Banoczy et al., 1979).

MANAGEMENT

Most cases of stomatitis areata migrans are asymptomatic. Patients complaining of burning tenderness or pain should be placed on a bland diet and use diphenhydramine (Benadryl) mouth rinses until the condition becomes asymptomatic.

ALLERGIES

Diffuse erythematous lesions may be seen on the oral mucosa as a result of allergies and also as toxic effects from drugs. These lesions take a variety of forms and have been classified as "erythema multiforme due to medication" (stomatitis medicamentosa) or as "lichenoid drug reaction" (lichen planus due to medication). The clinical presentation is identical in erythema multiforme and lichen planus, and the diagnosis is made by a careful history. Cessation of drug therapy, with the concurrent administration of antihistaminic agents, will usually result in prompt resolution.

Topical reactions to agents used in the oral cavity are relatively unusual. Individual idiosyncrasies to agents used in preparations such as surgical dressings, mouth rinses, toothpaste, and chewing gums have been reported (Fig. 11-15 and Plate 4). A careful history is usually of assistance in making the diagnosis. The patient will frequently report changing from one brand of oral product to another immediately prior to development of the symptomatology. Prompt withdrawal of the etiologic agent is usually both therapeutic and diagnostic.

Patients and clinicians frequently confuse the irritating effects of poorly fitting prosthetic appliances with allergy to a denture base material. Denture base materials are rarely allergenic, but poorly fitting appliances may produce such pathologic changes as papillary hyperplasia. Appliances that are not kept clean may be associated with an increased incidence of intraoral candidiasis. Improperly cured acrylic materials and improperly used denture relining materials can also cause injury to the oral mucosa, but this is a "burn" rather than a true allergy.

POLYCYTHEMIA

Polycythemia is a chronic and sustained elevation of the number of erythrocytes and of hemoglobin. Both primary and secondary polycythemia occur. Primary polycythemia (polycythemia vera) is a neoplastic condition of the erythropoietic system analogous to leukemia. Transition between polycythemia and myelogenous leukemia has been reported. Secondary polycythemia is a sustained elevation of erythrocytes and hemoglobin, usually resulting from bone marrow stimulation caused by living at high altitudes or by chronic pulmonary diseases such as emphysema. It is also seen in untreated congenital heart disease.

The entire oral mucosa of patients with polycythemia has a deep red or purple color. This discoloration is particularly noticeable in the gingivae and soft palate. The gingivae usually are prone to easy bleeding and petechial hemorrhages may be seen on the palate and labial mucosa. These changes are much more frequently seen in polycythemia vera. Infarcts may occur in the smaller vessels due to the increased viscosity of the blood and may produce multiple ulcers in the dusky red mucosa. Laboratory tests indicating a marked increase in erythrocyte hemoglobin concentration and hematocrit values quickly establish the general diagnosis of polycythemia and thus separate this condition from all the other mucositides.

LUPUS ERYTHEMATOSUS

Lupus erythematosus (LE) is a connective tissue disease of unknown cause. However, recently a rickettsial organism was implicated. Nearly every organ in the body runs the risk of involvement, resulting in an impressive array of signs and symptoms. The term "discoid LE" has been applied to cases where there is only skin involvement, and this is usually a benign disease with a good prognosis. Chances of conversion of discoid lupus to systemic lupus are small. Skin lesions may also accompany systemic lupus (Braverman, 1970, pp. 144, 145).

Fig. 11-15. Reaction to periodontal dressing. Note erythematous reaction on superior aspect of buccal mucosa where it was in contact with the dressing. Note severe tissue destruction on lingual gingiva. Plate 4 shows another view of this case.

FEATURES

Lupus erythematosus occurs predominantly in females, and most are adults affected before the age of 40. Oral manifestations of discoid lupus erythematosus (DLE) occur in about 20% of patients. The oral lesions may occur with or without skin involvement, before skin lesions develop, after skin lesions develop, or simultaneously with the skin lesions. Oral lesions may also be seen in patients with systemic lupus.

Schiodt and co-workers (1978) studied 32 patients (26 females, 6 males) with LE lesions of the oral mucosa. The time of onset of the oral lesions ranged from 6 to 75 years with a mean of 41 years. The mean duration of the oral lesions was 4.2 years. Symptoms such as discomfort, burning, and pain with hot spicy food were present in 75% of the patients. The lesions were most often located on the buccal mucosa, the gingiva, labial mucosa, and vermilion border. The oral lesions were infected by yeast in over half the patients (Schiodt et al., 1978).

In Schiodt's study early lesions were characterized by erythema without striae. The classic well-developed discoid lesions were characterized by central erythema with white spots and a 2 to 5 mm wide border of white striae radiating from the center. Some lesions were white plaques such as in leukoplakia and still others had areas of Wickham's striae as in lichen planus, usually on a reddish base (Schiodt et al., 1978).

Microscopically the epithelium shows hyperorthokeratosis or parakeratosis or both, acanthosis, and pseudoepitheliomatous hyperplasia interspersed with atrophy. The basal layer shows liquefaction degeneration, and keratin plugs can be found. A lymphocytic infiltrate is present beneath the epithelial layer, may be concentrated around vessels, and may extend deeply into the subepithelial tissue. The microscopic study of lesions may be nonconclusive in some cases as demonstrated by Schiodt and Pindborg (1976). These researchers completed a blind study of biopsy specimens of oral lesions from 21 patients with LE and 21 patients with oral lichen planus and leukoplakia. The correct histologic diagnosis was made in less than half the cases. In one third of the cases differentiation between DLE and lichen planus could not be made on a histologic basis.

DIFFERENTIAL DIAGNOSIS

Multiple lesions on several surfaces are usually the rule in lupus erythematosus. When the lesions are mostly of the red variety then the following conditions need to be considered: lichen planus, lichenoid drug reaction, ectopic geographic tongue, psoriasis, diffuse leukoplakia with erythroplakic components, and electrogalvanic lesions. Oral lesions of LE may be differentiated from lichen planus on the basis of immunofluorescent studies of sera and biopsy specimens (Table 11-1).

MANAGEMENT

Treatment for lupus erythematosus consists of the administration of systemic steroids or antimalarials. Topical steroids may be used on symptomatic intraoral lesions.

RARITIES

The following generalized red conditions occur more rarely:

Actinomycosis
Acute gangrenous stomatitis
Agranulocytosis
Amyloidosis
Bullous pemphigoid
Cheilitis granulomatosa (Melkersson-Rosenthal syndrome)
Diabetic ulcerations
Epidermolysis bullosa
Gonococcal stomatitis
Granulomatous disease of the newborn
Hand-foot-and-mouth disease
Heavy metal poisoning
Hereditary mucoepithelial dysplasia
Hereditary telangiectasia
Herpangina
Histoplasmosis
Impetigo
Kaposi's sarcoma (multiple)
Major aphthous ulcerations
Measles
Metastatic hemangiosarcomas
Mycosis fungoides
Psoriasis (Fig. 11-16)
Psoriasis variants
   Pustular psoriasis
   Acrodermatitis continua
   Impetigo herpetiformis
Reiter's syndrome (Plate 4)
Scurvy
Streptococcal stomatitis
Thermal and chemical burns (mild, recent)
Ulcerative colitis
Uremic stomatitis (Fig. 11-17)
Varicella zoster (primary and secondary) (Fig. 11-18)
Vincent's angina
Vitamin B deficiencies (severe)

Fig. 11-16. Psoriasis (red macular areas) on palate. (From White, D. K., Leis, H. J., and Miller, A. S.: Oral Surg. **41:**174-181, 1976.)

Fig. 11-17. Uremic stomatitis. Note erythematous and eroded areas on the lateral border of the tongue. (Courtesy M. Lehnert, D.D.S., Minneapolis.)

Fig. 11-18. Herpes zoster. **A** and **B,** Same case showing involvement of the skin and mucous membrane in area innervated by the mandibular branch of the trigeminal nerve. **C,** Another case of herpes zoster. Note white vesicles on an erythematous base and the sharp demarcation at the midline. (Courtesy A. C. W. Hutchinson collection, Northwestern University Dental School Library, Chicago.)

SPECIFIC REFERENCES

Baat de la Faille-Kuyper, E. H., and Baat de la Faille, H.: An immunofluorescent study of lichen planus, Br. J. Dermatol. **90**:365-371, 1974.

Banoczy, J., Roed-Petersen, B., Pindborg, J. J., and Inovay, J.: Clinical and histologic studies on electrogalvanically induced oral white lesions, Oral Surg. **48**:319-323, 1979.

Bertram, V.: Xerostomia: clinical aspects, pathology, and pathogenesis, Acta Odontol. Scand. [Suppl.] **25**(49):1-126, 1967.

Beutner, E. H., Chorzelski, T. P., and Bean, S. T., editors: Immunopathology of the skin, ed. 2, New York, 1979, John Wiley & Sons.

Blozis, G. G., and Robinson, J. E.: Oral tissue changes caused by radiation therapy and their management, Dent. Clin. North Am. pp. 643-656, Nov. 1968.

Brandtzaeg, P.: Erythema multiforme exudativum: a review of the literature with special reference to oral manifestations, Odontol. Tidskr. **72**:363-390, 1964.

Braverman, I. M.: Skin signs of systemic disease, Philadelphia, 1970, W. B. Saunders Co.

Brightman, V. J., and Guggenheimer, J. G.: Herpetic paronychia—primary herpes simplex infections of the fingers, J. Am. Dent. Assoc. **18**:112-115, 1970.

Eisenberg, E.: Medical considerations: cardiovascular, respiratory, gastrointestinal, and hematologic systems, xerostomia, and irradiation. In Wood, N. K., editor: Treatment planning: a pragmatic approach, St. Louis, 1978, The C. V. Mosby Co., pp. 122-128.

F.D.A. Drug Bulletin: Vidarabine approved for herpes simplex virus encephalitis, Washington, D.C., Dec. 1978 and Jan. 1979, U.S. Government Printing Office.

Fulling, H. J.: Cancer development in oral lichen planus: a follow-up study of 327 patients, Arch. Dermatol. **108**:667-669, 1973.

Glickman, I., and Smulow, J. B.: Chronic desquamative gingivitis: its nature and treatment, J. Periodontol. **35**:397-405, 1964.

Graykowski, E., and Hooks, J.: Summary of workshop on recurrent aphthous stomatitis and Behçet syndrome, J. Am. Dent. Assoc. **97**:599-602, 1978.

Kerr, D. A., McClatchey, K. D., and Regezi, J. A.: Idiopathic gingivostomatitis, Oral Surg. **32**:402-423, 1971.

Lehner, T.: Oral thrush, or acute pseudomembranous candidosis, Oral Surg. **18**:27-37, 1964.

Lehner, T.: Oral candidosis, Dent. Pract. **17**:209-216, 1967.

McCarthy, P. L., and Shklar, G.: Disease of the oral mucosa: diagnosis, management and therapy, New York, 1964, McGraw-Hill Book Co., pp. 183-191.

Michael, B., and Sy, E. K.: Tissue fixed immunoglobulins in lichen planus. In Beutner, E. H., Chorzelski, T. P., Bean, S. T., et al., editors: Immunopathology of the skin: labeled antibody studies, Stroudsburg, Pa., 1973, Dowden, Hutchinson & Ross, p. 182.

Nisengard, R. J., Alpert, A. M., and Krestow, V.: Desquamative gingivitis: immunologic findings, J. Periodontol. **49**:27-32, 1978.

Nisengard, R. J., Jalonski, S., Beutner, E. H., et al.: Diagnostic importance of immunofluorescence in oral bullous diseases and lupus erythematosus, Oral Surg. **40**:365-375, 1975.

Nisengard, R. J., and Neiders, M.: Unpublished data, 1979.

Perry, H. O., Deffner, N. F., and Sheridan, P. J.: Atypical gingivostomatitis, Arch. Dermatol. **107**:872-878, 1973.

Rosenberg, F. R., Sanders, S., and Nelson, C. T.: Pemphigus: a 20-year review of 107 patients treated with corticosteroids, Arch. Dermatol. **112**:962-970, 1976.

Rowe, N. H.: Infectious lesions. Paper presented to Scientific Session in Oral Pathology at Annual Meeting of A.D.A., Miami Beach, Fla., 1977.

Schiodt, M., Halberg, P., and Hentzer, B.: A clinical study of 32 patients with oral discoid lupus erythematosus, Int. J. Oral Surg. **7**:85-94, 1978.

Schiodt, M., and Pindborg, J. J.: Histologic differential diagnostic problems for oral discoid lupus erythematosus, Int. J. Oral Surg. **5**:250-252, 1976.

Shillitoe, E., and Silverman, S.: Oral cancer and herpes simplex virus—a review, Oral Surg. **48**:216-224, 1979.

Shklar, G.: Lichen planus as an oral ulcerative disease, Oral Surg. **33**:376-388, 1972.

Shklar, G., and McCarthy, P. L.: Oral lesions of mucous membrane pemphigoid: a study of 85 cases, Arch. Otolaryngol. **93**:354-364, 1971.

Silverman, S., Jr., and Griffith, M.: Studies on oral lichen planus. II. Follow-up on 200 patients, clinical characteristics and associated malignancy, Oral Surg. **37**:705-710, 1974.

Silverman, S., and Lazada, F.: An epilogue to plasma-cell gingivostomatitis (allergic gingivostomatitis), Oral Surg. **43**:211-217, 1977.

Weathers, D. R., Baker, G., Archard, H. O., and Burkes, J.: Psoriasiform lesions of the oral mucosa (with emphasis on "ectopic geographic tongue"), Oral Pathol. **37**:872-888, 1974.

Wooten, J. W., Katz, H. I., Hoffman, S., and Link, J. F.: Development of oral lesions in erythema multiforme exudativum, Oral Surg. **24**:808-816, 1967.

GENERAL REFERENCES

Album, M. M., Gaisin, A. L., Lee, K. W. T., et al.: Epidermolysis bullosa dystrophica polydysplastica, Oral Surg. **43**:859-872, 1977.

Barnett, M. L., and Nisengard, R. J.: Effects of immunofluorescent transport solution on the ultrastructure of human biopsies, Oral Surg. **44**:430-436, 1977.

Bayer, D. B., Kalfayan, B., and Banasik, P. M.: Kaposi sarcoma: report of a case with initial involvement of the oral mucosa, J. Oral Surg. **36**:907, 1978.

Belding, J. H., and Tade, W. H.: Evaluation of epithelial maturity in hormonally related stomatitis, J. Oral Med. **33**:17-19, 1978.

Ben-Aryeh, H., Malberger, E., Gutman, D., et al.: Salivary IgA and serum IgG and IgA in recurrent aphthous stomatitis, Oral Surg. **42**:746-752, 1976.

Bernstein, M. L., and McDonald, J. S.: Oral lesions in Crohn's disease: report of 2 cases and update of the literature, Oral Surg. **46**:234-245, 1978.

Burry, J. N., and Kirk, J.: Lichenoid drug reaction from methyldopa, Br. J. Dermatol. **91**:475-476, 1974.

Clark, P. M., and Gamble, J. W.: Mikulicz disease of a minor salivary gland, J. Oral Surg. **36**(11):895, 1978.

Cohen, L., and Randell, S.: Erythema multiforme: report of a case, J. Oral Med. **33**(4):128, 1978.

Croley, T. E., and Miers, C.: Epithelial changes in the oral mucosa resulting from a variation in hormone stimulus, J. Oral Med. **33**:85-89, 1978.

Eversole, L. R., Kenney, E. B., and Sabes, W. R.: Oral lesions as the initial sign in pemphigus vulgaris, Oral Surg. **33**:354-361, 1972.

Fischman, S. L., Barnett, M. L., and Nisengard, R. J.: Histopathologic, ultrastructural, and immunologic findings in an oral psoriatic lesion, Oral Surg. **44**:253-260, 1977.

Fonseca, R. J., Patel, M. F., and Rapidis, A. D.: Behçet's syndrome: report of a case, J. Oral Surg. **35**:227-230, 1977.

Galil, K. A.: Xerostomia as a post-operative complication of vagotomy: case report, J. Oral Med. **31**:82-83, 1976.

Gilmore, H. K.: Early detection of pemphigus vulgaris, Oral Surg. **46**:641-644, 1978.

Goldstein, B. H., and Katz, S. M.: Immunofluorescent findings in oral bullous lichen planus, J. Oral Med. **34**:8-12, 1979.

Graykowski, E. A., and Hooks, J. J.: Summary of workshop on recurrent aphthous stomatitis and Behçets syndrome, J. Am. Dent. Assoc. **97**:599-602, 1978.

Greenspan, D., and Silverman, S., Jr.: Study of a bland dentifrice for persons with radiation-induced mucositis and vesicul-erosive disease, J. Am. Dent. Assoc. **99**:203-204, 1979.

Hasler, J. F.: The role of immunofluorescence in the diagnosis of oral vesiculobullous disorders, Oral Surg. **33**:362-374, 1972.

Hay, K. D., Muller, H. K., and Reade, P. C.: D-Pencillamine-induced mucocutaneous lesions with features of pemphigus, Oral Surg. **45**:385-395, 1978.

Hay, K. D., and Reade, P. C.: Methyldopa as a cause of oral mucous membrane reactions, Br. Dent. J. **145**:195, 1978.

Hicks, M. L., and Terezhalmy, G. T.: Herpesvirus hominis type 1: a summary of structure, composition, growth cycle, and cytopathogenic effects, Oral Surg. **48**:311-318, 1979.

Koshiba, H., Kimura, O., and Nakata, M.: A clinical and histologic observation of enamel hypoplasia in a case of epidermolysis bullosa hereditaria, Oral Surg. **43**:585-590, 1977.

Limongelli, W. A., Rothstein, S. S., Smith, L. G., and Clark, M. S.: Disseminated South American blastomycosis (paracoccidioidomycosis): report of case, J. Oral Surg. **36**:625-630, 1978.

Lindgren, S., Enerback, L., and Freiberg, N.: Oral acantholytic itching disease responding to Dapsone, Oral Surg. **42**:597-605, 1976.

Logan, T. E., McDonald, J. S., and Alpert, B.: Mikulicz syndrome secondary to lymphosarcoma, J. Oral Surg. **35**:719-720, 1977.

Lozada, F., and Silverman, S., Jr.: Erythema multiforme, Oral Surg. **46**:628-636, 1978.

McCarthy, F. P., McCarthy, P. L., and Shklar, G.: Chronic desquamative gingivitis: a reconsideration, Oral Surg. **13**:1300-1313, 1960.

Mishkin, D. J., Akers, J. O., and Darby, C. P.: Congenital neutropenia: report of a case and a biorationale for dental management, Oral Surg. **42**:738-745, 1976.

Nilsen, R., Livden, J., and Tunold, S.: Oral lesions of epidermolysis bullosa acquisita, Oral Surg. **45**:749-754, 1978.

Nisengard, R. J., Jablonska, S., Beutner, E. H., et al.: Diagnostic importance of immunofluorescence in oral bullous diseases and lupus erythematosus, Oral Surg. **40**:365-375, 1975.

Paravecchio, R.: Photosensitization of a patient with discoid lupus erythematosus by a dental operating light: report of a case, J. Am. Dent. Assoc. **94**:907-909, 1977.

Person, J. R., and Rogers, R. S., III: Bullous and cicatricial pemphigoid. Clinical, histopathologic, and immunopathologic correlations, Mayo Clin. Proc. **52**(1):54-66, 1977.

Pisanty, S., and Markitzio, A.: Sjogren's syndrome with secondary tubular acidosis, J. Oral Med. **34**:47-50, 1979.

Samit, A. M., and Greene, G. W., Jr.: Atypical benign migratory glossitis: report of a case with histologic and electron microscopic evaluations, Oral Surg. **42**:780-791, 1976.

Sapiro, S. M., and Eisenberg, E.: Sjogren's syndrome (sicca complex), Oral Surg. **45**:591-599, 1978.

Schiodt, M., Dabelsteen, E., and MacKenzie, I. C.: An improved technique in the diagnosis of pemphigus, Int. J. Oral Surg. **4**:211-213, 1975.

Segelman, A. E., and Doku, H. C.: Treatment of the oral complications of leukemia, J. Oral Surg. **35**(6):469-477, 1977.

Shklar, G.: Lichen planus as an oral ulcerative disease, Oral Surg. **33**:376-388, 1972.

Stanley, H. R.: Management of patients with persistent recurrent aphthous stomatitis and Sutton's disease, Oral Surg. **35**:174-179, 1973.

Witkop, C. J., White, J. G., Sauk, J. J., Jr., and King, R. A.: Clinical, histologic, cytologic, and ultrastructural characteristics of the oral lesions from hereditary mucoepithelial dysplasia, Oral Surg. **46**:645-657, 1978.

Zecha, J. J., Van Dijk, L., and Hadders, H. N.: Cheilitis granulomatosa (Melkersson-Rosenthal syndrome), Oral Surg. **42**:454-460, 1976.

Zegarelli, D. J., and Zegarelli, E. V.: Intraoral pemphigus vulgaris, Oral Surg. **44**:384-393, 1977.

12

Red conditions of the tongue

Norman K. Wood
George G. Blozis
Paul W. Goaz

The red conditions discussed in this chapter are the following:

Migratory glossitis
Median rhomboid glossitis
Deficiency states
Xerostomia
Rarities

All of the single red lesions of the oral mucosa discussed in Chapter 10 have been reported to occur on the tongue. Likewise all the generalized reddish conditions of the oral mucosa (Chapter 11) may involve the tongue. In some cases the tongue is involved first, in others different mucosal surfaces are initially affected, and in some patients one or more mucosal surfaces and the tongue are involved simultaneously.

However, this chapter is dedicated to red conditions that occur only on the tongue or else have a predisposition for that structure. Such conditions usually produce one or more bald reddish patches or affect the entire dorsal surface and margins of the tongue.

MIGRATORY GLOSSITIS

A plethora of terms (erythema migrans, glossitis areata migrans, glossitis areata exfoliativa, geographic tongue, wandering rash of the tongue, and annulus migrans) has been used to describe this condition. Although the cause is unknown, emotional stress may be one of several factors involved in the onset or exacerbation of this lesion (Redman et al., 1966; Sumner and Shklar, 1973).

FEATURES

Migratory glossitis is a relatively common condition, occurring in 1% to 2% of the population.

The lesions are usually asymptomatic and are discovered as an incidental finding during a routine examination. The patient may complain of a burning sensation that is made worse by spicy foods or citrus fruits. Migratory glossitis occurs most commonly in young or middle-aged adults but has been seen in patients ranging in age from 5 to 84 years. There is a reported predilection for females. The lesions are found more frequently on fissured tongues (Gorlin and Goldman, 1970, p. 31).

Although they have a rather typical appearance, the lesions of migratory glossitis may be extremely variable in size and duration. Initially they appear as small erythematous nonindurated atrophic areas bordered by a slightly elevated, distinct rim that varies in color from gray to white to light yellow (Fig. 12-1). Loss of the filiform papillae produces a pink to red, relatively smooth, shiny surface, except for the residual fungiform papillae. A more intense redness may be present near the advancing margin of a lesion.

Single or multiple lesions may occur in migratory glossitis, and when multiple, they frequently coalesce to produce large areas of involvement that encompass much of the tongue. They appear as irregular circinate areas that gradually widen, change shape, and migrate over the tongue (Fig. 12-1). The progression of the lesions is usually quite rapid, with the pattern changing in a few days, or the lesions may remain relatively static. The duration of an attack is also quite variable, ranging from a few weeks to months and on rare occasions it may prolong for years. However, recurrent episodes of involvement are the general pattern.

Most frequently the lesions are confined to the

Fig. 12-1. Migratory glossitis. **A,** Multiple lesions with distinct borders and an inflamed atrophic mucosa. **B,** A larger more diffuse lesion with less inflammatory change and residual fungiform papillae.

Fig. 12-2. Lesions resembling migratory glossitis. **A,** Bilateral areas of atrophic lichen planus. **B,** Focal red and white areas on the lateral border of the tongue of an anemic patient.

dorsal surface and lateral borders of the tongue, but they may extend to the ventral surface. Occasionally lesions similar to those seen on the tongue have been reported on other mucosal surfaces of the oral cavity (Weathers et al., 1974). These lesions are considered to be a more extensive involvement by the same process and have been referred to as stomatitis areata migrans or ectopic geographic tongue (Fig. 11-14).

The histopathology of the lesions shows a loss of the filiform papillae and a variable thinning of the mucosa. In some areas there is an epithelial hyperplasia. The epithelium shows spongiosis and infiltration by acute and chronic inflammatory cells.

DIFFERENTIAL DIAGNOSIS

A diagnosis of migratory glossitis is made on the basis of the clinical appearance and history of the lesion. Similar-appearing lesions are reported in psoriasis, Reiter's syndrome, ectopic geographic tongue, and occasionally in pityriasis rubra pilaris (Dawson, 1974; O'Keefe et al., 1973; Weathers et al., 1974). These authors report that the clinical and histologic appearances of these conditions are often identical to those of geographic tongue. Thus the possibility must be con-

sidered that these conditions may be closely related. As far as the diagnostic aspects are concerned, if the classic tongue lesions are the only finding the clinician is correct in establishing a working diagnosis of migratory glossitis. However, he should be alert to the possibility that this isolated finding could be the first manifestation of the more generalized diseases included in the differential diagnosis above.

Thus in cases where skin, ocular, tongue, and urethral lesions occur with arthritis the most likely diagnosis would be Reiter's syndrome.

On the other hand, if the patient has skin lesions of psoriasis (particularly of the generalized pustular type) then the tongue changes may represent intraoral psoriasis. Likewise if the patient has skin lesions of pityriasis rubra pilaris then the possibility that the "geographic tongue" might really be a manifestation of this disease must be considered.

Lichen planus may occasionally produce reddish patches on the tongue, which in the healing phase may resemble geographic tongue (Fig. 12-2). The absence of raised whitish-yellow rims in lichen planus helps to differentiate these lesions from geographic tongue. In addition, it would be very unusual for lichen planus to affect

Fig. 12-3. A, Tongue of a middle-aged woman with pseudomembranous candidiasis of the dorsal surface. After 2 weeks of nystatin applications the candidal lesion had almost completely healed as shown in **B.** In 3 weeks the white appearance had completely resolved and the resultant picture was that of median rhomboid glossitis.

only the tongue. Also at least one white keratotic area can almost always be found on one of the oral mucosal surfaces in lichen planus.

It is interesting that the use of strong mouthwash can produce a variety of clinical lesions, one of which resembles geographic tongue (Kowitz et al., 1976). The history of the frequent use of mouthwash followed by the disappearance of the lesions when the mouthwash is discontinued would differentiate this condition from geographic tongue.

Anemic conditions that produce a patchy baldness of the tongue may be confused with geographic tongue (Fig. 12-2). Again the absence of the characteristic raised yellowish-white border from the red patches of anemia will differentiate these conditions from geographic tongue. Careful blood studies will demonstrate whether the patient is anemic.

MANAGEMENT

Usually all that is required in migratory glossitis is reassuring the patient that the problem is not serious. If there is some discomfort, bland diets and topical steroids will provide symptomatic relief while the lesions run their usual course and resolve.

MEDIAN RHOMBOID GLOSSITIS (CENTRAL PAPILLARY ATROPHY OF THE TONGUE)

For years median rhomboid glossitis has been generally considered to be a developmental defect resulting from an incomplete descent of the tuberculum impar and entrapment of a portion of it between the fusing lateral halves of the tongue. Recently however it has been noted that there is not a single report of this entity in a child (Baughman, 1971). Thus other etiologies have been offered. Baughman (1971) suggested the possibility of inflammatory infections (*Candida*) or degenerative causes. Wright's study (1978) strongly supported a theory that implicated a chronic candidal infection. Farman and co-workers (1977), using the term "central papillary atrophy of the tongue" (CPA), suggested that this condition represents a clinical appearance only and that the underlying disease process may not be identical in all cases. Van der Wall and co-workers (1979) support this concept suggesting the possibility of several different etiologies. Farman (1976) showed that there was an increased incidence of CPA in diabetics and in 1977 postulated that in some cases of CPA the defective microvasculature, which is commonly found in diabetics, may predispose the patient to candidal infection and the resultant tongue lesion. Fig. 12-3, *A,* shows an interesting ulcerative white necrotic lesion from which smears showed abundant clumps of *Candida*. The lesion was treated with applications of nystatin ointment. Within a week the lesion became asymptomatic and by 2 weeks was almost completely healed, assuming the reddish macular appearance of median rhomboid glossitis (Fig. 12-3, *B*).

FEATURES

Although most reports have indicated that median rhomboid glossitis occurs more frequent-

Fig. 12-4. A small but relatively typical lesion of median rhomboid glossitis.

Fig. 12-5. Classic appearance of median rhomboid glossitis.

ly in males (Baughman, 1971) in Wright's recent study of 28 cases (1978) 23 were in women and five were in men. It has been reported in patients ranging from 15 to 84 years. The lesion is located on the dorsal surface of the tongue in the midline and anterior to the circumvallate papillae (Figs. 12-4 and 12-5). The surface is dusky red, completely devoid of filiform papillae, and usually smooth; however, nodular or fissured surfaces have been noted (Fig. 6-16, *E*). Rarely there may be some keratosis. The size and shape of the lesion are somewhat variable, at times causing confusion as to the diagnosis. The lesions are generally asymptomatic, but pain and ulceration have been reported.

The histologic changes include an epithelium devoid of filiform papillae and slightly thickened. There is elongation and branching of the rete ridges. The underlying connective tissue shows increased vascularity and a chronic inflammatory infiltrate.

DIFFERENTIAL DIAGNOSIS

Median rhomboid glossitis is easily recognized by its usual asymptomatic nature and its characteristic location. Nevertheless, according to the foregoing discussion the clinician should consider the possibility that such a patient may be a diabetic.

Such a lesion also could be a squamous cell carcinoma or could represent another type of glossitis.

MANAGEMENT

The completely asymptomatic lesion that looks smooth and is not indurated requires no treatment but should be checked periodically in case of change.

Burning or painful lesions should be investi-

gated for the presence of candidal organisms and if found the lesion should be treated with nystatin ointment.

DEFICIENCY STATES

It has been recognized for years that certain deficiency states can produce a glossitis of either a completely bald or a patchy bald type. Diagnosticians of bygone years prided themselves in their ability to diagnose the specific deficiency by recognizing minute differences in appearance. Now it is generally agreed that the glossal changes induced by specific deficiencies are so similar that a definitive diagnosis based on their differentiation is at least unlikely if not impossible.

FEATURES

Symptoms vary from tender to burning tongue to extreme glossodynia. Frequently the tongue is initially intensely red and then becomes smooth as either the filiform or both types of papillae atrophy (Fig. 12-6). Reports indicate that in some instances normal papillation returns when the patient's basic problem is successfully treated (Basker et al., 1978).

The following deficiency states have been reported to produce the type of glossitides being discussed here: iron deficiency anemia, pernicious anemia, Plummer-Vinson syndrome, sprue, vitamin B complex deficiencies, especially thiamine, riboflavin, nicotoinic acid, pyridoxine, pantothenic acid, and B_{12} (cyanocobalamin).

DIFFERENTIAL DIAGNOSIS

If the tongue in question is completely bald, the only other condition that needs to be considered is the bald tongue of xerostomia (Fig. 12-7). Xerostomia can usually be readily recognized by noting the absence of a salivary pool in the

Fig. 12-6. Generalized glossitis. **A,** Patient with iron deficiency anemia. **B,** Patient had an untreated case of pernicious anemia. **C,** This man was severely malnourished and had several vitamin deficiencies. (**A** and **B** courtesy J. Lehnert, D.D.S., Minneapolis. **C** courtesy J. Lavieri, D.D.S., Maywood, Ill.)

floor of the mouth or the sticking of a tongue blade to the oral mucosa during the oral examination.

If the tongue in question shows partial or patchy baldness then all the conditions mentioned previously should be considered: migratory glossitis, psoriasis, Reiter's syndrome, pityriasis rubra pilaris, changes caused by the use of mouthwash, atrophic lichen planus, and median rhomboid glossitis. The differential diagnosis of these entities may be reviewed under the differential diagnosis section of median rhomboid glossitis. A thorough discussion of the differential aspects of all the deficiency states that may produce a glossitis is well beyond the intended scope of this text.

Fig. 12-7. Xerostomia. Tongue changes in a patient with Sjögren's syndrome. The tongue appears dry and is almost completely devoid of papillae.

Fig. 12-8. Syphilitic glossitis. (Courtesy R. Gorlin, D.D.S., Minneapolis.)

MANAGEMENT

Once the deficiency state or states have been identified specific measures may be undertaken for their correction if such are available.

XEROSTOMIA

The oral changes found in cases of xerostomia are discussed in Chapter 11, "Generalized Red Conditions." The red tongue of xerostomia (Fig. 12-7) is rather easily differentiated from the other causes by the absence of the formation of a salivary pool in the floor of the mouth.

RARITIES

A host of specific infectious diseases can effect superficial red changes in the surface of the tongue, but these are very rare examples indeed. Fig. 12-8 illustrates a case of syphilitic glossitis.

SPECIFIC REFERENCES

Basker, R. M., Sturdee, D. W., and Davenport, J. C.: Patients with burning mouths: a clinical investigation of causative factors, including the climacteric and diabetes, Br. Dent. J. **145:**9-16, 1978.

Baughman, R. A.: Median rhomboid glossitis: a developmental anomaly? Oral Surg. **31:**56-65, 1971.

Dawson, T. A. J.: Tongue lesions in generalized pustular psoriasis, Br. J. Dermatol. **91:**419-424, 1974.

Farman, A. G.: Atrophic lesions of the tongue: a prevalence study among 175 diabetic patients, J. Oral Pathol. **5:**255-264, 1976.

Farman, A. G.: Atrophic lesion of the tongue among diabetic outpatients: their incidence and regression, J. Oral Pathol. **6:**396-400, 1977.

Farman, A. G., Van Wyk, C. W., Staz, J., et al.: Central papillary atrophy of the tongue, Oral Surg. **43:**48-58, 1977.

Gorlin, R. J., and Goldman, H. M.: Thoma's oral pathology, ed. 6, St. Louis, 1970, The C. V. Mosby Co., p. 31.

Kowitz, G. M., Lucatorto, F. M., and Cherrick, H. M.: Effects of mouthwashes on the oral soft tissues, J. Oral Med. **31:**47-50, 1976.

O'Keefe, E., Braverman, I. M., and Cohen, I.: Annulus migrans: identical lesions in pustular psoriasis, Reiter's syndrome, and geographic tongue, Arch. Dermatol. **107:**240-244, 1973.

Redman, R. S., Vanc, F. L., Gorlin, R. J., et al.: Psychological component in the etiology of geographic tongue, J. Dent. Res. **45:**1403-1408, 1966.

Sumner, M. S., and Shklar, G.: Stomatitis areata migrans, Oral Surg. **36:**28-33, 1973.

Van der Waal, I., Beemster, G., and van der Kwast, W. A. M.: Median rhomboid glossitis caused by *Candida,* Oral Surg. **47:**31-35, 1979.

Weathers, D. R., Baker, G., Archard, H. O., and Burkes, J. E.: Psoriasiform lesions of the oral mucosa (with emphasis on "ectopic geographic tongue"), Oral Surg. **37:**872-888, 1974.

Wright, B. A.: Median rhomboid glossitis: not a misnomer, Oral Surg. **46:**806-814, 1978.

13

Yellow conditions of the oral mucosa

Ronald E. Gier

Yellow lesions, with the exception of Fordyce's granules, rarely occur in the oral cavity. The variety of yellow lesions is also small.

Fordyce's granules
Superficial abscess
Superficial nodules of tonsillar tissue
Yellow hairy tongue
Acute lymphonodular pharyngitis
Lipoma
Lymphoepithelial cyst
Epidermoid and dermoid cysts
Pyostomatitis vegetans
Jaundice or icterus
Lipoid proteinosis
Carotenemia

Many potentially yellow lesions may not appear yellow because the covering mucosa masks their color.

Normal fat covered by a thin layer of mucosa will appear yellow. Salivary gland tissue infiltrated with fat appears yellow. This condition occurs most often in the soft palate. Bone and salivary stones covered by a thin mucosa may impart a yellowish tinge to the mucosa.

The thrombin clot over some ulcers and the pseudomembranes of several conditions may become stained by food or microorganisms or both and have a yellowish color.

FORDYCE'S GRANULES

Fordyce's granules (Plate 3) occur in the oral mucosa as multiple small slightly raised granules that vary in color from a whitish yellow to a distinct yellow. They may occur in clusters or may form plaquelike areas. They are considered to be a normal variation made up of collections of sebaceous glands covered with intact mucosa. The lobules of these glands may be quite distinct.

The patient is usually unaware of the presence of Fordyce's granules; and when he does become aware of their presence, he may be worried that they are early cancer. This is frequently the reaction of a patient with cancerphobia.

FEATURES

Fordyce's granules have been reported by Miles (1958) to increase rapidly in number at puberty and to continue to increase during adult life. There is no established hereditary pattern to their occurrence. Halprin and co-workers (1953) found that approximately 80% of the individuals in a series they studied had Fordyce's granules and there was no difference in the distribution according to sex. They found that under the age of 10 years, the granules were present in approximately 60% of the population they examined and in 88% of those over the age of 10.

Fordyce's granules occur most often in the buccal mucosa and are usually bilaterally symmetric. They are also found in the retromolar pad area and in the labial mucosa; occasionally they occur on the gingiva, frenum, and palate. They are sharply delineated, with surfaces that are smooth and not ulcerated, and the solid nodules give the involved area a slightly cheesy feeling.

The histologic features are the same as those of normal sebaceous glands in the skin. The glands have ducts that may be plugged with keratin, and frequently extrusions of sebum into the oral cavity will be found.

DIFFERENTIAL DIAGNOSIS

The differential diagnosis of Fordyce's granules should include the possibility that the granules might be focal collections of *Candida* and that the plaquelike areas could possibly be a *hyperkeratotic leukoplakia*.

There is no special laboratory test for the diagnosis of Fordyce's granules; however, the appearance and distribution of the condition are so distinctive that, once recognized, there is little probability that the granules could be confused with another entity.

MANAGEMENT

Since this entity is innocuous, the importance of the condition is exclusively in the differential diagnosis. The involved glands are normal; and, unless malignant changes occur, as on rare occasion they may in sebaceous glands, no treatment is indicated for this condition.

SUPERFICIAL ABSCESS

A superficial bacterial or mycotic abscess (Plate 3) may appear as a yellow lesion. The yellow color is imparted by the pus pooling below the thinned mucosa stretched over the enlarging abscess. If a fistula forms and allows the pus to discharge, however, the lesion will probably no longer be yellow.

FEATURES

Pain is usually the chief complaint in superficial abscesses; and the history and oral examination frequently reveal its origin.

Superficial abscesses may be single or multiple; they may occur at all ages in either sex and primarily in the tooth-bearing areas. A single abscess will be a raised sessile swelling with a smooth frequently reddened mucosa over the yellow pus. On palpation the abscess is fluctuant and, when aspirated, yields pus. The surface may ulcerate and complete the sinus from the initiating infection, resulting in a draining lesion.

Teeth most often are the precipitating cause of this condition and can usually be identified as such, for they are either badly broken down by caries or involved with large restorations that have produced pulpal disease. At times the offending tooth or teeth will be associated with a deep periodontal pocket in which a lateral periodontal abscess has developed.

DIFFERENTIAL DIAGNOSIS

When a painful fluctuant swelling is present and pus is close enough to the surface to give the swelling a yellow color, there is little question that the diagnosis is an abscess. It is especially certain if the swelling is opposite the apex of an elevated tooth that is sensitive to percussion.

MANAGEMENT

In general the management of these lesions involves treatment of the underlying cause of the infection. This may be accomplished by initially draining the abscess, either by opening the pulp chamber of the offending tooth, extracting it, or by opening the abscess. If circumstances permit, the tooth may be retained and the infection eliminated by root canal therapy.

SUPERFICIAL NODULES OF TONSILLAR TISSUE

It is not uncommon to find discrete yellowish-pink nodules distributed over the posterior wall of the oropharynx as well as occasionally on the oral mucosa. These are nodes of lymphatic tissue that supplement the major tonsils composing Waldeyer's ring, and they are discussed in detail in Chapter 7.

FEATURES

When the nodes of tonsillar tissue are present and situated in areas that are visible during a routine examination of the oropharynx, from one to ten may be apparent. They vary in size but are usually from 3 to 5 mm in diameter, and have a yellowish-pink sheen.

DIFFERENTIAL DIAGNOSIS

The appearance and distribution of superficial tonsillar nodules are so characteristic that these structures are readily identified as a variation in the normal distribution of lymphatic tissue surrounding the entrance to the digestive and pulmonary systems.

MANAGEMENT

Since the nodules do not represent a pathologic reaction, their importance relates only to the differential diagnosis.

YELLOW HAIRY TONGUE

The conditions contributing to the development and discoloration of a hairy tongue are described in Chapters 5 and 9. At this point in the discussion of yellow oral lesions, it suffices to say that the hypertrophied filiform papillae of a hairy tongue may be stained yellow by food, tobacco, medicines, or chromogenic microorganisms.

ACUTE LYMPHONODULAR PHARYNGITIS

Acute lymphonodular pharyngitis is manifested by whitish to yellowish papular lesions on the soft palate and oropharynx. The causative factor is the coxsackievirus A10, and the occurrence of this disease today is probably widespread.

FEATURES

The incubation period for the virus is approximately 5 days after exposure. The patients, who are primarily children and young adults, complain of a sore throat. There is an elevation of temperature from 38 to 41 C (100 to 105 F) along with headache and anorexia. The oral lesions appear on about the third day. The course of the disease runs from 4 to 14 days, and the oral lesions resolve in 6 to 10 days after the onset of the symptoms. No sexual predilection has been reported for the disease (Steigman et al., 1963).

The lesions are raised discrete papules 3 to 6 mm in diameter. The whitish to yellowish papules are surrounded by a narrow well-defined zone of erythema. Their surfaces are not vesicular and do not ulcerate. The nodules are extremely tender, completely superficial, and bilateral; and they generally occur as multiple lesions on the uvula, soft palate, anterior tonsillar pillars, and posterior oropharynx.

The histopathology of these lesions consists of densely packed nodules of lymphocytes. There may be some inclusion bodies in the overlying epithelium.

DIFFERENTIAL DIAGNOSIS

The differential diagnosis must include *herpangina,* although the lesions of lymphonodular pharyngitis are not vesicular and do not ulcerate.

MANAGEMENT

Since acute lymphonodular pharyngitis is self-limiting and causes few if any complications, no treatment other than supportive therapy to maintain the patient is recommended.

LIPOMA

The lipoma (Plate 3) is one of the most common benign neoplasms, but it rarely occurs in the oral cavity. It is a tumor of mature fat cells that is found in the subcutaneous tissue. There is no significant mechanical, dental, family or social history that is consistent with the occurrence of lipomas.

The lipoma is classified as an exophytic lesion in Chapter 7.

FEATURES

The lipoma has been reported to occur in individuals from 1.5 months of age to 21 years; most lipomas, however, are found after the age of 40, with the peak incidence at 50 years (Burzynski et al., 1971; Yoshimura et al., 1972). The patient is usually aware of a slow-growing mass that may have been present from 1 month to 30 years before treatment is initiated (Hatziotis, 1971; Pisanty, 1976). There does not appear to be a racial distribution of these lesions, and the sexual distribution seems to be approximately equal. Burzynski and co-workers (1971) reported 55 in men and 41 in women; and Seldin and co-workers (1967) found 14 in women and 10 in men.

The review by Burzynski and co-workers (1971) indicated that the buccal mucosa and mucobuccal fold are the most common areas of occurrence of lipoma, followed by the tongue, floor of the mouth, and lip; lipomas in the palate, gingiva, and other oral locations are rare.

The lipoma usually occurs as a solitary lesion that may be sessile, pedunculated, or submerged. It ranges in size from a small lesion approximately 1 cm in diameter to a massive tumor 5.0 × 3.0 × 2.0 cm (Seldin et al., 1967). The lesion varies in contour and shape, ranging from a well-contoured, well-defined, round swelling to a large, ill-defined, lobulated mass. The color, which often is yellow, will depend on the thickness of the overlying mucosa. The surface is smooth and nonulcerated except when the tumor occurs in an area that causes it to be subjected to trauma.

On palpation the lesion is nontender, soft, almost cheesy in consistency; but it may be fluctuant. It is usually relatively superficial, but it may infiltrate muscle and become fixed to the surrounding tissue and therefore not be freely movable. The deeper-occurring lesions may produce only a slight surface elevation and may be well encapsulated, more diffuse, and less delineated than the superficial variety. This more diffuse form gives the clinical impression of fluctuance. Most of the lesions reported have been solitary, but multiple lesions have been described. There is no tooth involvement with these lesions.

Microscopically the lipoma is mature fat enclosed within a connective tissue capsule. There is a fibrous stroma dividing the fat into lobules, and these septa contain small blood vessels. Cartilage formation has been reported in a lipoma of the lip (McAndrew and Greenspan, 1976).

DIFFERENTIAL DIAGNOSIS

Differential diagnosis of this lesion must include an *epidermoid* or *dermoid cyst* and a *lymphoepithelial cyst.*

MANAGEMENT

If the lesion is not imposing an inconvenience on the patient, it may be ignored. Otherwise the treatment should be surgical excision, making certain to completely remove the tumor. There is a reported 20% recurrence.

LYMPHOEPITHELIAL CYST

The lymphoepithelial cyst is relatively uncommon in the oral cavity. It is apparently the result of cystic degeneration of epithelial inclusions in lymphoid aggregates about the oral cavity. In this respect it is not unlike a branchial cyst in the cervical area—which also results from cystic degeneration of epithelial inclusions. Knapp (1970) described this entity as a pseudocyst of oral tonsil tissue.

FEATURES

Lymphoepithelial cysts are asymptomatic and nontender, so the patient is frequently not aware of how long they have been present. Lesions reported by Acevedo and Nelson (1971) were present for 1 to 10 years before treatment. There is no related social or family history.

The studies by Acevedo and Nelson (1971) and Bhaskar (1966) showed that lymphoepithelial cysts occur predominantly in men; all of Acevedo and Nelson's cases were in men and Bhaskar reported a 2:1 incidence in men. The age range of the patients included in these two studies was 15 to 65 years, and the most common area of occurrence was the floor of the mouth.

Clinically the lesion is solitary and appears as a raised yellowish nodule with a smooth surface. It is usually small, with a diameter of only a few millimeters, but it may range in size up to 2 cm in diameter. It is fairly mobile, usually superficial, soft in consistency, variably fluctuant, and sharply delineated.

Since these lesions occur predominantly in the floor of the mouth, no teeth are involved.

On aspiration the cyst will produce an amorphous coagulum composed predominantly of keratin.

Microscopic examination illustrates that the nodule is a cyst lined with a thin stratified squamous epithelium containing nucleated partially keratinized cells and keratin. Circumscribed lymphoid follicles are embedded in the walls.

DIFFERENTIAL DIAGNOSIS

The differential diagnosis of this lesion should include *lymph node, mucocele, sialolith, dermoid cyst, neuroma, lipoma,* and *other benign tumors of the floor of the mouth.*

MANAGEMENT

Lymphoepithelial cysts are treated by conservative excision; recurrence is improbable.

EPIDERMOID AND DERMOID CYSTS

Epidermoid and dermoid cysts are developmental anomalies. They are basically cystic teratomas, resulting primarily from trapped germinal epithelium. They occur in all areas of the body but are rare in the oral cavity. The usual complaint of the patient with an oral epidermoid or dermoid cyst is that there is a swelling in the floor of his mouth.

FEATURES

The floor of the mouth is the most common area in the head and neck for the epidermoid or dermoid cyst to occur, followed by the submaxillary and submental areas. These cysts may lie above or below the mylohyoid muscle: if above, the tongue will be displaced superiorly; if below, the soft tissue in the submental region will be distended. The cysts may be in the midline or located laterally. Although they have been reported to occur at any time from birth to age 72 years, they usually become apparent between the ages of 15 and 35 (Meyer, 1955). They may be slow growing, as reported by Meyer, or of sudden onset.

Epidermoid and dermoid cysts are nontender and range in size from a relatively small lesion to a $10 \times 5 \times 5$ cm mass (Chakavorty and Schatzki, 1975; New and Erich, 1937). There is no pertinent medical or dental history that is unique to patients with these lesions and no recognizable familial pattern of occurrence or sexual predilection.

The cyst is usually not fixed to the surrounding tissue. Its color varies, depending on the position of the cyst and the thickness of the overlying tissue. If the cyst is relatively superficial, it is yellow to white; and its surface is smooth and nonulcerated unless traumatized.

The cyst varies in consistency from soft to firm; it may be fluctuant and frequently is rubbery or cheesy, depending on the elements within it.[*] The lesion is usually sharply delineated and aspiration produces a variety of materials other than the typical straw-colored cyst fluid.

Since this is usually a midline structure, the teeth are not involved unless some dental structures are included in the cyst.

---

[*]The cyst may contain (1) only typical cyst fluid or only keratin, (2) sebaceous material and keratin, or (3) in the case of a lesion that represents a complex teratoma, keratin, sebum, bone, muscle, and gastrointestinal tissue (Shafer et al., 1974, p. 380).

The histopathology of this entity ranges from a simple cyst, usually lined with stratified squamous epithelium and showing some keratinization, to a cyst composed of other germ layers and various types of epithelium:

1. The lumen of the simple cyst will be filled with cyst fluid or keratin and no other specialized structure; such a cyst would be defined as an *epidermoid cyst*.
2. On the other hand, the lumen may contain other elements, depending on the germinal potential of the originating epithelium; consequently, in the case of these more complex cysts, the lumen may be filled with sebum, hair, and even teeth.
   a. If the lumen contains sebaceous material as well as keratin, the lesion would be a *dermoid cyst*.
   b. If the lumen contains elements from various germinal layers such as bone, muscle, or teeth, the entity would be called a *teratoma*.

DIFFERENTIAL DIAGNOSIS

The differential diagnosis should include *ranula, thyroglossal duct cyst, cystic hygroma, branchial cleft cyst, cellulitis, tumors,* and *fat masses*.

MANAGEMENT

The treatment for epidermoid and dermoid cysts is surgical removal; the cyst usually does not recur.

PYOSTOMATITIS VEGETANS

The oral lesions of pyostomatitis vegetans are composed of large numbers of small closely set papillary projections with a broad base and usually on an intensely erythematous mucosa. Although the small projections are red to red-pink, they may show tiny yellow pustules beneath the epithelium. These lesions were first described by McCarthy (1949) as a rare inflammatory disease of the oral mucosa. The cause of the disease is unknown, but McCarthy and Shklar (1963) suggested that psychosomatic factors may be involved. The chief complaint is usually "eruptions in the mouth."

The lesions may be present for months before the patient seeks professional attention, and occasionally they may be found on routine examination. McCarthy and Shklar (1963) suggested that pyostomatitis vegetans is part of a syndrome that includes ulcerative colitis.

FEATURES

The lesions of pyostomatitis vegetans are painless, and there is little if any lymphadenitis. They occur in any area of the mouth and are usually multiple; however, few appear on the tongue. When the condition is present, the buccal and labial mucosal lesions have many folds and the papillary projections develop on these folds. The erythema surrounding the lesions on the buccal mucosa is generally not as intense as in the rest of the mouth.

The yellow vesicles that develop on the papillary projections resemble pustules and, if opened, discharge small amounts of purulent material.

No sexual predilection has been reported for this disease, and the patients whom McCarthy (1949) and McCarthy and Shklar (1963) described ranged in age from 15 to 47 years.

Histologically the involved mucosal tissue is characterized by a chronic inflammatory infiltration, with occasional localized accumulations of polymorphonuclear leukocytes. The lymphocytic infiltration is arranged in patterns of small abscesses or is spread diffusely throughout the tissue. Basophils are predominant in the early lesions.

Bacterial studies have not demonstrated consistent findings in pyostomatitis vegetans. Only microorganisms of the normal oral flora are isolated from the lesions, so the disease is not believed to be infectious.

DIFFERENTIAL DIAGNOSIS

A diagnosis is possible only if the following can be ruled out: *generalized papillomatosis* of the oral mucosa, the group of vesicular eruptions that includes *pemphigus vegetans, viral* and *fungal infections, systemic drug reactions,* and allergic reactions such as *erythema multiforme*.

MANAGEMENT

In most cases the lesions are completely resistant to any kind of therapy, including antibiotics. Those lesions that are concomitant with ulcerative colitis frequently improve when the colitis is controlled; and an exacerbation of the colitis is followed by a similar change in the oral lesions. Topical steroids have proved to be of some benefit for the oral lesions.

JAUNDICE OR ICTERUS

Jaundice or icterus is a condition that is recognized by the yellowish discoloration of the skin, mucous membranes, and sclerae of the eyes. The discoloration is produced by an increase in the blood level of bilirubin and the deposition of this bile pigment in the tissues. The jaundice appears when the serum concentration exceeds 2 to 3 mg/dl (Jeffries, 1971, p. 1389). The hyperbilirubinemia is caused by one of several mechanisms:

1. Excessive pigment production
2. Reduced hepatic uptake
3. Decreased transport, conjugation, and biliary excretion of bilirubin

Hemolysis is the most common cause of excessive production of bilirubin. It is a feature of a number of diseases such as thalassemia, sickle cell anemia (Chapter 22), pernicious anemia, polycythemia, and neonatal jaundice. There is a reduced conjugation of bilirubin in the liver in neonatal jaundice and in some other rare syndromes caused by the immaturity of the hepatoexcretory system.

Reduced uptake of bilirubin in the liver is usually the result of a defect in the transport of plasma bilirubin to the liver cells. Such a defect occurs in Gilbert's syndrome, acute viral hepatitis, and congestive heart failure and follows portacaval shunt surgery. Some drugs interfere with bilirubin uptake.

The reduced excretion of the conjugated bilirubin is found in cases of hepatocellular injuries such as in viral hepatitis or in inflammatory granulomatous or neoplastic infiltration of the liver, resulting in an obstruction of the biliary tree or bile ducts.

FEATURES

The physical manifestation of jaundice includes a yellow tinge of the eyes, skin, and oral mucous membranes. Icterus is frequently the first, and sometimes the only, manifestation of liver disease. The appearance of bilirubin in the urine, however, may precede for some time the development of clinical jaundice. The discoloration of the oral mucosa is most often seen first at the junction of the hard and soft palates. This may be due to the accentuation of the yellow color by the fat in this area.

Depending on the cause of the jaundice, there may be pruritus, pain, and an enlarged liver. The feces will be very light in color if there is partial, intermittent, or total biliary obstruction; and the urine will be darker.

DIFFERENTIAL DIAGNOSIS

Jaundice must be distinguished from the other causes of yellow pigmentation of the skin such as *carotenemia* and *quinacrine therapy*.

MANAGEMENT

A patient with icterus who is suspected of having liver disease and/or one of the hemolytic diseases should be referred to a physician for consultation and treatment.

LIPOID PROTEINOSIS

Lipoid proteinosis is a rare disease that severely affects the oral cavity, with the formation of characteristic yellowish-white papular plaques on the oral mucosa. The same type of plaques also develops on the skin. The disease is thought to be a disturbance of the mucopolysaccharide metabolism or an alteration in the formation of lipoprotein, and it is transmitted as an autosomal recessive trait (Gorlin, 1969).

The chief complaint with lipoid proteinosis is an inability to cry as a baby, a husky voice from birth on, and scarring maculopapular eruptions on the skin. Calcification of the hippocampal gyri may occur; and when it does it is pathognomonic of this disease (Bearn, 1971, p. 1703).

FEATURES

Lipoid proteinosis is present from birth, and lesions occur on the lips, oral mucosa, face, neck, hands, axillae, scrotum, perineal areas and intergluteal cleft, eyelids, knees, and elbows. Lesions also occur on the epiglottis, the aryepiglottic folds, and the interarytenoid region. The patient may have a recurrent painful parotitis.

The yellowish-white lesions are multiple and appear to occur in all races; no sexual predilection has been reported for this disease. The lesions are characteristically raised waxy nodules that are whitish to yellow and have smooth nonulcerated surfaces. They may be of varying size, from 2 mm to 0.5 cm in diameter, and they will be solid in consistency and firmly fixed to the underlying tissue. They increase in number and prominence from childhood into adult life. Congenital absence of teeth and enamel hypoplasia have been reported to accompany this disease. Hofer and Bergenholtz (1975) were unable to substantiate these associated tooth anomalies.

Histologically there is hyalinosis of the connective tissue of the upper layer of the corium in the plaques. Small blood vessels are affected much like those in diabetes mellitus. The hyalin material stains intensely with the periodic acid–Schiff stain.

DIFFERENTIAL DIAGNOSIS

The lesion may be mistaken for an unusual *scar formation,* but the nature of the plaques can be determined by a biopsy.

MANAGEMENT

The treatment for this disease is symptomatic. Corticosteroids have been employed, but there is no convincing evidence that they are effective.

CAROTENEMIA

Carotenemia is an extremely rare condition in which there is a generalized yellowness of the skin and mucosa. It is produced by an excessive deposition of carotenoid (lipochrome), which is the result of a high intake of foods containing carotene pigments (Blankenhorn, 1960; Jeghers, 1943; Josephs, 1944). There is usually no other systemic problem, but increased yellowness is seen in hyperlipemia, diabetes, nephritis, and hypothyroidism, and in conditions in which the conversion of carotene to vitamin A is impaired by an inborn metabolic error or by hepatic disease (Ebling and Rook, 1968, p. 1111).

FEATURES

Carotenemia is a generalized yellowness of the skin and mucous membrane. There is no unusual statistical relationship between the occurrence of this phenomenon and the sex or age of the individual. The history usually discloses that the patient has an extremely high intake of food containing relatively large amounts of carotene (e.g., carrot juice, oranges, halibut, liver oil).

DIFFERENTIAL DIAGNOSIS

The differential diagnosis must include *jaundice,* which can be ruled out by clinical laboratory tests showing a high serum level of the carotenoid pigments. (If equal parts of serum, alcohol, and petroleum ether are shaken together, the carotenoids will be absorbed by the ether.) Also most of the laboratory tests that give elevated values in jaundice are within the normal limits in carotenemia. In addition, since the carotenoids have a great affinity for fat and bilirubin has a great affinity for elastic tissue, there is an early involvement of the sclera in jaundice whereas the eye is not discolored in carotenemia.

MANAGEMENT

The treatment involves restricting the dietary intake of food containing carotenoids.

SPECIFIC REFERENCES

Acevedo, A. E., and Nelson, J. F.: Lymphoepithelial cysts of the oral cavity: report of nine cases, Oral Surg. **31:**632-636, 1971.

Bearn, A. G.: Lipoid proteinosis. In Beeson, P. B., and McDermott, W., editors: Cecil-Loeb textbook of medicine, ed. 13, Philadelphia, 1971, W. B. Saunders Co.

Bhaskar, S. N.: Lymphoepithelial cysts of the oral cavity: report of twenty-four cases, Oral Surg. **21:**120-126, 1966.

Blankenhorn, D. H.: The infiltration of carotenoids into human atheromas and xanthomas, Ann. Intern. Med. **53:**944-954, 1960.

Burzynski, N. J., Sigman, M. D., and Martin, T. H.: Lipoma of the oral cavity: literature review and case report, J. Oral Med. **26:**37-39, 1971.

Chakravorty, R. C., and Schatzki, P. F.: Lateral sublingual dermoid, Oral Surg. **39:**862-866, 1975.

Ebling, F. J., and Rook, A.: Disorders of skin color. In Rook, A., Wilkinson, D. S., and Ebling, F. J., editors: Textbook of dermatology, Philadelphia, 1968, F. A. Davis Co.

Gorlin, R. J.: Genetic disorders affecting mucous membrane, Oral Surg. **28:**512-525, 1969.

Halprin, B., Kolas, S., Jefferis, K. R., et al.: The occurrence of Fordyce spots, benign migratory glossitis, median rhomboid glossitis and fissured tongue in 2,487 dental patients, Oral Surg. **6:**1072-1077, 1953.

Hatziotis, J. C. H.: Lipoma of the oral cavity, Oral Surg. **31:** 511-524, 1971.

Hofer, P., and Bergenholtz, A.: Oral manifestations in Urbach-Wiethe disease (lipoglycoproteinosis; lipoidproteinosis; hyalinosis cutis et mucosae), Odont. Revy **26:**39-58, 1975.

Jeffries, G. H.: Diseases of the liver. In Beeson, P. B., and McDermott, W., editors: Cecil-Loeb textbook of medicine, ed. 13, Philadelphia, 1971, W. B. Saunders Co.

Jeghers, H.: Medical progress; skin changes of nutritional origin, N. Engl. J. Med. **228:**678-686, 1943.

Josephs, H. W.: Hypervitaminosis A and carotenemia, Am. J. Dis. Child. **67:**33-43, 1944.

Knapp, M. J.: Pathology of oral tonsils, Oral Surg. **29:**295-304, 1970.

McAndrew, P. G., and Greenspan, J. S.: Lipoma of the lip with cartilage formation, Br. Dent. J. **140:**239-240, 1976.

McCarthy, F. P.: Pyostomatitis vegetans: report of 3 cases, Arch. Dermatol. Syph. **60:**750-764, 1949.

McCarthy, P., and Shklar, G. A.: A syndrome of pyostomatitis vegetans and ulcerative colitis, Arch. Dermatol. **88:**913-919, 1963.

Meyer, I.: Dermoid cysts (dermoids) of the floor of the mouth, Oral Surg. **8:**1149-1164, 1955.

Miles, A. E. W.: Sebaceous glands in the lip and cheek mucosa of man, Br. Dent. J. **105:**235-248, 1958.

New, E. B., and Erich, J. B.: Dermoid cysts of the head and neck, Surg. Gynecol. Obstet. **65:**48-55, 1937.

Pisanty, S.: Bilateral lipomas of the tongue, Oral Surg. **42:**451-453, 1976.

Seldin, H. M., Seldin, S. D., Rakower, W., and Jarrett, W. J.: Lipoma of the oral cavity: report of 26 cases, J. Oral Surg. **25:**270-274, 1967.

Shafer, W. G., Hine, M. K., and Levy, B. M.: A textbook of oral pathology, ed. 3, Philadelphia, 1974, W. B. Saunders Co.

Steigman, A. J., Lipton, M. M., and Braspennickx, H.: Acute lymphonodular pharyngitis: a newly described condition due to Coxsackie A virus, J. Pediatr. **61:**331-336, 1963.

Yoshimura, Y., Miyagi, K., Shoju, M., et al.: Lipoma in the infant and child: report of cases, J. Oral Surg. **30:**690-693, 1972.

GENERAL REFERENCES

Brooke, R. I.: Traumatic herniation of buccal pad of fat (traumatic pseudolipoma), Oral Surg. **45:**689-691, 1978.

Messenger, K. L., and Cloyd, W.: Traumatic herniation of the buccal fat pad: report of case, Oral Surg. **43:**41-43, 1977.

Vindenes, H.: Lipomas of the oral cavity, Int. J. Oral Surg. **7:**162-166, 1978.

14

Masses in the neck

Raymond L. Warpeha

The more common masses occurring in the neck are listed below and are ranked in approximate order of frequency.

Anatomic structures
Benign lymphoid hyperplasia
Acute lymphadenitis
Fibrosed lymph nodes
Sebaceous cysts
Space abscesses
Salivary gland inflammations
Lipomas
Salivary gland tumors
Thyroid gland enlargements
Benign systemic lymph node enlargements (infectious mononucleosis and viral diseases)
Epidermoid and dermoid cysts
Metastatic tumors
Thyroglossal cysts
Cystic hygromas
Lymphomas
Branchial cysts
Rarities
    Actinomycosis
    Cat-scratch disease
    Laryngocele
    Ludwig's angina
    Primary tumors of mesenchymal tissue
    Sarcoidosis
    Subcutaneous emphysema
    Tuberculosis

In other chapters lesions are discussed sequentially, in the same order as they are listed. In this chapter, however, it was considered more useful to group the neck lesions according to the regions where they predominantly occur. Thus the discussion of pathologic masses of the neck will be divided into the following segments:

1. Masses of nonspecific location
2. Masses in the submandibular region
3. Masses in the parotid region
4. Masses in the median-paramedian region
5. Masses in the lateral neck region

The identification of a particular mass in the neck involves a reasoning process that combines the information obtained from the medical history and the physical examination of the mass and then evaluates it in relation to the normal structures and their positions in the neck. In addition, further information from laboratory and radiographic studies may be required. After the foregoing information is analyzed, a clinical diagnosis or a group of likely diagnoses *(differential diagnosis)* can be formulated. Although a clinical diagnosis might suffice in some instances, a definitive (microscopic) diagnosis is frequently required for proper treatment. For this determination, tissue for microscopy or material for culture is necessary. The obtaining of tissue or tissue products for study may involve certain additional insult and when done ineptly may compromise therapy or perhaps even hinder the cure of a malignant neoplasm. For these reasons, then, the most definitive step in diagnosis—microscopic study—may be reserved for final consideration.

PHYSICAL EXAMINATION AND ANATOMY OF THE NECK

Physical examination of a region involves inspection, palpation, percussion, and auscultation. Palpation plays the major role in the examination of neck masses. Although auscultation of bruits within blood vessels is a necessary part of a complete neck examination, auscultation and percussion are seldom the focal measures in evaluating neck masses.

So that one may detect subtle changes in the contour of the neck, he must know the normal topography of this region. Good lighting and total exposure of the neck with the shoulders bared

Fig. 14-1. A, Submandibular region. **B,** Parotid region. **C,** Median-paramedian region. **D,** Lateral region. See text for the description of the boundaries of each region.

are necessary for proper visualization. Most visible neck masses cause asymmetries that rapidly focus the examiner's attention to such masses.

Certain normal skeletal and soft tissue structures of the neck are readily identified by palpation. Familiarity with the usual size, contour, consistency, and mobility of these structures is necessary both to readily identify them and to distinguish the normal from the pathologically palpable masses.

Skin and subcutaneous tissues within the neck

The investing cervical fascia is attached to the readily palpable lower border of the mandible, mastoid process, hyoid bone, and clavicles. It forms a heavy membrane over the deep structures of the neck, placing a screen between these

structures and the examiner's fingers. The mobile skin and subcutaneous tissues are superficial to the investing fascia. Thus masses arising within this layer exhibit the mobility of the layer unless fibrosis or a malignancy has secondarily fixed the layer to deeper structures.

Specific regions of the neck and their palpable anatomic structures

SUBMANDIBULAR REGION

The boundaries of the submandibular region are easily recognized, with the lower border of the mandible from its angle to the canine region forming the superior margin and the bellies of the digastric muscle constituting the anterior and posterior limits of the inferior border of the region (Fig. 14-1, *A*). These muscular bellies are palpable only when they are stiffened by func-

Fig. 14-2. Major cervical lymph node areas. *1,* Submental; *2,* submandibular; *3,* subparotid; *4,* subdigastric; *5,* bifurcation; *6,* jugulo-omohyoid.

tion. Therefore the examiner is able to define the limits of this region by asking the patient to open his jaw against resistance (the examiner holding the jaw shut) while the examiner palpates the rising ridges of the digastric muscle.

The submandibular gland lies within this region on the extremely mobile mylohyoid muscle, which forms a hammock between the hyoid and the inner aspect of the mandibular body. Although most of the gland lies superficial to the mylohyoid muscle and consequently occurs in the neck, a small part insinuates itself around the free posterior border of the muscle and therefore lies in the posterior floor of the mouth.

If the examiner merely palpates the gland externally, only a vague impression of its dome is appreciated. If, however, the patient is asked to push with his tongue against his anterior teeth, greater definition of the gland's circumference can be attained because the tightening of the floor of the mouth (mylohyoid muscle) creates a rigid base for palpation.

Bimanual palpation offers the greatest opportunity to feel the entire structure and is a mandatory step in any physical examination. This is accomplished by the examiner inserting two or three fingers into the patient's mouth to support the distensible mylohyoid muscle while palpating the submandibular gland externally with the fingers of the opposing hand (Chapter 3).

The submandibular gland does not occupy the entire submandibular region. Numerous lymph nodes are also found within the areolar tissue of this region but are not ordinarily palpable (Fig. 14-2).

PAROTID REGION

The parotid gland fills the parotid region (Fig. 14-1, *B*). This is the area bounded anteriorly by the posterior border of the ascending mandibular ramus and posteriorly by the external auditory canal, mastoid process, and upper portion of the sternocleidomastoid muscle. The gland overlaps the mandibular ramus and masseter muscle for a short distance beyond their posterior borders. Also the inferior tip of the gland extends 1 to 2 cm below the projected line of the inferior border of the mandible (Fig. 14-1, *B*).

Palpation of the parotid gland is more difficult to carry out than of the submandibular gland because the firm adherent investing fascia normally prevents the precise identification of the normal gland's margins. In addition, bimanual examination is difficult to perform because of the presence of the interposed pharyngeal structures and ramus and because of the gag reflex. In some cases, however, bimanual palpation of the parotid region is mandatory to establish certain clinical findings and may be accomplished by resorting to either topical or general anesthesia.

Lymph nodes are found within and superficial to this gland in the subcutaneous tissues of the preauricular area and at the lower pole of the gland (Fig. 14-2). Consequently pathoses of these structures must also be considered in the differential diagnosis of any mass in the parotid region.

MEDIAN-PARAMEDIAN REGION

This area is bounded superiorly by the lower border of the mandible and laterally by the attachments of the anterior bellies of the digastric muscles. The posterior boundary is delineated by the posterior extremities of the hyoid bone and the thyroid and cricoid cartilages. The medial parts of the clavicles and superior margin of the manubrium form the inferior boundaries of the region (Fig. 14-1, *C*).

The most important structure in the median-paramedian region is the butterfly-shaped thyroid gland, which has two lateral lobes connected by a narrow isthmus that crosses the trachea at a variable distance below the palpable ridge produced by the cricoid cartilage. Like the submandibular and parotid glands the thyroid gland lies deep to the investing cervical fascia, and its features are partially masked from palpation. Its lateral lobes, forming the greater part of the thyroid mass, are further concealed by the overlying infrahyoid strap muscles and the bulky sternocleidomastoid muscle. Thus the normal thyroid gland is not palpable in the usual sense but rather is recognized by a feeling of fullness to the touch. The left lobe frequently imparts a greater fullness because this lobe is regularly larger than the right.

Masses within or an enlargement of the lateral lobes of the thyroid gland are best appreciated by manipulation of the overlying sternocleidomastoid muscle. While one hand stabilizes the gland by insinuating the fingers behind the posterior border of that muscle, the palpating fingers of the opposite hand characterize the lateral lobe. The isthmus is palpated near the midline below the prominent ringlike cricoid cartilage and is best felt during a swallowing motion since the gland is attached to the trachea and moves upward with this structure during deglutition. Verification that a mass is in a lateral lobe is likewise accomplished by palpating it while the patient swallows. In such a case the intrinsically attached mass will likewise move with the thyroid gland.

The palpable hyoid bone and thyroid cartilages are also present within the median-paramedian region. The mobility of these structures requires bimanual fixation similar to that used in examining the submandibular and thyroid glands. The greater cornu of the hyoid bone and superior cornu of the thyroid cartilage are occasionally mistaken for stony-hard lymph nodes in the upper cervical chain, which would clinically imply malignant metastasis. The two cornua are normal structures anterior to the cervical node chain, however, and their morphology is identified by their presence bilaterally and their upward displacement during swallowing.

In the median-paramedian region, lymph nodes are found above the hyoid bone in the submental area and in front of the cricothyroid membrane. Normally these nodes are not palpable, and consideration of such masses in the neck will be dealt with in the ensuing discussion.

LATERAL REGION

The lateral neck region is that portion of the neck remaining after the preceding regions have been defined. It is the area posterior to the hyolaryngotracheal conduit, below the posterior belly of the digastric muscle and tip of the parotid gland, and extends down to the clavicle (Fig. 14-1, *D*). It is crossed obliquely by the sternocleidomastoid muscle, which obliterates the detail of the central structures in this region.

The contents of this region include the large vessels and nerves of the neck just anterior to the bodies and transverse processes of the cervical vertebrae. The transverse processes of the first and seventh cervical vertebrae are vaguely palpable as immovable hard masses below the tip of the mastoid and in the supraclavicular area, respectively. They become more apparent in the thin and emaciated patient and are prominent in the postsurgical patient after radical neck dissection with removal of the sternocleidomastoid muscle and soft tissues of the lateral neck region.

The carotid pulse can be felt on the prominent bulge marking the carotid bifurcation. This structure lies below the posterior belly of the digastric muscle, level with the angle of the mandible, and is frequently mistaken for a pathologic mass by the unwary examiner. Just as the greater cornu of the hyoid bone, superior cornu of the thyroid cartilage, or transverse processes of either the first or the seventh cervical vertebra may be mistaken for disease, so in the elderly patient, calcification within the arterial wall at the carotid bifurcation may be misinterpreted as a hard node of metastatic cancer. Careful manipulation of the artery, however, and determination of whether the carotid pulse can be detected through the hard mass will identify the mass as part or not part of the artery.

A vertical groove can be felt in the middle third of the neck immediately behind the sternocleidomastoid muscle between the anterior and middle scalene muscles in all patients but the very obese. It contains the cervical and brachial plexus nerve roots after they exit the intervertebral foramina. Although the individual nerve roots cannot be detected by touch, pathologic masses associated with these structures would be found along this line. An example would be the amputation neuromas that sometimes form on the nerve stumps after a radical neck dissection.

The lateral neck region carries the greatest number of lymph nodes found in the neck (Fig. 14-2). This area is also the most common site of lymph node metastases from head and neck cancer because the lymph from several of the common primary cancer sites drains first to nodes in this area. As in other regions, normal lymph nodes of the lateral neck region are not plapable. The distribution and drainage areas of the nodes in this and other regions of the neck are described next.

Lymph nodes of the neck

A capillary plexus of endothelial tubes is found below the epidermis and oral mucosa of the head and neck. It collects the fluid from the interstitial spaces for return to the large venous trunks at the base of the neck. Between a given capillary plexus and the veins are increasingly larger channels, the lymphatics, with one or more lymph nodes in their course. Within each of these lymph nodes, the lymph fluid must again pass capillary-sized channels before proceeding through to the efferent lymphatic channel.

The first lymph node encountered in a channel draining a particular submucosal or subepidermal lymph capillary plexus is called the "first-echelon node," because it is here that pathogenic organisms or free tumor cells within the lymph fluid meet their first resistance to travel.

The first-echelon nodes are also found in the preauricular (superficial to the parotid gland and investing fascia), postauricular, and suboccipital areas. With the submental and submandibular nodes they form a collar about the face and scalp, filtering the drainage from the subepidermal lymph plexuses of the skin in this region.

GENERAL CHARACTERISTICS OF PATHOLOGIC MASSES

Before the discussion of specific masses by region begins, it is appropriate to review some of the characteristics of abnormal masses since the presence or absence of certain features often directs the clinician to the correct disease or group of diseases. These characteristics are common to abnormal masses no matter where the masses are found in the body.

Degree of tenderness

Tenderness usually indicates inflammation or infection or both within the tissues affected. Benign or malignant tumors and cysts are usually nontender. Painful tumors are usually the result of frank invasion of a nerve, but pain may also reflect rapid growth and simple compression of sensory nerves. In other cases a secondary inflammatory process or abscess or both within a tumor or cyst may be the cause of tenderness.

Consistency

Solid masses impart a feeling of firmness, whereas cysts and abscesses are soft to rubbery. Fluctuation may be masked by a surrounding zone of inflammation or fibrous tissue, or a fluid-filled mass may be situated so deep in the tissues that fluctuance is not demonstrable. Although other signs of the inflammatory process are generally present, whether an abscess is fluctuant or not will depend on its stage of development.

In the early stage before a pool of pus forms,

Fig. 14-3. Large lymphoma. This child had a rapidly growing rubbery mass. (Courtesy O. H. Stuteville, D.D.S., M.D., St. Joe, Ark.)

the swelling is due to inflammation only; so the mass is not fluctuant but is firm in consistency. Later, if a pool of pus does form, the swelling becomes fluctuant. Still later, in the regressing stage, the fluctuance disappears as the pus is eliminated.

Malignant tumors and their metastases to lymph nodes are frequently described as stony hard, although lymph nodes involved by lymphoma have a distinctly rubbery feeling (Fig. 14-3). Tuberculosis characteristically produces a caseation necrosis of several nodes, resulting in a matted type of mass.

Degree of mobility

Each structure of the neck has its own range of motion when manipulated. A decrease in mobility may be associated with fixation of the structure to less mobile ones.

Lymph nodes are ordinarily freely movable but become fixed in certain pathologic conditions. Usually fixation of a node is the result of an inflammatory process that has penetrated the node's capsule and caused fibrosis to the surrounding immovable structures. Less frequently, in cases of metastatic spread, the malignant cells may penetrate the capsule and invade the surrounding tissue.

PATHOLOGIC MASSES

Aside from masses originating in the skin, the majority of neck masses may be categorized into the following general types: (1) enlarged lymph nodes, (2) enlarged submandibular, parotid, and thyroid glands or masses within these glands, (3) congenital cysts of specific origin and location, and (4) derivatives of vessels and nerves in the lateral neck region. Other distinctive masses in the neck not falling into this classification will be discussed with those occurring in specific regions of the neck.

Masses of nonspecific location

Commonly occurring masses, although not specific to the neck region (e.g., the lipoma), will not be classified or discussed. Also it is obvious that some masses are not peculiar to certain regions of the neck but may occur anywhere in the neck; these most frequently originate in the skin or lymph nodes and will be referred to as masses of nonspecific location.

ENLARGED LYMPH NODES

Enlarged lymph nodes are by far the most common pathologic masses found in the neck. The majority of the enlarged cervical lymph nodes are the result of an acute or chronic response to an infectious organism (lymphadenitis), the growth of a metastatic tumor, or a primary malignant neoplasm (lymphoma). These three main groups of lymph node pathosis are listed according to frequency of occurrence, with the most common group noted first.

A lymphadenitis is by definition an inflammation and/or infection of a lymph node and frequently occurs when there is an infection in the tissues that are drained by the particular node's pathway. Pathoses of this type may be divided into acute or chronic, solitary or multiple, local or disseminated, and specific or nonspecific.

As with the same process in other organs and tissues, the sequelae of a lymphadenitis will depend on the modifying factors. If the adenitis is short lived, the node may subsequently return to practically normal size and architecture. If, on the other hand, the infection is acute, the node may become painful, necrotic, and liquefied and may lead to a space abscess.

In more chronic cases a permanent hyperplasia of the lymph node may result, and such a pathosis is referred to as a benign lymphoid hyperplasia. In some instances of chronic lymphadenitis, scarring replaces the node architecture and the enlarged node remains as a permanently fibrosed mass. Clinically, then, there are two distinct types of benign node enlargement: (1) nontender and (2) tender or painful.

Fig. 14-4. Benign lymphoid hyperplasia. This unusually large example in the submental region was firm, nontender, and freely movable. (Courtesy S. Svalina, D.D.S., Maywood, Ill.)

Nontender lymphoid hyperplasia. The majority of nontender benign enlargements of the cervical lymph nodes are nontender lymphoid hyperplasias (Fig. 14-4). At least one or two such enlarged nodes are found in the routine palpation of the neck of almost every patient examined. Nontender lymphoid hyperplasias represent either a persistent chronic lymphadenitis or a permanently enlarged node after an acute or chronic lymphadenitis.

Features. The patient is usually unaware of the enlarged node, but in some cases he may recount the presence of a previous painful swelling in the region and perhaps identify the primary infection site. The nodes are solitary, discrete, asymptomatic, and usually freely movable. The submandibular, submental, and subdigastric groups are the nodes most frequently affected (Fig. 14-4).

Differential diagnosis. The nontender lymphoid hyperplasia is by far the most common pathologic mass to occur in the neck.

The fact that this benign enlargement is painless differentiates it from the less frequently encountered *acute lymphadenitis.*

As a general rule it can be differentiated from *secondary carcinoma* by the fact that the carcinoma is bony hard and often fixed whereas the hyperplasia is firm and usually freely movable. A complete head and neck examination and evaluation are necessary, however, before benign lymphoid hyperplasia can be affected as the final diagnosis because occasionally a metastatic tumor in an enlarged lymph node will manifest a softer consistency.

Management. If there is any doubt in the clinician's mind concerning the diagnosis, the patient should be reexamined at 2-week intervals to see whether there are perceptible changes in the mass. If the mass continues to be asymptomatic and does not enlarge, it is almost certainly a nontender node of lymphoid hyperplasia. If doubt still exists, removal of the node with subsequent microscopic study is advised.

Acute lymphadenitis. This is the second most common pathologic cervical mass and the most common painful enlargement found in the neck. The primary infection may be in the oral cavity, the nasal cavities, the tonsils, or the pharynx. Frequently minor mucosal erosions or shallow ulcers permit the entrance of sufficient bacteria to produce a regional lymphadenitis. Depending on the location of the tooth (Fig. 14-5), a periapical abscess, periodontal abscess, or pericoronitis-type infection may cause painful swollen nodes in the submental, submandibular, or subdigastric area (Fig. 14-13, C). With tonsillar inflammation the subdigastric node is most commonly involved and has thus become known as the "tonsillar node." Rapid regression of the inflammation may result in the node's returning to normal, being nonpalpable. In more chronic cases the node will become fibrosed or persist as an asymptomatic lymphoid hyperplasia. In either circumstance the node is enlarged, firm, and usually freely movable.

Features. Acute lymphadenitis will be tender or quite painful to palpation. Single affected nodes will be round, firm, and discrete and may be either movable or fixed. Several nodes in one region may be involved, and in such cases an accompanying inflammation in the adjacent soft tissues will cause a firm swelling that will prevent palpation of the individual nodes (Fig. 14-13, C). Microscopically the node will be enlarged and have more numerous germinal centers; and acute inflammatory cells will be present. Such a condition is termed a "nonspecific adenitis." The architecture of nodes affected by a severe inflammation may be almost obliterated by the inflammatory process, even to the point of necrosis and liquefaction.

Differential diagnosis. Acute lymphadenitis must be differentiated from infected cysts and Ludwig's angina.

Ludwig's angina is usually a nonpurulent hemolytic streptococcal infection of the floor of the mouth and submental and submandibular areas. The classic location of this entity, along with the serosanguineous fluid obtained on incision, is almost pathognomonic.

Infected cysts of the neck, except for the sebaceous type, which is very superficial, may be suspected in certain locations; in other words, branchial and thyroglossal cysts characteristically occur in the lateral neck and midline regions, respectively.

Management. In most cases, when the primary mucosal infection is eliminated, the secondary acute lymphadenitis soon regresses. Adequate doses of antibiotics administered for at least 5 days are usually employed. Cases of generalized

Fig. 14-5. Lymphatic drainage areas of the oral cavity (exclusive of the tongue) and pharynx showing first-echelon lymph nodes for various regions.

lymphadenitis in which lymph nodes are uniformly and symmetrically enlarged in all accessible areas, such as the axillae, groin, and neck, are not rare; and such a condition usually suggests a viremia. Thus in cases of multiple and bilateral nodes in the neck, a careful examination of other nodal areas and the spleen as well as a complete history and physical examination is necessary to determine whether the enlarged neck nodes are a manifestation of a local or a systemic disease.

Rare varieties of specific lymphadenitis. The majority of cases of cervical lymphadenitis result from primary infections by garden-variety bacteria or viruses. Microscopically there is nothing characteristic that relates to these "common" organisms since only a nonspecific adenitis is seen. Specific diagnostic changes may occur in some rare diseases, however, and the situation is then referred to as a specific adenitis (Robbins, 1967, p. 665).

The specific lesions within lymph nodes generated by tuberculosis, histoplasmosis, sarcoidosis, and infectious mononucleosis are similar to the lesions in other tissues infected by these specific organisms. Except for infectious mononucleosis, these are relatively uncommon in the neck; but the examiner must realize that occasionally pathologic lymph nodes that might initially appear to be of the nonspecific variety (Fig. 14-6) prove on biopsy to be caused by one of the specific infections.

Metastatic carcinoma to cervical nodes. The cervical lymph nodes are more frequently the

Fig. 14-6. Tuberculous adenitis. The nodular enlargement in the parotid region was tender and moderately soft to palpation. The patient also had pulmonary tuberculosis. (Courtesy O. H. Stuteville, D.D.S., M.D., St. Joe, Ark.)

site of metastatic carcinomas than of primary tumors (lymphomas). The majority of these secondary tumors are the result of metastatic spread from primary tumors in the head and neck, especially those in the oral and pharyngeal cavities. In unusual cases, however, they may represent secondary tumors from primary sites below the clavicles.

In addition to the common sites of origin of squamous cell carcinoma of the mouth and oropharynx, other mucosal surfaces, particularly of the larynx and vocal cords, develop tumors that metastasize to regional nodes. The first-echelon nodes for metastatic tumors occurring inferior to the oropharynx are located roughly opposite the primary tumor site in the jugular chain.

Since squamous cell carcinoma constitutes the preponderance of primary malignancies of the head and neck (95% of all oral malignancies are squamous cell carcinomas), it is by far the most common tumor spreading to the cervical nodes (Fig. 14-9, C). Adenocarcinoma of the salivary glands, occasionally squamous cell carcinoma from the skin, and melanoma are the next most common tumors that metastasize to the cervical nodes. Sarcoma characteristically spreads by the blood channels but on a rare occasion will involve a lymph node.

The lymphatic trunks draining the upper extremities and the rest of the body below the clavicles converge in the base of the lateral neck region, the supraclavicular area. Hence solitary metastatic nodes in this area are mostly from primary tumors located in areas other than the head and neck. The breasts, lungs, and stomach are common sites for such primary tumors. A complete history, physical examination, and specific laboratory studies will usually reveal the primary tumor.

Features. Metastatic tumors in lymph nodes are almost always painless and thus are not detected by the patient until they reach considerable dimensions. The smaller nodes are usually detected on routine examination; they characteristically feel stony hard and are freely movable until the tumor cells penetrate the node capsule and invade the surrounding tissue. Then they become fixed, and the expanding tumor may amalgamate surrounding nodes into one larger stony-hard fixed mass. In the majority of cases, the primary tumor is readily evident, especially if the primary site is in the oral cavity. Small tumors in the nasal cavities, nasopharynx, and larynx, however, may go undetected—the only evidence of their presence being the metastatic tumor. The submandibular and subdigastric nodes are the most frequent sites of early metastatic spread from primary tumors within the oral cavity.

Differential diagnosis. The differential diagnosis of metastatic lymph node tumors will be considered later with the discussion of pathologic masses occurring in specific regions.

Small metastatic nodes may be confused with *fibrosed nodes* or nodes that have undergone *nontender lymphoid hyperplasia,* however, because these entities are quite firm and may even be fixed to the surrounding tissue by fibrosis resulting from a previous infection; but in such cases the history relating to a severe infection in the region would probably direct the clinician to the likely diagnosis of benign lymphoid hyperplasia.

It is also necessary to differentiate between a secondary tumor and a *lymphoma;* but the fact that a metastatic tumor is usually stony hard, whereas the lymphoma is more rubbery, is helpful in making this differentiation.

Management. Various combinations of resection, radiation, and chemotherapy are used, with inconsistent results; however, the prognosis for a patient with lymph node metastasis is grave.

Lymphoma. Lymphoma is a neoplastic proliferation within the reticuloendothelial system that occurs as a primary tumor of lymph nodes but is not as common as a metastatic tumor (Batsakis, 1974, p. 346). There are several types of lymphoma, which vary in behavior.

At one time lymphomas were classified as giant follicle lymphoma, reticulum cell sarcoma, lymphosarcoma, and Hodgkin's disease. More recently, disagreement resulting from intensive study, however, has resulted in the development of a more complicated classification, which more accurately reflects the behavior of the specific tumor; but a detailed discussion of this newer classification is beyond the scope of the text.

Lymphomas may be solitary or multiple. Although it is generally accepted that they reflect a systemic disease, about 10% of the time the initial finding is a mass in the neck (Rosenberg et al., 1961).

Features. The nodes involved may be solitary or multiple and unilateral or bilateral; they are usually rubbery in consistency and may be a single discrete mass or several nodes joined together (Fig. 14-3). In advanced cases the patient may be quite ill with fever; and the total and differential leukocyte counts may be markedly changed, indicating that the increased production of mononuclear cells has spilled over into the blood. Other node groups such as the axillae, groin, and mediastinum are frequently involved in these advanced cases.

Differential diagnosis. Advanced and disseminated lymphomas (Hodgkin's disease) are readily differentiated from other tumors on a clinical basis.

For a discussion of the clinical differentiation between a *metastatic carcinoma* and a *lymphoma,* the reader is referred to the differential diagnosis section of metastatic carcinoma to cervical nodes in the preceding column.

Multiple and disseminated nodal involvement may also occur with certain *viral diseases* and in *mononucleosis.* In these diseases, however, the nodes are tender and painful; and a Paul-Bunnell heterophil test is positive in infectious mononucleosis.

Management. Radiation and various chemotoxic drugs as well as steroids are used, with varying results, to treat patients who have malignant lymphoma. Solitary nodes are amenable to surgical excision.

SEBACEOUS CYSTS

Sebaceous cysts occur in hair-bearing areas and are found in the neck with some regularity. They are superficial, dome-shaped masses and are usually detectable on visual examination (Figs. 14-9, *B,* 14-10, *A,* 14-12, *C,* and 14-13, *B*).

Features. Sebaceous cysts grow slowly and are painless unless secondarily infected. They range from a few millimeters to a few centimeters in diameter. The smaller cysts may have a dimple or enlarged pore on the surface. If situated in the anterior two thirds of the neck, they will be movable over the deeper structures because considerable mobility is imparted to masses arising within the dermis in this area. The skin of the posterior neck region is more adherent to the underlying fascia, however, and cysts arising in the posterior third of the neck may appear to be fixed to the underlying structures.

Aspiration of a thick material from such a mass is indicative of this type of cyst. Secondary infection is quite common and produces pain, induration, and fixation. Recurrent episodes of infection with periodic painful enlargement of the cyst and purulent drainage are a common sequence of events.

Differential diagnosis. The sebaceous cyst may be differentiated from the *epidermoid* and *dermoid cysts* by the fact that most often it is superficially located in the skin. Thus it usually cannot be moved independently of skin over the deeper structures. On the other hand, the epidermoid cysts are deeper and freely movable unless involved with inflammation and resultant fibrosis.

Although numerous *solid benign* and *malignant tumors* of a primary and occasionally metastatic nature occur in the skin, their firm consistency would differentiate them from a sebaceous cyst.

Management. Because of the simplicity of removal and the tendency toward secondary infection, excisional biopsy is recommended. This will also correctly identify the occasional skin tumor that could be clinically mistaken for a cyst. Suitable antibiotics should be administered if the sebaceous cyst is infected.

• • •

The majority of pathologic masses in the neck occur in four specific regions: submandibular, parotid, median-paramedian, and lateral. Thus the masses will be discussed according to the region in which they occur.

Masses in the submandibular region

The majority of all masses in the submandibular region originate in the lymph nodes or the submandibular salivary gland. The first step in diagnosis is to distinguish between submandibular gland and nonsubmandibular gland tissues by careful bimanual, intraoral, and extraoral palpation.

MASSES SEPARATE FROM THE SUBMANDIBULAR GLAND

A mass may be assumed to be an enlarged lymph node if it is determined not to be the sub-mandibular salivary gland. In such a case all possible sites in the mouth (Figs. 14-5 and 14-7), on the face, and in the nasal vestibule should be carefully examined to detect a source of infection or a primary tumor.

Tender nodes. If the node is tender, whether the constitutional signs of infection such as fever are present or not, and an obvious source of infection such as an abscessed tooth is found, the working diagnosis of lymphadenitis should be made. Such a case is managed by treating the patient with antibiotics or tooth extraction or both. If no primary site of infection can be found, an antibiotic effective against staphylococcal and streptococcal infections should be administered and the patient frequently reexamined to determine whether changes in size and tenderness of the mass have occurred.

If the tender mass subsides, it is assumed to have been an acute nonspecific nonsuppurative lymphadenitis. The specific adenitis of tuberculosis will appear, in rare cases, as a tender mass in children. Such a mass will not respond to ordinary antibiotic treatment; and a general workup, including skin test and chest radiograph, that is positive for tuberculosis should alert the clinician to the possibility of tubercular adenitis. An excisional biopsy would establish the diagnosis if the process is tuberculosis.

If the tender mass expands with or without softening and this change is accompanied by some reduction in pain and tenderness, the mass is assumed to be an abscess forming; incision and drainage are then indicated. In the adult it is wise to do a biopsy of the abscess wall during the drainage procedure if a primary infection is not

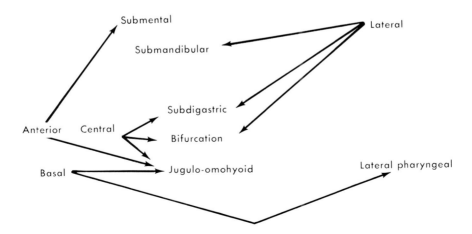

Fig. 14-7. Lymphatic drainage areas of the tongue showing first-echelon lymph nodes.

found or if the usual signs of inflammation are minimal. Such a precaution is necessary because lymph node metastases from occult carcinomas may undergo necrosis and abscess formation.

A staphylococcal node abscess may be manifested in a fussy neonate or young child as a hard submandibular (or submental or suboccipital) swelling (Fig. 14-8, A). A primary infection in the mouth or in the skin might not be obvious because the hardness of the swelling and the lack of constitutional symptoms frequently distract

Fig. 14-8. A, Staphylococcal submandibular space abscess. This enlarging hard tender mass was present for 4 days in a fussy and mildly febrile child. No primary oral or skin infections were found. **B,** Submental and submandibular space abscess secondary to infected mandibular incisors.

the clinician from the infectious origin of the mass. Usually the abscess matures after a few days, however, and the diagnosis becomes readily apparent.

A submandibular abscess may form by the direct extension of a preexisting infection or abscess in the mouth. This pathosis appears as a diffuse tender fluctuant swelling (Fig. 14-8).

The following sequence is typical in the formation of such an abscess:

1. A pericoronitis of a mandibular third molar develops with pus formation.
2. The pus extends into the pterygomandibular space, causing trismus.
3. From the pterygomandibular space the pus breaks through the connective tissue barrier around the anterior margin of the medial pterygoid muscle and gains access to the submandibular space.
4. When this happens, a space abscess is produced.

The history and physical findings are diagnostic, and treatment consists of incision, drainage, and irrigation of the abscess and eradication of the primary infection.

Nontender nodes. The majority of nontender nodes in the submandibular region represent either benign lymphoid hyperplasias or fibrosed nodes resulting from a previous oral infection. If a nontender node of short duration is detected, however, especially in a patient over 40 years of age, the clinician must be aware of the increased possibility that it may be a secondary malignant tumor.

Such a case requires a thorough physical and radiographic examination of the head and neck to detect a possible primary malignancy. If a primary tumor is located, a biopsy of the node is done immediately and a frozen section is examined. If the enlarged node proves to be a typical metastasizing malignancy, a neck dissection of the cervical lymph nodes is done concurrently with the definitive treatment of the primary lesion. In some institutions a combination of irradiation and surgical resection is utilized; in others irradiation is the sole method of treatment.

When no primary tumor can be located but the clinician suspects that a submandibular mass may be malignant, an excisional biopsy of the mass should be done to determine whether or not it has the stony-hard characteristic of a metastatic tumor. The patient is informed that the mass will be microscopically evaluated for malignancy during the biopsy procedure and that a neck dissection will be completed if the mass proves to be malignant. This policy seems justified since a substantial increase in the cure rate has been observed when neck resection is undertaken even though the primary site was not detected prior to removal of the lymph nodes. In over half these patients no primary site is ever discovered (Batsakis, 1974, p. 173).

Multiple nontender nodes occurring unilaterally in the neck without an overt primary cause should be managed the same as a single nontender node.

The occurrence of bilateral multiple nontender cervical nodes with or without generalized lymphadenopathy should prompt a complete medical examination for the detection of systemic disorders.

In the adult, excisional biopsy may be necessary for diagnosis; but it should await the results of other diagnostic tests, which might preclude the necessity for this step.

In the child, multiple enlarged bilateral neck nodes of inflammatory origin are common whereas metastasizing neoplasms are rare. Contrariwise, lymphomas are more common in children than are secondary tumors. Although it would not be feasible to do biopsies of all asymptomatic nodes in children with multiple and bilateral cervical lymphadenopathy, any unusually large node in a child that shows progressive growth or is rubbery or stony hard should be excised and microscopically examined.

MASSES WITHIN THE SUBMANDIBULAR GLAND

If a mass is within the submandibular gland, the gland should be removed intact and histologically examined at the time of the surgery. A total excision of the gland is required because (1) there is a high ratio of submandibular tumors that are malignant (50%) and (2) the most common tumor in this gland, the pleomorphic adenoma, does not have a restricting capsule (Fig. 14-9, A). Furthermore, a wide local resection of the surrounding tissues and occasionally a radical neck dissection at the time of the excisional biopsy may be necessary. For a more complete discussion of salivary gland tumors, the reader is referred to Batsakis (1974, pp. 1-51).

SUBMANDIBULAR GLAND SIALADENITIS

A painful enlargement of the submandibular gland (sialadenitis) may be produced by two different circumstances: (1) an inflammation or infection of the gland due to ductal occlusion and (2) an infection not preceded by ductal obstruction.

When there is obstruction of the duct, pain and swelling in the gland are associated with eating—the secretions accumulating behind the obstruction. The pain and swelling tend to subside somewhat between meals and are minimal on waking in the morning. The clinician can determine whether the duct is patent or not if milking the submandibular gland causes the expression of saliva at Wharton's papilla. He may discover a sialolith in the submandibular duct by palpating the floor of the mouth bimanually. About 90% of the time, a sialolith will be dense enough to show on a radiograph (Figs. 27-14 and 27-15).

If the results of these examinations are equivocal, a sialogram with a radiopaque substance will disclose whether the duct is patent or not. The advantage of this procedure, however, must be weighed against the hazard of precipitating a retrograde infection. Also, the injection of the disclosing material into the inflamed gland will cause the patient additional discomfort.

Obstruction of the duct may also result from other causes such as changes in the floor of the mouth produced by a malignant tumor or postoperative scarring. Under these circumstances the obstructive process is frequently insidious; and, although the gland is enlarged and firm, tenderness is frequently not a feature.

Elimination of the obstruction by removal of the stone, tumor, or cicatrix is the indicated treatment. If may be necessary to completely remove the gland when much fibrosis is present in a chronic case or when the stone is situated near or within the gland.

Sialadenitis without prior ductal obstruction. Sialadenitis without prior ductal obstruction is caused by either viral or bacterial infection.

Mumps is the most common type of viral sialadenitis occurring in childhood; and, although primarily a disease of the parotid glands, it may also affect the submandibular glands. The diagnosis is usually made by confirming a history of contact with an infected person. When such information is lacking, the demonstration of mumps antibodies in the serum will establish the diagnosis.

Other viruses may cause a sialadenitis. Zollar and Mufson (1970) showed the association of coxsackievirus A and echovirus in cases of parotitis that were serologically negative for mumps virus. Although such a viral relationship has not been established in submandibular gland adenitis, such a cause might be considered in uncommon cases of enlarged tender unobstructed glands.

Fig. 14-9. Submandibular masses. **A,** Pleomorphic adenoma of the submandibular salivary gland. **B,** Sebaceous cyst. **C,** Metastatic squamous cell carcinoma to the submandibular and subdigastric nodes. The primary tumor was located in the left floor of the mouth. The mass was painless, firm, and fixed to the surrounding structures. **D,** Metastatic melanoma from a primary lesion on the palate. **E,** Actinomycosis. **F,** Tuberculous adenitis. (**A** courtesy E. Kasper, D.D.S., Maywood, Ill.)

A suppurative sialadenitis is produced almost exclusively by a retrograde bacterial infection in patients experiencing reduced salivary secretion. Such a reduction may be due to dehydration or the use of parasympathetic blocking drugs and also to partial occlusion of a major duct. The retrograde infection occurs because oral bacteria are able to ascend the duct to the gland in the absence of the duct-cleansing salivary flow.

Pus-producing sialadenitis seldom occurs in the major glands but is more common in the parotid gland. In the submandibular gland it is usually associated with a ductal stone; and the

clinical and radiographic examinations previously described should be completed. The use of sialography is contraindicated in suppurative sialadenitis.

Clinically the gland is firm and painful. Pressure over the gland will cause the expression of pus from the opening of Wharton's duct if the duct is not completely obstructed. A specimen of pus should be collected and sent for culture and sensitivity tests so an effective antibiotic may be administered. Systemic problems as well as any local factors causing occlusion of the duct should be eliminated. Occasionally a child or an adult will have recurrent bouts of nonobstructive sial-adenitis, and such a condition is described as chronic recurrent sialadenitis (Batsakis, 1974, p. 55).

In rare instances a branchial cleft cyst may project into the submandibular region. Also a ranula of the sublingual gland may insinuate itself around the posterior border of the mylohyoid muscle and cause a cystlike mass in this region as well. Thus these entities must be considered when cystic masses are encountered in this region.

Masses in the parotid region

The numerous masses that commonly occur in the parotid region are similar to those that were described in the submandibular region. This is to be expected since the chief structures occupying both regions are the major salivary glands and the lymph nodes. Thus a complete discussion will not be repeated for each of the masses dealt with previously; only those lesions peculiar to the parotid region will be detailed here. Concerning the previously discussed masses, only differences in emphasis will be made.

When a mass is discovered in the parotid region, the clinician must first determine whether it is superficial or deep to the investing fascia of the salivary gland. The majority of masses superficial to the investing fascia will be enlarged lymph nodes, whereas those within the gland will usually be either parotid masses or enlarged intraparotid nodes. Masses within the parotid gland are fixed beneath the confines of the investing fascia and capsule of the gland.

ENLARGED MASSES SUPERFICIAL TO THE PAROTID FASCIA

Various lymph nodes are present in the loose connective tissue superficial to the parotid gland and fascia. The preauricular node is found immediately anterior to the external auditory meatus. It is quite mobile unless fixed to the surrounding tissues as a result of penetrating pathoses.

An enlarged *firm, tender,* or *painful mass* that can be moved over the deeper structures in this superficial region is most likely an *acute lymphadenitis* resulting from a furuncle or other infection of the scalp, upper face, conjunctiva, or external auditory canal.

An infected *congenital preauricular cyst* or *sebaceous cyst* must also be considered because either may be found superficial to the parotid fascia (Fig. 14-10, *A*). The rubbery consistency

and fluctuance of these masses, however, will help to differentiate them from an acute lymphadenitis. Also erythema and edema of the overlying skin are more characteristic of an infected cyst than of an acute lymphadenitis.

Painless superficial masses are usually benign lymphoid hyperplasias, parotid gland tumors occurring superficial to the gland, or preauricular or sebaceous cysts.

The *preauricular* or *sebaceous cysts* will be moderately soft (rubbery) in consistency and fluctuant, whereas the other two entities will be firm.

An *extraparotid tumor* cannot be differentiated clinically from a *benign lymphoid hyperplasia* since both may be firm and demonstrate some mobility; however, the former pathosis is quite rare whereas the latter is quite common. Should the firm mass continue to grow while remaining painless, it is most likely an extraparotid tumor and should be surgically excised and microscopically studied.

Lymph nodes in the preauricular area are seldom the site of a *lymphoma.* Also rare in this group of nodes is a *metastatic carcinoma,* which may originate from a primary carcinoma or a melanoma in the skin of the region drained.

Whether a mass located at the inferior tip of the parotid lobe is superficial to or within the parotid gland is frequently difficult to determine. In such an instance a primary site for possible tumors or inflammatory lesions is sought on the appropriate skin surfaces of the scalp and face or the mucosal surfaces of the oral cavity, pharynx, and nasal cavities. Because of the distinct possibility that this mass may be a secondary or a salivary gland tumor, if the examination of the frozen section indicates that it is malignant, the mass should be excised and more extensive surgery completed at the same operation.

MASSES WITHIN THE PAROTID GLAND

The majority of masses occurring within the parotid gland are salivary gland tumors. Approximately 70% of these are benign, most being benign mixed tumors that are characteristically slow growing and produce a noticeable firm swelling in the parotid area (Fig. 14-10, *B*). Malignant mixed tumors, on the other hand, usually grow more rapidly, may be stony hard, and may cause a unilateral paralysis of the muscles of facial expression. The types of salivary gland tumors are listed in Chapter 7. Although the clinician may develop an impression of whether the tumor is benign or malignant, the definitive

Fig. 14-10. Masses in the parotid region. **A,** Sebaceous cyst. **B,** Benign mixed tumor. The mass was firm and slow growing. **C,** Malignant mixed tumor. This mass was firm and rapidly enlarging. **D,** Parotid space abscess resulting from a dental infection. **E,** Hemangioma. (**D** courtesy V. Barresi, D.D.S., DeKalb, Ill.)

diagnosis must be made microscopically in every case.

Management. Besides parotid gland tumors, a mass within the parotid gland may be an enlarged node, a simple cyst, a cyst of the first and second branchial arches, or a hamartoma. Although the diagnosis of each of these entities is occasionally suspected on the basis of clinical features, the physical examination is not sufficiently definitive to rule out a tumor. Therefore biopsies must be done of all masses detected within the parotid gland.

If at surgery the mass proves to be a tumor, the complete superficial lobe of the gland is excised, leaving the facial nerve intact. The complete lobe is sacrificed because the most common lesions, the pleomorphic adenoma, frequently penetrates its pseudocapsule and a high recurrence rate results if an attempt is made to merely enucleate the lesion.

When a mass is found to extend into or originate in the deep parotid lobe, the entire gland is removed for biopsy. Cases of malignant tumors that characteristically metastasize to the cervical lymph nodes or show clinical evidence of metastasis will require resection of the cervical lymph nodes in addition to removal of the primary lesion.

In rare instances primary lesions arising in the mouth or oropharynx may metastasize to the nodes within the parotid gland, so these regions should be examined carefully prior to the biopsy procedure. A wide variety of tumors are found within the parotid gland, and these are characterized in detail by Batsakis (1974, p. 433).

SIALADENITIS OF THE PAROTID GLAND

The various types of disturbances causing a sialadenitis have been discussed with regard to sialadenitis of the submandibular gland. The types and characteristics are similar in the parotid gland, so a discussion of these will not be repeated for parotid sialadenitis (Fig. 14-11, *A*). The following points are peculiar to the parotid gland, however:

1. Salivary stones (calculus) in Stensen's duct occur much less frequently than in Wharton's duct, and those that do develop are frequently poorly calcified and radiolucent.
2. Bimanual palpation of much of the duct is impossible because of the ramus of the mandible.
3. The greater susceptibility of the parotid gland to secondary infection frequently prolongs the period of enlargement, pain, and tenderness, in contrast to the short symptomatic attacks characteristic of obstruction of the submandibular duct.
4. Scar tissue, intraductal tumor, and external ductal compression rarely cause obstruction of the parotid duct.

BILATERAL PAROTID ENLARGEMENT

An *asymptomatic* bilateral enlargement of the parotid glands due to a benign lymphoepithelial lesion with or without enlargement of the submandibular and lacrimal glands has been classically referred to as "Mikulicz's disease" (Fig. 14-11, *B*). When a variety of systemic diseases such as lymphoma and sarcoidosis are associated with these findings, the symptom complex is termed "Mikulicz's syndrome." The association of symptoms, including xerostomia, combined with conjunctivitis and coupled with a connective tissue disease such as rheumatoid arthritis is called "Sjögren's syndrome." In all these disorders the parotid swelling may be bilateral or unilateral. Attempts have been made to interrelate this group of diseases, but the specific pathogenetic relationships currently remain unclear.

Fig. 14-11. Bilateral parotid swelling. **A,** Painful bilateral suppurative parotitis ("surgical mumps"). There was postoperative staphylococcal infection of the parenchyma of both glands. Pus could be expressed from Stensen's papillae. **B,** Mikulicz's disease. Note the bilateral parotid swelling, which was asymptomatic. (**A** courtesy O. H. Stuteville, D.D.S., M.D., St. Joe, Ark. **B** courtesy P. Akers, D.D.S., Chicago.)

The identification of an asymptomatic parotid enlargement as one of the aforementioned diseases will depend on clinical and laboratory findings. The diagnosis of *Sjögren's syndrome* is strengthened by the demonstration of focal lymphocytic infiltrates in the labial minor salivary glands.

Bilateral parotid swelling has been noted in a variety of nutritional and metabolic disorders (Batsakis, 1974, p. 60). *Enlargement due to drugs* (e.g., iodine, certain heavy metals) is infrequent but must be considered in the differential diagnosis of parotid swelling. Finally, swelling of the major salivary glands may occur *after radiation* and is usually painful.

Masses in the median-paramedian region

Pathoses of the thyroid gland and its developmental derivatives account for the majority of pathologic masses in this region.

TENDER ENLARGEMENT OF THE THYROID GLAND

The thyroid gland may undergo inflammatory changes that produce an enlarged tender gland frequently accompanied by dysphagia and voice chances. Suppuration resulting from a bacterial infection is rare; but if it occurs, treatment consists of administering antibiotics in conjunction with surgical drainage.

An *acute nonsuppurative* form of thyroiditis with persistent signs and symptoms of inflammation occurs. Although the cause of this type of thyroiditis is still obscure, the thyroid glands of these patients usually show a decreased capacity for iodine uptake. Corticosteroids and analgesics have been used to treat the symptoms, but irradiation or surgery is necessary to eliminate the underlying disease (Schwartz, 1969).

Hashimoto's disease is a chronic disorder characterized by an enlarged tender thyroid gland. The disease is thought to be due to an autoimmune process in which the patient's thyroid gland is sensitive to its own thyroglobulin. The diagnosis is made by laboratory means (Schwartz, 1969, p. 1445). When nodular glands are present in Hashimoto's disease, a complete biopsy may be necessary to rule out thyroid tumor. Treatment is controversial and ranges from the administration of thyroid hormone to surgical excision of the gland.

NONTENDER ENLARGEMENT OF THE THYROID GLAND

The *simple* goiter is the most common type of diffuse enlargement of the thyroid gland—having a variety of causes, such as familial enzyme defect and iodine deficiency. In some cases there may be multiple nodules with the goiter, and this condition presents a dilemma to the clinician since the nodular architecture could be masking

a tumor. Laboratory studies, including radioactive iodine uptake to evaluate thyroid function, are necessary in the diffusely enlarged or nodular glands. Treatment of the goiter may be medical or surgical, depending on the cause, symptoms, and nodularity. For further details the reader is referred to Schwartz (1969, p. 1445).

MASSES WITHIN THE THYROID GLAND

Benign and malignant tumors and cysts occur as masses within the thyroid gland.

If a mass is found within the thyroid gland (Fig. 14-12), it is excised with the lateral lobe of the gland. The excision is done to determine whether the mass is malignant, and the involved lateral lobe is completely excised to prevent transection of a tumor during the removal of the mass.

An uncommon entity known as *Riedel's thyroiditis* develops as a fixed and hard mass, thus clinically mimicking a malignant neoplasm. If the diagnosis of Riedel's thyroiditis is established, the treatment of choice is with thyroid hormone, surgery being reserved for patients who require relief of tracheal and esophageal constriction.

When a thyroid mass is found, careful examination of the cervical lymph nodes is required to detect the infrequent but possible occurrence of metastatic tumor. Furthermore, metastatic tumor from a primary lesion in either the thyroid gland or the lower larynx may be present in an enlarged lymph node located on the cricothyroid membrane. The preoperative diagnostic workup in the patient with a thyroid mass is discussed in detail by Schwartz (1969).

THYROGLOSSAL CYSTS

Cystic masses arising from remnants of the embryonic thyroglossal duct are found in the midline anywhere from the base of the tongue to the sternum (Fig. 14-13, *D*). The duct may persist in postnatal life as a draining tract or as a cystic mass. A pathognomonic sign is the upward thrust of the mass when the patient protrudes his tongue, which demonstrates the connection of the thyroglossal duct and the tongue.

A thyroglossal cyst most commonly occurs below the hyoid bone and is usually readily visualized as a dome-shaped mass. These cysts may also be found submentally above the hyoid bone (Fig. 14-13, *D*) and within the musculature of the tongue. On rare occasion, thyroid tumors may develop in the walls of these cysts. Treatment consists of total excision of the cyst and the entire tract to the base of the tongue.

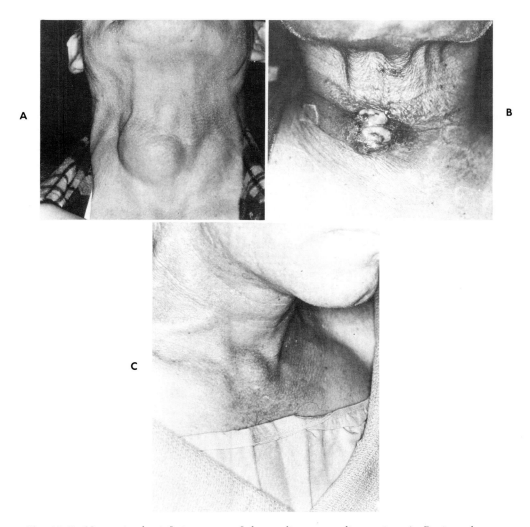

Fig. 14-12. Masses in the inferior aspect of the median-paramedian region. **A,** Benign adenoma of the thyroid gland. The mass was firm and smooth and arose from the right lobe of the gland. Swallowing caused the mass to be elevated. **B,** Anaplastic carcinoma of the thyroid gland. This mass was firm and fixed to the surrounding tissues. **C,** Sebaceous cyst. The cyst was just superficial to the isthmus of the thyroid gland.

SUBMENTAL MASSES

As stated in the preceding discussion, a *thyroglossal cyst* in a suprahyoid position will be found as a submental mass.

Although it is uncommon, an *epidermoid* or *dermoid* cyst may occur in this area (Fig. 14-13, *E*), lying in the midline; and, although it is fluctuant, its doughy consistency will help the clinician to differentiate it from the more rubbery thyroglossal cyst.

Excision of these two types of submental cystic masses with subsequent microscopic study will establish the diagnosis and is the recommended treatment.

Submental lymph nodes drain the regions of the lips and are subject to all the acute, chronic, inflammatory, and neoplastic changes described for nodes of the submandibular and parotid regions (Fig. 14-13, *A* and *C*); and the differential diagnosis and management of lymph node patho-

Fig. 14-13. Submental masses. **A,** Unusually large lymphoid hyperplasia. The mass was firm and freely movable. **B,** Sebaceous cyst. The mass was nontender, soft, fluctuant, and obviously attached to the skin. **C,** Diffuse submental acute lymphadenitis secondary to an infection of the lower lip. **D,** Thyroglossal cyst. This soft to rubbery fluctuant mass was elevated as the patient protruded his tongue. **E,** Dermoid cyst. This mass was doughy, fluctuant, and freely movable. **F,** Plunging ranula. This unusual lesion was painless, soft, and fluctuant. (**A** courtesy S. Svalina, D.D.S., Maywood, Ill. **B** courtesy P. Akers, D.D.S., Chicago.)

ses will be dictated by the same considerations as were discussed for such conditions in the submandibular and parotid regions.

Masses in the lateral neck region
LYMPH NODES

Most masses in the neck are enlarged lymph nodes extending along the linear path of the internal jugular vein from the angle of the mandible to the clavicle. The information concerning lymph nodes in other regions is especially perti-

nent to those in the lateral neck region since the preponderance of cervical nodes occur in this segment.

First-echelon nodes for the common cancer sites of the tongue, floor of the mouth, tonsil, and larynx are distributed along the jugular vein from the digastric to the omohyoid muscle (Figs. 14-5 and 14-7). In cancer patients the alternate lymphatic chain of nodes residing along the course of the accessory nerve, posterior to the posterior border of the sternocleidomastoid muscle, must

Fig. 14-14. Masses in the lateral neck. **A,** Metastatic squamous cell carcinoma in the subdigastric lymph nodes. This mass was stony hard and fixed. The primary tumor was located in the left side of the nasopharynx. **B,** Branchial cleft cyst. **C,** Cystic hygroma. **D,** Carotid body tumor. The mass was movable only in a lateral direction.

also be carefully examined for lymphadenopathy. Diagnostic and therapeutic measures for dealing with the masses presumed to be enlarged lymph nodes in the region follow the general principles detailed in the previous sections.

MASSES DISPLACING THE UPPER REGION OF THE STERNOCLEIDOMASTOID MUSCLE

The normal structures lying deep to the upper section of the sternocleidomastoid muscle are lymph nodes that drain large submucosal plexuses, the carotid artery, the internal jugular vein, the vagus nerve, and the cervical sympathetic trunk.

A bulging mass in this area may represent a metastatic carcinoma to the jugulodigastric and bifurcation nodes (Fig. 14-14, *A*), a branchial cyst of the second arch (Fig. 14-14, *B*), a carotid body tumor (Fig. 14-14, *D*), or a neurogenic tumor of

vagus nerve or cervical sympathetic trunk origin.

Lymph node metastasis in this region is usually from a primary lesion at the base of the tongue or elsewhere in the oropharynx. As the mass enlarges, it displaces the superior aspect of the sternocleidomastoid muscle laterally. If necrosis occurs, the mass may become fluctuant and painful, causing the inexperienced clinician to misdiagnose it as a primary abscess; however, a clinical diagnosis of primary abscess should not be considered likely without a history of an antecedent oropharyngeal infection. To further ensure the detection of a possible malignancy in such a case, a biopsy should be completed at the time the mass is drained to identify the presence of a possible metastatic tumor. If the primary tumor is discovered, treatment of the primary and secondary lesion is undertaken simultaneously.

Branchial cleft cyst. A cystic mass in this area

Fig. 14-15. Pan-neck infection. **A,** Elderly man with an infected left upper molar of 5 days' duration and only moderate upper neck swelling. The swelling subsequently became generalized. A chest radiograph showed gas in the mediastinum, and a culture of the region revealed *Bacteroides*. The infection traveled from the upper neck into the mediastinum through the areolar connective tissues. **B,** Pan-neck infection of dental origin. The patient had severe diabetes. (Courtesy O. H. Stuteville, D.D.S., M.D., St. Joe, Ark.)

will usually prove to be of branchial cleft origin. Branchial cleft cysts may occur at any level in the neck and frequently lie under the sternocleidomastoid muscle (Fig. 14-14, *B*).

If a sinus is present, its opening usually occurs at the anterior border of the sternocleidomastoid muscle. If a cyst and sinus of the second branchial cleft are present, the tract will lead to the tonsillar fossa. Complete excision of the cyst is the indicated treatment.

Frequently microscopic lymph node follicles are seen in the walls of a branchial cyst. Secondarily infected cysts are often mistaken for abscesses; and if these cysts are incised and drained, a cutaneous sinus will usually persist.

Carotid body tumors and neurogenic tumors. Carotid body tumors and to a lesser extent neurogenic tumors of cervical sympathetic origin occur under the anterosuperior aspect of the sternocleidomastoid muscle as solid masses (Fig. 14-14, *D*).

Because these masses are affixed to the nerves and vessels, they characteristically are mobile in a lateral direction but not in a vertical direction. Excision of these slow-growing and usually benign tumors is the required treatment, and the final diagnosis is made from the biopsy. For further details on these tumors, the reader is referred to Batsakis (1974, pp. 280-286).

MISCELLANEOUS MASSES OF THE LATERAL NECK REGION

Pan-neck infection. When all or most of the potential spaces of the neck are abscessed, the patient is said to have a pan-neck infection (Fig. 14-15). Such a patient may experience two very grave complications: respiratory obstruction and spread of the infection to the mediastinum.

Much has been written about the grave complication of a dental or tonsillar infection reaching the mediastinum through the neck. Although fascial planes play a prominent role in the passage of pus from one potential space in the head and neck to another, it appears more likely that the transmission of infection from the upper neck to the mediastinum is through the areolar tissues in general. The virulence of the organism and the resistance of the patient are frequently more important considerations for the prognosis of the infection than is the size or extent of the abscess.

This means that, although he may have minimal swelling (Fig. 14-15, *A*), the patient with a pan-neck infection may be at the brink of death. The key to the gravity of the case is the degree of systemic toxicity, which is reflected in the patient's vital signs. Radiographs of the neck and chest may provide clues as to the type of infection; for example, when a gas-forming organism such as *Bacteroides* is responsible for the infection, radiographs may reveal the presence of gas in the tissues.

The treatment for pan-neck infections is the wide surgical opening of all the planes at the base of the neck and drainage of the mediastinum when involved. Specific antibiotic therapy is unquestionably lifesaving in the advanced infections.

Cystic hygroma. This is a developmental benign cystic dilatation of lymphatic vessel aggregates at variable ages after birth. The characteristically soft swelling may occur at any point in the neck from the base of the skull down to the mediastinum (Fig. 14-14, *C*), and frequently it enlarges at an alarming rate. The cystic mass may be solitary or multiple and may infiltrate into and around muscle and nerve, making excision extremely difficult and hazardous.

Few other entities occur in the child as soft compressible masses of indistinct dimensions, so recognition of the cystic hygroma is seldom in question. Also fluid aspirated from the mass froths readily on agitation—indicative of a cystic hygroma because lymph fluid has a high fat content.

A cystic hygroma frequently occurs at an age when respiratory complications from the mass or from the surgical excision carry a high mortality. Unfortunately there is also a danger in the infant of sudden enlargement with obstruction of the airway. Thus management in the small child presents a dilemma: Does the surgeon remove the cystic hygroma to prevent a possible airway obstruction and risk death resulting from the surgery, or does he wait until the child is older hoping that in the interim the mass will not suddenly enlarge and cause death by suffocation?

SPECIFIC REFERENCES

Batsakis, J. G.: Tumors of the head and neck, Baltimore, 1974, The Williams & Wilkins Co.

Robbins, S. L.: Textbook of pathology, ed. 3, Philadelphia, 1967, W. B. Saunders Co.

Rosenberg, S. A., Diamond, H. D., Jaslowitz, B., and Craver, L. F.: Lymphosarcoma: a review of 1,269 cases, Medicine **40**:31-84, 1961.

Schwartz, S. I.: Principles of surgery, New York, 1969, McGraw-Hill Book Co.

Zollar, L. M., and Mufson, M. A.: Parotitis of non-mumps etiology, Hosp. Pract. **5**:93-96, 1970.

GENERAL REFERENCES

Berger, J. S., Tideman, H., and Bronkhorst, F. B.: Adenoid cystic carcinoma of the parotid gland: report of case, J. Oral Surg. **36**:390-393, 1978.

Briggs, P. C.: Submandibular duct stenosis as a complication of Ludwig's angina, Oral Surg. **47**:14-15, 1979.

Cardo, V. A., Jr., Mooney, J. W., and Stratigos, G. T.: Iatrogenic dental-air emphysema: report of a case, J. Am. Dent. Assoc. **85**:144-147, 1972.

Friedlander, A. H., Schwartz, S., Mazzarella, L., and Kisner, A.: Radiographic marker as an aid in evaluation of neck masses, J. Oral Surg. **37**:440, 1979.

Gross, B. D., and Chase, D.: Cat scratch disease, Oral Surg. **43**:698-701, 1977.

Hanna, D. C., and Clairmont, A. A.: Submandibular gland tumors, J. Plast. Reconstr. Surg. **61**:198-203, 1978.

Kaban, L. B., Mulliken, J. B., and Murray, J. E.: Sialadenitis in childhood, Am. J. Surg. **135**:570-576, 1978.

Kreller, J. S., Carr, R. F., and Quinn, J. H.: Cystic hygroma in a 17-year-old patient: report of a case, J. Oral Surg. **36**:808-810, 1978.

Narang, R., and Dixon, R. A.: Surgical management of submandibular sialadenitis and sialolithiasis, Oral Surg. **43**:201-210, 1977.

Nickel, A. F., Jr., and Roser, S. M.: Carotid body tumors, J. Oral Med. **32**:64-66, 1977.

Nitzan, D., and Azaz, B.: Submandibular lymph gland manifestation with unsuspected sarcoidosis, Oral Surg. **40**:728-731, 1975.

Pesavento, G., and Ferlito, A.: Benign mixed tumors of heterotopic salivary gland tissue in the upper neck, J. Laryngol. Otol. **90**:577, 1976.

Richardson, G. S., Clairmont, A. A., and Erickson, E. R.: Cystic lesions of the parotid gland, Plast. Reconstr. Surg. **61**:364-370, 1978.

Spaulding, C. R.: Soft tissue emphysema, J. Am. Dent. Assoc. **98**:587-588, 1979.

Towns, T. M.: Actinomycosis: case report, Oral Surg. **46**:615-617, 1978.

Part III

BONY LESIONS

Adherence to the following general guidelines is essential for accurate radiographic interpretation and the development of a differential diagnosis:

1. Radiographs must be of good quality.
2. The radiograph represents only a portion of the available clinical data relative to a particular pathologic process or change.
3. The proper evaluation of radiographic information necessitates an intimate working knowledge of osseous and soft tissue anatomy, radiographic anatomy, and the basic nature and varieties of the pathologic processes that affect the tissues in the areas of concern.
4. A differential diagnosis leading to a working diagnosis is as necessary in evaluating bony lesions as it is in evaluating soft tissue lesions.

Good-quality radiographs

Even at the risk of its wearing effect, the fact that good-quality radiographs are essential must be stressed. There is little doubt that quality is frequently disregarded, apparently on the grounds of inconvenience—in other words, to determine the proper radiographic techniques and then apply them just does not seem to be convenient.

Corroborative data

The radiographic evaluation must in every case be qualified on the basis of information obtained from the complete examination of the patient. Basing an opinion on radiographic findings alone is risky and often leads to error. Thus, when a radiolucency is discovered on a radiograph, the patient must be questioned in an attempt to outline the onset and course of the suspected lesion and to obtain other pertinent historical facts. Furthermore, the adjacent soft tissue, the cortical plates of the bone, and any teeth in the region must be examined. This examination should include a thorough inspection and a systematic tissue-knowledgeable palpation.* The clinician will thereby be able to determine much about the lesion, such as whether the process in the bone has enlarged sufficiently to expand or erode the cortical plates and possibly invade the adjacent soft tissue.

Basic knowledge necessary for diagnosis

A further explanation of the third guideline mentioned relates to the clinician's basic preparation for the evaluation of radiologically detectable changes in the bone. To become accomplished in this area of diagnosis, he must acquire and utilize a general knowledge of anatomy, pathology, and radiology. The pertinence of such a contention is well illustrated by the wide variability that anatomic structures can manifest and yet be considered to fulfill the requirements of the normal order. Consequently the clinician must be not only aware of the potential for deviation from the usual morphology but also familiar with the altered radiographic appearances these irregularities can assume. The true nature of many normal

---

*In Chapter 3 the manner in which careful palpation of a pathologic area, swelling, or mass can provide considerable definitive information is described. Therefore, when a lesion is suspected or discovered in a bone, all the physical characteristics of the region must be considered.

anatomic variations has often been recognized only during the surgery for their intended removal.

After the student has become quite familiar with the normal radiographic appearances and variations that anatomic structures can assume, he is ready to study the radiographic changes produced by disease states. The breadth of this information may appear awesome at first encounter because of the multitudinous lesions that may occur in bone. Fortunately, however, a comprehension of these diseases is facilitated by the fact that practically all bony lesions can be categorized into three groups, depending on whether their radiographic appearances are any of the following:

Completely radiolucent

Mixed radiolucent-radiopaque

Totally radiopaque

To emphasize this concept, Part III is divided into three sections. In addition, each section is divided into chapters that represent a subclassification of the lesions based on more subtle radiographic differences—periapical radiolucencies, cystlike radiolucencies, etc. (Fig. 1).

A factor complicating this simplified scheme is that frequently a lesion will occur with two or even three different images, usually representing different stages of maturation. Thus it has been necessary to include some entities in more than one chapter. Appendix A lists the more common bony lesions that are appropriately placed in two or more of the basic categories (radiolucent, mixed, radiopaque).

Differential diagnosis

In most cases the microscopic examination of biopsy tissue will provide the final diagnosis. Yet prior to biopsy the clinician is without such explicit information but nevertheless must formulate his own list of possibilities supported by the results from physical, radiologic, and laboratory examinations. To emphasize the need for a carefully formulated working diagnosis, imagine the chagrin and the problems encountered by the credulous clinician who finds himself well into a surgical procedure on an unsuspected vascular tumor. In summary, when osseous lesions are being studied, the formulation of a differential diagnosis—with the disease entities arranged in decreasing order of probability, as indicated by the strength of their supporting clinical evidence—is just as necessary as it is for the study of soft tissue lesions.

Furthermore, when studying a radiolucent lesion, the clinician must be cognizant of the possibility that such a lesion may have developed in the overlying mucosa and subsequently extended into the bone rather than have originated in the bone. A careful clinical examination of the patient in conjunction with the radiographic findings will usually indicate the correct inference. This distinction is, of course, important when a list of pertinent pathoses is being considered since the soft tissue entities can usually be deemphasized if the evidence suggests an origin in bone. A rare exception would be concomitant lesions—one originating in bone, and another in the adjacent soft tissue.

Careful adherence to these principles will ensure that the clinician approach lesions of the bone in a logical manner.

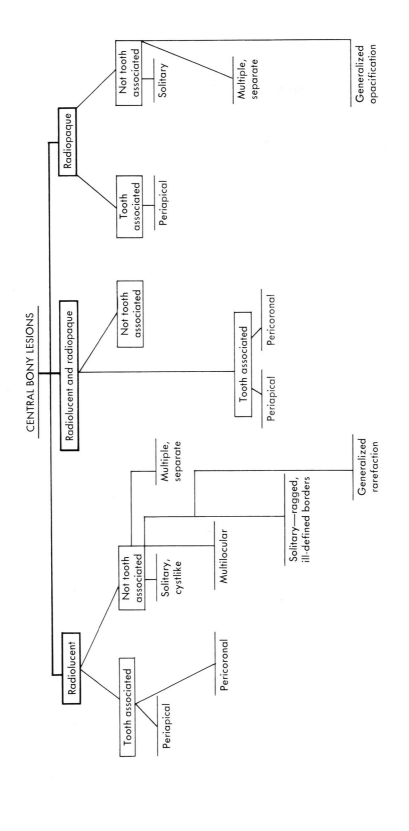

CENTRAL BONY LESIONS

Radiolucent

Tooth associated
Periapical
Pericoronal

Not tooth associated
Solitary, cystlike
Multilocular
Multiple, separate
Solitary—ragged, ill-defined borders
Generalized rarefaction

Radiolucent and radiopaque

Tooth associated
Periapical
Pericoronal

Not tooth associated

Radiopaque

Tooth associated
Periapical

Not tooth associated
Solitary
Multiple, separate
Generalized opacification

15

Anatomic radiolucencies

Norman K. Wood
Paul W. Goaz

The following structures produce anatomic radiolucencies:

Structures peculiar to the mandible
Mandibular foramen
Mandibular canal
Mental foramen
Lingual foramen
Airway shadow
Submandibular fossa
Mental fossa
Midline symphysis

Structures peculiar to the maxilla
Intermaxillary suture
Incisive foramen, incisive canal, and superior foramina of incisive canal
Nasal cavity
Naris
Nasolacrimal duct or canal
Maxillary sinus
Greater palatine foramen

Structures common to both jaws
Pulp chamber and root canal
Periodontal ligament space
Marrow space
Nutrient canal
Developing tooth crypt

In view of the foregoing comments relative to the diagnosis of radiographically apparent lesions, any consideration of the differential diagnosis of pathologic radiolucencies of bones should be prefaced by a discussion of the normal anatomic radiolucencies and their variations.

The usual procedure of discussing entities—in the order of their decreasing frequency of occurrence—followed in the other chapters of this book is not generally appropriate for these entities since they are normal and are to be expected in most adequate radiographs of the anatomic regions considered.

Some circumstances may seem to contradict the above comment, however, and require mention. These relate to the mitigating factors that alter the nature and radiographic reproduction of the usual normal landmarks.

For example, the presence or absence of certain normal radiolucencies is related to age. The developing tooth crypts in persons under 16 years of age are usually not present in older individuals. Likewise pulp chambers, root canals, and periodontal ligament spaces decrease in size with age and are, of course, not present at all in edentulous persons. There is also considerable variation in the frequency of occurrence and radiographic representation of the lingual foramen, but this variability does not appear to be related to age. Nutrient canals are another example of radiolucencies that may be prominent in the radiographs of some patients but difficult to identify or find at all in others. Consequently only an arbitrary decision accounts for the order of the following discussion: first, the radiolucencies of the mandible; second, those of the maxilla; and, finally, those that are common to both jaws.

Structures peculiar to the mandible

MANDIBULAR FORAMEN (INFERIOR DENTAL FORAMEN)

The mandibular foramen is usually situated just above the midpoint in the medial surface of the ramus and just posterior to the midpoint between the anterior and posterior borders (Hayward et al., 1977). It receives the inferior dental nerve and artery after they traverse the pterygomandibular space. Because of its position in the

293

Fig. 15-1. Mandibular foramen (arrows). **A,** Lateral oblique projection. **B** and **C,** Dry specimens. Note the mandibular canal leading anteriorly from the foramen. (**B** has been retouched.)

ramus, this foramen is seldom seen on periapical films; but it may often be identified on panographic and lateral oblique films, in which its outline varies from triangular to oval to funnel shaped and its definition varies from faint to prominent (Fig. 15-1).

The radiographic image of the mandibular foramen is seldom larger than 1 cm in diameter; and the foramen can be positively identified by its bilateral occurrence and its association with the relatively radiolucent mandibular canal, which passes from it in an anteroinferior direction. Frequently the lingula can be detected as a triangular radiopacity of variable density at the foramen's anterior border. These associated structures, the mandibular canal and the lingula, can be mistaken for pathologic entities.

MANDIBULAR CANAL (INFERIOR DENTAL CANAL)

The outline of the mandibular canal, the largest of the nutrient canals in the jaws, is usually readily seen on a panographic or periapical view of the molar region. The canal appears as a relatively radiolucent channel, bounded by definite thin radiopaque lines (cortical bone) throughout its length (Fig. 15-2). Its course can be followed from the mandibular foramen anteroinferiorly to

a point where it frequently appears to sweep upward to meet the mental foramen. Occasionally it is seen to extend some distance anteriorly and inferiorly from the mental foramen (Fig. 15-3).

There is great variation between persons as to width and prominence of the mandibular canal, but in any individual the bilateral appearance is usually quite similar. There is some variation also in the position of the canal within the body of the mandible; some canals are near the inferior border whereas others lie just below the apices of the molars. The curvilinear course is normally rather gentle; and abrupt changes in outline, whether narrowing, broadening, discontinuity, or alteration of direction, are suggestive of pathosis (Fig. 15-4).

MENTAL FORAMEN

The mental foramen permits the exit of the mental branches of the mandibular artery and nerve to the soft tissue in the area of the chin, lower lip, and labial gingiva. It can usually be located on a radiograph of the area, generally in the vicinity of the premolar apices (Fig. 15-5).

The relative definition of the foramen may vary, however, because the mental canal does not often meet the buccal cortical plate at a right angle. When the angle approaches 90°, the resultant

Fig. 15-2. Mandibular canal delineated by two thin radiopaque lines. **A,** In an edentulous jaw. Note the mental foramen (arrow) at the anterior terminal of the canal. **B,** In a dentulous jaw.

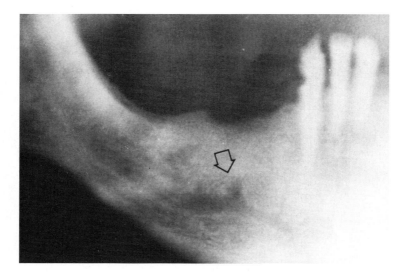

Fig. 15-3. Note the continuation of the mandibular canal anterior to the mental foramen (arrow).

Fig. 15-4. Lateral oblique view of a mandible fractured at the angle. Note the interrupted course of the canal caused by displacement of the fragments. (Photograph has been retouched.)

Fig. 15-5. A, Mental foramen (arrows). **B,** Occasionally the mental foramen will be confused with an adjacent foramenlike marrow space (arrow), as illustrated in this radiograph.

Fig. 15-6. This prominent image of the mental foramen is a result of directing the x rays parallel to the mental canal.

Fig. 15-7. Mental foramen (arrows). Occasionally the foramen will be projected near or over the roots of adjacent teeth and may be misinterpreted as periapical pathosis. This happens especially when the pulps of the teeth are suspect.

radiographic image is the most conspicuous because the beam is directed parallel to the canal (Fig. 15-6).

Since this foramen frequently occurs at the apices of the premolars, there is a tendency for the unwary clinician to confuse it with periapical pathosis (Fig. 15-7).

LINGUAL FORAMEN

The lingual foramen can often be seen on periapical views of the lower central incisors. It is located well below the apices of these teeth in the midline, is generally surrounded by a prominent radiopaque ring of cortical bone, and is variable in frequency, size, and appearance (Fig. 15-8, *A*). It seldom is more than 1 or 2 mm in diameter. Occasionally two or more foramina are present (Fig. 15-8, *B*). Terminal branches of the inferior dental artery (incisive branches) exit at this point to supply the lingual incisive gingiva.

AIRWAY SHADOW

An airway shadow is bilateral, relatively radiolucent, and especially well recorded on cephalometric and lateral oblique radiographs.

This image, which runs in an inferoposterior direction across the angle of the mandible just posterior to the molar region, is frequently troublesome to the inexperienced clinician (Fig. 15-9). It results from the lack of intervening soft tis-

Fig. 15-8. Lingual foramen. **A,** A single foramen (arrow) is accentuated by the radiopaque projections of the geniotubercles that usually encircle it. **B,** This radiographic view shows a double foramen.

Fig. 15-9. Airway shadow. *1,* Nasopharyngeal airway; *2,* oropharyngeal airway. **A,** Panograph. **B,** Cephalometric view.

Fig. 15-10. Submandibular fossa. **A,** The fossa appears as a poorly defined radiolucency below the apices of the molars. **B,** The prominent mylohyoid ridge (arrows) in this view accentuates the fossa.

sue between the posterodorsal surface of the tongue and the soft palate and posterior pharynx region.

SUBMANDIBULAR FOSSA

The submandibular fossa is a concave area on the lingual side of the mandible below the molar area. It accommodates the submandibular salivary gland and usually appears as a poorly defined relatively radiolucent area (Fig. 15-10, *A*). Often its contrast is enhanced by a prominent radiopaque mylohyoid ridge that runs across the top of the depression, thus making its radiolucency more pronounced (Fig. 15-10, *B*).

MENTAL FOSSA

The image of the mental fossa is similar to the image produced by the submandibular fossa. The mental fossa is situated on the labial aspect of the midline of the mandible just above the mental tubercle. Radiographs of the area often show such a relative radiolucency over the incisor roots that this fossa may be mistaken for periapical pathosis (Fig. 15-11).

MIDLINE SYMPHYSIS

The mandibular midline symphysis is present on radiographs at the midline of the mandibles of very young persons and is represented by a radiolucent line that may be misinterpreted as a fracture (Fig. 15-12). The symphysis usually fuses and ossifies by the age of 1 year and is then no longer apparent. Consequently it is not frequently encountered by the dental clinician on radiographs since few patients have cause to be radiographically examined at this young age.

Fig. 15-11. Mental fossa. This radiograph showing a generalized radiolucency in the periapical incisor region illustrates the thinning of the bone due to the mental fossa.

Fig. 15-12. This radiograph of a stillborn child shows the mandibular symphysis at birth. The structure has been erroneously identified as a fracture.

Structures peculiar to the maxilla

INTERMAXILLARY SUTURE

The intermaxillary suture, between the right and left maxillary bones, can be identified as a thin vertical radiolucency in the midline between the central incisors (Fig. 15-13). It is usually delineated by two thin vertical radiopaque lines (cortical bone). It generally fuses later in life and is then no longer represented on the radiograph.

INCISIVE FORAMEN, INCISIVE CANAL, AND SUPERIOR FORAMINA OF INCISIVE CANAL

The incisive foramen (incisive fossa, anterior palatine foramen) frequently shows as a well-defined round, oval, diamond- or heart-shaped radiolucency on occlusal films; and less often, on periapical films, especially of the central incisors, it appears as a rounded to ribbon-shaped poorly defined radiolucency. The variation in size of this foramen also parallels its nonuniformity in shape. The position of the foramen on the radiograph ranges from between the roots of the

Fig. 15-13. The intermaxillary suture can be identified as a vertical radiolucent line in the central incisor region. It becomes less distinct with age.

Fig. 15-14. The incisive foramen (arrows) represents the oral terminal of the incisive canal. It is frequently projected onto the central incisor region near the crest of the alveolar process. **B,** Note the presence of the foramen of a nutrient canal immediately inferior to the incisive foramen.

Fig. 15-15. Incisive canals (arrows).

central incisors, close to the alveolar ridge, to the level of the apices (Fig. 15-14).

This variability in the position of the foramen on radiographs relates to the angulation of the rays used to expose the film as well as to the position of the foramen itself. The location of the foramen, which is in the midline, may range from the crest of the alveolar ridge to some distance posteriorly.

The incisive canals (nasopalatine or anterior palatine canal) that end at the incisive foramen will occasionally be seen on periapical films of the central incisors. Their radiolucency on the film is more apparent than real—emphasized by the contrast with their relatively sharp opaque lateral walls, which actually delineate the canals (Fig. 15-15). The images vary greatly in width and length and may be seen to converge from the nasal fossa toward the foramen, but they usually become indistinct before reaching this terminal (Fig. 15-17).

The images of the superior foramina of the incisive canals are found on periapical films of the maxillary central and lateral incisors and canines, especially if the vertical angle is increased sharply (Fig. 15-16). These foramina are seen on the floor of the nasal fossa bordering the septum. On the periapical films their radiolucent images may be projected over the apices of any of the incisor teeth, prompting an impression of periapical pathosis.

NASAL CAVITY (NASAL FOSSA)

The inferior aspect of the nasal cavities is often seen on periapical radiographs of the incisor and

Fig. 15-16. Arrows indicate the nasal terminals of the incisive canals.

canine regions, especially if the horizontal angulation is increased. These cavities appear as twin radiolucencies separated by the radiopaque septum and are delimited by radiopaque cortical bone (Fig. 15-17). The inferior border of the cavities is often projected above the apices of the incisors and canines.

NARIS

The image of the nose is sometimes projected over the image of the alveolar bone on anterior periapical films. The density of this soft tissue added to the density of the bone results in a radiographic impression of increased bone density in the area of the superimposition.

Contrariwise, the images of the nares project onto this area of increased density as relative radiolucencies that frequently appear over or on the maxillary incisor region (Fig. 15-18). The nares may then be misinterpreted by the uninitiated diagnostician as evidence of periapical pathosis.

NASOLACRIMAL DUCT OR CANAL

The nasolacrimal duct on each side is usually enclosed in such a thin tube of cortical bone that it is seldom discernible on the usual periapical radiograph (Fig. 15-19, A). The orbital extreme of the structure, however, does appear on the maxillary occlusal radiograph—projected onto

Fig. 15-17. The paired radiolucencies at the superior border represent the nasal cavities. Note the divergent branching (arrows) of the incisive canals toward their nasal terminals.

Fig. 15-18. The faint image of the nose and outlines of the nares (arrows) are seen in this periapical view of the maxillary incisor region.

A

B

Fig. 15-19. Nasolacrimal canal (arrows). **A,** This structure is not usually projected on a periapical film. **B,** On maxillary occlusal films the nasolacrimal canals are frequently misinterpreted as the greater palatine foramina. Note the nasal cavities, *1,* and the maxillary sinuses, *2.*

the posterior hard palate at about the first or second molar area as a relatively large bilateral radiolucency that is well defined by sharp radiopaque borders (Fig. 15-19, *B*).

On the well-centered radiograph the image of each duct is usually at the junction of the radiopaque lines representing the maxillary sinuses and the nasal fossa. These radiopaque lines are situated lateral to and roughly parallel with the midsagittal plane, where the median suture may be seen if it is still radiographically apparent before fusion.

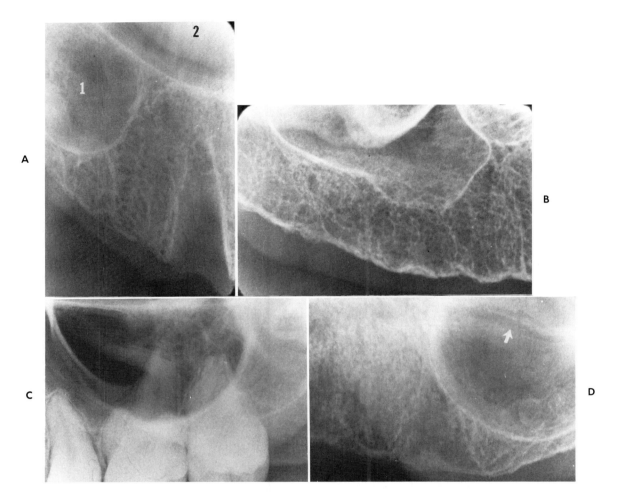

Fig. 15-20. Maxillary sinus. **A,** This periapical view of the canine region shows the maxillary sinus, *1,* the nasal cavity, *2,* and the antral Y. **B,** Maxillary sinus in an edentulous molar region. **C,** Maxillary sinus, showing complex contours and unusual extensions. **D,** Maxillary sinus with a cystlike configuration. A nutrient canal (arrow) in the sinus wall aids in differentiating the sinus from a cyst.

MAXILLARY SINUS

The maxillary sinus on each side appears as a well-defined radiolucency with thin sharp radiopaque borders (Fig. 15-20). The radiolucency may be crisscrossed by one or more thin radiopaque lines that represent bony septa appearing to subdivide the sinus. The sinus occurs bilaterally over the molars and premolars and may vary in anteroposterior extent from tuberosity to canine root, or even to the lateral incisor root.

Each maxillary sinus may appear to border or overlap the nasal fossa, depending on the angle of exposure. In the adult the inferior aspect of each sinus lies below the level of the floor of the nasal fossa; frequently nutrient canals are seen in the sinus wall and, when present, help to distinguish this anatomic structure from a cyst or other pathosis.

GREATER (MAJOR) PALATINE FORAMEN

Occasionally the greater palatine foramen can be identified on each side as a round to ovoid ill-defined radiolucency over or between the apices of the maxillary second and third molars (Fig. 16-7).

Structures common to both jaws

PULP CHAMBER AND ROOT CANAL

The shadows of pulp chambers and root canals, along with the variations in these anatomic structures, are of great importance in restorative dentistry and in root canal therapy but are beyond the scope of this text.

PERIODONTAL LIGAMENT SPACE

Clinicians are well oriented to the radiographic appearance of the smooth radiolucent outline of the periodontal ligament spaces; and dental students are equally well drilled in its appearance. When the spaces are superimposed over anatomic radiolucencies, however, the resultant radiographic images can simulate a broadening of the spaces and occasionally be mistaken for disease.

MARROW SPACE

The marrow spaces between the trabeculae of spongy bone appear as radiolucent areas whose size, shape, and distribution vary greatly from person to person as well as throughout the jaws of the same individual (Fig. 15-21). In general, however, the radiographic representations of these structures throughout the maxilla are relatively uniform in size; this is in contrast to the mandible, where the marrow spaces are smaller and more numerous in the anterior portion and tend to be larger in the posterior areas.

In some persons the trabecular spaces about and below the roots of the molars are so large and the trabeculae so sparse that the combined appearance may resemble and be misinterpreted as cysts, traumatic bone spaces, rarefying osteitis, or other such pathoses. In areas where trabeculae are few and marrow spaces are large, the thinly scattered trabeculae are often relatively dense. It is pertinent to emphasize that the size of the marrow spaces is not a particularly reliable criterion for evaluating the status of the jawbone.

NUTRIENT CANAL

The nutrient canals appear as linear ribbonlike radiolucencies of fairly uniformly width that are most often found between the roots of teeth (Figs. 15-14, *B*, and 15-22). These interdental canals,

Fig. 15-21. Marrow space. **A,** This pattern occurs with some frequency adjacent to the mandibular molar roots. **B,** Large marrow space (arrows) that was mistaken for a lesion. **C,** Large marrow spaces (arrow) frequently occur in the bifurcation of the mandibular molars. These variations must be differentiated from periodontal involvement in the bifurcation. **D,** A large marrow space (arrow) in the coronoid process was mistaken for a lesion. Note the relatively small marrow spaces in the maxilla as compared with those usually occurring in the posterior region of the mandible.

which are most frequently observed on radiographs of the mandibular incisor region, become less numerous in the mandibular premolar area; and the bone supporting the maxillary premolars is the third most likely area in which they will be found.

Occasionally a relatively large nutrient canal, carrying the posterior superior alveolar artery and traversing the lateral wall of the maxillary sinus, will be apparent on a maxillary posterior radiograph (Fig. 15-20, *D*). Although nutrient canals are rarely seen in the anterior region of the maxilla and are seldom recognized below or between the mandibular molars, infrequently one will be found in the mandibular posterior region where the trabeculae are few in number and the marrow spaces large. In this region a canal or two may be apparent and accentuated by its fine radiopaque walls.

In all the regions of both jaws, the canals become much more marked when the teeth are missing. If the beam of the radiograph is directed parallel to a canal and through its foramen in the cortical bone, the canal appears as a small

Fig. 15-22. Nutrient canal. **A,** These canals are frequently prominent between the roots of the mandibular incisors and they terminate as small foramina on the crest of the interseptal bone. **B,** The prominent nutrient canal (arrow) in this view could be mistaken for a fracture. **C,** The prominence of this unusually large nutrient canal or accessory foramen (arrow) is produced by directing the x rays parallel to the canal.

Fig. 15-23. Developing tooth crypt of a third molar. This cystlike radiolucency may be correctly identified by its position in the jaw, its bilateral occurrence, the age of the patient, and serial radiographs.

round radiolucency (Fig. 15-22, C). These radiolucencies technically are accessory canals and foramina. Occasionally, however, they will be confused with pathologic radiolucencies.

DEVELOPING TOOTH CRYPT

Tooth crypts are seen on radiographs of developing dentitions, so they are seldom present in patients over 15 years of age. If the developing tooth is uncalcified, the crypt will appear as a roundish homogeneous radiolucency and be mistaken for a cyst by the uninitiated diagnostician (Fig. 15-23). If just the tips of the cusps have calcified, the radiographic appearance will be of a well-defined radiolucency containing radiopaque foci.

SPECIFIC REFERENCE

Hayward, B. S., Richardson, E. R., and Malhotra, S. K.: The mandibular foramen: its anteroposterior position, Oral Surg. **44:**837-843, 1977.

GENERAL REFERENCES

Bachman, L. H.: Pedodontic radiography, Dent. Radiogr. Photogr. **44:**51-56, 1971.

Beideman, R. W.: Pitfalls in interpreting radiographs of developing mandibular third molars, J. Am. Dent. Assoc. **86:** 870-871, 1973.

Calman, H. I., Eisenberg, M., Grodjesk, J. E., and Szerlip, L.: Shades of grey: radiographic interpretive challenges, Dent. Radiogr. Photogr. **40:**27-45, 1967.

Crawford, B. E., and Weathers, D. R.: Osteoporotic marrow defects of the jaws, J. Oral Surg. **28:**600-603, 1970.

Farman, A. G., Nortje, C. J., and Grotepas, F. W.: Pathological conditions of the mandible: their effect on the radiographic appearance of the inferior dental (mandibular) canal, Br. J. Oral Surg. **15:**64-74, 1977.

Grier, D. C.: Radiographic appearance of the greater palatine foramen, Dent. Radiogr. Photogr. **43:**34-38, 1970.

Knight, N.: Anatomic structures as visualized on the Panorex radiograph, Oral Surg. **26:**326-331, 1968.

Poyton, H. G.: Methodical approach to radiographic interpretation, Dent. Radiogr. Photogr. **40:**71-77, 1967.

Poyton, H. G.: Maxillary sinuses and the oral radiologist. Dent. Radiogr. Photogr. **45:**43-59, 1972.

Silha, R. E.: Special radiographic surveys, Dent. Radiogr. Photogr. **45:**23-32, 1972.

Standish, S. M., and Shafer, W. G.: Focal osteoporotic bone marrow defects of the jaws, J. Oral Surg. **20:**123-128. 1962.

16

Periapical radiolucencies

Norman K. Wood
Paul W. Goaz
Marie C. Jacobs

Periapical radiolucencies include the following:

Anatomic periapical radiolucencies (false)
> Marrow spaces
> Dental papillae
> Maxillary sinus
> Incisive foramina and canals
> Nasolacrimal duct
> Naris
> Greater palatine foramen
> Mental foramen
> Submandibular fossa
> Mandibular canal

True periapical radiolucencies
Periapical radiolucencies — sequelae of pulpitis
> Granuloma
> Radicular cyst
> Scar
> Chronic and acute dentoalveolar abscesses
> Surgical defect
> Cholesteatoma
> Osteomyelitis
Dentigerous cyst
Periapical cementomas
Periodontal disease
Traumatic bone cyst
Non-radicular cysts
Malignant tumors
Rarities
> Ameloblastic variants
> Ameloblastoma
> Aneurysmal bone cyst
> Benign nonodontogenic tumors
> Cementifying and ossifying fibromas
> Cementoblastoma — early stage
> Gaucher's disease
> Giant cell granuloma
> Giant cell lesion of hyperparathyroidism
> Histiocytosis X
> Lingual salivary gland depression
> Odontoma — early stage
> Osteoblastoma — early stage
> Solitary and multiple myeloma

Radiolucent shadows are cast over the periapical regions of teeth in practically all oral radiographic surveys of dentulous patients. Some of these periapical radiolucencies represent innocent anatomic variations, whereas others are caused by benign conditions and require treatment to preserve the associated teeth; still others represent systemic disease conditions that many times will become the responsibility and obligation of the dental clinician to recognize and bring to the attention of the patient's physician. The dental clinician should in every case afford whatever cooperation facilitates the most effective treatment.

Malignancies represent a small group of these periapical shadows; and early detection, recognition, and treatment currently represent the only hope the patient has of being cured.

The high incidence and broad spectrum of conditions causing periapical radiolucencies combine to make it imperative that all dental clinicians acquire a broad and comprehensive working knowledge of the conditions listed at the beginning of and/or discussed in this chapter.

True or false periapical radiolucencies

All periapical radiolucent shadows may be readily divided into one of two categories: true or false. *True* periapical radiolucencies represent lesions that are truly located in contact with the apex of a tooth. Hence their shadow cannot be shifted from the periapex by taking additional radiographs at different angles. In contradistinction *false* periapical radiolucencies are produced by anatomic cavities or lytic bony lesions that do not contact the apex of a tooth. Hence these radiolucent shadows may be shifted from the periapex by taking additional radiographs at different angles.

Classifying a periapical radiolucency as being *true* or *false* is very useful in the differential diagnosis process because if it can be clearly demonstrated that the radiolucency in question is truly periapical in location then it is most likely that the lesion has resulted from a pulpitis. On the other hand, if the radiolucency can be shifted from the apex it most likely is produced by an anatomic cavity or space.

ANATOMIC PERIAPICAL RADIOLUCENCIES

Anatomic radiolucencies are projected over the periapical regions in almost every radiograph of jawbone-bearing teeth. Different views of the area in question (e.g., a panographic, occlusal, or Waters projection) will frequently aid in differentiating the normal anatomic shadows from periapical radiolucencies that result from disease processes. Also radiographs of suspect periapical regions made with the central beam directed from at least two different angles will cause structures not in the periapical region to be displaced in succeeding films.

Thus the shadow of a distant anatomic structure may be demonstrated to overlie the image of the apex and thereby create a radiolucent area. Furthermore, a complete examination—including the patient history and clinical, laboratory, and pulp tests—will aid in this differentiation. If the radiolucencies are anatomic in origin, a comparison with the radiographs of the opposite side will frequently reveal an identical situation. Clinicians should be not only aware of the normal location and appearance of the anatomic cavities, canals, and foramina that will produce innocent periapical radiolucencies but also familiar with the normal ranges and variations of these structures.

The normal structures which may be responsible for radiolucencies that could be confused with those caused by disease processes are discussed in some detail in Chapter 15. Therefore anatomic radiolucencies that may appear on periapical films are only listed here with their illustrations for convenience:

Marrow spaces (Fig. 16-1)
Dental papillae (Fig. 16-2)
Maxillary sinus (Fig. 16-3)
Incisive foramina and canals (Fig. 16-4)

Fig. 16-1. Periapical marrow spaces (arrows).

Fig. 16-2. Dental papillae (radiolucencies) at the apices of the second molar.

Fig. 16-3. Maxillary sinus projected as a periapical radiolucency (arrows). (**D** courtesy M. Smulson, D.D.S., Maywood, Ill.)

Fig. 16-4. Incisive foramina projected as periapical radiolucencies.

Fig. 16-5. Nasolacrimal duct as a radiolucency at the apex of the first premolar (arrow).

Fig. 16-6. Naris (arrow) projected as a periapical radiolucency over the apex of the central incisor.

Fig. 16-7. Greater palatine foramen (arrow).

Fig. 16-8. Mental foramen (arrows).

Fig. 16-9. A radiolucency near the apices of the second molar proved to be the submandibular fossa. (Courtesy L. Schwartz, D.D.S., Maywood, Ill.)

Fig. 16-10. Mandibular canal superimposed over apices of the third molars (arrows).

Nasolacrimal duct (Fig. 16-5)
Naris (Fig. 16-6)
Greater palatine foramen (Fig. 16-7)

Mental foramen (Fig. 16-8)
Submandibular fossa (Fig. 16-9)
Mandibular canal (Fig. 16-10)

PERIAPICAL RADIOLUCENCIES— SEQUELAE OF PULPITIS (PULPOPERIAPICAL PATHOSES)

The seven pathologic entities included in the group of pulpoperiapical pathoses initially share a common cause: irritating inflammatory products from a pulpitis. These products escape from the pulp canal and initiate a local inflammatory response in the periapical area. Currently it is thought that antigen-antibody reactions may play an important initiating role (Torabinejad and Kettering, 1979). Various factors (e.g., host resistance, presence, number, and virulence of bacteria, amount of antigenic material and other toxins emanating from the canal, degree of tooth function, extent of other trauma, presence of epithelial rests of Malassez, thickness of adjacent cortical plates, nature of previous treatment) will determine the type of sequelae.

Interventional treatment might include any of the following:

1. Pulp capping (Jordan et al., 1978)
2. Preparation and obliteration of the canal with or without a root resection or apical curettage or both
3. Establishment of drainage either via the pulp canal or through the soft tissues
4. Administration of drugs through the pulp canal or systemically
5. Extraction

Such measures will frequently modify the sequelae of pulpal infection, in contrast to what might result from an uninterrupted sequence of pathologic events.

Thus the information provided by the history of the circumstances attending a periapical radiolucency—including the response to previous treatment—plus the information gained from clinical and radiographic examinations will be necessary for the development of a working diagnosis. The final diagnosis of an asymptomatic radiolucency, however, can be determined only by microscopic examination of the periapical tissue.

Until recently it has been believed that without exception periapically involved teeth included in this group have nonvital pulps. It has been recognized for years that occasionally one root of a multirooted tooth will contain a gangrenous pulp and have a periapical radiolucency whereas the other root(s) may remain vital. Such a tooth will frequently give a vital reaction with the electrical pulp tester.

Recently, however, it has been suggested and partially substantiated that radiographically discernible periapical lesions may occur at the apex of those teeth that have a localized area of pulpitis in the coronal portion of the pulp. Such a pulp is vital and would give positive responses to electrical pulp testing. Block and co-workers (1976) explain the process in this manner: "One could assume that the accumulated disintegration products and bacterial toxins travel from their place of origin through the lymph vessels of the remaining vital pulp and gather in the periapical tissue. This would explain the seemingly illogical appearances of a remaining nearly unaltered pulp tissue between two areas of severe inflammation." The study by Jordan and co-workers (1978) lends credence to this general concept. These investigators treated, by indirect pulp capping, 24 vital posterior teeth that had deep carious lesions and radiographically demonstrable periapical lesions. Eleven of these teeth showed apparent resolution of periapical pathology, absence of pain, and continued vitality in the posttreatment follow-up.

The periapical lesions in this group share several clinical characteristics as well as a similar cause:

1. The periapical lesion is radiolucent.
2. The roots associated with the lesion usually contain nonvital pulps that will be clinically apparent on instrumentation.
3. The crown may often be discolored and/or show deep caries or have a restoration that is close to the pulp.
4. The crown may be partially or completely missing because of a traumatic incident; this is more frequently seen in anterior teeth.
5. A history of painful pulpitis, which heralded the death of the pulp some time before the radiolucency formed, may be reported by or can be elicited from the patient.

Teeth with a dens in dente have an increased incidence of pulp death and also an increased incidence of pulpoperiapical lesions (Fig. 16-11).

In the discussion of the differential diagnosis of lesions that follows, it must be understood that frequently the clinician will be unable to clearly differentiate between a granuloma, a radicular cyst, a scar, a surgical defect, and a cholesteatoma on the basis of the history or by the clinical and radiographic findings alone. The final diagnosis can be decided by the microscopic examination of the periapical tissue.

The foregoing statement notwithstanding, it is possible in most cases of periapical radiolucencies for the astute diagnostician to develop a

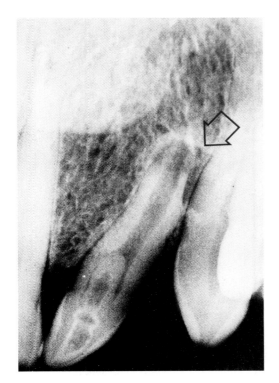

Fig. 16-11. Pulpless lateral incisor tooth in a 22-year-old patient with a nonvital pulp, an extensive dens in dente, and a pulpoperiapical radiolucent lesion. Note the arrested development of the pulp canal.

working diagnosis or impression from a well-conceived differential diagnosis. The fact that approximately 90% of the pathologic periapical lesions are either granulomas or cysts greatly aids the clinician in the development of a valid differential diagnosis.

Sequence of events after pulp death

As a consequence of pulpitis with or without pulp death, from whatever cause, one or a combination of sequelae can be expected at the periapex.

First, not any (or at most a very limited amount) of the irritating products of pulp necrosis may reach the periapical tissues. As a result no periapical pathosis will be induced and no such change will be suggested by the patient's history or be clinically or radiographically detectable.

Second, irritating products may arrive at the periapex but in such moderate amounts that the host's defenses will be able to effectively combat and localize their effects. The resultant inflammation in the circumscribed area will be of a

chronic nature, and a "primary-type"* periapical granuloma will develop.

Third, in teeth with contaminated gangrenous pulp(s), the number and virulence of the bacteria passing from the root canal(s) may be sufficient to overwhelm the defenses of the periapical tissue and consequently an acute periapical abscess will develop.

Fourth, the resultant infection may be partially controlled by the body's defenses, by surgically induced drainage, and/or by antibiotic therapy. The most probable result, however, will be the development of a chronic periapical periodontitis or chronic alveolar abscess.

The dental granuloma may in turn evolve into one of several entities, depending on the presence and interaction of certain factors.

If the odontogenic epithelial rests of Malassez (present in the periodontal ligament and frequently identified in periapical granulomas) proliferate and become cystic, a *radicular cyst* will result. If bacteria of sufficient virulence and in sufficient numbers to counteract the host resistance are introduced into the granuloma or cyst, an *acute periapical abscess* will develop.

If, in the course of the infection of a cyst or granuloma, the correct antibiotics are administered in adequate amounts or the abscess is drained, the infection will be aborted and the periapical lesion may regress into a "secondary-type"† *dental granuloma* or *cyst*. If a sinus develops from the abscess to the surface, the lesion will become a *chronic alveolar abscess*.

Another possible sequence of events that may influence the course of a dental granuloma is the effective treatment of the associated tooth's root canal(s)—resulting in the ultimate disappearance of the granuloma and the complete resolution of the radiolucency to normal bone. If the granuloma has been subjected to repeated exacerbations of inflammation as a result of periodic contact with irritants from the root canal, however, areas of it may become fibrosed during the quiescent interludes. Then, if the tooth is successfully treated by conservative endodontic techniques, the remaining inflammation and granula-

---

*In the present discussion the term "primary-type" or "virgin-type" granuloma refers to the lesion that is the first pathologic entity developing at the apex. This is in contrast to the granuloma that replaces another periapical entity, such as a cyst converted by infection or mechanical disruption ("secondary type").

†In contrast to the primary-type granuloma, the secondary type replaces another periapical entity such as a cyst or a primary granuloma that has been converted by acute infection or mechanical disruption or both.

tion tissue will resolve, leaving only the fibrosed area. Such entities are referred to as periapical scars and frequently remain for many years, during which time they may be repeatedly observed unchanged as a periapical radiolucency.

Granuloma

The periapical granuloma represents the most common type of pathologic radiolucency, accounting for approximately 50% of such lesions. Recent studies suggest that a much higher percentage of these pulpoperiapical lesions are granulomas. For instance, Block and co-workers (1976) reported that a microscopic evaluation of 230 cases of pulpoperiapical radiolucent lesions treated by apicoectomy revealed that approximately 94% were granulomas and 6% were cysts. These investigators did not mention whether any of the lesions could be classified as periapical scars or not.

Basically the periapical granuloma is the result of a successful attempt by the periapical tissues to neutalize and confine the irritating toxic products that are escaping from the root canal. The continual discharge of chronic irritating products from the canal into the periapical tissue is, however, sufficient to maintain a low-grade inflammation in these tissues; and this inflammatory reaction continues to induce the proliferation of vascular granulation tissue, which makes up the entity.

In addition, the granuloma represents a stage in the repair process which is altering the defect that has resulted from the lysis of bone in the immediate vicinity of the root end. Consequently the clinician should consider the presence of a periapical granuloma as an indication that the natural defenses have contained the insult from the related diseased root canal.

The microstructure of the granuloma consists of proliferating endothelial cells, capillaries, young fibroblasts, a minimal amount of collagen, and chronic inflammatory cells (lymphocytes, plasma cells, macrophages) (Fig. 16-12). Occasionally nests of odontogenic epithelium, Russell bodies, foam cells, and cholesterol clefts are present.

Classically more inflammation is seen in the center of the lesion, where the apex of the tooth is usually located, because at this point the irritating substances from the pulp canal are most concentrated. At the periphery of the lesion, fibrosis (healing) may already have begun since the irritants will be quite diluted and neutralized some distance from the apex. Practically, though,

Fig. 16-12. Periapical granuloma. **A,** The pulp of the first molar was nonvital. **B,** Photomicrograph.

the orderly picture just described may not often be found.

FEATURES

Radiographically the lesion is a rather well-circumscribed radiolucency somewhat rounded in shape and surrounding the apex of the tooth (Fig. 16-12). This periapical radiolucency may or may not have a thin radiopaque (hyperostotic) border. Radiographs of the involved tooth may reveal the presence of deep restorations, extensive caries, fractures, or a narrower pulp canal than in the contralateral tooth. All these features would lead the clinician to suspect the presence of pulp pathosis. A periapical granuloma cannot be differentiated from a radicular cyst by radiographic appearance alone; however, when a periapical radiolucent lesion has attained a diameter of 1.6 cm or larger the likelihood of its being a radicular cyst is much greater (Lalonde, 1970). Few granulomas ever become larger than 2.5 cm in diameter. In our opinion any granuloma reaching a size greater than 2.5 cm in diameter probably represents a resolving chronic alveolar abscess rather than a primary-type granuloma.

The response of the patient when the offending tooth is subjected to electrical and thermal pulp testing will usually indicate that the pulp is nonvital. The tooth is completely asymptomatic, including usually an absence of sensitivity to percussion. The crown may have a darker color than that of its neighbors due to blood pigments that have diffused into the empty dentinal tubules. Swelling or expansion of the cortical plates over the area of the apex is most unusual since periapical granulomas rarely reach a size to produce such an effect.

DIFFERENTIAL DIAGNOSIS

The discussion of a differential diagnosis for a periapical granuloma is included in the corresponding section under radicular cyst (p. 319).

MANAGEMENT

The management of a periapical granuloma is discussed under the management section of radicular cyst.

Radicular cyst

The radicular cyst is the second most common pathologic periapical radiolucency after the dental granuloma. It constitutes approximately 40% of all periapical radiolucent lesions although recent studies suggest a much smaller figure. For instance, only 6% of a series reported by Block and co-workers (1976) were radicular cysts. The radicular cyst may be classified as an inflammatory cyst because this process is thought to initiate the growth of the epithelial component. It may also be classified as an odontogenic cyst because of its origin in the cell rests of Malassez, which are remnants of Hertwig's root sheath—the latter, in turn, a product of the odontogenic epithelial layers (the inner and outer enamel epithelia).

Practically all radicular cysts originate in pre-existing periapical granulomas, and their pathogenesis is dependent on an inflammatory reaction. Hence they are also classified as inflammatory cysts. A significant number of granulomas contain epithelial remnants (Block and co-workers [1976] reported that 20% do), that may start to proliferate because of the irritation* that induced the proliferation of the granuloma. As the masses of proliferating epithelial nests increase in size,

---

*The inflammatory products are suspected of causing a shift in the oxidative metabolism of the rests of Malassez, which permits them to proliferate in the milieu of the granulation tissue while apparently the quiescent cells are maintained by the aerobic pathway (Grupe et al., 1967).

the central cells start to degenerate and liquefy because they are actually being physically removed from an adequate blood supply in the surrounding connective tissue and because the capillaries in the tissue surrounding the developing cyst are being compressed. This sequence of events leads to the formation of a liquid-filled cavity lined with epithelium (i.e., a cyst). The cyst continues to grow because of a combination of factors. The products from cell lysis are probably irritating and may provide a growth stimulus. In addition, epithelial cells (their products as well as the contents of the degenerating cells) are discharged into the cyst lumen and thus increase the protein content and the osmotic pressure of the cyst fluid. The result is that more water diffuses into the lumen, further expanding the cyst. The pressure exerted by the enlarging cyst on the alveolar bone induces osteoclastic action and resorption of the peripheral bone.

FEATURES

The patient's history and the clinical and radiographic findings associated with a pulpless asymptomatic tooth that has a small well-defined periapical radiolucency at its apex are identical whether the lesion is a periapical granuloma or a radicular cyst.

This statement notwithstanding, the more pronounced the hyperostotic border of the lesion, the more likely is the lesion to be a cyst (Fig. 16-13). Studies by Lalonde (1970) showed that such a lesion is more likely to be a radicular cyst if the periapical radiolucency measures at least 1.6 cm in diameter. When it is encountered, an untreated cyst may slowly enlarge and cause expansion of the cortical plates. In these instances the expansion can be observed clinically as a domelike swelling on the alveolus over the periapical region of the involved tooth.

The swelling may develop on either the buccal or the lingual side of the alveolar process and will be covered with normal-appearing mucosa. Initially it will be bony hard to palpation, but later it may demonstrate a crackling sound (crepitus) as the cortical plate becomes thinned. Usually the cortical plates remain intact, although numerous cases have been encountered in which a radicular cyst completely resorbed the overlying cortical bone (Fig. 16-13). In these cases the clinical swelling is rubbery and fluctuant because of the cyst fluid within. Large cysts may involve a complete quadrant with some of the teeth occasionally mobile and some of the pulps nonvital. Root resorption is also seen. Neither the causative

Fig. 16-13. Radicular cyst. E, Note the erosion of the labial cortex. F, Photomicrograph.

tooth nor the alveolar swelling produced by an expanding cyst is painful in sterile cysts. If such a cyst becomes infected, however, the tooth and swelling will develop all the painful symptoms of an abscess.

Microscopically the radicular cyst is classically described with a connective tissue wall that may vary in thickness from region to region and from cyst to cyst. This wall may also vary in character throughout its width. Peripherally it is fibrous, although its inner regions may be composed of

granulomatous tissue. Within the wall, and especially within its granulomatous portions, foci of chronic inflammatory cells, foam cells, Russell bodies, and cholesterol slits may be found. The wall surrounds the fluid-filled lumen; and its lumen side is usually covered with various types of epithelium, which may also vary greatly in form, thickness, and continuity.

Although the lumen lining is usually stratified squamous epithelium, occasionally ciliated pseudostratified columnar and even keratinizing epithelium will be found, whether the cyst is in the mandible or the maxilla (Fig. 16-13). Practically, however, these layers of tissue do not often occur so uniformly; inflammation may be present in some areas, resulting in the destruction of the epithelial lining in that region. Frequently the radicular cyst is, in fact, a combination of dental granuloma and radicular cyst. Aspiration of a noninfected radicular cyst will produce a light straw-colored fluid, usually containing an abundance of shiny granules (cholesterol crystals).

DIFFERENTIAL DIAGNOSIS

When the clinician encounters a periapical radiolucency, he must consider that it could represent any of the entities discussed or listed in this chapter.

If a well-defined radiolucency is at the apex of an untreated asymptomatic tooth with a nonvital or diseased pulp and if anatomic structures can be ruled out, then in approximately 90% of the cases it will be either a *dental granuloma* or a *radicular cyst*. Although these two entities cannot be distinguished by radiographic features alone, if the radiolucency measures 1.6 cm or more in diameter, it is more likely to be a cyst.

Occasionally, however, tissue obtained from large periapical lesions will be diagnosed by the pathologist as a *periapical granuloma*. Our experience with these cases has led us to expect such a report, especially when the tooth in question has precipitated repeated episodes of pain and alveolar swelling, has spontaneously developed intermittent drainage, or has been incised and drained a number of times. By way of explanation of this apparent contradiction, the history of the involved tooth is reasonably good evidence that the larger granuloma is not the primary type but is the secondary type—which has perhaps proliferated in an infected cyst whose epithelium was destroyed by acute inflammation and necrosis and has just resolved to the healing granulomatous stage.

Many attempts have been made to develop a technique that will consistently differentiate between a periapical granuloma and a radicular cyst without resorting to biopsy.

The radiographic examination of periapical radiolucencies after the injection of a radiopaque contrast medium, either directly into the area or through the root canals, has been proposed but has not proved to be dependable.

More recently preliminary electrophoretic studies of fluid from root canals of pulpless teeth with periapical radiolucencies are showing promise.

The fluid from teeth that were subsequently found to have radicular cysts gave a segment characteristic of serum globulin; but this segment was not given by fluid from teeth that had periapical granulomas.

Aspiration of straw-colored fluid via the extracanalicular approach has long been recognized as indicating the presence of a cyst rather than a granuloma. In practice, however, it is not necessary to differentiate between small periapical granulomas and cysts since either lesion responds quite well to conservative root canal therapy.*

Periapical scars and *surgical defects* are frequently confused with a periapical granuloma or cyst. In teeth that have received nonsurgical endodontic treatment for granulomas and cysts and are assumed to be well sealed, a persistent asymptomatic nonenlarging radiolucency is most likely a periapical scar. Similarly an asymptomatic radiolucency that persists after root resection can be either a scar or a surgical defect; but it is unlikely to be any type of residual pathosis if the tooth remains asymptomatic and the radiolucency does not increase in size.

The *periapical cementoma* in its early lytic fibroblastic stage cannot be distinguished radiographically from a periapical granuloma or cyst. In the tooth with a cementoma, however, the pulp is vital and healthy whereas the tooth with a granuloma or cyst has a nonvital pulp. On rare occasion a pulpless tooth may have a concomitant early cementoma at the apex, so the criterion of pulp vitality would be confusing; however, periapical cementomas most frequently involve the lower teeth (in a ratio of about 9:1), most often the incisors.

Although a *traumatic bone cyst* in a periapical area may be mistaken for a dental granuloma or cyst, as with a cementoma, the pulps of the associated teeth will usually be vital. Also a traumatic bone cyst differs from a periapical cyst and a granuloma since approximately 90% of traumatic bone cysts occur in the mandible, where they are most frequently seen in the molar, premolar, and incisor regions (in that order). On the contrary, periapical cysts and granulomas have no predilection for the lower jaw.

When a patient's history indicates a *systemic disorder* (e.g., hyperparathyroidism, primary ma-

---

*The term "conservative root canal therapy" encompasses all the procedures required to properly obliterate the root canal(s) but does not include any direct surgical intervention in the periapex.

lignant tumor, multiple myeloma), obviously the working diagnosis of periapical granuloma or cyst must be broadened to include these more serious entities.

The periapical lesion associated with periodontal disease usually will show moderate to severe crestal bone loss. According to Brynolf (1978) this is coupled with a pattern of periapical bone loss that is morphologically distinct from that usually produced by pulpitis.

MANAGEMENT

A small periapical cyst or granuloma may be treated in either of two ways:

1. The clinician may decide the offending tooth will not facilitate his plans for restoring the dentition, and he may extract it. The periapical soft tissue in this case should be removed and examined microscopically.
2. He may decide the tooth should be retained. In this case most clinicians prefer to resort to conservative root canal therapy alone and observe the lesion radiographically every 6 months to ensure that it is not enlarging but hopefully is regressing.

Reported clinical experience has shown that routine root canal obliteration is the indicated treatment for most small lesions whether granulomas or cysts. It will be interesting during the next decade to observe whether Dr. Jordan's method of indirect pulp capping will be utilized in more of the cases that have periapical lesions in combination with vital but diseased pulps.

Why should cysts respond so well to nonsurgical endodontic treatment? Several theories have been proposed.

One suggests that instrumentation beyond the apex in these nonvital cases permits the cyst to drain into the canal and produces an inflammatory reaction that results in the lysis of the cystic epithelial cells. Currently the overinstrumentation approach has few adherents (Block et al., 1976).

Another theory holds that when the root canal is sealed the irritating products from the gangrenous pulp are no longer present and the inflammation subsides. Healing then commences at the periphery, where such dense collagen is laid down that the blood supply to the epithelial lining becomes impaired and the epithelial cells necrose. The products from these degenerating epithelial cells are responsible for the inflammatory reaction that stimulates the proliferation of granulation tissue; and the tissue, in turn, fills the cystic space. The resulting granuloma then regresses since the inflammation-inducing material is no longer draining into the area from the root canal or being produced in the area by degenerating cystic epithelia.

In general, then, a radicular cyst is initiated in a granuloma and may be subsequently replaced by the granuloma in a sequence of events that attend its healing. Regardless of the mechanism responsible, apparently many small cysts are successfully treated by nonsurgical root canal therapy. When a conservative type of endodontic therapy has been employed, it is imperative that the clinician observe his patient radiographically at regular intervals to be certain that the radiolucency is resolving or at least is not enlarging.

This close supervision of the area is of utmost importance, because a final definite diagnosis has not been verified by such a nonsurgical approach and the clinician must be cognizant that the radiolucency could represent a more serious entity (e.g., a malignant tumor). If there did prove to be an enlarging radiolucency, the clinician would then know that he must obtain a biopsy via a buccal window to determine the nature of the lesion. Frequently an enlarging lesion is demonstrated to be an expanding granuloma or cyst due to an inadequate root canal seal and the continued irritation of the periapex by degradation products.

Although management varies somewhat with the clinician, some believe that apical curettage or a more extensive root resection procedure is indicated for periapical radiolucencies measuring 2 cm in diameter or larger since most of these are radicular cysts. Conditions also arise that dictate the surgical approach for smaller lesions; for example, when a patient cannot be available for three or four appointments and a direct root canal filling with surgical curettage and periapical retrograde sealing might be the best way to manage the case; or if the root canal was found to be nonnegotiable, a surgical approach to facilitate a retrograde filling of the canal and periapical curettage might be indicated.

On occasion large radicular cysts that have destroyed a consider amount of bone are encountered. Currently six approaches may be utilized for the management of such lesions. These are described in detail in Chapter 17:

1. Surgical enucleation
2. Surgical enucleation and restoration of the defect with a graft, preferably autogenous bone
3. Marsupialization
4. Decompression

5. Decompression with delayed enucleation
6. Creation of a common chamber with the maxillary sinus or the nasal cavity (used occasionally for large maxillary cysts)

Sequential postsurgical radiographs to ensure that the defect is regressing are essential no matter which method is employed. The average healing time for cysts measuring over 10 mm in diameter is approximately 2½ years. Incomplete removal of the cyst lining may result in the formation of a residual cyst or in rare instances a more aggressive type of pathosis.

Scar

The periapical scar is composed of dense fibrous tissue and is situated at the periapex of a pulpless tooth in which usually the root canals have been successfully filled. This entity is represented by a periapical granuloma, cyst, abscess, or cholesteatoma whose healing has terminated in the formation of dense scar tissue (cicatrix) rather than bone in the defect (Fig. 16-14). From 2% to 5% of all periapical radiolu-

Fig. 16-14. Periapical scars. **A** and **B,** The periapical lesions had become markedly smaller in these two asymptomatic teeth following conservative root canal therapy. **C,** Photomicrograph showing dense fibrous tissue that makes up the periapical scar.

cent lesions are estimated to be periapical scars, although there is little information in the literature concerning this entity.

Scar tissue represents one of the possible endpoints of healing, whether it occurs on the surface of the body or in the deeper tissues (e.g., at the periapex). The sequence of events is as follows:

If the introduction of the irritant into the inflamed area is continued, as might be possible from the apex of an untreated pulpless tooth, chronic inflammatory cells accumulate, young fibroblasts, endothelial cells, and capillaries proliferate, and subsequently a granuloma is formed. Grossly the granulation tissue is soft, compressible, and reddish in color.

Fluctuations in the severity of the irritant are paralleled by cyclic changes in the associated inflammation. In periods of minimal irritation and inflammation, some portions of the granulation tissue mature, being transformed into a more dense connective tissue (scar) instead of replaced by bone (if that is the normal tissue of the area, and it is in the case of a periapical scar).

When the tooth is successfully treated by nonsurgical endodontic techniques, the irritants from the root canal are eliminated and the periapical granuloma or cyst frequently resolves, being replaced by bone, and is no longer apparent on the radiograph. In some instances, however, the granulation tissue slowly organizes, with the production of more and more collagen fibers, and eventually a dense contracted connective tissue scar results, which is quite permanent.

Microscopically a mature periapical scar shows a few spindle-shaped fibroblasts scattered throughout dense collagen bundles; and the collagen bundles often show an advanced degree of hyalinization. Inflammatory cells are not a feature, and vascularity is quite meager (Fig. 16-14, C).

In our experience a significant percentage of lesions diagnosed microscopically as periapical granulomas have contained isolated areas of scar tissue as well as regions of granulation tissue. Such lesions are in reality mixed lesions and probably should be thought of as scarring periapical granulomas or perhaps as relatively young less dense scar that is experiencing intermittent inflammation. Since a substantial portion of periapical granulomas microscopically examined are found to be such mixed lesions, the contention would seem to be substantiated that if the lesions are properly treated by nonsurgical (conservative) procedures their granulomatous portion will

readily resolve and their reduced area may persist as periapical scar tissue.

Serial radiographs of such lesions would be expected to show a decrease in the size of the periapical radiolucency proportional to the amount of granulation tissue present at the time the endodontic treatment was initiated.

It would seem, then, that the majority of persisting radiolucencies at the apex of asymptomatic teeth whose canals have apparently been successfully sealed by nonsurgical endodontic procedures are periapical scars. Of course, since there is little justification, few of these apparent periapical areas are surgically explored or their contents microscopically examined. Consequently evidence bearing on this question is extremely limited. Periapical scars also frequently occur in patients initially treated by periapical curettage or root resection (Arwill et al., 1974).

FEATURES

The periapical scar causes a well-circumscribed radiolucency that is more or less round and radiographically resembles the periapical granuloma and cyst (Fig. 16-14). It is frequently smaller than either of these two entities. The tooth and associated radiolucency are asymptomatic; and, if observed radiographically over the years as it should be, the scar will be seen to remain constant in size or perhaps diminish slightly. Such a history is, of course, dependent on the establishment and maintenance of a good apical seal.

The periapical scar occurs most often in the anterior region of the maxilla. The majority of the involved teeth have been treated endodontically. Occasionally such a scar will be located at the periapex of a pulpless tooth that has not been endodontically treated, however; and in these cases the natural defenses of the body are assumed to have completely neutralized the irritants emanating from the root canal after an initial successful inflammatory response to the irritants. In other cases the root canal may have sealed itself off, thus restricting the irritants within the canal.

DIFFERENTIAL DIAGNOSIS

The differential diagnosis of these lesions is included in the differential diagnosis section under periapical surgical defects (p. 327).

MANAGEMENT

When it is associated with an asymptomatic root canal–filled tooth, the periapical scar requires no treatment. Such a tooth presents a problem to the clinician who is contemplating extensive restorative procedures, however, since he cannot clinically or radiographically differentiate between a dental granuloma or cyst and the scar. The tooth in question may appear to have an adequate root canal filling but in fact not have a good apical seal, which would cause the cyst or granuloma to persist.

The asymptomatic root canal–filled tooth, of course, imposes the potential of an acute inflammatory reaction that may not be evidenced until after extensive restorative work has been completed; and at this time the inflammatory reaction can be successfully treated only by procedures that will adversely alter the restoration. If the tooth has remained asymptomatic since the root canal filling and the periapical area has not increased in size, then the radiolucency can be safely assumed to be a periapical scar.

As a general rule a tooth that is to be used as an abutment but has a periapical radiolucency should be observed radiographically for about 6 months after endodontic treatment so that its status can be ascertained.

Chronic and acute dentoalveolar abscesses

Abscesses make up approximately 2% of all pathologic periapical radiolucencies. In the context of this chapter, the periapical or dentoalveolar abscesses are subdivided as follows, according to whether they are radiolucent or not:

1. *Primary or neoteric abscesses* are pulpoperiapical inflammatory conditions associated with teeth that have not developed apparent periapical radiolucent lesions; they are usually described as an acute apical periodontitis or an acute periapical abscess.
2. *Secondary or recrudescent abscesses* develop in a previously existing asymptomatic periapical radiolucent lesion (e.g., granuloma, cyst, scar, cholesteatoma).

The primary (neoteric) abscess develops in a radiographically normal periapical region. The infection is almost always acute and exudative, involving the periodontal tissues at the apex of a tooth with a necrotic pulp. The canal contains large numbers of virulent bacteria that rapidly spread to the periapical tissues and cause an acute periodontitis, a very sensitive tooth, and perhaps alveolar swelling. The onset and course of the infection are so sudden that resorption of bone has not yet occurred; hence a periapical radiolucency is not a feature. Frequently the infection and inflammation in the apical area cause a swelling of the periodontal ligament and force the tooth slightly from its socket, thus creating an increased periodontal ligament space around the entire root. The increased space is usually apparent on the radiograph; but because a periapical radiolucency is not a feature of the neoteric abscess, a detailed discussion is not presented in this chapter.

The secondary (recrudescent) abscess may be either of the chronic or the acute type, depending on various factors—the number and virulence of the invading organisms, the resistance of the host, and the type and timing of the treatment instituted. Although various strains of staphylococci and streptococci are the most frequent causative microorganisms, a wide variety of other microorganisms have been found to be offenders in certain instances.

FEATURES

The primary lesion in which the infection occurs may be a granuloma, cyst, scar, or cholesteatoma; thus a periapical radiolucency is a feature of the secondary abscess. The radiolucency may vary in size from small to quite large and may involve much of the jaw. The initial periapical lesion may have even caused an expansion of the cortical plate.

If the acute infection is discovered soon after its onset, and depending on its duration, acuteness, or chronicity, the margins of the radiolucency may vary from well defined with possibly a hyperostotic border to poorly defined in chronic cases (Fig. 16-15). Sometimes the radiolucency will be represented as a blurred area of somewhat lessened density than the surrounding bone. Radiographs of the related tooth will frequently show such features as deep restorations, caries, narrowed pulp chambers, or canals—which suggest that the pulp is nonvital. The roots of these teeth may also show resorption at the apex.

Microscopically the picture varies somewhat, depending on the stage of the infection, but basically it consists of a central region of necrosis containing a dense accumulation of polymorphonuclear leukocytes surrounded by an inflamed connective tissue wall of varying thickness. A chronic resolving abscess may have fewer polymorphonuclear leukocytes, less necrosis, and more lymphocytes, plasma cells, macrophages, and granulation tissue (Fig. 16-15). On the contrary, an acute abscess may contain only necrotic and unidentifiable soft tissue.

Fig. 16-15. Chronic periapical abscess. **A** and **B,** Note the ill-defined ragged borders. **C,** Parulis resulting from a chronic draining abscess at the apex of the pulpless left central incisor. **D,** Microscopy of a chronic abscess surrounded by granulation tissue.

Clinically the tooth with an acute abscess will be very painful to percussion; and if it is in occlusion, the patient will complain that it seems "high" when it occludes with the opposing tooth. As a rule it will not respond to electrical pulp tests. The application of ice, however, will relieve the pain somewhat—in contrast to heat, which will intensify the pain. The tooth may demonstrate increased mobility.

If permitted to progress without treatment, the abscess may penetrate the cortical plate at the thinnest and closest point to the apex and form a space infection in the adjacent soft tissues. The space abscess will be painful, and the surface of the skin or mucosa over the abscess will feel warm and rubbery to palpation and will demonstrate fluctuance. The systemic temperature may be elevated. Aspiration will usually produce yellowish pus. Regional lymph nodes may become enlarged and painful.

Serial, total, and differential leukocyte counts are valuable in determining the course and nature of the infection. If circumstances are unfavorable, such as lowered host resistance combined with virulent multiplying organisms and inadequate early treatment, serious complications may ensue—osteomyelitis, septicemia, septic emboli, asphyxia from a Ludwig's angina or other space infection that compromises the airway, cavernous sinus thrombosis—any of which could be fatal.

A chronic infection will ensue when the virulence and number of the organisms are low and the host resistance is high. If untreated, the chronic abscess will frequently form a sinus tract, permitting the pus to drain to the surface. A small proliferation of granulomatous tissue often forms on the surface and is referred to as a parulis (Fig. 16-15, *C*).

When drainage is established, the tooth and

associated swelling are no longer painful since the pain-producing pressure of the abscess is reduced.

DIFFERENTIAL DIAGNOSIS

When a painful fluctuant swelling is present, there is little question that the diagnosis is *abscess*. When the abscess is determined to be of the secondary type, however, the original periapical lesion may not be easy to identify. Actually such an identification is often impossible because the histomorphology has been destroyed by the infection.

If the abscess is a sequela of pulpitis, whether it was a cyst, granuloma, scar, or cholesteatoma is not of practical concern; but the clinician must always be alert to the possibility that the apical radiolucency might be either a *secondarily infected primary* or a *secondary malignant tumor*.

In addition, any of the nonodontogenic cysts (e.g., incisive canal, globulomaxillary, median) may become infected and be projected radiographically over the apices of teeth with vital pulps, simulating an infected *radicular cyst*. Thus teeth could be unnecessarily compromised if the clinician fails to recognize this possibility and to establish the exact location of the radiolucency in question.

It is also necessary to consider the fact that all abscesses involving teeth are not of pulpal origin. The *periodontal abscess,* originating in a deep periodontal pocket, is a common lesion and can be distinguished from the incited periapical abscess by proper radiographic procedures showing the absence of a periapical radiolucency and usually the presence of a periodontal pocket. In addition, the pulps of teeth with such periodontal abscesses are almost always vital.

MANAGEMENT

The acute abscess should be treated aggressively to alleviate the patient's pain and to ensure that untoward sequelae do not occur. In our opinion it is better to immediately establish drainage if possible since this will speed the resolution of the abscess.

Drainage may be established in some cases by opening the pulp chamber and passing a file through the canal into the periapical region. When drainage cannot be established in this manner, a trephination procedure is indicated; that is, an opening is made through the mucosa and bone to the abscess at the apex. When a vestibular palatal or lingual space abscess has

formed, a through-and-through drain* may be placed in the abscess and frequently irrigated with a solution of hydrogen peroxide and saline.

A sample of pus should be obtained for culture and sensitivity tests. In more severe cases penicillin therapy should be instituted immediately (not less than 500 mg q.i.d. for at least 5 days) since many of the microorganisms responsible for odontogenic infections are sensitive to penicillin (if the infection is not by one of the resistant strains indigenous to many hospitals). Nevertheless, before the antibiotic therapy is initiated, the patient must be questioned to determine whether he is allergic to penicillin; and if he is or if there is some question that he might be, then erythromycin should be substituted. Later the type and dosage of antibiotic may be tailored as indicated by the results of the culture and sensitivity tests.

It is generally deemed unwise to extract a severely abscessed tooth (especially if much surgical manipulation will be required) unless the patient has been adequately treated with antibiotics to ensure an effective blood level that will protect against the bacterial shower in the circulation produced by surgical manipulation in an abscessed area.

Patients with severe abscesses are frequently discovered to have a decreased resistance caused by a debilitating systemic disease, such as diabetes. Thus it is mandatory to effect a good medical evaluation, including the history and a physical and laboratory examination of the patient. If an underlying systemic disease is found, the patient's physician can undertake treatment of the concomitant medical problem—thus increasing the patient's resistance and aiding in the management of the abscess.

If it is advantageous to retain the offending tooth once the acute phase of the infection has been controlled, then routine endodontic treatment may be performed with or without a root resection.

When there is a chronic abscess with a draining sinus, the exact origin of the abscess must be located. This can usually be accomplished by inserting a gutta-percha cone to the extent of the sinus and making a radiograph of the area. The image of the cone will be pointing to the abscess. The procedure may not only direct attention to

---

*An appliance of nonabsorbent material, such as a perforated tube or strip of rubber dam material, is passed through the abscess to maintain a passage for irrigation by injecting fluid into one opening and letting it escape through another.

Fig. 16-16. Periapical surgical defects.

the offending tooth but also demonstrate whether the abscess is of pulpal or periodontal origin. Sinus defects usually close when the infection has been eradicated and the root canals properly obliterated. These treated teeth must be radiographically reexamined at 6-month intervals to ascertain that the periapical radiolucency is regressing, because treatment with apparent healing does not provide a definite diagnosis of the original periapical lesion.

Surgical defect

A surgical defect in bone is an area that fails to fill in with osseous tissue after surgery. It is frequently seen periapically after root resection procedures, especially when both labial and lingual plates have been destroyed. Approximately 45% of all periapical radiolucencies treated surgically require from 1 to 10 years for complete resolution, and another 30% take longer than 10 years. In the remaining 25%, the surgical defects resulting from root resection procedures, complete healing does not occur. The post–root resection defect represents an area where the cortical plate is entirely lacking.* There may also be a periapical scar present in addition to the defect in the cortical plate.

FEATURES

The periapical radiolucency produced by a surgical defect is rounded in appearance and smoothly contoured, and it has well-defined borders. It accounts for about 3% of all the periapical radiolucencies. It usually does not measure more than 1 cm in diameter and is frequently smaller. The radiolucent shadow may be projected directly over the apex or a few millimeters beyond the apex of the resected root of the endodontically treated tooth (Fig. 16-16). If a time-sequence series of radiographs is available, from the time of the resection, the radiolucency will usually show a decrease in size. Frequently it will resolve to a certain size and then remain constant.

---

*This circumstance is illustrated by the radiographic examination of experimental bone destruction. Bone loss in the mandible is difficult to detect radiographically unless the lingual or buccal cortical bone is eroded or destroyed. Even though the entire cancellous portion of the mandible is removed, radiographs of the area do not demonstrate any change unless at least the junctional trabeculae on the cortical plates are removed (Bender, 1961; Ramadan and Mitchell, 1961). More recently, however, Shoha and co-workers (1974) have shown that in the premolar region (more than in the molar region) radiographic change cannot be detected without involvement of the junctional or cortical bone.

The tooth and periapical area will be completely asymptomatic. A careful clinical examination may reveal the mucosal scar from the previous surgery. If the defect is large enough, it may be detected by palpation.

DIFFERENTIAL DIAGNOSIS

The periapical radiolucency produced by a surgical defect may be confused with any of the periapical lesions included in this chapter, especially the granuloma, radicular cyst, secondary abscess, and periapical scar.

The entity most likely to be confused with the surgical defect is the *periapical scar*. The periapical scar, however, would not be displaced from the apex by radiographic localization techniques.

A history of root resection combined with the radiographic appearance of a resected asymptomatic endodontically treated tooth containing a well-defined periapical radiolucency not larger than 1 cm and a small depression in the mucosa over the apical area will alert the clinician to the probability that the lesion is not an *abscess, cyst, or granuloma*.

If changing the angle of the beam shifts the radiolucent shadow about in the periapical area, this can be taken as additional presumptive evidence that the entity in question is not at the periapex but rather is in the cortical plate. If the shadow is caused by a surgical defect, it should show a reduction in size as it is periodically reexamined, especially during the first 6 months after surgery.

MANAGEMENT

Correct identification and periodic surveillance with radiographs are required for the management of periapical surgical defects.

Cholesteatoma

The cholesteatoma accounts for less than 1% of all periapical pathologic radiolucencies. It commences with the formation of a few localized cholesterol crystals, which form as a result of fatty degeneration in a dental granuloma or within the wall of a radicular cyst. Although these localized accumulations of cholesterol crystals commonly occur in dental granulomas and radicular cysts, sometimes the formation of cholesterol is so outstanding that the majority of the lesion is composed of cholesterol crystals and the lesion is referred to as a cholesteatoma.

Several authors consider the term "cholesteatoma" to be inappropriate for oral lesions, but its descriptive value in this setting would appear to justify its application here.

FEATURES

The history and the clinical and radiographic features of the cholesteatoma are similar to those of the dental granuloma and radicular cyst (Fig. 16-17). Occasionally the radiolucent image of the cholesteatoma appears somewhat less distinct and cloudy because of the increased density of the accumulated cholesterol crystals. Microscopically excessively large and numerous cholesterol clefts are seen. The clefts contain cholesterol crystals that are dissolved and removed during the tissue processing. Varying amounts of granulation tissue, chronic inflammatory cells, and foreign body giant cells are found surrounding the clefts. If the lesion commenced as a cyst, seg-

ments of the epithelial lining may still be present (Fig. 16-17).

DIFFERENTIAL DIAGNOSIS

Except for the occasionally detectable increase in radiographic density, the differential diagnosis of the periapical cholesteatoma is similar to that discussed for the *dental granuloma* and *radicular cyst*. Clinical differentiation is usually not possible.

MANAGEMENT

The rationale and resulting management of the cholesteatoma are the same as those for granulomas and cysts.

Fig. 16-17. Periapical cholesteatoma. **B** and **C,** Histopathology.

Osteomyelitis

Occasionally a periapical abscess will develop into an acute or chronic osteomyelitis, especially in patients who have an underlying systemic disease that has depressed their systemic resistance or who have received large doses of radiation therapy to the jaws. Osteomyelitis is defined as an infection of bone that involves all three components: periosteum, cortex, and marrow. On this basis, the periapical abscess can be considered a localized type of osteomyelitis (Chapter 20).

Although the terms "osteomyelitis" and "osteitis" are often used interchangeably, the latter actually describes the more localized condition and the former describes the more active diffuse conditions. We believe this distinction of nomenclature should be made because, although the pathologic processes may be fundamentally similar, there are clinical and radiographic differences between the entities and a difference in the regions of the jaw involved. Furthermore, the differences in the architecture, circulation, and character of the marrow between the alveolus and the body of the jawbone are apparently responsible for the usual localized restricted nature of the osteitis—in contrast to the diffuse almost unrestricted spread of the infection through the medullary spaces of the jawbone in an osteomyelitis. Differing responses to treatment also aid in the delineation of the two entities: an osteitis may be readily managed whereas an osteomyelitis often proves difficult to eradicate. Inasmuch as osteomyelitis is discussed in detail in Chapter 20, only a brief description in relation to periapical radiolucencies will be presented here.

Acute osteomyelitis is similar to an acute primary alveolar abscess since the onset and course may be so rapid that bone resorption does not occur and thus a radiolucency may not be present. Chronic osteomyelitis, on the other hand, represents a low-grade infection of bone, which if untreated follows a protracted course of bone destruction and produces a radiolucent lesion. Chronic osteomyelitis may demonstrate four distinct radiographic pictures: completely radiolucent, mixed radiolucent and radiopaque, completely radiopaque, and Garré's. This last can be recognized as a somewhat opaque layering of the periosteum, with bone proliferating peripherally. In the present discussion only the chronic destructive type, causing a periapical radiolucency, is considered.

FEATURES

Osteomyelitis is seldom observed in the maxilla, probably because of the comparatively rich blood supply; but when it does occur, it may be a much more fulminating infection than in the mandible, where it occurs predominantly.

The exciting tooth will usually contain a nonvital pulp, may be sensitive to percussion, and may have been previously associated with an acute or chronic periapical abscess. There will be a periapical radiolucency—somewhat rounded in shape—resembling the image seen in a periapical cyst, granuloma, or abscess. Frequently, however, the borders of the radiolucency will be poorly defined and ragged in contour (Fig. 16-18). Such an appearance is characteristic of infections in bone and results from the irregular extensions

Fig. 16-18. Chronic osteomyelitis. **A,** Note the radiolucencies around the roots of the first molar. **B,** Sinus draining extraorally. **C,** Note the nonvital bony trabeculae (empty lacunae), the inflammatory infiltrate, and the necrotic material. (**A** courtesy R. Moncada, M.D., Maywood, Ill.)

of the inflammation through marrow spaces and channels in the bone.

The bony course of a draining tract traversing the body of the jawbone may be seen as a radiolucent band from the periapical radiolucency through the cortical plate beneath the sinus opening on the mucosa or skin (Fig. 16-18). The course of this tract will be deeper or longer than that seen with a pointed chronic alveolar abscess since it will be traversing the body of the jaw in contrast to the shorter course through the alveolar process characteristic of the draining restricted alveolar process.

If a sequestrum (segment of dead bone) is present and large enough, it will show as a radiopacity within a radiolucency. The patient will complain of malaise and may have a fever, and there will be a concomitant swelling on the bone and mucosa around the osteomyelitis that may vary from slight to moderate. The swelling will be firm, painful, and hot to palpation; and pressure on the swelling or tooth may cause pus to be discharged from the sinus opening. Cultures of the purulent drainage will usually demonstrate varieties of streptococci or staphylococci.

Microscopically the picture will be identical with that produced by a chronic alveolar abscess: necrotic tissue containing polymorphonuclear leukocytes and also regions of granulation tissue. More dead bone (spicules with empty lacunae) will be seen in osteomyelitis than in a chronic alveolar abscess (Fig. 16-18). Although such spicules may be found in the radiolucent lesions, they are not large enough to show on the radiographs.

DIFFERENTIAL DIAGNOSIS

The entities that should be included in the differential diagnosis are osteomyelitis, chronic alveolar abscess, an infected malignant tumor, Paget's disease complicated with osteomyelitis, and eosinophilic granuloma. If the draining sinus involves the body of the jawbone and courses through the marrow, then the prognosis for the lesion is less favorable than for a chronic alveolar abscess.

If the area of bone destruction is large and the region not painful, then *eosinophilic granuloma* must be considered. A biopsy will establish the final diagnosis.

An *osteomyelitis superimposed on a malignant tumor* of bone may completely disguise the more serious lesion, which becomes apparent again only after successful treatment of the osteomyelitis. Thus valuable time may be lost in the treatment of the malignancy. Since the concomitant occurrence of an osteomyelitis and a malignancy of bone is not common, such an entity would be assigned a low ranking in the differential diagnosis.

The suspicion that a lesion may be an osteomyelitis can be qualified in light of the following circumstances:

1. If only the alveolar portion of the jawbone is infected, the diagnosis is *alveolar abscess*.
2. On the other hand, if the tooth suspected of precipitating the condition is in a fracture line, the diagnosis of *chronic osteomyelitis* is strengthened.* This diagnosis is also supported if an accompanying uncontrolled systemic disease such as diabetes is present.
3. Also an attending bone disease, such as *Paget's disease,* or previous radiation therapy—along with some pathognomonic symptoms of infection—would tend to strengthen the impression of osteomyelitis. Paget's disease would be evident when several bones were found to have the classic cotton-wool appearance.

When considering Paget's disease, the clinician must remember that there is an increased incidence of osteosarcoma in this disease and the radiographic appearance of the disease and osteogenic sarcoma can be confused with that of chronic sclerosing osteomyelitis.

MANAGEMENT

The management of osteomyelitis is discussed in detail in Chapter 20. The clinician must predicate any treatment he may be inclined to administer on the premise that the patient has an uncontrolled systemic disease so the osteomyelitis may be difficult to eliminate. Usually the best treatment will be to extract the offending tooth rather than attempt to conserve it by endodontic procedures.

DENTIGEROUS CYST

Although a dentigerous cyst may form adjacent to the crown of an unerupted tooth, sometimes the position of the crown of the involved tooth and the extension of the cyst will be such that the pericoronal radiolucency is projected over the apex of a neighboring tooth (Fig. 16-19, *A*). On rare occasion the radiolucency will be projected over the apex of the same tooth especially in cases

---

*The occurrence of teeth in the fracture line and the failure to remove them in patients with poor oral hygiene may cause complications in the management of jaw fractures.

Fig. 16-19. Dentigerous cysts seen as periapical radiolucencies. **A,** The pulps of the canine and first premolar tooth tested vital. **B,** Unusual radiographic shadow of a circumferential dentigerous cyst, which gives the illusion that the cyst is associated with the root rather than the crown. (**B** couresty R. Latronica, D.D.S., Albany, N.Y.)

of a circumferential or lateral dentigerous cyst (Fig. 16-19, *B*). In such situations whether the radiolucency is pericoronal or periapical may not be immediately apparent; and the confusion will be compounded if the tooth over whose apex the image of the follicular cyst is cast has a nonvital pulp. Dentigerous cysts are discussed in detail in Chapter 17.

PERIAPICAL CEMENTOMAS

The periapical cementomas, cementifying and/or ossifying fibromas, and benign cementoblastomas arise from elements in the periodontal ligament. As a result an increasing number of oral pathologists currently consider these lesions to be related. Within the versatile periodontal ligament are mature osteoblasts and cementoblasts as well as precursor cells possessing the capacity to form cementum, alveolar bone, or fibrous tissue.

Periapical cementomas are by far the most common of this group of lesions and have been called many names: periapical cemental dysplasia, periapical osteofibroma, and periapical osteofibrosis. Periapical cementomas are thought to arise on a reactive basis rather than on a neoplastic basis like their "cousins," the cementifying and ossifying fibromas.

These periapical lesions have three stages in their development, which are radiographically apparent:

1. The early (osteolytic or fibroblastic) stage is radiolucent; and the microstructure consists chiefly of a cellular fibroblastic stroma that may contain a few very small foci of calcified material (Fig. 16-20).

2. As these lesions mature, they pass through an intermediate stage, which is indicated by a radiolucent area containing radiopaque foci.

3. The third and final stage is referred to as the mature lesion; the cementoma has become almost completely calcified and appears as a well-defined solid rather homogeneous radiopacity surrounded in most cases by a thin radiolucent border.

The calcified material in periapical lesions may seem to be entirely cementum, both cementum and bone, or all bone; however, to differentiate between cementum and bone by routine microscopic techniques is usually quite difficult if not impossible. It has been suggested that such distinction can be made by means of polarizing microscopy on the basis that the patterns of cemental fibers are distinctive from those of bone (Waldron and Giansanti, 1973).

In this chapter, which deals with the periapical radiolucencies, only the osteolytic (fibroblastic)

Fig. 16-20. Periapical cementomas (early stage). **A** to **D,** All incisors were vital and all patients were over 30 years of age.

or radiolucent stage of the lesion will be discussed.

FEATURES

In the early stage of development, the periapical cementomas occur as radiolucencies that are usually somewhat rounded, have well-defined borders, and are associated with teeth having vital pulps (Fig. 16-20). Blacks are more com-

monly affected than whites; and 80% of the lesions occur in women. The lesions are seldom seen before the fourth decade of life.

Although any tooth may be affected, approximately 90% of periapical cementomas occur in the mandible, where the periapical region of the incisors is the most frequently involved site. The lesions may be solitary or multiple, are completely asymptomatic, and seldom exceed 1 cm in diam-

Fig. 16-20, cont'd. E, Photomicrograph of an early cementoma showing a few small droplets of cementum in a fibroblastic field.

eter. It is unusual for a periapical cementoma to become large enough to produce a detectable expansion of the cortical plate.

DIFFERENTIAL DIAGNOSIS

The osteolytic or early stage of the periapical cementoma could be confused with the periapical radiolucencies that are related to pulpal disease, and the unalert clinician might needlessly extract or institute endodontic treatment on a tooth with a normal pulp. There is little excuse for this type of error, however, because the lesions can usually be readily recognized.

The cementoma is totally asymptomatic, the pulp of the involved tooth is usually vital, and the lesion most frequently affects the mandibular incisors. These features are in contrast to those of a *pulpoperiapical lesion,* which is associated with pulp disease or pulp death in a tooth that is frequently (or has been) sensitive to pressure or percussion or both. The two lesions cannot be differentiated radiographically while the cementoma is at the radiolucent stage. In some instances, however, although not always, the apex of a tooth with a cementoma will give the appearance of having been sharpened in a pencil sharpener (Fig. 16-20, *C*).

A *traumatic bone cyst* may be projected over the apex of a tooth with a vital pulp and may be confused with a periapical cementoma; but it is usually much larger and is characteristically

found in a younger age group. If its identity is in doubt, however, radiographs taken at a later date will reveal the developing calcifying foci within the radiolucency if the lesion is a cementoma. In the intermediate stage differentiating the cementoma from pulpoperiapical pathosis is also easier because of the radiopaque areas present at this time within the radiolucent area.

The *cementoblastoma* in its early stage may also be confused with an early cementoma; but the former is a rare lesion that occurs almost exclusively at the periapices of the mandibular molars (Fig. 16-28, *C*). Furthermore, it characteristically extends higher on the root.

MANAGEMENT

Once the clinician has established a working diagnosis of periapical cementoma, it is sufficient to observe the lesion radiographically. In the rare instance in which a cementoma reaches a sufficient size to expand the cortical plate and become infected because of ulceration of the mucosa, the lesion must be enucleated surgically and the material examined microscopically.

The development of a cementoma is not apparently related to the condition of the pulp; and although the entity classically occurs at the apex of a vital tooth, this does not preclude the subsequent or concomitant development of a gangrenous pulp and an inflammatory reaction attending a cementoma. Such a case could present a confusing diagnostic problem; but the significance of such an episode would be only academic since treatment would necessarily be directed at the inflammatory process. Conservative endodontic intervention would be the initial choice of treatment in such a case.

PERIODONTAL DISEASE

As stated in the preface, a discussion of periodontal disease is not within the purview of this text. Nevertheless, periodontal disease must be considered here because it occasions a relatively common periapical radiolucency. Such a radiolucency is usually caused by advanced periodontal bone loss involving one tooth much more severely than teeth immediately adjacent. The entire bony support of the involved tooth may be completely destroyed and the tooth appear to be floating in a radiolucency (Fig. 16-21). Sometimes a narrow vertical pocket will extend to the apex and appear to be a fairly well-defined periapical radiolucency, which in one projection will seem to be completely surrounded by bone (Fig. 16-21). Brynolf (1978) described specific characteristics that she considered useful in differentiating between periodontal disease–produced periapical radiolucencies and pulpoperiapical radiolucencies. However, these findings remain to be substantiated by other investigators.

This situation may lead the unwary clinician to a false conclusion of pulpoperiapical pathosis if the diagnosis is not based on clinical as well as radiographic evidence. A misdiagnosis of the condition can usually be obviated by a clinical examination of the supporting structures through identifying and probing all periodontal pockets. Pocket depth relative to the root length of associated teeth can be demonstrated by placing gutta-percha points in the pockets to their full depths and then taking a radiograph of the area with the points in place.

Teeth with advanced periodontal destruction are usually quite mobile and sensitive to percussion; but surprisingly many remain vital, and the demonstration of such vitality will aid the clinician in determining the correct diagnosis.

Extraction of the tooth is the indicated treatment. The soft tissue must be curetted from the region of the apex and sent for microscopic examination to establish the final diagnosis and rule out the more serious diseases that can cause a similar pattern of bone loss.

TRAUMATIC BONE CYST

Although the traumatic bone cyst (hemorrhagic bone cyst, extravasation cyst, simple bone cyst, solitary bone cyst, progressive bony cyst, blood cyst) is discussed in detail in Chapter 18, it should also be included in this series since it may present a difficult diagnostic problem when it occurs as a periapical radiolucency. The traumatic bone cyst is classified as a false cyst of bone because it does not have an epithelial lining. Its cause has not been definitely established although some authors favor trauma as the provoking factor.

Fig. 16-21. Periodontal disease. Periapical radiolucencies caused by periodontal disease. The teeth tested vital.

FEATURES

A history of trauma may or may not be elicited. The lesion is usually discovered on routine radiographs and is asymptomatic except when it occasionally reaches a size sufficient to cause expansion of the jaw. In such instances cortical plates are expanded rather than eroded and this produces a bony hard bulge on the jaw. Sometimes the lesion will involve half the mandible. The mandible is involved much more frequently than the maxilla. The premolar-molar region is the most common location, but the symphysis is also involved with some frequency (Fig. 16-22).

Teeth involved with this type of periapical radiolucency are vital, and the lamina dura is intact. Tipping, migration of teeth, and root resorption are not features. Traumatic bone cysts are usually found in patients under 25 years of age.

Radiographically a traumatic bone cyst is a well-defined (cystlike) radiolucency above the mandibular canal either predominantly round and positioned somewhat symmetrically about the periapex of a root (Fig. 16-22) or more elongated and oriented in a mesiodistal direction extending superiorly between the premolar and molar roots and producing a scalloped appearance. The lateral and inferior borders of the elongated variety have smooth regular contours (Fig. 16-22).

Aspiration will usually be fruitless, but in some cases serosanguineous fluid or even a small quantity of blood may be obtained. At surgery scanty tissue may be found, which on microscopic examination proves to be loose or dense fibrous connective tissue containing some hemosiderin.

DIFFERENTIAL DIAGNOSIS

The traumatic bone cyst that is projected around and between the roots of teeth is most frequently mistaken for a *radicular cyst*. The fact that the pulps of the associated teeth are vital in traumatic bone cysts, however, makes the distinction between the two entities clear-cut in most cases.

Differentiating between a periapical traumatic bone cyst and a relatively large early-stage *periapical cementoma* may pose a diagnostic problem, since the pulps of the associated teeth in both cases should be vital (barring a concomitant nonrelated pulpal problem). In distinguishing between these two, the clinician can take a clue from the size of the lesion: the periapical cementoma is seldom more than 0.7 cm in diameter whereas the traumatic bone cyst is usually

Fig. 16-22. Traumatic bone cyst. All teeth tested vital. (**B** courtesy M. Kaminski, D.D.S., Chicago.)

larger than 1 cm. Also the traumatic bone cyst usually occurs in individuals under 25 years of age whereas the cementoma is seen in patients over 30 years of age. Periodic radiographs will show the maturation changes of the radiolucent cementoma—through the mixed radiopaque-radiolucent stage to the mature radiopaque stage—and thus permit the identification of the lesion as a cementoma.

A traumatic bone cyst may also be confused with the rare *median mandibular cyst*. Both entities have similar features. The surrounding teeth have vital pulps. Both can occur in this region and both may project between the teeth, although the median mandibular cyst will frequently cause a separation of the teeth whereas the traumatic bone cyst will not. Both are usually asymptomatic. Even though expansion of the cortical plates is an unusual finding in either case, such a deformity is even less common in the traumatic bone cyst. Aspiration may produce similar and confusing results.

When the characteristics of a lesion in the symphysis of the mandible do not tend to delineate one lesion or the other and establishing a priority between the entities is difficult, the traumatic bone cyst should be given a higher ranking since the mandibular developmental cyst is quite rare. The microscopic examination of surgical specimens from a median mandibular cyst would reveal a substantial cyst wall lined with epithelium whereas the tissue from a traumatic bone cyst would consist of only a few strands of connective tissue.

MANAGEMENT

In our opinion the traumatic bone cyst cannot be positively identified on the basis of the patient's history and the clinical and radiographic features alone. Thus we do not recommend that a lesion suspected of being a traumatic bone cyst be managed by periodic radiographic examination. This contention is based on the possibility that such a cystlike radiolucency could represent many types of serious pathosis so a final definite diagnosis must be established. In addition, if the radiolucency has reached a fair size, it will predispose the jaw to pathologic fracture.

The treatment of choice is to open the area surgically, establish a diagnosis of traumatic bone cyst, remove the tissue debris present, curette the walls of the bony cavity to induce bleeding, and close the soft tissue flap securely. The patient should be protected with antibiotics since the clinician has in effect produced an intrabony hematoma. This mode of treatment has proved to be quite successful, with bone filling the defect after the clot has organized.

An alternate method of treatment has been suggested when the clinician is confident of his diagnosis; it involves injecting venous blood into the bony defect. Although good results have been obtained, a serious objection to this injection technique is that it precludes establishing a firm diagnosis. Consequently the clinician may discover in periodic radiographic follow-up examinations that the radiolucency is not resolving subsequent to the injections but rather is expanding. In such instances he may have lost valuable time for the treatment of a more serious lesion.

NONRADICULAR CYSTS

On occasion nonradicular cysts may be projected over the apices of teeth. Their description is thus appropriate in a discussion of periapical radiolucencies.

The following cysts are the most common offenders: incisive canal cyst, midpalatal cyst, median mandibular cyst (refer to foregoing discussion of traumatic bone cyst), and primordial cyst (Fig. 16-23). With the exception of primordial cysts, these occur in specific regions of the jawbones. In general, they must be differentiated from anatomic shadows, radicular cysts, periapical granulomas, traumatic bone cysts, early cementomas, and other less common entities.

Changing the angle at which the radiograph is taken will frequently project the radiolucent image of the nonodontogenic cyst away from the apices that may be superimposed over it, and this will differentiate the nonodontogenic from the radicular cyst and from the dental granuloma or other pulpoperiapical lesions. Also the teeth seemingly associated with these nonradicular cysts will usually be vital.

DIFFERENTIAL DIAGNOSIS

If a 2 cm cystlike radiolucency is present over the apex of a vital maxillary incisor and can be projected away from the apex by changing the horizontal angle at which a second radiograph is taken, then the most likely diagnosis for the lesion is *incisive canal cyst*.

If a cystic area at the periapex of a maxillary first molar on a periapical film is shown on an occlusal film to involve the whole palate and if all the maxillary teeth are vital, then the most appropriate diagnosis is *midpalatal cyst*.

MALIGNANT TUMORS

Malignant tumors may be found as a single periapical radiolucency mimicking a more com-

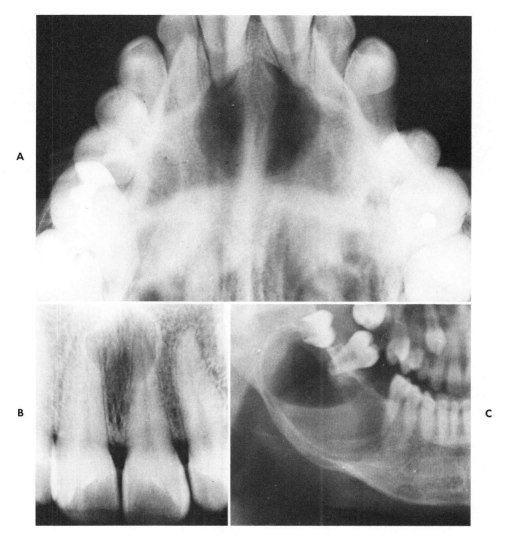

Fig. 16-23. Nonradicular cyst. **A** and **B,** Incisive canal cysts. **C,** Primordial cyst. (Courtesy N. Barakat, D.D.S., Beirut, Lebanon.)

mon benign lesion. This is a fact that unfortunately the clinician sometimes ignores. Malignant tumors may be either primary or secondary. Primary malignancies that cause radiolucent lesions are discussed in detail in Chapter 20. Metastatic tumors of the jaws often produce a variable radiographic appearance, and those that resemble benign conditions most often escape early diagnosis.

The discussion of malignant tumors will be limited to their appearance as periapical radiolucencies. The most commonly occurring malignancies producing this image are the squamous cell carcinoma, malignant tumor of the minor salivary glands, (Figs. 16-24 and 16-25), metastatic tumors, osteolytic sarcoma, chondrosarcoma, melanoma, fibrosarcoma, reticulum cell sarcoma, and multiple myeloma.

Secondary tumors metastasizing to the jaws include malignant tumors of the lungs, the gastrointestinal tract, the breasts, the prostate and thyroid glands, and the kidneys.

Malignant tumors (e.g., the squamous cell carcinoma, the malignant salivary gland tumor originating on or in the surface mucosa) usually erode much alveolar crest bone before they arrive at the apex, so they generally do not produce an isolated periapical radiolucency. Rather, the apical area of the tooth will be included in a large radiolucency with ragged borders, represent-

Fig. 16-24. Periapical radiographs showing bony destruction and periapical radiolucencies at the apices of the premolar and molar teeth all caused by squamous cell carcinoma of the maxillary sinus. (Courtesy R. Copeland, D.D.S., Libertyville, Ill.)

Fig. 16-25. Adenoid cystic carcinoma. **A,** Periapical radiograph showing the existing periapical radiolucency prior to endodontic treatment. **B,** Periapical radiograph taken 4 months later showing enlargement of the radiolucency. Surgery and microscopic study established the diagnosis. (From Burkes, J.: J. Endodont. **1:**76-78, 1975. Copyright by the American Dental Association. Reprinted by permission.)

ing a large area of bone destruction (Fig. 16-26). On the other hand, a low-grade slow-growing malignant salivary gland tumor that has destroyed some cortical bone may project over the periapex as a rather discrete well-defined radiolucency. Mesenchymal malignant tumors and metastatic tumors originating within bone are more apt to produce a more localized periapical radiolucency than a peripheral squamous cell carcinoma, which almost always originates in the surface and erodes through the alveolar bone to arrive at the apex. However, a squamous cell carcinoma originating within a cyst could be seen as a localized periapical radiolucency.

In summary, malignant periapical radiolucen-cies may be indicated by any one of the following images:

1. A well-defined periapical radiolucency
2. A poorly defined periapical radiolucency
3. A large ragged well-defined radiolucent tumor that has destroyed a large segment of the surface bone and has involved the apex of a tooth

Root resorption may be a feature accompanying any of the three images.

FEATURES

The signs and symptoms of most malignancies of the oral cavity and jaws have much in common. The age range in which these tumors occur

Fig. 16-26. Malignant periapical radiolucencies. **A,** Chondrosarcoma. **B** and **C,** Osteogenic sarcoma. (Note the bandlike widening of the periodontal ligament spaces around the incisor roots in **B.**) **D,** Adenoid cystic carcinoma on the posterolateral hard palate. **E,** Metastatic carcinoma from the pancreas.   *Continued.*

includes the young, the middle-aged, and the old. Pain may or may not be a feature. The involved teeth may retain their vitality. If the tumor is advanced, there may be migration, loosening, tipping, and spreading of teeth. There may also be gingival bleeding. Paresthesia or anesthesia of the soft tissues is sometimes present.

Expansion of the jaw is a feature in advanced lesions. With the exception of squamous cell carcinoma, at first this expansion has a smooth surface covered with normal-appearing mucosa. Later in the course of the tumor's growth, the mucosa breaks down because of chronic trauma, ulcerates, and then develops into a fulminating necrotic growth of tissue because the surface is continually traumatized.

DIFFERENTIAL DIAGNOSIS

The advanced lesions are readily recognized as malignancies, so a differential diagnosis is not so important in these cases—except as it may help to arrive at a definitive diagnosis. The earlier lesions, however, do present a problem because they may mimic the benign conditions just discussed; and, unless other subtle telltale symptoms are recognized, the clinician will not be alerted to the seriousness of the case.

A well-defined rounded radiolucency produced by a malignant tumor may resemble a *radicular cyst, granuloma, scar, cholesteatoma, cementoma,* or *traumatic bone cyst,* whereas an ill-defined periapical radiolucency will resemble a *chronic alveolar abscess* or an *osteomyelitis* (radiolucent type). The diagnostic problem blends with the philosophy of treatment of all periapical radiolucencies.

MANAGEMENT

Fortunately two basic principles are employed by clinicians who manage periapical radiolucencies:

First, if the lesion and tooth are treated with conservative endodontics only, the tooth and the area in question are observed with periodic

Fig. 16-26, cont'd. F, Hemangiosarcoma. Note the radiolucencies at the apices of the molar and the bandlike widening of the periodontal ligament spaces on all teeth shown. **G,** Metastatic rhabdomyosarcoma at the periapex of a molar. **H,** Metastatic carcinoma at the apices of the central incisors. (**A** courtesy O. H. Stuteville, D.D.S., M.D., St. Joe, Ark. **B** and **G** courtesy R. Goepp, D.D.S., Zoller Clinic, University of Chicago. **C** from Curtis, M.: J. Oral Surg. **32:**125-130, 1974. Copyright by the American Dental Association. Reprinted by permission. **F** courtesy D. Skuble, D.D.S., Maywood, Ill. **H** courtesy R. Oglesby, D.D.S., Chicago.)

clinical and radiographic examination. Thus if a small malignant periapical radiolucency has been misdiagnosed and treated as a pulpal sequela, this error will soon become apparent as a result of the clinician's continued surveillance.

Second, if the clinician chooses to do a root resection in addition to the root canal filling, the tissue he recovers from the periapex is routinely sent for microscopic study. Thus the malignancy will be diagnosed immediately and the more extensive procedures such as surgical resection, radiation, and/or antitumor medication may be instituted at the discretion of the local tumor board.

RARITIES

The following list, although not complete, includes pathologic entities that at times occur as periapical radiolucencies. Thus the clinician must be aware that even though these lesions are either rare or rarely present primarily as peri-

apical radiolucencies a specific lesion under study could indeed be one of them:

    Ameloblastic variants
    Ameloblastoma
    Aneurysmal bone cyst
    Benign nonodontogenic tumor
    Cementifying and ossifying fibroma
    Cementoblastoma—early stage
    Gaucher's disease
    Giant cell granuloma
    Giant cell lesion of hyperparathyroidism
    Histiocytosis X
    Lingual salivary gland depression
    Odontoma—early stage
    Osteoblastoma—early stage
    Solitary and multiple myeloma

Specific points obtained from the patient's history or by clinical, radiographic, or laboratory examination would presumably direct the examiner to the lesion most likely responsible for the patient's periapical radiolucency (Figs. 16-27 to 16-29).

Fig. 16-27. Rare periapical radiolucencies. **A** to **C,** Giant cell granuloma involving teeth that were vital. **D** and **E,** Ameloblastoma. **F** and **G,** Histiocytosis X. (**F,** Radiolucency at the apex of the lateral incisor and canine in an adult patient; **G,** three periapical radiolucent lesions [arrows] in a 14-year-old boy.) **H,** Periapical lesion in a 62-year-old woman with multiple myeloma. The lesions in myeloma usually have smoother contours than shown. (**A** courtesy N. Barakat, D.D.S., Beirut, Lebanon. **B** and **F** courtesy R. Goepp, D.D.S., Zoller Clinic, University of Chicago. **C** courtesy J. Ireland, D.D.S., and J. Dolci, D.D.S., Mundelein, Ill. **D** courtesy P. Akers, D.D.S., Chicago. **E** courtesy O. H. Stuteville, D.D.S., M.D., St. Joe, Ark.) *Continued.*

Fig. 16-27, cont'd. For legend see p. 341.

Fig. 16-28. Uncommon or rare benign fibro-osseous lesions of periodontal origin. **A,** Ossifying fibroma at apex of a vital mandibular canine tooth. **B,** Radiograph taken 9 months after root canal therapy, root resection, and enucleation of the lesion. **C,** Cementoblastoma in the early radiolucent stage associated with the root of an unerupted third molar tooth. Note that the lesion is in contact with a considerable length of the root. Periapical cementomas seldom extend to this extent in a cervical direction. (**A** and **B** courtesy N. Barakat, D.D.S., Beirut, Lebanon. **C** courtesy P. Pullen, D.D.S., St. Louis.)

Fig. 16-29. Periapical radiograph showing well-defined radiolucency projected over the apex of the mandibular canine tooth. This radiolucency was produced by an anterior lingual mandibular bone concavity. (From Connor, M. S.: Oral Surg. **48:**413-414, 1979.)

SPECIFIC REFERENCES

Arwill, R., Persson, G., and Thilander, H.: The microscopic appearance of the periapical tissue in cases classified as "uncertain" or "unsuccessful" after apiectomy, Odontol. Revy **25:**27-42, 1974.

Bender, I. B.: Roentgenographic and direct observation of experimental lesions in bone. I, J. Am. Dent. Assoc. **62:**152-160, 709-716, 1961.

Block, R. M., Bushell, A. Rodridgues, H., and Langeland, K.: A histopathologic, histobacteriologic, and radiographic study of periapical endodontic surgical specimens, Oral Surg. **42:** 656-678, 1976.

Brynolf, I.: Radiography of the periapical region as a diagnostic aid. I. Diagnosis of marginal changes, Dent. Radiogr. Photogr. **51:**21-39, 1978.

Connor, M. S.: Anterior lingual mandibular bone concavity. Report of a case, Oral Surg. **48:**413-414, 1979.

Grupe, H. E., Jr., Ten Cate, A. R., and Zander, H. A.: A histochemical and radiobiological study of *in vitro* and *in vivo* human epithelial cell rest proliferation, Arch. Oral Biol. **12:** 1321-1329, 1967.

Jordan, R. E., Suzuki, M., and Skinner, D. H.: Indirect pulpcapping of carious teeth with periapical lesions, J. Am. Dent. Assoc. **97:**37-43, 1978.

Lalonde, E. R.: A new rationale for the management of periapical granulomas and cysts: an evaluation of histopathological and radiographic findings, J. Am. Dent. Assoc. **80:** 1056-1059, 1970.

Ramadan, A. E., and Mitchell, D. F.: Roentgenographic study of experimental bone destruction, Oral Surg. **15:**934-943, 1961.

Shoha, R. R., Dowson, J., and Richards, A. G.: Radiographic interpretation of experimentally produced bony lesions, Oral Surg. **38:**294-303, 1974.

Torabinejad, M., and Kettering, J. D.: Detection of immune complexes in human dental periapical lesions by anticomplement immunofluorescence techniques, Oral Surg. **48:**256-261, 1979.

Waldron, C. A., and Giansanti, J. S.: Benign fibro-osseous lesions of jaws: a clinical-radiologic-histologic review of sixty-five cases. II. Benign fibro-osseous lesions of periodontal ligament origin, Oral Surg. **35:**340-350, 1973.

GENERAL REFERENCES

Ahlstrom, U., Johnson, C. O., and Lantz, B.: Radicular cysts of the jaws: a long term roentgenographic study following cystectomies, Odontol. Revy **20:**111-117, 1969.

Bender, I. B.: A commentary on General Bhaskar's hypothesis, Oral Surg. **34:**469-476, 1972.

Bhaskar, S. N.: Non-surgical resolution of radicular cysts, Oral Surg. **34:**458-468, 1972.

Cherrick, M. H., and Demkee, D.: Metastatic carcinoma of the jaws, J. Am. Dent. Assoc. **87:**180-181, 1973.

Cunningham, J. C., and Penick, E. C.: Use of a roentgenographic contrast medium in the differential diagnosis of periapical lesions, Oral Surg. **26:**96-102, 1968.

Dutta, B. B.: A pilot study of periapical radiolucencies, J. Indian Dent. Assoc. **43:**237-240, 1971.

Eversole, L. R., Sabes, W. R., and Brandebura, J.: Medullo-

blastoma: extradural metastasis to the jaw, Oral Surg. **34:** 634-640, 1972.

Freeland, J. B.: Conservative reduction of large periapical lesions, Oral Surg. **29:**455-464, 1970.

Hall, D. H., Phillips, R. M., and Chase, D. C.: Bone grafts of large cystic defects in the mandible, J. Oral Surg. **29:**146-150, 1971.

Harris, M., and Pannell, G.: Fibrinolytic activity in dental cysts, Oral Surg. **35:**818-826, 1973.

Horton, P. S., Sippy, F. H., Kerber, P. E., and Poule, C. L.: Analysis of interpretations of full mouth and panoramic surveys, Oral Surg. **44:**468-475, 1977.

Kramer, J. R., White, R. P. and Berkowitz, R. P.: A surgical approach to the large maxillary cyst, J. Oral Surg. **27:**665-668, 1969.

Lineberg, W. B., Waldron, C. A., and Delanne, G. F.: A clinical roentgenographic and histopathologic evaluation of periapical lesions, Oral Surg. **17:**467-472, 1972.

Mau, R. B., and McKean, T. W.: Hand-Schüller-Christian disease: report of case, J. Am. Dent. Assoc. **85:**1353-1357, 1972.

Morse, D. C., Patnik, B. S., and Schacterle, G. R.: Electrophoretic differentiation of radicular cysts and granulomas, Oral Surg. **35:**249-264, 1973.

Nakajima, T., Yagata, H., Kato, H., and Tokiwa, N.: Surgical treatment of chronic osteomyelitis of the mandible resistant to intraarterial infusion of antibiotics: report of case, J. Oral Surg. **35:**823-827, 1977.

Patterson, S. S., and Hillis, P. D.: Scar tissue associated with the apices of pulpless teeth prior to endodontic therapy, Oral Surg. **33:**450-457, 1972.

Patterson, S. S., Shafer, W. G., and Healey, J. J.: Periapical lesions associated with endodontically treated teeth, J. Am. Dent. Assoc. **68:**191-194, 1964.

Regan, J. E., and Mitchell, D. F.: Evaluation of periapical radiolucencies found in cadavers, J. Am. Dent. Assoc. **68:**529-533, 1963.

Roane, J. R., and Marshall, J. F.: Osteomyelitis: a complication of pulpless teeth, Oral Surg. **34:**257-261, 1972.

Salman, L., and Harrigan, W. F.: Decompression of a median mandibular cyst: report of case, J. Oral Surg. **30:**503-505, 1972.

Sanders, B.: Current concepts in the management of osteomyelitis of the mandible, J. Oral Med. **33:**40-43, 1978.

Seward, M. H., and Seward, G. R.: Observations on Snowden's technique for the treatment of cysts in the maxilla, Br. J. Oral Surg. **6:**49-59, 1969.

Sigalla, J. L., Silverman, S., Brody, H. A., and Kushner, J. H.: Dental involvement in histiocytosis, Oral Surg. **33:**42-48, 1972.

Stanback, J. S.: The management of bilateral cysts of the mandible, Oral Surg. **30:**587-591, 1970.

Stene, T., and Pedersen, K. N.: Aberrant salivary gland tissue in the anterior mandible, Oral Surg. **44:**72-75, 1977.

Ten Cate, A. R.: The epithelial rests of Malassez and the genesis of the dental cyst, Oral Surg. **34:**956-964, 1972.

Tucker, M. W., Pleasants, J. E., and MacComb, W. S.: Decompression and secondary enucleation of a mandibular cyst, J. Oral Surg. **30:**669-673, 1972.

17

Pericoronal radiolucencies

Norman K. Wood
Paul W. Goaz
Leon J. Schwartz

The entities producing pericoronal radiolucencies include the following:

Pericoronal or follicular space
Dentigerous cyst
Mural ameloblastoma
Ameloblastoma
Calcifying odontogenic cyst
Adenomatoid odontogenic tumor
Ameloblastic fibroma
Rarities
    Ameloblastic variants
    Calcifying epithelial odontogenic tumor
    Ewing's sarcoma
    Extrafollicular dentigerous cyst
    Odontogenic carcinoma
    Odontogenic fibroma
    Odontogenic myxoma
    Odontoma (early stage and in supracoronal
      position)
    Pseudotumor of hemophilia
    Salivary gland tumors (central)
    Squamous cell carcinoma
    Squamous odontogenic tumor

PERICORONAL OR FOLLICULAR SPACE

The crowns of unerupted teeth are normally surrounded by a follicle—a soft tissue remnant of the enamel organ that is frequently referred to as the reduced enamel epithelium.

Microscopically the follicle is shown to be composed of soft myxomatous to dense collagenous fibrous tissue containing nests or cords of odontogenic epithelium (Fig. 17-1).

Radiographically the follicle appears as a homogenous radiolucent halo with a thin outer radiopaque border (Fig. 17-2) representing compact bone that is continuous with the lamina dura in the area of the cementoenamel junction. This halo, which appears as a space, merges with the periodontal ligament space and varies in breadth because of the varying thicknesses of the follicles and/or the accumulation of fluid between the capsule of the reduced epithelium and the crown of the tooth.

Teeth that have been impacted for some years frequently show a meager pericoronal space (Fig. 17-3). By contrast, the unerupted maxillary canines frequently have an enlarged follicular space, especially when their eruption has been delayed (Fig. 17-4). Because cystic change can take place in such follicles and effect delayed eruption and/or displacement of unerupted teeth, it is important to identify any developing pathosis. Unfortunately these entities are usually painless and there is no specific criterion that will enable the dentist to distinguish between a normal and an abnormal (enlarging) follicle.

It is interesting that some children have generalized enlargement of their follicular spaces. Fig. 17-5 illustrates such a case. Almost all the follicular spaces surrounding the unerupted teeth were "abnormally" large but only the largest one, which surrounded the crown of the mandibular left first premolar tooth, represented a lesion (a dentigerous cyst). The clinicians in charge of this case observed the boy closely to ensure that tooth eruption was not delayed.

Fig. 17-1. Low magnification, **A,** and high-magnification, **B,** photomicrographs of a pericoronal follicle. Note the nests and cords of odontogenic epithelium (arrows), which are found throughout the fibrous and myxomatous stroma.

Fig. 17-2. Normal follicular space. **A,** Mandibular premolars. **B,** Maxillary canine. **C,** Mandibular second molar. **D,** Impacted mandibular canines.

Fig. 17-3. Meager follicular space associated with an impacted premolar. Diminished follicular spaces are frequently seen with impacted teeth of long standing.

Fig. 17-4. Pericoronal spaces surrounding maxillary canines frequently achieve these proportions and are often misdiagnosed as follicular cysts.

Fig. 17-5. Enlarged follicular spaces within normal limits. Panorex radiograph of an 8-year-old child showing multiple enlarged follicular spaces around unerupted permanent teeth. Surgery and microscopic study demonstrated a dentigerous cyst associated with the crown of the lower left first premolar tooth. Follow-up examinations showed the eruption of the remainder of the teeth without surgical intervention. (Courtesy J. Dolce, D.D.S., and J. Ireland, D.D.S., Mundelein, Ill.)

The following guidelines for distinguishing between a normal and an abnormal follicle have been utilized:

Worth (1963, p. 76) suggested that when an asymptomatic follicular radiolucency becomes about 2.5 cm in diameter and the surrounding cortical plate is poorly defined this is strongly suggestive of disease.

Stafne (1969, p. 149) contended that if the pericoronal space reaches 2.5 mm in width on the radiograph this is presumptive evidence that fluid is collecting within the follicle and pathosis is present in 80% of the cases.

In our experience the contention of Stafne (1969) has not proved useful for evaluating the pericoronal spaces of upper canines, which are consistently larger than those surrounding other erupting teeth.

DIFFERENTIAL DIAGNOSIS

For a discussion of the differential diagnosis of a pericoronal or follicular space, refer to the differential diagnosis section at the end of this chapter.

MANAGEMENT

In the absence of clinical symptoms, it is advisable to radiographically examine equivocally enlarged or enlarging follicles at least every 6 months or until it becomes apparent that eruption is being delayed, the tooth is being displaced, or the tooth actually erupts. If eruption is being delayed, surgical intervention is indicated.

DENTIGEROUS (FOLLICULAR) CYST

After the radicular cyst, the dentigerous cyst is the most common odontogenic cyst. Dentigerous cysts are associated with the crowns of unerupted or developing teeth.

FEATURES

The dentigerous cyst is the most common pathologic pericoronal radiolucency. It has a lumen lined with epithelium derived from the enamel organ or from other remnants of the dental lamina (Fig. 17-6). Various types of epithelial linings may be observed, and occasionally keratinizing epithelial linings occur. In these cases the lesion may be either an odontogenic keratocyst or a keratinizing odontogenic cyst.

The teeth most frequently affected are the mandibular third molars, the maxillary canines, the mandibular premolars, and the maxillary third molars (in that order). The highest incidence occurs during the second and third decades.

If multiple dentigerous cysts are found, the patient should be examined for either multiple basal cell nevus syndrome or cleidocranial dysostosis. In the latter condition there are many supernumerary teeth, and thus multiple impactions with increased possibilities of dentigerous cyst formation.

It has been reported that 2.6% of patients with one or more unerupted teeth have dentigerous cysts (Mourshed, 1964). The cysts vary greatly in size, from less than 2 cm in diameter to mas-

Fig. 17-6. This follicular cyst wall is lined with stratified epithelium. The thick wall consists mostly of dense fibrous connective tissue.

sive expansions of the jaws (Fig. 17-7). The expansion may in turn produce gross deformity of the region involved.

Although a slowly expanding cyst may markedly thin the cortical plates, it seldom erodes them. This, however, is by no means a hard and fast rule; and when the cortical plates are eroded, palpation will reveal a rubbery fluctuant non-emptiable mass (in contrast to the crepitus or crackling quality of the sensation when the expanded and very thin bony cyst walls are manually examined).

Aspiration, a very useful and well-recognized procedure, may be utilized in the examination of cystic or cystlike lesions. Odontogenic cysts frequently yield a straw-colored thin liquid and usually cholesterol crystals, which may be seen in the aspirate when the syringe is slowly rotated be-

Fig. 17-7. Dentigerous cyst. **A,** Molar impactions showing, *1,* a follicular space and, *2,* a dentigerous cyst. Microscopic examination confirmed this impression. **B** and **C,** Dentigerous cysts associated with impacted mandibular third molars. **D,** Dentigerous cyst surrounding an impacted second molar. **E** and **F,** Two views of the same cyst surrounding the crowns of impacted second and third molars. This case illustrates the importance of obtaining adequate radiographs to grossly determine the extent of the lesion. (**C** courtesy D. Skuble, D.D.S., Hinsdale, Ill.)

fore a relatively strong light. The introduction of contrast medium into the evacuated cyst lumen will occasionally provide additional diagnostic information since the outline and extent of the cystic defect are sometimes made more distinct.

Because a cyst is usually painless, delayed eruption of a tooth may be the only clinical sign suggesting pericoronal pathosis. A painful cyst generally indicates the presence of infection. Rarely will a dentigerous cyst expand so rapidly that it presses on a sensory nerve and causes pain. When this does occur, however, the pain may be referred to any part of the face and is frequently described as headache. Paresthesia, anesthesia, or mobile teeth are almost never produced.

One exception to the foregoing comments relative to pain is the occurrence of a particular type of eruption cyst, usually involving a premolar below a deciduous molar. This circumstance has been observed to precipitate a severely painful condition, possibly resulting from the pressure of the cyst on the unprotected pulp of the resorbing deciduous tooth. The situation may be relieved by removing the deciduous tooth, whose loss is usually not considered premature in view of the position of the permanent tooth when the condition develops.

The eruption cyst is a dentigerous cyst that has developed, or is discovered, when the associated tooth is near the surface. It may be found immediately below the gingiva, producing a domelike swelling on the ridge. The eruption cyst should not be considered a separate entity. It is described in greater detail in Chapter 9.

Pathologic fracture is an inherent danger associated with a large cyst that has destroyed an extensive segment of the jaw. The jaw may become so weakened that it must be splinted before surgery to prevent fracturing during the enucleation. The splint is placed on the teeth.

DIFFERENTIAL DIAGNOSIS

For a discussion of the differential diagnosis of a dentigerous cyst, refer to the differential diagnosis section at the end of this chapter.

MANAGEMENT

The position of a cyst should be confirmed before surgery by the Clark technique (studying several radiographs of the area taken from various angles) and by careful clinical examination. Since ameloblastic change may happen in islands of odontogenic epithelium that occur in the cyst lining or that extend from the epithelial lining itself, complete enucleation must be accomplished.

Such a precaution reduces the possibility that potentially dangerous cells will remain in the region after surgery.

To ensure that these latently dangerous foci are specifically noticed by the pathologist, the surgeon should carefully examine the lumen of any cyst he has removed and identify suspicious areas before the specimen is sent for frozen section evaluation. Most follicular cysts have smooth uniformly thin walls, but some have smooth thick walls. If, on examination of a cyst lining, a local thickening or elevation projecting into the lumen is noted, the attention of the pathologist can be directed to the area by a suture placed in the specimen to identify the region of special interest (Fig. 17-9, B). Should microscopic examination of the frozen section show that the elevation is a tumor (most likely an ameloblastoma) and that it has penetrated the cyst wall, the surgeon must recognize the corresponding area in the bony defect. This procedure will enable him to return to the appropriate place and excise more tissue from the area to be certain that all traces of tumor are removed.

Enucleation and primary closure are quite successful in treating smaller cysts; and the defect resulting from the removal of a larger cyst can be repaired with a graft, preferably utilizing autogenous cancellous bone. Some surgeons prefer to use surgical dressings, which are changed and reduced as the bony cavity decreases in size by secondary intention healing. The treated area must be periodically examined radiographically since there is no way the surgeon can be certain that all the epithelium was removed at operation.

Marsupialization (or the Partsch procedure) is a conservative approach to the treatment of especially large cysts. It is accomplished by removing just the roof of the cyst, making the defect saucer shaped (the overhanging bony edges cut away until the cavity is shallow with gradually sloping walls), and then suturing the cyst membrane to the oral mucosa around the periphery of the opening.

Decompression is another approach used in treating bony cysts. A small acrylic button or short section of rubber tubing is placed in a preformed surgical opening in the cyst; this button keeps the opening patent and permits drainage. The procedure effects a slow diminution in size of the cyst defect, which slowly fills with bone.

The main disadvantage of both marsupialization and decompression is that the surgeon does not have an opportunity to grossly or microscopically examine the epithelial lining in the deeper extremes of the cyst. Hence ameloblastic change or worse if present in the lining can go unnoticed. Such procedures then impose the liability of leaving the potentially dangerous cystic epithelial lining in situ.

When there is no clinical evidence of mural tumors, however, and a cyst is of such proportions that enucleation may result in pathologic or iatrogenic fracture, and if the condition of the patient precludes extensive grafting procedures, then marsupialization or decompression may be the treatment of choice.

Another situation in which marsupialization or decompression may be applied to advantage is in the treatment of large dentigerous cysts that occur in tooth-bearing areas of children. Enucleation in children may result in the unnecessary loss of permanent teeth. This technique is utilized most frequently when a dentigerous cyst is preventing the eruption of a tooth and the tooth appears not to be impacted but to be ready to erupt once it is relieved of the cyst. The operation can also be used for the patient who appears to be a poor surgical risk and not likely to tolerate the more traumatic procedure of total enucleation and bone grafting.

Occasionally a cyst bordering on the maxillary sinus has been treated by anastomosing with the sinus, which thus enlarges the sinus. This approach has proved successful, but it positions the sinus so near the crest of the ridge that a worrisome situation may be created.

MURAL AMELOBLASTOMA

The ameloblastoma that forms in the wall of a dentigerous cyst ranks next to the dentigerous cyst as the most frequently occurring pathologic pericoronal radiolucency.

Shteyer and co-workers (1978) reviewed some 80 cases of mural ameloblastoma and reported that this entity represents approximately 5% of all ameloblastomas. These two types of ameloblastoma are similar in predilections for sex (M ~ F) and site (mandibular third molar region). However, they differed markedly in average age of patient affected: 21.8 years for the mural ameloblastoma vs 38.9 years for the ameloblastoma. Eighty-five percent of mural ameloblastomas were associated with dentigerous cysts, all of which were discovered before 30 years of age. Other cyst types associated with mural ameloblastoma are residual, radicular, globulomaxillary, and primordial cysts.

Various studies have shown that between 15% and 30% of all ameloblastomas form in the wall of a follicular cyst (Kane, 1951; Mehlisch et al., 1972). It should be noted, however, that Stanley

and Diehl (1965) found the ameloblastomatous potential of follicular cysts to decline markedly after 30 years of age.

Gorlin (1970, p. 484) stated that only rarely does an ameloblastoma arise from a nonneoplastic cyst. From the clinician's viewpoint, however, the identification of a radiolucent cystlike area as a nonneoplastic entity must await surgery and microscopic examination since the clinical and radiographic appearances of the early mural ameloblastoma are identical with those of the follicular cyst (Fig. 17-8). Nevertheless, if the latter entity enlarges and remains untreated, it will develop all the locally invasive characteristics of the ameloblastoma. The clinical characteristics of the larger ameloblastoma are detailed in Chapters 18 and 19.

FEATURES

Sufficient to the present discussion is the recognition that a localized thinning and haziness of the hyperostotic radiopaque rim of the pericoronal radiolucency should prompt the clinician to suspect that a mural ameloblastoma may have penetrated the fibrous capsule of a follicular cyst and is initiating the invasion of bone between trabeculae.

The mural ameloblastoma, which occurs with greatest frequency under age 30 years (average age at discovery is 21 years), will be asymptomatic and unsuspected and will go undetected until the pericoronal radiolucency is seen on the routine radiograph. As the lesion slowly enlarges, however, a slight nontender swelling will become clinically apparent. This swelling is the result of an expansion of the cortical plates of the jaw and can be identified by palpation as hard and bony. With enlargement of the tumor, the overlying cortical plates will be thinned to the point of destruction and palpation will disclose softer areas, some of which may be fluctuant cystic spaces. Other softer areas will be firm but not bony hard and represent solid masses of tumor or fibrous tissue that has extended through the eroded bone.

DIFFERENTIAL DIAGNOSIS

For a discussion of the differential diagnosis of a mural ameloblastoma, refer to the differential diagnosis section at the end of this chapter.

MANAGEMENT

Before a surgeon undertakes the treatment of a pericoronal radiolucency, he should develop a differential diagnosis that includes the mural ameloblastoma. Subsequently, at surgery, if he discovers a distinct mass in the cyst wall project-

Fig. 17-8. A, Mural ameloblastoma in a young adult, seen as a pericoronal radiolucency associated with the impacted mandibular third molar tooth. **B,** Orthopantograph showing another case of a mural ameloblastoma seen as a pericoronal radiolucency. (**A** courtesy D. E. Cooksey, D.D.S., Los Angeles. **B** courtesy E. Casper, D.D.S., Chicago.)

ing into the lumen, he should mark it with sutures to enable the pathologist to concentrate on this mass as the area of greatest concern. Such a discrepancy on the surface of the lining may prove to be any of the following:

1. Heavy localized deposits of cholesterol (Fig. 17-9, *A*)

2. Fibrous tissue nodule (Fig. 17-9, *B*)
3. Granulation tissue nodule (Fig. 17-9, *C*)
4. An area showing ameloblastic change (Fig. 17-9, *D*)
5. A mural ameloblastoma (Fig. 17-9, *E*)
6. Another type of odontogenic tumor (Figs. 17-11, *B* and *C*, and 17-12)

Fig. 17-9. Mural nodules on follicular cyst walls. **A,** Mural cholesteatoma found in a follicular cyst wall (low and high magnification). **B,** Mural nodules (arrows) are composed of fibrous tissue.

Continued.

Fig. 17-9, cont'd. C, A mural nodule composed of granulation tissue. **D,** A mural nodule contains odontogenic epithelial nests, which are undergoing ameloblastic change.

7. Salivary tumor (Breitenecker and Wepner, 1973)
8. Central squamous cell carcinoma

Should the pathologist's examination establish the mass to be a tumor that has penetrated the capsule, the surgeon will moderately excise more bone or soft tissue from the area of the bony de-fect that corresponded to the irregularity in the cyst lining.

The foregoing information emphasizes the re-quirement that the surgeon must develop a tech-nique which will enable him to identify the point on the wall of the cyst defect that corresponds to the suspicious thickening in the cyst lining. If a

Fig. 17-9, cont'd. E, This mural nodule proved to be a follicular ameloblastoma.

cyst lining proves to be unusually adherent at a certain point, this site should be closely examined for the presence of a mural ameloblastoma. Some mural ameloblastomas do not show as an elevation but are situated in the periphery of the wall, and the adherent lining may be the only clue the clinician has that another pathosis is present. All adhesions will not necessarily prove to be ameloblastomas, however, since inflammatory areas are often adherent too.

The study of Shteyer and co-workers (1978) revealed that the frequency of recurrence after simple enucleation of cysts containing mural ameloblastomas is considerably lower than for ameloblastomas in general that have been treated in a similar manner. These investigators recommended that further and more extensive surgery for mural ameloblastoma be done only in the event of recurrence. In our opinion the management of each case should be determined after weighing all findings of that individual case.

The discussion thus far has related to the treatment of pericoronal radiolucencies. The management of large ameloblastomas is described in Chapter 18.

AMELOBLASTOMA

It is important to consider that the pericoronal radiolucency under investigation may prove to be a "garden-variety" ameloblastoma at surgery and microscopic study. In other words the radiolucent cavity may be completely filled by ameloblastoma that has infiltrated peripherally into the bony margins. Presumably such examples may represent mural ameloblastomas that have had sufficient time to develop into full-blown ameloblastomas. At any rate these should be recognized as locally aggressive lesions that require more extensive surgery. The ameloblastoma is discussed in detail in Chapter 18 as a solitary cystlike radiolucency and in Chapter 19 as a multilocular radiolucency.

CALCIFYING ODONTOGENIC CYST

On first thought the calcifying odontogenic cyst should be included with the mixed radiolucent-radiopaque lesions in Chapters 23 and 24 but not here. However, we have observed a wide variation in the amount of calcified material in these lesions ranging from very small foci that can only be seen at the microscopic level to moderate-sized foci that can readily be seen as white flecks in the cystic radiolucency (Fig. 23-11) to lesions where the calcified component is so large that it almost completely obliterates the radiolucency. Hence it is apparent that in its early stage the calcifying odontogenic cyst will appear as a completely radiolucent cystlike lesion. A significant number of these occur as pericoronal radiolucencies and so are included here (Fig. 17-10).

Fig. 17-10. A, Calcifying and keratinizing odontogenic cyst. **A,** Panorex radiograph showing a pericoronal radiolucency in association with an impacted mandibular molar tooth. The calcified areas in this case were so small that they failed to be seen in the radiograph as radiopaque flecks. **B,** Photomicrograph of an early lesion prior to calcification showing the ghost cells with keratinization. Arrows indicate the basal cell layer of the cyst wall.

We are unaware of any difference in site or age predilection or in behavior between this lesion and the "garden-variety" dentigerous cyst. The calcifying odontogenic cyst is discussed in greater detail in Chapter 23 as a mixed radiolucent-radiopaque lesion.

ADENOMATOID ODONTOGENIC TUMOR (ADENOAMELOBLASTOMA)

The adenomatoid odontogenic tumor (AOT) is somewhat uncommon, is benign, and makes up approximately 3% of all odontogenic tumors according to the study reported by Regezi and

Fig. 17-11. Adenomatoid odontogenic tumor. **A,** Maxillary occlusal radiograph showing a large radiolucency involving and displacing the maxillary right canine. **B,** Low-power photomicrograph of an adenomatoid odontogenic tumor showing fingers of tumor tissue projecting into the lumen. **C,** Higher-power photomicrograph of an adenomatoid odontogenic tumor showing the typical picture of pseudoducts and pseudoacini. Note the small areas of calcification (arrow) that were not large enough to show as radiopaque foci on the radiograph of this lesion. **D,** Note the expansion of the alveolar process and vestibule in the upper right canine region in a 14-year-old black with an adenomatoid odontogenic tumor. This tumor had destroyed the labial plate. **E,** Surgical specimen from this patient. Note the smooth regular periphery, which permitted ready separation from the surrounding bone. The root tip of the permanent canine is protruding from the mass. **F,** Bisected specimen from the same patient. Note the papillomatous projections from the wall into the lumen of this cystic tumor. (**A, D, E,** and **F** courtesy W. Smith, D.D.S., M.D., San Diego.)

co-workers (1978). The origin of the AOT is still in dispute, but it seems certain that it arises from residual odontogenic epithelium. Some authorities suggest that instead of classifying the AOT as a benign tumor it might be better to consider it a hamartoma of residual odontogenic epithelium (Courtney and Kerr, 1975). At any rate it is important to distinguish the AOT from the ameloblastoma. Actually these two lesions differ radically in clinical, radiographic, microscopic features and behavior, and so the AOT must not be considered as a type of ameloblastoma.

Some pathologists have described the adenomatoid odontogenic tumor as passing through definite stages of maturation (early, middle, and mature). Although this concept is still unproved, two distinct radiographic appearances are known to exist—depending on whether sufficient calcification is present in the tumor to be radiographically evident.

1. In one stage, perhaps representing an early period, the tumor is completely radiolucent (Fig. 17-11, *A*). Macroscopically it may be solid or may contain large cystlike areas (Fig. 17-11, *B*). Histologically it has an acinar pattern and in many areas shows nodules, cords, and swirls in addition to ductlike structures lined with cuboidal or columnar epithelial cells (Fig. 17-11, *C*). Minute calcifications are also apparent in the microscopic picture of this stage, although the degree and extent of the calcification are not sufficient to produce radiopacities.
2. In the more advanced stage sufficient calcification has occurred to produce clusters of radiopaque foci within the radiolucency.

Although no apparent difference may be observable in the clinical behavior of the tumors that could be related to their histologic or radiographic picture or both, the clinician nevertheless might suspect that the more radiopaque the tumors the less active they would be.

The adenomatoid odontogenic tumor is twice as common in women and usually occurs in the second decade of life, with the average age being 16 years. At least 75% occur in association with unerupted teeth or in the walls of dentigerous cysts. Several of the tumors have been reported in areas where teeth failed to develop, suggesting that they could have arisen from primordial cysts or directly from the enamel organ before the development of the hard dental structures. About 90% have occurred in the anterior portions of the jaws; and they are about one and one-half times more frequent in the maxilla than in the mandible.

The order in which unerupted teeth are most frequently associated with this tumor is as follows: maxillary canine, lateral incisor, mandibular premolar. The lesions are slow growing, and the radiolucent type just described is similar to a dentigerous cyst in both growth pattern and appearance (Fig. 17-11, *A*). Thus the tumor may be small and show no clinical signs or symptoms. Conversely, continued slow growth may expand the cortical plates and produce a clinical swelling and asymmetry but not cause invasion of the soft tissues (Fig. 17-11, *D*).

MANAGEMENT

The adenomatoid odontogenic tumor is best treated by conservative surgical removal, for it separates easily and cleanly from its bony defect, has an extremely low recurrence rate, and shows no evidence of metastatic tendency (Fig. 7-11, *E*). Its behavior is much more benign than that of the simple ameloblastoma.

The surgical specimen may be solid or cystic, and on gross inspection elevations of varying size and shape may be found projecting from the lining into the fluid-filled lumen (Fig. 17-11, *F*). Some areas of the cystic wall will be thinner and smooth, however, and are in essence segments of typical dentigerous cyst wall. An examination of frozen sections should be undertaken at the time of surgery so a definite diagnosis can be established. Also this will permit the surgeon to remove more tissue if the biopsy report so indicates.

AMELOBLASTIC FIBROMA

The ameloblastic fibroma is a true mixed odontogenic tumor, containing nests and strands of odontogenic and ameloblastic epithelium in a primitive dental papillalike connective tissue (Fig. 17-12, *B*). Calcified dental structures are not present. It is usually found as a well-defined unilocular radiolucency, although occasionally multilocular lesions will occur surrounding the crowns of unerupted teeth or in tooth-bearing regions where teeth have failed to develop (Fig. 17-12, *A*).

FEATURES

The ameloblastic fibroma is not as frequently associated with an unerupted tooth as is the adenomatoid odontogenic tumor, however, although both are usually found in the same age group (under 20 years of age).

The ameloblastic fibroma does not demonstrate a predilection for either sex. More than 70% oc-

Fig. 17-12. Ameloblastic fibroma. **A,** This very large well-defined radiolucency displacing the mandibular canine and expanding the cortical plates proved to be an ameloblastic fibroma. **B,** Low and high magnification of the histology of an ameloblastic fibroma showing ameloblastic nests in a pulplike stroma. (**A** courtesy O. H. Stuteville, D.D.S., M.D., St. Joe, Ark.)

cur in patients who are under 20 years of age, and the average age has been reported as 14 years (Gorlin et al., 1961) and 15.5 years (Trodahl, 1972). While this tumor may arise in either jaw the vast majority occur in the mandible, and the highest incidence is in the premolar-molar region. This mixed odontotenic tumor grows slowly by expansion of the cortex and usually does not invade bone.

Radiographically the ameloblastic fibroma may appear as a unilocular or multilocular radiolucency that may or may not show cortical expansion (Fig. 17-12). The tumor is often associated with unerupted teeth and may spread roots of adjacent teeth (Hager et al., 1978).

MANAGEMENT

The treatment suggested for the ameloblastic fibroma by most surgeons is conservative enucleation. The tumor readily separates from the bone; and since the ameloblastic cells generally do not invade the connective tissue capsule, few recurrences are observed. The recurrence rate is higher for this tumor than for the adenomatoid odontogenic tumor, however, and in rare instances there have been several recurrences.

Fig. 17-13. Calcifying epithelial odontogenic tumor (Pindborg tumor) seen as a well-defined pericoronal radiolucency involving the impacted third molar in a 30-year-old white woman. (From Smith, R. A., Roman, R. S., Hansen, L. S., et al.: J. Oral Surg. **35:**160-166, 1977. Copyright by the American Dental Association. Reprinted by permission.)

Fig. 17-14. Ragged ill-defined pericoronal radiolucency involving the impacted mandibular right second premolar tooth. Biopsy in this 15-year-old adolescent revealed Ewing's sarcoma. (Courtesy N. Barakat, D.D.S., Beirut, Lebanon.)

Consequently periodic radiographic reexamination of the operated area is a necessary precaution. Ameloblastic fibrosarcomas have been reported.

RARITIES

Almost any pathologic process may occur about the crowns of unerupted teeth, including primary and metastatic malignant tumors. Although these processes are rare and do not generally produce well-defined radiolucent lesions, nevertheless under this category of rarities, it is appropriate to mention the odontogenic fibroma and the odontogenic myxoma—which do occur (infrequently) about unerupted teeth and indeed can displace associated teeth from their normal position. Both tumors may enlarge and produce expansion and thinning of the cortical plates but rarely do they destroy the plates.

An incomplete list of lesions that rarely produce a pericoronal radiolucent lesion is as follows:

Ameloblastic variants
Calcifying epithelial odontogenic tumor (Fig. 17-13)
Ewing's sarcoma (Fig. 17-14)
Extrafollicular dentigerous cyst
Odontogenic carcinoma
Odontogenic fibroma
Odontogenic myxoma (Fig. 17-15)
Odontoma in pericoronal location (premineralized stage)
Ossifying fibroma (Fig. 17-16)
Pseudotumor of hemophilia (Fig. 17-17)
Salivary gland tumors (central)
Squamous cell carcinoma
Squamous odontogenic tumor

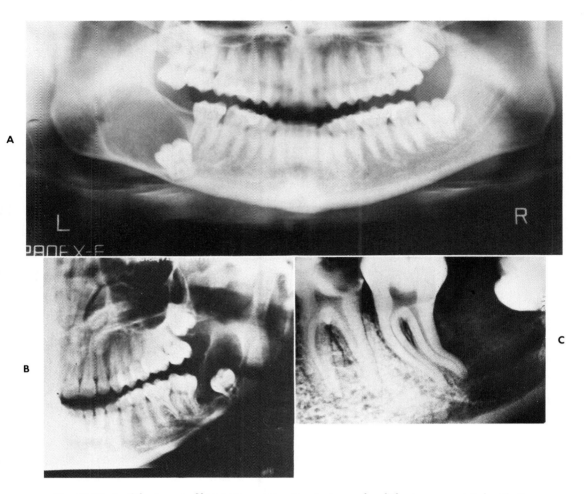

A

B

C

Fig. 17-15. **A,** Odontogenic fibromyxoma seen as a pericoronal radiolucency associated with the impacted left mandibular third molar. **B** and **C,** Another case of fibromyxoma seen as a pericoronal radiolucency. **B,** Panoramic film. **C,** Periapical film. (Courtesy D. E. Cooksey, D.D.S., Los Angeles.)

Fig. 17-16. Ossifying fibroma. Note the large radiolucent area that appears to contact the crown of the displaced mandibular third molar. Note also the thin radiopaque borders of the lesion. The increased buccolingual thickness of the ramus composed of dense fibrous tissue imparts a hazy semiradiopaque appearance to this lesion that contained minimal foci of calcification.

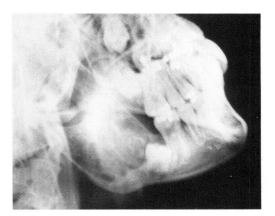

Fig. 17-17. Pseudotumor of hemophilia seen as a pericoronal radiolucency in this lateral oblique radiograph of a young man with a hereditary deficiency of factor VIII. (Courtesy G. Blozis, D.D.S., Columbus, Ohio.)

Table 17-1. Pericoronal radiolucencies*

	Predominant sex	Peak age (years)	Most frequent jaw involved	Most frequent area of jaw involved	Most frequent tooth involved	Signs or symptoms	Recurrence
Follicular spaces Developing teeth		4-12				None	—
Impacted teeth	M ~ F†	Over 18	Mandible	Posterior	Mandibular third molar	Delayed eruption of tooth	Recurs as cyst or ameloblastoma
Dentigerous cysts	?	Over 18	Mandible	Posterior	Mandibular third molar	Delayed eruption of tooth Swelling; asymmetry	Recurs as cyst or ameloblastoma
Mural ameloblastomas	M ~ F	85% before 30 (avg. 21)	Mandible	Posterior	Mandibular third molar	Delayed eruption of tooth Swelling; asymmetry	Occasional
Ameloblastoma	M ~ F	Avg. 38.9	Mandible	Posterior	Mandibular third molar	Delayed eruption of tooth Swelling	Significant
Adenomatoid odontogenic tumors	$\frac{F}{M} = \frac{2}{1}$	10-21 (avg. 16.5)	Maxilla	Anterior = 90%	Maxillary canine = 60%	Delayed eruption of tooth Swelling; asymmetry	Unusual
Ameloblastic fibromas	M ~ F	70% under 20 (avg. 14-15.5)	Mandible	Posterior	Mandibular molar and premolar	Delayed eruption of tooth Advanced swelling; asymmetry	Unusual

*Entities listed according to frequency of occurrence.
†~Approximately equal.

DIFFERENTIAL DIAGNOSIS OF PERICORONAL RADIOLUCENCIES

When the clinician is confronted by a pericoronal radiolucency, he must prepare his surgical team for the anticipated procedure. This is best accomplished by the formulation of a list of possible diagnoses arranged in order of probability, with the most probable lesion heading the list, as the basis of a working diagnosis. Thus, if all the discernible features of the pathosis under study give ameloblastoma a low level of probability, the need to prepare the surgical team for an extensive procedure (e.g., a block resection with bone graft) is obviated.

As an example to illustrate the usefulness of formally developing a differential diagnosis, the circumstances attending a 50-year-old woman with a well-defined pericoronal radiolucency associated with an impacted lower right third molar will be analyzed.

The lesion was discovered on a routine radiographic survey. It was asymptomatic and measured 2 cm in diameter with an intrafollicular space measuring 1 cm. Because normal follicular spaces usually decrease in size with age, it was initially recognized, on the basis of its proportions, as not a simple enlarged uncomplicated follicle but rather a pathologic process.

Although the lesion under investigation occurred in the mandibular third molar area, a frequent site of the *mural ameloblastoma,* this entity was not assigned a prominent rank since it seldom occurs in persons over 30 years of age (Stanley and Diehl, 1965).

The *odontoma* and its *ameloblastic variants* commonly occur in a supracoronal position in close approximation to the occlusal surface of an unerupted tooth. Thus in radiographs these lesions in their unmineralized stages could be seen as pericoronal radiolucencies. However, the chances of the lesion in question representing an odontoma or one of its ameloblastic variants is quite remote because these lesions develop at the same time as the dentition and so would have already passed into the completely radiopaque stage in a patient who is 50 years old.

The *calcifying odontogenic cyst* may occur as a pericoronal radiolucency and be unsuspected until small radiopaque foci appear. Inasmuch as its management is identical to that of the uncomplicated dentigerous cyst extensive attempts at ranking are academic rather than practical.

Although the *ameloblastic fibroma* is four times more common in the mandible, the choice of this entity as the working diagnosis was inappropriate since this mixed odontogenic tumor occurs most frequently in the mandibular premolar–first molar area and seldom is seen in patients over 20 years of age.

Also none of the lesion's characteristics (e.g., location, age) suggested an *adenomatoid odontogenic tumor* since these entities show a predilection for the anterior region of the jaws of young persons.

Thus the working diagnosis—or the condition assigned the highest rank in the differential diagnosis for this radiolucent lesion—was dentigerous cyst. The possibility that any of the other pericoronal radiolucencies might be found at operation was quite remote; but nevertheless the mural ameloblastoma was a distant second on the formulated list.

SPECIFIC REFERENCES

Abrams, A. M., Melrose, R. J., and Howell, F. J.: Adeno-ameloblastoma: a clinical pathological study of ten new cases, Cancer **22:**175-185, 1968.

Breitenecker, G., and Wepner, F.: A pleomorphic adenoma (so-called mixed tumor) in the wall of a dentigerous cyst, Oral Surg. **36:**63-71, 1973.

Courtney, R. M., and Kerr, D. A.: The odontogenic adenomatoid tumor, Oral Surg. **39:**424-435, 1975.

Gorlin, R. J.: Odontogenic tumors. In Gorlin, R. J., and Goldman, H. M., editors: Thoma's oral pathology, ed. 6, St. Louis, 1970, The C. V. Mosby Co., vol. 1.

Gorlin, R. J., Chaudhry, A. P., and Pindborg, J. J.: Odontogenic tumors, classification, histopathology and clinical behavior in man and domestic animals, Cancer **14:**73-101, 1961.

Hager, R. C., Taylor, C. G., and Allen, P. M.: Ameloblastic fibroma: report of case, J. Oral Surg. **36:**66-69, 1978.

Kane, J. P.: Odontogenic tumors: a statistical and morphological study of 88 cases. Thesis, Georgetown University, Washington, D.C., 1951.

Mehlisch, D. R., Dahlin, D. C., and Masson, J. K.: Ameloblastoma: a clinicopathologic report, J. Oral Surg. **30:**9-22, 1972.

Mourshed, F.: A roentgenographic study of dentigerous cysts. I. Incidence in a population sample, Oral Surg. **18:**47-53, 1964.

Regezi, J. A., Kerr, D. A., and Courtney, R. M.: Odontogenic tumors: an analysis of 706 cases, J. Oral Surg. **36:**771-778, 1978.

Shteyer, A., Lustmann, J., and Lewin-Epstein, J.: The mural ameloblastoma: review of the literature, J. Oral Surg. **36:**866-872, 1978.

Stafne, E. C.: Oral roentgenographic diagnosis, ed. 3, Philadelphia, 1969, W. B. Saunders Co.

Stanley, H. R., and Diehl, D. L.: Ameloblastoma potential of follicular cysts, Oral Surg. **20:**260-268, 1965.

Trodahl, J. N.: Ameloblastic fibroma, a survey of cases from the Armed Forces Institute of Pathology, Oral Surg. **33:**547-558, 1972.

Worth, H. M.: Principles and practice of oral radiologic interpretation, Chicago, 1963, Yearbook Medical Publishers.

GENERAL REFERENCES

Albright, C. R., and Henning, G. H.: Large dentigerous cyst of the maxilla near the maxillary sinus: report of case, J. Am. Dent. Assoc. **83:**1112-1115, 1971.

Battle, R. J. V., and Winstock, D.: Adamantinoma of the mandible rising in the dentigerous cyst, Br. J. Plast. Surg. **13:** 349-353, 1961.

Berk, R. S., Baden, E., Ladov, M., and Williams, A. C.: Adeno-ameloblastoma (odontogenic adenomatoid tumor): report of case, J. Oral Surg. **30:**201-208, 1972.

Cahn, C. R.: The dentigerous cyst is a potential adamantinoma, Dent. Cosmos **75:**889-893, 1933.

Carr, R. F., Halperin, V., Wood, C., et al.: Recurrent ameloblastic fibroma, Oral Surg. **29:**85-90, 1970.

Christ, T. F., Cavalaris, C. J., and Crocker, D. J.: Papilliferous ameloblastic fibroma, Oral Surg. **34:**806-810, 1972.

Cramer, J. R., White, R. P., Jr., and Berkowitz, R. P.: A surgical approach to the large maxillary cyst, J. Oral Surg. **27:** 665-668, 1969.

Eversole, L. R., Tomich, C. E., and Cherrick, H. M.: Histogenesis of odontogenic tumors, Oral Surg. **32:**569-581, 1971.

Franklin, C. D., and Hindle, M. O.: The calcifying epithelial odontogenic tumor—report of four cases; two with long-term follow-up, Br. J. Oral Surg. **13:**230-238, 1976.

Giansanti, J. S., Someren, A., and Waldron, C. A.: Odontogenic adenomatoid tumor (adenoameloblastoma): survey of 111 cases, Oral Surg. **30:**69-86, 1970.

Gillette, R., and Weinmann, J. P.: Extrafollicular stages in dentigerous cyst development, Oral Surg. **11:**638-645, 1958.

Goldman, L., and Franzen, M.: Orientation of small biopsies, Arch. Dermatol. **103:**407-408, 1971.

Goracy, E., and Stratigos, G. T.: Adenoameloblastoma: report of a case, J. Am. Dent. Assoc. **86:**672-674, 1973.

Hall, D. H., Phillips, R., and Chase, D. C.: Bone grafts of large cystic defects in the mandible, J. Oral Surg. **29:**146-150, 1971.

Halperin, V., Carr, R. F., and Pettier, J. R.: Follow-up of adeno-ameloblastomas: review of thirty-five cases from the literature and a report of two additional cases, Oral Surg. **24:**642-647, 1967.

Hutton, C. E.: Occurrence of ameloblastoma within a dentigerous cyst, Oral Surg. **24:**147-150, 1967.

Josell, S. A., Reiskin, A. B., and Gross, B. D.: Dentigerous cyst with mural ameloblastoma, J. Am. Dent. Assoc. **99:**634-636, 1979.

Lee, F. M. S.: Ameloblastoma of the maxilla with probable origin in a residual cyst, Oral Surg. **29:**799-805, 1970.

Leider, A. S. Nelson, J. F., and Trodahl, J. N.: Ameloblastic fibrosarcoma of the jaws, Oral Surg. **33:**559-569, 1972.

Lubar, R. L., Williams, R. F., and Henefer, E. P.: Mural ameloblastoma of mandible with post-extraction fracture and repair by iliac cancellous bone graft: report of a case, J. Oral Surg. **29:**674-680, 1971.

Madan, R.: Ameloblastoma developing from a dentigerous cyst, Oral Surg. **13:**781-786, 1960.

Martinelli, C., Melhado, R. M., and dos Santos-Pinto, R.: Adenoameloblastoma: histologic and histochemical study in one case, Oral Surg. **28:**534-538, 1969.

Mehlisch, D. R., Dahlin, D. C., and Masson, J. K.: Ameloblastoma: a clinicopathologic report, J. Oral Surg. **30:**9-22, 1972.

Minderjahn, A.: Incidence and clinical differentiation of odontogenic tumors, J. Maxillofac. Surg. **7:**142-150, 1979.

Novince, W. M., and Grau, W. H.: Ameloblastic fibroma, J. Oral Surg. **35:**150-152, 1977.

Paul, J. K., Fay, J. T., and Stamps, P.: Recurrent dentigerous cyst evidencing ameloblastic proliferation: report of case, J. Oral Surg. **27:**211-214, 1969.

Philipsen, H. P., and Brin, H.: The adenomatoid odontogenic tumor. Adenomatoid tumor or adenoameloblastoma, Acta Pathol. Microbiol. Scand. **75:**375-398, 1969.

Pullon, P. A., Shafer, W. G., Elzay, R. R., et al.: Squamous odontogenic tumor: report of six cases of a previously undescribed lesion, Oral Surg. **40:**616-630, 1975.

Quinn, J. H., and Fournet, L. F.: Dentigerous cyst with mural ameloblastoma: report of a case, J. Oral Surg. **27:**662-664, 1969.

Rittersma, J., Hadders, H. N., and Feenstra, K.: Early unicystic ameloblastoma: report of case, J. Oral Surg. **37:**747-750, 1979.

Salman, L., and Harrigan, W. F.: Decompression of a median mandibular cyst: report of case, J. Oral Surg. **30:**503-505, 1972.

Seward, M. H.: Eruption cyst: an analysis of its clinical features, J. Oral Surg. **31:**31-35, 1973.

Stafne, E. C.: Oral roentgenographic diagnosis, ed. 3, Philadelphia, 1969, W. B. Saunders Co.

Stanley, H. R., and Diehl, D. L.: Ameloblastoma potential of follicular cysts, Oral Surg. **20:**260-268, 1965.

Szerlip, L.: Displaced third molar with dentigerous cyst—an unusual case, J. Oral Surg. **36:**551-552, 1978.

Tanaka, S., Mitsui, Y., Mizuno, Y., and Emori, S.: Recurrent ameloblastic fibroma: report of a case, Oral Surg. **33:**944-950, 1972.

Taylor, R. N., Callins, J. F., Menell, H. B., et al.: Dentigerous cyst with ameloblastomatous proliferation: report of case, J. Oral Surg. **29:**136-140, 1971.

Trodahl, J. N.: Ameloblastic fibroma: a survey of cases from the Armed Forces Institute of Pathology, Oral Surg. **33:**547-558, 1972.

Tsaknis, P. J., Carpenter, W. M., and Shade, N. L.: Odontogenic adenomatoid tumor: report of case and review of the literature, J. Oral Surg. **35:**146-149, 1977.

Tucker, W. M., Pleasants, J. E., and MacComb, W. S.: Decompression and secondary enucleation of a mandibular cyst: report of case, J. Oral Surg. **30:**669-673, 1972.

Vickers, R. A., and Gorlin, R. J.: Ameloblastoma: delineation of early histopathologic features of neoplasia, Cancer **26:** 699-710, 1970.

Warson, R. W., and Whitehead, R. G.: Dentigerous cyst of the nasal cavity and maxillary sinus: report of a case, J. Am. Dent. Assoc. **85:**652-653, 1972.

Wilson, D. L., and Roche, W. C.: Dentigerous cyst with ameloblastomatous change: report of case, J. Oral Surg. **18:**173-174, 1960.

Wine, W. M., Welch, T. J., and Graves, R. W.: Marsupialization of a dentigerous cyst of the mandible: report of case, J. Oral Surg. **29:**742-745, 1971.

Worth, H. M.: Principles and practice of oral radiologic interpretation, Chicago, 1963, Year Book Medical Publishers.

18

Solitary cystlike radiolucencies not necessarily contacting teeth

Norman K. Wood
Paul W. Goaz
Sol Goldman

In this chapter the cystlike radiolucencies that usually do not involve the teeth are presented.

Anatomic patterns
    Marrow spaces
    Maxillary sinus
    Early stage of tooth crypts
    Mandibular foramen
Postextraction socket
Residual cyst
Traumatic bone cyst
Developmental bone defect of the mandible
    (salivary)
Primordial cyst
Odontogenic keratocyst (OKC)
Ameloblastoma
Surgical defect
Giant cell granuloma
Giant cell lesion of hyperparathyroidism
Incisive canal cyst
Fissural cysts
    Globulomaxillary cysts
    Midpalatal cyst
    Median mandibular cyst
Cementifying and ossifying fibromas (early stage)
Benign nonodontogenic tumors
Rarities
    Adenomatoid odontogenic tumors
    Ameloblastic variants
    Aneurysmal bone cyst
    Aneurysms in bone
    Calcifying epithelial odontogenic tumor
    Cementoma
    Central hemangioma of bone
    Central squamous cell carcinoma in cyst
      lining
    Desmoplastic fibroma
    Histiocytosis X
    Lateral periodontal cyst
    Low-grade metastatic carcinoma
    Minor salivary gland tumor in bone
    Myxoma
    Odontogenic fibroma
    Odontoma (early stage)
    Osteoblastoma (early stage)
    Plasmacytoma
    Squamous odontogenic tumor

The term "cystlike radiolucency" describes a dark radiographic shadow that is approximately circular in outline and usually smoothly contoured with well-defined borders. On occasion the radiolucency may be somewhat elongated, especially in the horizontal plane, and thus appear more elliptic in shape. It is sometimes accentuated by a narrow radiopaque rim that is cast by a thin hyperostotic layer of bone.

When the unwary less perceptive clinician is confronted by such radiographic evidence, he is inclined to immediately conclude that he has encountered a cyst, disregarding the myriad other possibilities that may appear cystlike. His lack of discernment may well precipitate an unpleasant experience if he surgically enters the cystlike radiolucency without conducting a careful examination or developing an adequate differential diagnosis. Such preliminary procedures not only will assure the appropriate therapeutic approach but also will help obviate the possibility of an unexpected encounter with any of the potentially dangerous cystlike lesions. This group includes the imposing spectrum of entities from normal anatomic spaces to cysts of various types, benign tumors, ameloblastomas, dangerous intrabony hemangiomas, and malignancies (e.g., slow-growing metastatic tumors, squamous cell carcinomas within cysts).

Consequently it cannot be overemphasized that all cystlike radiolucencies in the jaws must be given careful consideration before they are treated.

The radicular, lateral, and follicular cysts are not discussed here but are taken up in other chapters. Some lesions included in this chapter (e.g., traumatic bone cysts, early cementomas) will also occur as periapical radiolucencies and so are included in Chapter 16; but since these entities also occur with some frequency independent of the roots of teeth, they satisfy the criterion for inclusion in the present chapter.

Furthermore, cysts, giant cell granulomas, giant cell lesions of hyperparathyroidism, ameloblastomas, aneurysmal bone cysts, myxomas, metastatic carcinomas, and hemangiomas may all have more than one radiographic appearance, so they are also included in other chapters.

Finally, lesions such as metastatic carcinoma are not discussed here but are merely listed in the rarities section because they do not commonly cause a cystlike radiolucency. They are dealt with in other chapters, however, in which their more common appearances are discussed.

ANATOMIC PATTERNS

The anatomic radiolucencies found in radiographs of the jawbones are discussed in some detail in Chapter 15. Consequently their consideration here will be restricted to a brief comment on the four entities: marrow spaces, maxillary sinus, early tooth crypts, and the inferior dental (mandibular) foramen.

Marrow spaces

There is great variation among the patterns of marrow spaces from person to person and also between the jaws in the same person. When they occur as larger than normal somewhat rounded radiolucencies with borders that appear to be hyperostotic and not contacting teeth, marrow spaces may be mistaken for any of the cystlike radiolucencies included in this chapter (Fig. 18-1).

Such unusual marrow space patterns occur quite frequently in the mandible but are seldom seen on radiographs of the maxilla. When the

Fig. 18-1. Cystlike marrow space (arrow).

clinician encounters what he interprets as an uncommon marrow space pattern, a comparison with the spaces in the same area on the opposite side of the jaw will usually show a similar picture if indeed he is dealing with an anomalous condition. This finding, coupled with an absence of local or systemic symptoms, is usually sufficient to permit him to arrive at the correct diagnosis.

It should be borne in mind, however, that if the contralateral areas being compared are subject to different magnitudes of stress, as might be the case when the occlusion on one side has been altered by the loss of teeth, such a comparison will not be valid without some qualification in light of these extenuating circumstances. Furthermore, some abnormal changes in size of the marrow spaces occur with certain systemic disorders and these changes are usually bilateral. Thus comparison of contralateral patterns might be misleading.

Nevertheless, if the clinician is in doubt as to the diagnosis, he should reexamine the area radiographically at regular intervals to ascertain that it is not enlarging. On the contrary, if symptoms that can be related to the region in question are present, a careful examination and complete differential diagnosis must be formulated and a biopsy of the area performed.

Maxillary sinus

Frequently a cystlike outpouching of the maxillary sinus occurs on a radiograph of an edentulous upper jaw, and this normal variation presents a difficulty in differentiation from a pathologic process (Fig. 18-2). Radiographs of the area taken from different angles (Clark technique), however, will often show a connection between such an outpouching and the larger maxillary sinus cavity and will resolve the question of iden-

Fig. 18-2. A, Cystlike maxillary sinus. **B,** Cystlike outpouching of the maxillary sinus. **C,** Large nasolacrimal duct (arrow).

tity. Large nutrient canals in the walls of the sinus will also contribute to a tentative identification.

Although the maxillary sinuses are frequently asymmetric, comparing their configurations may be helpful in the correct interpretation of a cystlike projection. Again, however, as is true of the changes in marrow space patterns in response to altered function, the sinus may expand and its shape be altered when stresses are reduced as a result of the loss of maxillary posterior teeth on the corresponding side.

Finally, if the clinician cannot satisfy his doubts as to the nature of the structure in question, periodic radiographs will demonstrate whether the radiolucency is changing. As a last resort, aspiration of air from the cavity will identify it as the maxillary sinus.

Early stage of tooth crypts

The radiographic picture of a tooth crypt in the early stages of development before calcification will be round, smooth, and well defined and will have a radiopaque rim identical with that of a cyst (Fig. 18-3).

Since periapical radiographs of younger dentitions are not often made when the developing crypts of the permanent canines and premolars

Fig. 18-3. Early molar crypt.

are in the radiolucent stage, these teeth do not usually cause a diagnostic problem. Furthermore, the clinician who is familiar with the chronologic development and calcification of the permanent dentition will readily identify such areas as developing tooth crypts and will verify their identity by relating to the contralateral sites in the jaw. Nevertheless, a single tooth may be delayed in its development as compared with the corresponding tooth in the opposite quadrant and may present a diagnostic problem. The diagnosis of primordial cyst will then be assigned a high rank in the order of possible entities.

The clinician can differentiate between the two entities (delayed calcification or primordial cyst) by periodically examining the region radiographically for about 6 months.* if the radiolucent area is a retarded developing tooth, radiopaque foci representing the initiation of mineralization at the cusp tips will soon be found. If no calcification is detected within 6 months to 1 year, the discontinuity in the bone is most likely a primordial cyst that began within the odontogenic epithelium of the tooth bud before calcification was initiated.

Mandibular foramen

The mandibular foramen, which provides the entrance for the inferior dental vessels and nerve into the mandibular canal, is usually apparent on lateral oblique and panoramic views of the jaws. It is located on the medial surface of the ramus at the approximate center and can be readily identified by its position and by the presence of the mandibular canal, which runs anteroinferiorly from it. The mandibular canal, however, may not be radiographically diagnostic; and in such instances the round to ovoid to funnel-shaped radiolucency of the inferior dental foramen may be mistaken for a lesion in the ramus.

As is usual with anatomic structures, however, a comparison with the opposite side will aid in making the correct diagnosis. Occasionally the triangular-shaped lingula will be projected over the shadow of the foramen in such a manner as to give the illusion of a mixed radiolucent-radiopaque lesion.

POSTEXTRACTION SOCKET

Sometimes after an extraction the socket will resemble a cystlike radiolucency and present a difficult problem in developing a working diagnosis. This situation usually occurs in edentulous molar areas of the mandible but is also seen in the mandibular incisor region (Fig. 18-4).

Questioning the patient will frequently yield the information that there has been a recent extraction in the region—which may be verified by a clinical examination revealing a depressed area on the ridge. Sockets at extraction sites will sometimes remain uncalcified for years as unchanging cystlike radiolucencies, but a check of other eden-

*The clinician should be alert, however, to the fact that occasionally teeth are unusually slow in developing. Cunat and Collard (1973) described premolars that developed 5 to 8 years later than normal.

Fig. 18-4. Extraction site (arrow) 3 years after tooth removal.

tulous areas will usually reveal similar-appearing sockets.

In such cases the history of an extraction is of little value to the differential diagnosis since the patient with a *residual cyst* would give the same history of an extraction from the area.

If the examiner is reasonably certain that a cystlike radiolucency is indeed an old extraction wound, then periodic radiographic examination of the area is indicated to confirm this impression. If the clinician has serious doubts as to the true nature of the radiolucency, however, he should surgically explore the area and remove tissue for examination regardless of whether or not a typical cyst aspirate is obtained.

RESIDUAL CYST

A residual cyst, as the name implies, is a radicular, lateral, or dentigerous cyst that has remained after its associated tooth has been lost. In practice, to determine whether it was present at the time of extraction or developed later in the residual rests of Malassez (residual odontogenic epithelial nests from Hertwig's root sheath) is not possible unless a radiograph showing it was present before the extraction can be obtained. The residual cyst appears as a rounded radiolucency with well-defined borders (Figs. 18-5 and 18-6).

Sometimes, because of the resistance of the cortical plates, the cyst will enlarge in a more elliptic shape. Its borders will frequently be accentuated by a thin radiopaque line that is produced by hyperostosis resulting from the minimal pressure of the expanding cyst. There are no radiographic features that will permit differentiation between this type of cyst and any of the other lesions included in this chapter.

Fig. 18-5. **A** and **B,** Residual cysts. **C,** Midline cyst of the mandible; type not identified (could be a residual, primordial, or true midline cyst). (Courtesy F. Prock, D.D.S., Joliet, Ill.)

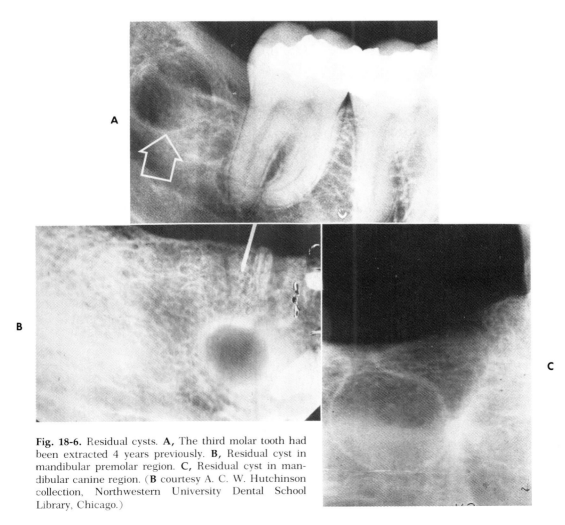

Fig. 18-6. Residual cysts. **A,** The third molar tooth had been extracted 4 years previously. **B,** Residual cyst in mandibular premolar region. **C,** Residual cyst in mandibular canine region. (**B** courtesy A. C. W. Hutchinson collection, Northwestern University Dental School Library, Chicago.)

FEATURES

The residual cyst occurs in the alveolar process and body of the jawbones in edentulous areas, but it may also be found in the lower ramus area. Patients over 20 years of age show the highest incidence of residual cysts, the average age being 52 years. The male-female ratio is 3 : 2, and the maxilla is more commonly involved than the mandible (Cabrini et al., 1970). The cyst seldom reaches more than 0.5 cm in diameter but may at certain times be large enough to cause jaw expansion and asymmetry. Its symptoms, clinical characteristics, and histopathology are identical with those of the other odontogenic cysts discussed in Chapters 16 and 17.

DIFFERENTIAL DIAGNOSIS

All the entities included in this chapter must be considered when a residual cystlike radiolucency is found; but the *cystlike anatomic patterns, primordial cyst, keratocyst,* and *traumatic bone cyst* are the entities most likely to cause confusion. A discussion of the differential diagnosis for these entities is detailed under keratocysts (p. 377).

MANAGEMENT

The treatment of a residual cyst is identical with that of any other intrabony odontogenic cyst except that in these cases the offending teeth have already been lost. Such circumstances as the patient's age, systemic condition, and size of the cyst may prompt the utilization of one of the following methods in preference to the others:

1. Complete enucleation of the cyst wall with its epithelium and primary closure of the mucoperiosteal flap
2. Complete enucleation of the cyst tissue with the placement of a surgical pack, which is slowly withdrawn as the defect fills in
3. Complete excision and replacement with autogenous particulate bone or a single segment of bone fixed in place
4. Marsupialization
5. Decompression
6. Decompression combined with delayed enucleation

Just prior to surgical intervention, aspiration of the area with at least an 18-gauge needle is a wise precautionary measure and will circumvent the unpleasant surprise of encountering a more serious lesion than the surgeon anticipated (e.g., solid tumor, intrabony hemangioma, or aneurysmal bone cyst).

A more thorough discussion of the management of cysts is given in Chapter 16 under radicular cysts.

TRAUMATIC BONE CYST

The traumatic bone cyst (hemorrhagic bone cyst, extravasation cyst, simple bone cyst, solitary bone cyst, progressive bony cyst, blood cyst) occurs in other bones as well as the jaws and is classified as a false cyst because it does not have an epithelial lining.

A substantial percentage of traumatic bone cysts are found in the inferior portion of the alveolar process adjacent to the apices of teeth, although not actually contacting the apices (as evidenced by an intact lamina dura and the persistence of pulp vitality). Such examples will not be discussed further here because they are included in Chapter 16 with the periapical radiolucencies. This ordering was necessary to compare and differentiate them from the periapical radiolucencies, which are sequelae of pulpal involvement.

On the contrary, the traumatic bone cyst occurs with some frequency in the basal bone of the jaws and may then be clearly seen on radiographs as separate from the apex of the tooth (Figs. 18-7 and 18-8). Consequently it is included in this chapter since it satisfies the criteria for cystlike radiolucencies dissociated from teeth. It is frequently round to oval and, in contrast to cysts in the alveolar bone, has a scalloped superior margin produced by its molding around the roots of the mandibular premolars or molars (Fig. 18-7 and 18-8).

The cause of the traumatic bone cyst has not been conclusively established. Some pathologists favor the theory that the lesion is a sequela of a trauma-induced intrabony hematoma; others believe that it represents a burned-out cyst; still others contend that it is a cyst whose lining is so membrane thin that the surgeon does not detect it but nevertheless the inflammation he induces is sufficient to destroy this epithelial lining and account for the resolution of the lesion; and, finally, a theory of tumor degeneration has been proposed.

FEATURES

The traumatic bone cyst is frequently found unexpectedly on routine radiographs. When questioned about the lesion, half the patients will give a history of trauma to the region. The cyst is usually totally asymptomatic, pain being experienced by only a few of the patients, and

Fig. 18-7. Traumatic bone cyst. **C,** Note the pseudomultilocular appearance and cortical expansion of this large lesion. (**A** and **C** courtesy M. Kaminski, D.D.S., and S. Atsaves, D.D.S., Chicago. **B** courtesy R. Goepp, D.D.S., Zoller Clinic, University of Chicago.)

only occasionally does the jaw show regional expansion.

The mandible is involved in the majority of reported cases—with the premolar-molar area, the inferior region of the ramus, and the incisor region being affected in this order of frequency. Paresthesia is not a feature of the entity. The lesion seldom occurs in the maxilla (Winer and Doku, 1978) and seldom in a person over 25 years of age. It is found slightly more frequently in men. Multiple lesions have been reported in the same person. Furthermore, although jaw expansion has been observed in some patients, pathologic fractures have not been reported when expansion has been described. The surface has been smoothly contoured, and the covering mucosa has been normal in appearance.

Generally the lesion does not measure over 3 cm in diameter, but examples have been reported in which there was involvement and expansion of almost the entire ramus and body (Fig. 18-7, C). Aspiration may yield a little straw-colored or even serosanguineous fluid, although on occasion copious amounts have been reported. Microscopic examination of the lesion will usually reveal sparse shreds of fibrous tissue along with small deposits of hemosiderin.

DIFFERENTIAL DIAGNOSIS

For a discussion of the differential diagnosis of a traumatic bone cyst, refer to the differential diagnosis section under keratocysts (p. 377). Fig. 18-8, *D*, shows an intrabony hemangioma that resembles a traumatic bone cyst.

MANAGEMENT

It is important not to rely on the radiographic image or the usual clinical features to establish a final diagnosis of traumatic bone cyst. These radiolucencies of the jaws should be positively identified.

Even after carefully evaluating all the radio-

Fig. 18-8. A to **C,** Traumatic bone cysts. **A,** Lesion is in the symphysis region, where it has projected over the apices of the incisor teeth. **B,** Lesion is in the first molar region. **C,** Lesion is in the premolar region. **D,** Central cavernous hemangioma of bone, which resembles a traumatic bone cyst. Note the "wormhole" appearance sometimes seen in bony hemangiomas. (**A** courtesy P. Akers, D.D.S., Evanston, Ill. **B** courtesy J. Lehnert, D.D.S., Minneapolis. **C** courtesy W. Heaton, D.D.S., Chicago. **D** from Zalesin, H. M., Rotskoff, K., and Silverman, H.: J. Oral Surg. **33:**877-884, 1975. Copyright by the American Dental Association. Reprinted by permission.)

graphic and clinical evidence he might obtain from a complete examination, including the results from any indicated laboratory tests, the clinician should not conclude that a particular cystlike radiolucency is unquestionably a traumatic bone cyst or other kind of cyst. Before surgically entering any such defect, he must rule out by aspirating the area the remote possibility that the lesion could be a dangerous vascular tumor. When he opens the region of a traumatic bone cyst, he will discover either an empty bony cavity or, on occasion, a cavity containing some friable loose brownish material. A thin lining of the bony walls is sometimes observed.

Since this lesion must be surgically explored to ensure the correct diagnosis, the subsequent enucleation and curettement, which produces hemorrhage into the cavity, usually assures a successful regression of the defect as it is slowly obliterated by bone. The healing period should be closely observed radiographically.

PRIMORDIAL CYST

A primordial cyst is thought to develop as the result of some influence causing cystic degeneration in the odontogenic epithelium of the tooth germ before mineralization has been initiated. The involved tooth bud may be of either the regular permanent dentition or of a supernumerary tooth. The radiographic picture is nonspecific, showing only a cystlike radiolucency.

The patient with a primordial cyst will usually have a missing permanent tooth because of failure of the tooth to develop. When a permanent tooth is not missing but the patient shows a tendency for the development of supernumerary teeth, the clinician must consider that a cystlike radiolucency is possibly a primordial cyst developing in the germ of a supernumerary tooth. In practice, however, it is often difficult to establish with certainty whether a particular missing tooth has been extracted, because frequently the tooth (e.g., 6-year molar) may have been removed at an early age and the patient failed to realize that a permanent tooth had been lost. Consequently the examiner often must determine the true nature of the situation through an intuitive process involving such considerations as the state of the patient's oral health, the particular permanent teeth missing, and the frequency with which the teeth in question are congenitally absent in the appropriate population.

FEATURES

The primordial cyst shows no sexual predilection and occurs most frequently between the ages of 10 and 30 years. The mandibular molar region, especially the third molar and the area just distal to it, represents the most frequent site of development (Fig. 18-9). These cysts demonstrate all the usual features of cysts and seldom cause cortical expansion. Microscopically they are usually keratocysts, which are discussed next. Thus on aspiration the clinician will frequently obtain a thick yellowish granular fluid composed primarily of exfoliated cells and keratin.

DIFFERENTIAL DIAGNOSIS

The differential diagnosis of this lesion is discussed under the section dealing with keratocysts (p. 377).

MANAGEMENT

The management of the primordial cyst is the same as that for other intrabony odontogenic cysts. Because a significant percentage of primordial cysts appear microscopically as odontogenic keratocysts, which have a high recurrence

Fig. 18-9. Primordial cyst. The permanent tooth failed to develop in each case.

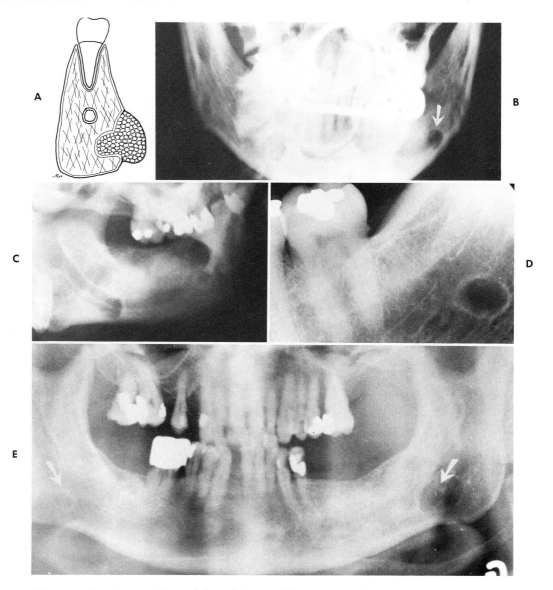

Fig. 18-10. Developmental bone defect of the mandible. A, Diagram of a cross section of the mandible showing part of the submandibular gland within the defect. B to D, Radiographs of several different cases. E, Bilateral defects (arrows). (B and C courtesy O. H. Stuteville, D.D.S., M.D., St. Joe, Ark. E courtesy N. Barakat, D.D.S., Beirut, Lebanon.)

Fig. 18-11. Developmental bone defects of the mandible.

rate, they require more vigorous curettement and vigilant postsurgical attention than do other types of bony cysts.

DEVELOPMENTAL BONE DEFECT OF THE MANDIBLE (STAFNE'S CYST)

The developmental bone defect of the mandible (known also as static bone cyst or defect, latent bone cyst or defect, idiopathic bone cavity, developmental submandibular gland defect of the mandible, aberrant salivary gland defect in the mandible, and lingual mandibular bone concavity) is a depression in the medial surface of the mandible in the third molar–angle area. Azaz and Lustmann (1973), examining dry mandibles, reported that 8% of their specimens had either anterior or posterior lingual depressions (Figs. 18-10 and 18-11).

Because a lobe of the submandibular salivary gland has been found to extend into this bony depression in several cases, the defect is generally believed to be caused by the mandible's developing around the lobe of the gland during embryonic life. Rarely the sublingual gland may produce a similar invagination in the canine and premolar region.

In a report of an interesting case, Hansson (1980) described a lingual mandibular bone cavity in an 11-year-old boy. Serial radiographs revealed that the radiolucency appeared between 11 and 12½ years of age, expanded, and became more prominent over the next 5 years.

FEATURES

The pouch extending through the lingual plate of the mandible produces a well-circumscribed radiolucency surrounded by a heavy radiopaque border (Fig. 18-10). This border is the result of x rays passing parallel through the relatively greater thickness of cortical bone that makes up the walls of the defect.

The radiolucency may vary in size from 1 to 2 cm in diameter and be oval, elliptic, round, or semicircular in shape. On occasion the defect is completely enclosed by bone. Sometimes bilateral defects have been described (Fig. 18-10).

The developmental bone defect of the mandible is completely asymptomatic and usually found on routine radiographic surveys. It is generally located near the angle of the mandible between the mandibular canal and the inferior border. It does not contact the apices of molars whose pulps are vital unless concomitant caries has produced gangrenous pulps. Statistical reports indicate that it is observed radiographically more frequently in women and occurs in about one out of every 250 patients.

DIFFERENTIAL DIAGNOSIS

The position and appearance of this radiolucency are all but diagnostic. Occasionally when the defect is small and situated in a more superior position in a region where teeth are present or have only recently been extracted, it may be mistaken for a *radicular* or *residual cyst.* Confusion more frequently occurs in the anterior variety because the entity is often cast over the apices of the teeth (see Fig. 16-29).

Some clinicians use the following procedure to strengthen their impression of developmental bone defect: a curved needle, of about 16 gauge for rigidity, is advanced into the tissue either intraorally or extraorally until the medial surface of the mandible is encountered; thus the lingual surface of the mandible can be explored by walking the needle along the surface of the bone; if a recess is found on the medial wall, the diagnosis of developmental bone defect is quite certain provided all the other findings concur. Also sialography may show the distribution of dye in the radiolucency, since a portion of the submandibular salivary gland usually lies within this bony pocket.

MANAGEMENT

Recognition of this entity is all that is necessary. In our opinion these defects should no longer be surgically explored unless the clinician has reason to suspect a more serious diagnosis. It must not be forgotten, however, that *salivary gland tumors* have been reported to occur within these defects.

ODONTOGENIC KERATOCYST

The odontogenic keratocyst (OKC) has been recognized and classified as distinct from other types of bony cysts on the basis of its somewhat different clinical behavior and its distinct and unique microscopic structure.

The OKC cuts across the usual classification of cysts because its diagnosis depends entirely on its microscopic features and is independent of its location. For example, a primordial cyst, a follicular cyst, or a radicular cyst may prove to be a keratocyst on microscopic examination of the specimen. Interestingly the primordial cyst, the lateral periodontal cyst, and the multiple jaw cysts of the basal cell nevus syndrome are predominantly OKCs. Also a reported 7.8% of all jaw cysts, 8.5% of all dentigerous cysts, and 0.9% of all radicular cysts are OKCs (Payne, 1972). In

Shafer's series (1978) 45% of primordial cysts were OKCs.

Radiographically the OKC cannot be distinguished from other intrabony cysts. On occasion its lumen, densely filled with keratin, will cause the usual radiolucent cystlike image to have a hazy appearance (Fig. 18-12). Sometimes also it will have scalloped borders and may even occur with a multilocular appearance.

In this chapter the discussion of OKCs will be limited to those that do not contact teeth, representing about 28% of these cysts.

FEATURES

The symptoms produced by the OKC are identical with those of the other bony cysts. The cyst may occur in all age groups, but its peak incidence falls in the second and third decades and shows a gradual decline through the later years; 56.9% occur in males; and 65% are found in the mandible (Brannon, 1976).

Although multiple OKCs of the jaws have been reported, only some of these were accompanied by the basal cell nevus syndrome. Occasionally the cyst will expand the cortical plates and perforate; and when palpated, it will demonstrate a firmer fluctuance than the usual bony cyst that has perforated the bony plates because the lumen of the OKC is filled with keratin having a somewhat doughy consistency.

For this reason the clinician should use a large-bore needle when attempting to aspirate these cysts to recover the thick cheesy yellow substance that fills the lumen. The OKC differs from other bony cysts in showing a recurrence rate of approximately 12% after removal (Brannon, 1976). This investigator reported a 36.4% recurrence rate in syndrome OKCs. Forssell and co-workers (1974a) reported that in their series more recurrences occurred in men and in young patients. Also they reported that fewer recurrences occurred in cases where the cyst was extirpated totally in one piece. Recurrences are rare with other bony cysts.

Microscopically the keratocyst also presents a characteristic picture and must be distinguished from a keratinizing odontogenic cyst, which seldom recurs. Its lumen is frequently filled with keratin produced by an epithelial lining whose appearance is distinct from that of the usual stratified squamous keratinizing epithelium and is peculiar to this type of cyst (Fig. 18-12). The wall is frequently thin and has a similarly thin epithelial lining deficient in rete ridges. The basal cells are either columnar or cuboidal and are arranged in a well-defined palisading row. The prickle cells are often vacuolated, usually sparse, and sometimes absent altogether in certain regions. The stratum corneum may be atypical in appearance, with the keratinized cells generally

Fig. 18-12. Odontogenic keratocyst. **A,** Note the hazy appearance. **B,** Note the scalloped margins. **C,** Characteristic histopathology.

retaining their nuclei; hence the keratinization is predominantly of the parakeratotic type. A buddinglike proliferation from the basal layer is frequently seen in recurrent OKCs. Brannon (1977) published an extensive paper on the histology of the OKC. Wilson and Ross (1978) discussed the ultrastructure of the OKC.

DIFFERENTIAL DIAGNOSIS

Because of its unusually high recurrence rate, the OKC must be distinguished from all other cystlike radiolucencies listed in this chapter.

For example, a cystlike radiolucency measuring 1 cm in diameter is found on a radiograph of an edentulous third molar region of the mandible in a 21-year-old white man. The entity is completely asymptomatic, and there are no related clinical signs. On the radiograph the mandibular canal appears to be displaced inferiorly by the lesion.

Less likely. An assessment of the circumstances surrounding the discovery of a cystlike radiolucency will undoubtedly lessen the probability that any of the entities in this group warrant further consideration in the differential diagnosis. Nevertheless, the fact that they do have some features in common with the lesion under investigation will compel the clinician to include them in his list of possibilities albeit they represent unlikely choices.

Benign nonodontogenic tumors of the mandible are quite uncommon and hence would be assigned a low ranking in the list of possibilities.

The *cementifying* or *ossifying fibroma* is not a common lesion.

Although a *developmental bone defect* might occur in the third molar region, it would almost never be found superior to the mandibular canal and would not cause displacement of the canal—except (rarely) when an expanding soft tissue tumor in the submaxillary space protruded into it, causing it to enlarge.

Fissural cysts do not occur in the third molar region.

The *giant cell reparative granuloma* is usually found in the anterior regions of the jaws.

The *giant cell lesion of hyperparathyroidism* can often be ruled out by examination of the serum chemistry.

Although the third molar region is a likely location for an *ameloblastoma*, the young age of the patient and the less frequent occurrence of this odontogenic tumor would characterize it as less likely.

The possibility that the radiolucency is a *third molar tooth crypt* is not great because the calci-

fication of this tooth is usually initiated in the eighth year and the tooth is fully formed by age 21. Also the contralateral third molar area can be used for a comparison if delayed calcification is suspected. Radiographs taken 6 months later will confirm the presence of the calcifying crown; but taking radiographs again in 6 months' time would not be a suitable practice if the clinician strongly suspects that the lesion represents a serious pathologic condition.

Comparing the bone trabeculation in the remainder of the jaws will aid in determining whether the entity is a *cystlike marrow space*, for a single marrow space of this size and shape without similar areas elsewhere in the jawbone would be quite unusual.

More likely. The clinician's attention is now directed to the following more likely entities, which are similar in several respects and are appropriate for inclusion in the working diagnosis (ranked in descending order of frequency):

Residual cyst
Traumatic bone cyst
Primordial cyst
Odontogenic keratocyst—primordial type
Ameloblastoma

All these entities show a predilection for the third molar area and, except for the ameloblastoma (which usually occurs in an older age group), for patients in their early to mid 20s. The patient's medical history may produce some clues that will aid in arranging the entities in a differential diagnosis, but more often than not it will add to the confusion.

Although the mandibular third molar region is a characteristic site for the *ameloblastoma*, this tumor should not be given a high ranking in this 21-year-old patient if paresthesia is not present.

Aspiration may be helpful in developing a working diagnosis. If the procedure produces an amber-colored fluid, a *primordial cyst*, a *residual cyst*, or a *cystic ameloblastoma* would be suggested. Conversely, if a thick yellow cheesy material is collected, a *keratocyst—primordial type* would be inferred. If aspiration proved to be nonproductive, the area could then be a *tooth crypt*, a *traumatic bone cyst*, or one of the *solid* entities listed at the beginning of the chapter.

If the cystlike radiolucency shows a haziness within a hyperostotic border, the increased opacity could be caused by keratin packed in the lumen and be suggestive of a diagnosis of *keratocyst*.

If the clinician can determine that the third molar failed to develop in the affected quadrant, the *developing tooth crypt* or the *primordial cyst* should be considered as the most likely diagnosis. A patient who has had several posterior teeth extracted over a period of years, however, can seldom be relied on to give sufficiently accurate information regarding whether a third molar ever developed, especially if the other molars are present. Also, if the first permanent molar was extracted relatively soon after its eruption, the patient will quite often become confused and report that a deciduous tooth was lost. Furthermore, the second molar frequently erupts into the position of the first molar and the third molar drifts into the position of the second molar.

The rarer *myxoma* also must be considered in such a circumstance because this lesion is compatible with the history of a tooth that failed to develop and may be seen as a cystlike radiolucency.

If the patient informs the clinician that a tooth was extracted from the area and a cyst was associated with the tooth, the impression that the radiolucent area is a *residual cyst* is reinforced—unless there is otherwise conflicting evidence.

A previous radiograph showing a tooth present and associated with a cyst, whether radicular, lateral, or follicular, would add credence to the choice of *residual cyst*.

Forssell and co-workers (1974b) indicated that the following findings are highly suggestive of the diagnosis of OKCs: (1) a cystlike radiolucency in the third molar region or mandibular ramus, (2) a diameter of more than 3 cm, (3) a unilocular cystlike radiolucency with scalloped margins, (4) a multilocular cyst, and (5) odorless creamy or caseous contents.

MANAGEMENT

The OKC should be approached in the same manner as that recommended for other bony cysts (Chapters 16 and 17) with the following exceptions:

1. When the clinician encounters a cystic lumen filled with yellow, cheesy, granular keratin, he must curette the bony walls in a more vigorous and thorough manner than usual since the recurrence rate of the keratocyst is approximately 40%.
2. After the microscopic examination confirms the working diagnosis of OKC, a more careful than usual postsurgical radiographic follow-up is indicated.

An intense curetting is employed to help ensure the complete enucleation and/or removal of the epithelial buds, which are frequently present deep in the walls of this cyst and which, if left

behind, can be expected to cause a recurrence. The unusual epithelial budding phenomenon, causing the high recurrence rate, usually precludes the more conservative approaches such as marsupialization and decompression. Lurie and co-workers (1976) favor the use of a bone scan in order to more precisely define the extent of the lesion presurgically.

If other factors persuade the clinician that either marsupialization or decompression should be employed, he must maintain a careful vigilance of the region both during and after the course of treatment.

AMELOBLASTOMA

The ameloblastoma is an odontogenic tumor usually described as a locally malignant lesion and thought to arise from ameloblasts. It represents approximately 11% of odontogenic tumors (Regezi et al., 1978). It may cast a unilocular cystlike radiolucency or a multilocular image. When it occurs in the maxilla, it is mostly unilocular; and when it occurs in the mandible, it is more evenly divided between unilocular and multilocular. Either way the radiographic appearance is not diagnostic. The multilocular appearance of this tumor is emphasized in Chapter 19.

FEATURES

The ameloblastoma is painless and slow growing; it can cause migration and loosening of teeth as well as root resorption and paresthesia of the lip. Struthers and Shear (1976) reported that in their series 81% of ameloblastomas contacting roots showed root resorption radiographically (dentigerous cysts showed resorption in 55% of cases). It may expand the cortical plates, but frequently it erodes them and then invades the adjacent soft tissue. True metastasis is rare and, of course, indicates that the particular lesion in question is malignant. The cystlike appearance on the radiograph is identical with that of the other entities discussed in this chapter (Fig. 18-13).

Ameloblastomas are found with approximately equal frequency in men and women (Minderjahn, 1979). The incidence peaks between 20 and 50 years of age (approximate average 40 years). The tumors occur five times more frequently in the mandible than in the maxilla (Regezi et al., 1978) and most commonly in the posterior part of the lower jaw, a propitious feature since the thick compact bone of the mandible tends to restrict their extension. The maxilla, on the other hand, lacks the limiting barriers

Fig. 18-13. Ameloblastoma. **A** to **F,** Four cystlike ameloblastomas. In **E** the entity produced an exophytic lesion. **F,** A radiograph of the lesion in **E. G** to **K,** Histologic types of ameloblastoma: **G,** alveolar; **H,** plexiform; **I,** acanthomatous; **J,** granular cell; **K,** spindle cell. (**A** courtesy O. H. Stuteville, D.D.S., M.D., St. Joe, Ark. **B** and **C** courtesy D. Skuble, D.D.S., Hinsdale, Ill. **D** courtesy J. Lehnert, D.D.S., Minneapolis. **E** and **F** courtesy D. Bonomo, D.D.S., Flossmoor, Ill.)

Continued.

of compact bone; and tumors in this area are close to the nasal cavity, paranasal sinuses, orbital contents, pharyngeal tissues, and vital structures leaving and entering the base of the skull—which contributes to the unfavorable prognosis of expanding tumors occurring in the maxilla.

The early ameloblastoma is asymptomatic; but later, as it expands and/or perforates the cortical plates, it becomes clinically discernible and palpable. A particular ameloblastoma may feel firm if it is of the solid type* or soft and fluctuant if it has undergone cystic degeneration. If it is a cystic type, straw-colored fluid will be aspirated, thus prompting the incorrect impression of a cyst. To distinguish between the solid and the cystic type radiographically is not possible.

Microscopically there are at least five histologic types of true ameloblastoma: simple (alveolar),

---

*Gross and scanning microscopic examinations disclose two distinct physical types, the solid and the cystic. The *solid* type is composed of a solid mass of tumor along with varying amounts of fibrous tissue; clinically such a tumor has a fine, granular, firm consistency. If the tumor is of the *cystic* type, cystic areas of varying sizes will be clinically evident on the surface of or within the specimen and histologically cystic degeneration of the stellate reticulum–like tissue will be apparent.

plexiform, acanthomatous, spindle cell, and granular cell (Fig. 18-13). To date, a difference in invasive properties or recurrence rates among these five types has not been shown. The very cellular ameloblastomas, however, may prove to be more aggressive than the less cellular types—which are composed of more fibrous tissue or large cystic spaces.

DIFFERENTIAL DIAGNOSIS

So as not to be surprised at surgery, the surgeon must consider that every cystlike radiolucency of the jawbones could be an ameloblastoma. The differential diagnosis of the lesion is discussed under that of the odontogenic keratocyst (p. 377).

MANAGEMENT

The relatively radical surgical treatment of ameloblastomas is predicated on their high frequency of recurrence, which is due to their tendency to develop small projections that extend beyond their apparent margins.

Consequently the area from which an ameloblastoma has been removed must be suspected

Fig. 18-13, cont'd. For legend see p. 379.

for an extended period and regularly reexamined if an undetected recurrence is to be precluded.

Mehlisch and co-workers (1972) aptly describe the successful treatment of an ameloblastoma as that which achieves an acceptable prognosis and causes minimal disfigurement. Their criteria are based on a compromise among such variables as the age and general health of the patient and the size, location, and duration of the tumor. In light of these guidelines, judging whether treatment of an ameloblastoma is successful or not depends on the distinctive features of the tumor in question. The complete spectrum of approaches, ranging from conservative incision to wide block resection, has been practiced over the years. Wide block resection, with placement of a bone graft, has produced the lowest recurrence rate.

We do not say, however, that radical resection is always the treatment of choice since less radical treatment appears to be effective for tumors located in the anterior part of the jaw and measuring less than 5 cm in diameter. Also small lesions in older patients whose poor general health precludes resection have been well managed by vigorous curettement in conjunction with cautery, Ameloblastomas occurring in the anterior region of either jaw have the lowest recurrence rates. Marciani and co-workers (1977) recommended the use of cryotherapy in selected cases.

SURGICAL DEFECT

Defects of a transitory or permanent nature result from the enucleation or resection of lesions occurring within bone. The majority of these defects possess well-defined borders; and when they are round or ovoid in shape, they have a cystlike appearance on radiographs (Fig. 18-14).

Usually a radiolucency may be recognized as a surgical defect when the patient informs the clinician of the prior surgery. Occasionally a surgical defect will be permanent in nature usually because relatively large areas of cortical bone, along with the periosteum and marrow, have been lost; hence there is a deficiency of the bone-forming elements. When a patient with such a deformity is seen by a different clinician some years after the surgery, the cystlike radiolucency may present a dilemma. Is it a surgical defect or a recurrence of the original condition; or is it a new lesion? If a series of postsurgical radiographs have been taken over the years and are available to the new clinician, he will readily be able to tell whether the area is decreasing, remaining constant, or enlarging in size.

If it has remained constant or is decreasing

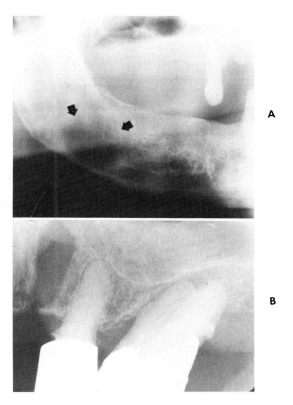

Fig. 18-14. Surgical defect. **A,** Twenty years after cystectomy. **B,** One year after a traumatic extraction.

slightly in size, it is most likely a surgical defect. If it is increasing in size, however, it must be considered a recurrence of the original pathologic process or possibly a new lesion. For example, if a dentigerous cyst was removed some years before, an ameloblastoma may have developed from remnants of the epithelial lining.

If the clinician encounters an asymptomatic radiolucency in an area of the jaw that according to the patient's history was the site of previous surgery, and if the original diagnosis can be obtained, he will have some insight as to the possibility that the image is a quiescent defect or a recurrence of disease.

If postsurgical radiographs of the area are not available, the size and shape of the asymptomatic radiolucency should be monitored every 6 months. Even though the original diagnosis was a benign condition (i.e., a cyst), this does not relieve the clinician of the obligation to periodically reexamine the presumed surgical defect until its innocent status has been convincingly demonstrated. Such a demonstration would be indicated by a constant or diminishing size in subsequent radiographs. If an increase in size is noted on successive radiographs, the area must be investigated to determine the cause of the change.

Palpation of the jawbone may reveal a depression on the medial or lateral surface in a position corresponding to the location of the radiolucency. Such a finding will contribute to the description of the defect's true nature.

CENTRAL GIANT CELL (REPARATIVE) GRANULOMA

The central giant cell granuloma may occur initially as a solitary cystlike radiolucency (Fig. 18-15); but as it grows larger, it frequently develops an architecture that cause a soap bubble type of mutlilocular radiolucency. Although trauma was thought to be the causative factor, many pathologists now believe that this is not the case; and the cause is in doubt.

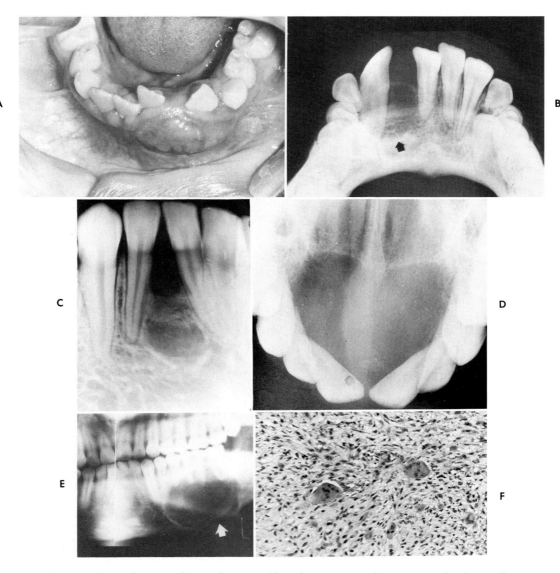

Fig. 18-15. Central giant cell granuloma. **A,** Clinical appearance of an anterior alveolar swelling in a 9-year-old boy. **B,** Radiograph of the lesion. **C** to **E,** Additional cystlike central giant cell granulomas. **F,** Photomicrograph showing giant cells in the fibrovascular stroma. (**C** courtesy F. Prock, D.D.S., Joliet, Ill. **D** courtesy N. Barakat, D.D.S., Beirut, Lebanon. **E** courtesy J. Ireland, D.D.S., and J. Dolci, D.D.S., Mundelein, Ill.)

FEATURES

The central giant cell granuloma occurs most frequently in women under 30 years of age, and two out of three lesions are found in the mandible. The portion of the jaws anterior to the molars is the usual site of involvement. Paresthesia is not a feature. In Raibley and Shafer's series (1979) of 90 central giant cell granulomas the mean age was 26.3 years, 65.5% occurred in patients under 30 years of age, and 32% occurred in the second decade of life. The sex ratio was 2.4:1 in favor of females. Female predilection in the 20s was 8:1. Of the lesions 70.4% occurred in the mandible and 95.6% were situated anterior to the second molar teeth. Concerning appearance on radiographs, 71% were reported as being unilocular and 17.5% as multilocular.

The lesion is painless and grows slowly by expanding and thinning the cortical plates, but it seldom perforates into the soft tissue. Thus the clinician usually finds a hard expansion demonstrating some flexibility. If the cortical plates are perforated, however, the swelling will be moderately soft to palpation (Fig. 18-15). This is to be expected because microscopically the lesion consists of multinucleated giant cells scattered throughout a vascular granulomatous tissue stroma that contains a minimum of collagen (Fig. 18-15).

Hemosiderin is often scattered throughout the tissue and, with the high vascularity, may impart a bluish cast to a lesion that has extended peripherally through the cortical plates and lies just beneath a thin mucosal surface. The covering mucosa appears normal unless traumatized. An expanding lesion may cause some migration of teeth, but root resorption is not the rule.

DIFFERENTIAL DIAGNOSIS

All the cystlike lesions discussed in this chapter must be considered in the differential diagnosis of giant cell granuloma. The clinical characteristics of the lesion in question should be compared with those listed for each entity at the end of the chapter.

Whenever a diagnosis of giant cell granuloma is reported by the pathologist, the serum chemistry must be studied to exclude the possibility of a *giant cell lesion of hyperparathyroidism.*

MANAGEMENT

Surgical enucleation of the lesion with curettement is the treatment of choice. Recurrences are not common; but when they do happen, the possibility that the lesion is a giant cell lesion of hyperparathyroidism must be considered. Such a suspicion can be rejected or confirmed only by a study of the patient with emphasis on serum examination.

The serum should be analyzed particularly for calcium, phosphorus, and alkaline phosphatase to rule out hyperparathyroidism. Such steps are imperative since the giant cell granuloma cannot be differentiated from this giant cell lesion on the basis of a clinical, radiographic, or microscopic examination.

GIANT CELL LESION (HYPERPARATHYROIDISM)

The clinical, radiographic, and microscopic characteristics of the giant cell lesion of hyperparathyroidism are identical with those of the giant cell granuloma just discussed. This lesion occurs as a unilocular or a multilocular radiolucency and is found in patients with primary, secondary, or tertiary hyperparathyroidism. If the jaws show rarefaction (a possible finding in advanced hyperparathyroidism), the giant cell lesion will appear to have poorly demarcated borders because of the osteoporosis of the surrounding bone (Fig. 18-16). The establishment of its true identity is dependent on demonstrating the concomitant parathyroid, kidney, or other systemic disorder.

SECONDARY HYPERPARATHYROIDISM

Secondary hyperparathyroidism is discussed before the primary type because it is detected more frequently. One of the causative pathologies is impaired kidney function from disease (e.g., an ascending infection), which induces a shift in the ionic balance of the blood that ultimately causes

Fig. 18-16. Giant cell lesion of hyperparathyroidism (arrow). Note the poorly defined borders of the tumor caused by the generalized rarefaction of the jawbone. (Courtesy O. H. Stuteville, D.D.S., M.D., St. Joe, Ark.)

a lowered level of serum calcium. The mechanism of this shift is not yet a subject of complete agreement.

The reduced serum calcium level then leads to parathyroid hyperplasia and an increased production of parathyroid hormone, which in turn causes bone to resorb and return calcium to the blood to maintain serum calcium at normal levels. In moderate to severe cases, enough mineral is removed from the bones that the bones become rarefied and this rarefaction is radiographically discernible (i.e., osteitis fibromsa cystica generalisata, Chapter 22). The same phenomenon is observed in patients who are on prolonged dialysis.

In severe cases of hyperparathyroidism, the cortical plates are especially thinned and the lamina dura around the roots of the teeth may not be apparent on radiographs. Central giant cell lesions (brown tumors) are prone to occur in these patients with hyperparathyroidism and are found with some frequency in the jaws (Fig. 18-16). They are identical with the central giant cell granuloma in clinical, radiographic, and histologic features; but they differ insofar as the giant cell lesion of hyperparathyroidism may demonstrate a high recurrence rate if the systemic problem is not alleviated. Rao and co-workers (1978) reported on several cases of brown tumors associated with chronic renal failure.

PRIMARY HYPERPARATHYROIDISM

Clinically detectable primary hyperparathyroidism is less common than the secondary type and is caused by a functioning adenoma (less often by a carcinoma) of one of the parathyroid glands. The increased parathyroid hormone stimulates bone resorption and thus increases the serum calcium. Concomitantly it induces an increased excretion of phosphate by the kidney. The skeletal changes and giant cell lesions are identical with those of the secondary type.

DIFFERENTIAL DIAGNOSIS

Primary and secondary hyperparathyroidism may be differentiated on the basis of history and laboratory findings.

Patients with *primary hyperparathyroidism* will usually be in a younger age group, between 30 and 60 years and may complain of polydipsia and polyuria because of the increased diuresis. Women are seven times more frequently involved than men. Serum values in advanced primary hyperparathyroidism are as follows: increased calcium levels, decreased phosphorus levels, and increased levels of alkaline phosphatase (which is characteristically elevated during increased bony resorption or apposition).

A patient with *secondary hyperparathyroidism* will have the symptoms and usually a history of kidney disease and will likely have a decreased renal output. An older age group (50 to 80 years) is involved, and women are only twice as often afflicted as men. Laboratory tests reveal an inverted relationship of the serum calcium and phosphorus levels as compared with those found in the primary disease (i.e., the serum calcium levels are normal or decreased whereas the serum phosphate and alkaline phosphate levels are increased).

MANAGEMENT

If the primary medical problem is corrected, the giant cell lesions often regress without surgery and the rarefaction disappears. Surgical excision of the parathyroid gland with its adenoma is the treatment for the primary type and is quite successful. The treatment of the kidney defect in the secondary type is usually more complicated.

INCISIVE CANAL CYST

Cysts of the incisive canal and of the palatine papilla are subclassifications of nasopalatine cysts originating in nests of epithelium that remain after the disintegration of the nasopalatine duct, an early epithelial fetal structure that is present in the area of the incisive canal (Fig. 18-17).

This bilateral epithelium-lined duct structure runs superiorly through the incisive canal area to become Jacobson's organ, which is bilaterally positioned on the lateral aspects of the nasal septum. These lateral structures disintegrate in later fetal life, but nests of epithelium remain and are sometimes stimulated to produce cysts of the incisive canal and palatine papilla.

The incisive canal cyst is situated within bone and thus shows as a cystlike radiolucent enlargement of the canal (Fig. 18-17). It is the most common nonodontogenic cyst of the maxilla and is reported to occur in one of every 100 persons. A cyst of the palatine papilla is located in soft tissue, so it usually does not produce a radiolucency.

FEATURES

The incisive canal cyst is evident as a cystlike radiolucency on occlusal and periapical radiographs of the maxillary central incisor area (Fig. 18-17). Frequently its image is projected over the apices of the central incisors and must be differ-

Fig. 18-17. A, Transverse section of a 15-week-old human embryo showing the incisive canal (inverted V-shaped structure). Note the bilateral epithelial nasopalatine ducts. **B** to **D,** Radiographs of incisive canal cysts. **B,** If one or both of the central incisors are nonvital one would suspect a pulpoperiapical lesion. (**B** and **C** courtesy R. Goepp, D.D.S., Zoller Clinic, University of Chicago.)

entiated from a radicular cyst. Often the anterior nasal spine is seen over the superior portion of the cyst as a radiopaque shadow, thus producing a heart-shaped radiolucency (Fig. 18-17).

On occasion, the cyst will form in a superior aspect of one of the incisive canals at a point where the canals are discernibly divergent, in which case it will be positioned slightly to one side of the midline and the displacement will be perceptible on radiographs. Sometimes also two separate cysts will develop simultaneously in the left and right branches of the canal and cause paired cystlike radiolucencies. The appearance of separate cysts, however, may be an illusion resulting from a cyst at the juncture of canals extending superiorly into the separate branches of the incisive canal.

A cyst of the papilla palatinae may be clinically evident as a nodular fluctuant mass involving the area of the papilla; but it will not be demonstrable on radiographs since it is primarily of soft tissue and extends into the soft tissue more readily than into bone; bony destruction in the incisive foramen therefore does not usually result. On occasion, however, an incisive canal cyst at the oral limits of the bony canal will bulge out of the canal into the soft tissue papilla and produce a nodular swelling that clinically appears to be a cyst of the papilla palatinae but can be correctly recognized from the obvious bony destruction that is apparent on the radiograph. A cyst in the canal may also erode the bone posterior to the canal, bulge into the mucosa posterior to the papilla, and create the clinical impression of a midpalatal cyst (Fig. 18-20, C).

The majority of incisive canal cysts are small, asymptomatic, and found on routine radiographic surveys. Frequently the patient will complain of a salty taste in his mouth, produced by a small sinus or a remnant of the nasopalatine duct that permits cystic fluid to drain into the oral cavity. Besides drainage, a feeling of fullness and a burning and numbness of the palatal mucosa over the papilla are frequent complaints.

When a sinus is not present and the cyst slowly enlarges, the patient usually observes a palatal swelling just posterior to the maxillary central incisors. This swelling will become painful if it is in a position that permits it to be traumatized during mastication or if it becomes secondarily infected. The swelling will be fluctuant as soon as it projects through the bone. Aspiration may yield the typical amber-colored fluid. On occasion, a very large cyst will be seen to produce an obvious facial swelling in the region of the philtrum-lip junction.

Other cysts may bulge into the nasal cavity and extend so far posteriorly as to appear to be midline cysts of the palate (Fig. 18-20, C).

The microscopic structure of the incisive canal cyst is similar to that of other cysts, although the epithelium lining the lumen is occasionally of the respiratory type and mucous glands are frequently present in the cyst wall.

DIFFERENTIAL DIAGNOSIS

Several types of cysts may occur in the anterior maxillary region and be projected over the apices of the incisors. Also it is important to be aware that the incisive canal and foramen may normally vary greatly in size. Consequently the clinician may have great difficulty distinguishing between a large incisive canal and a small asymptomatic incisive canal cyst on the basis of radiographic evidence alone. Some clinicians follow the rule of thumb that radiolucencies of the incisive canal measuring less than 0.6 cm should not be considered cystic in the absence of other symptoms (Fig. 18-18).

A diagnostic problem frequently arises when a cystlike radiolucency is projected over the apex of a maxillary central incisor. The clinician must distinguish whether this is an incisive canal cyst or a radicular cyst (Fig. 18-17, B).

If the lesion is an *incisive canal cyst,* the radiolucency in many instances may be projected away from the apex of the tooth in question by changing the horizontal angulation of the x-ray tube. Also if the pulps prove to be vital, the possibility of a *radicular cyst* will be eliminated.

When an *incisive canal cyst* has reached large proportions and extended posteriorly, destroying most of the hard palate, or has contacted and perhaps resorbed the roots of the incisors, the correct diagnosis will often prove difficult. In such situations the lesion may be confused with a *midline palatal cyst* or a *radicular cyst,* respectively.

Occasionally a *primordial cyst,* arising in a supernumerary tooth bud, occurs in the midline and must be differentiated from a radicular and an incisive canal cyst. Radiographs taken at different angles and vitality tests of the adjacent teeth will aid in the distinction.

Some older texts describe a *midalveolar cyst* that was thought to occur in the anterior midline and to arise from epithelial remnants left in the midfusion line of the median nasal process. Clearly, however, the median nasal process is not a paired structure so it does not have a fusion line. These cysts were most likely examples of primordial cysts.

Fig. 18-18. A, Large incisive canal. No pathosis was found at surgery. Note the two small bilateral radiolucent shadows lying within the larger radiolucency, which are cast over the apices of the left and right central incisor teeth (white arrows). These are the canals of Scarpa. **B,** Large incisive canal cyst in a Panorex radiograph.

MANAGEMENT

Surgical excision is the treatment of choice for small incisive canal cysts; and if possible, the defect should be entered from the palate to avoid devitalization of the adjacent incisor teeth. The nasopalatine nerve is frequently severed during surgery, and as a result the small patch of mucosa surrounding the incisive papilla and including the lingual incisive gingivae is numb for some time. Because the nasopalatine nerve innervates such a small area of palatal mucosa, numbness in the area is readily accepted by the patient, especially if he is informed of this possibility before surgery.

Occasionally large cysts have been treated by marsupialization.

FISSURAL CYSTS
Globulomaxillary cyst

The origin of the epithelial nests that form the globulomaxillary cyst is still a matter of dispute (Christ, 1970; Little and Jakobsen, 1973). Some pathologists favor the theory that epithelial nests are left in the fusion line between the embryonic maxillary processes. Others believe that these primitive processes merge rather than fuse and, since there is no fusion line, there cannot be nests of epithelium entrapped.

Most recent embryonic studies have illustrated, however, that both mechanisms (fusion and merging) are involved and that epithelial nests could easily be trapped in the bottom of the grooves during obliteration of the nests by the merging processes. Another reasonable school of thought is that globulomaxillary cysts are really primordial cysts that have occurred in supernumerary tooth buds in the area.

To further complicate the issue, many radicular cysts positioned between the lateral incisor and the canine have been misdiagnosed as globulomaxillary cysts. It is therefore important that the vitality of adjacent teeth be assured before the diagnosis of globulomaxillary cyst is made. This will rule out the possibility that the cyst is pulpal in origin.

The classic radiographic picture is of a more or less inverted pear–shaped or tear-shaped well-defined radiolucency between the roots of the lateral incisor and canine (Fig. 18-19). Furthermore, a careful examination of the radiograph will

Fig. 18-19. A, Globulomaxillary cyst. **B,** Lateral radicular cyst from a pulpless lateral incisor simulating a globulomaxillary cyst. **C,** Anatomic depression between the lateral incisor and canine suggesting a globulomaxillary cyst. **D,** Surgical defect simulating a globulomaxillary cyst. (**A** courtesy F. Prock, D.D.S., Joliet, Ill. **B** courtesy T. Emmering, D.D.S., Maywood, Ill. **D** courtesy R. Goepp, D.D.S., Zoller Clinic, University of Chicago.)

disclose that the lamina dura about the roots of both teeth is intact.

FEATURES

The globulomaxillary cyst will often be asymptomatic and discovered on routine radiographic examination. As it becomes larger and expands the cortical plate buccally, the patient may complain of swelling or of pain—especially if it becomes secondarily infected. The astute examiner will notice that the contact point between the lateral incisor and canine has shifted toward the incisal edges of these teeth because of rotation of the crowns by the spreading roots. The mucosa over the buccal swelling will be normal in appearance, and palpation of the surface will produce crepitus if the cortical plate is still intact but fluctuance if not. Aspiration will often yield typical amber-colored cyst fluid. The microscopic picture is similar to that seen in other cysts.

DIFFERENTIAL DIAGNOSIS

When an inverted tear-shaped radiolucency is found on the radiographs of a patient, the clinician must be especially careful not to make an impulsive diagnosis.

An *odontogenic cyst*, a *giant cell granuloma*, an *adenomatoid odontogenic tumor, surgical defects*, and even *anatomic variations* have masqueraded as a globulomaxillary cyst (Fig. 18-19).

If the clinician finds an amber-colored fluid on aspiration, he can be reasonably sure that he is dealing with a *cyst* or that there is a remote chance the lesion is a *mural or cystic ameloblastoma*.

Having determined a working diagnosis of cyst, he must then establish whether it is a *lateral periodontal*, a *radicular*, or a *globulomaxillary cyst*. This distinction must be made before treatment is initiated, because the root canals of the involved teeth will have to be treated and filled prior to surgery if the pulps are nonvital. Pulp vitality tests will aid in establishing whether the radiolucency is a sequela of a nonvital pulp.

In our experience the most common cause of a radiolucency between the maxillary canine and lateral incisor tooth is a normal anatomic depression in the labial plate in this region. This trough can be readily identified by visual inspection and also by palpation. In contradistinction almost all pathologic bony lesions would not produce a depression but would expand the jaws as soon as growth was sufficient to do so. In our experience the second most common cause of radiolucencies is pulpoperiapical lesions perhaps positioned

laterally because of the presence of lateral canals. Zegarelli and Zegarelli (1973) have published a very worthwhile paper on radiolucent lesions in the globulomaxillary region as also have Taicher and Azaz (1977).

MANAGEMENT

The management of this cyst is identical with that described for other bony cysts in Chapters 16 and 17. Special care must be taken during surgery to avoid devitalizing the adjacent teeth. As with other cysts, the lining must be carefully investigated to ascertain that no mural tumors are present. The surgical site must be observed radiographically until the defect has completely resolved or until time has lessened concern for recurrence.

Midpalatal cyst

The midpalatal cyst is an uncommon bony cyst that develops in the midline of the palate posterior to the palatal papilla. It originates in residual embryonic epithelial nests in the fusion line of the lateral palatal shelves. Radiographically a unilocular radiolucency will be seen in the midline of the palate (Fig. 18-20). Large cysts may completely destroy the bony palate.

FEATURES

The patient with a midpalatal cyst may complain of a painless bulging in the roof of his mouth that is increasing in size. If the cyst is not traumatized or secondarily infected, the dome-shaped mass will be nontender and covered with normal mucosa, which will perhaps appear more glossy than usual. The mass will be situated over the midline of the palate posterior to the incisive papilla (Fig. 18-20).

Because the bone inferior to the cyst is so thin, the cortical plate is rapidly perforated as the cyst grows; consequently the swelling will be soft and fluctuant but nonemptiable by digital pressure unless a sinus is present. If, as sometimes happens, the bony floor of the nose is completely eroded, the cyst may be slightly displaced superiorly by digital pressure. Aspiration will produce an amber-colored fluid.

The microscopic picture is identical with that of other cysts. The epithelial lining may be of the respiratory type (with goblet cells).

DIFFERENTIAL DIAGNOSIS

Although many lesions occur on the palate with some frequency, it seems reasonable to limit the differential diagnosis to soft lesions: midpalatal

Fig. 18-20. A, Radiographs of a midpalatal cyst injected with radiopaque dye. **B,** Clinical appearance of a midpalatal cyst. **C,** Palatal swelling from an incisive canal cyst that destroyed the posterior bony boundary of the canal and simulated a midpalatal cyst. **D,** Palatal space abscess from a pulpless premolar. (**A** courtesy D. Skuble, D.D.S., Hinsdale, Ill.)

cyst, incisive canal cyst, radicular cyst, palatal space abscess, lipoma, plexiform neurofibroma, mucocele, papillary cyst adenoma, and mucoepidermoid tumor (low grade).

Occasionally an early *low-grade mucoepidermoid tumor* will appear clinically as a mucocele when much mucus is produced by the mucous cells—which are the predominant cell type in the low-grade variety; but minor salivary gland tumors and retention phenomena are seldom seen in the midline of the hard palate since there is a paucity of minor salivary glands in this region. These tumors may be seen more in the lateral aspect of the posterior palate in the region of the anterior palatine foramen. The clinician would therefore assign a low rank to mucoepidermoid carcinoma, *papillary cyst adenoma,* and *mucocele* in the differential diagnosis for a soft midpalatal swelling.

Furthermore, although both the low-grade mucoepidermoid tumor and the mucocele might demonstrate fluctuance and not be emptiable by digital pressure—characteristics similar to those of cysts—unlike cysts, on aspiration they would not yield a typical amber-colored fluid but a viscuous, clear, sticky liquid (concentrated mucus).

The *plexiform neurofibroma* is the only peripheral nerve tumor that is soft and fluctuant. It is the usual type that occurs in von Recklinghausen's disease, so it would be a likely choice if the patient had this disease. Also it could be readily differentiated from a cyst since aspiration of a plexiform neurofibroma would not produce an aspirate.

A *lipoma* is not common in the oral cavity, and like the neurofibroma it could be readily distinguished from cysts by aspiration.

A *palatal space abscess* will be somewhat soft and fluctuant and will yield pus on aspiration. It is generally associated with the palatal roots of nonvital posterior teeth or a vital or nonvital tooth with a lateral periodontal abscess on the lingual aspect of a palatal root. Consequently a palatal space abscess will seldom be located in the posterior midline but will be displaced into the area adjacent to the tooth that gave rise to the infection (Fig. 16-15)—in contrast to an abscess resulting from a secondarily infected midpalatal cyst, which would be more symmetrically situated in the midline.

A *radicular cyst* involving a canine or a premolar will only rarely perforate the denser cortical bone of the lingual plate; rather this type of cyst will extend through the thinner buccal plate into the buccal vestibule. Further vitality tests and periapical radiographs would aid in the differentiation of the midpalatal cyst from the odontogenic palatal space abscess.

The *incisive canal cyst* is easily differentiated from the midpalatal cyst in most cases because it occurs in the canal above the palatine papilla whereas the midpalatal cyst occurs in the midline of the palate posterior to the papilla. When either an incisive canal cyst or a midpalatal cyst expands and destroys the posterior limits of the incisive canal, however, distinguishing with certainty between the two is usually impossible (Fig. 18-20).

MANAGEMENT

After the working diagnosis of midpalatal cyst has been established and the possibility of more serious entities ruled out by all appropriate diagnostic techniques, including aspiration, an acrylic stent should be fabricated on a revised cast to cover the entire hard palate. A mucoperiosteal flap should then be raised from the anterior, including the entire palatal mucosa, by incising along the gingival sulci around the lingual necks of all the teeth from the first molar on the right to the first molar on the left. This will ensure good access and permit complete removal of the cyst. If the full thickness of the bony palate has been destroyed, care should be taken to avoid perforating the nasal mucosa because such a perforation may well result in an oronasal fistula. The flap should be closed with sutures and the prefabricated stent placed securely in position. Clinical and radiographic follow-up is mandatory.

Median mandibular cyst

The median mandibular cyst occurs in the symphyseal region of the lower jaw. It is uncommon, and its origin is in dispute. Some authorities contend that it is a *true fissural cyst* originating from epithelium trapped in the fusion and/or merging of the paired mandibular processes during the fourth week of embryonic life. Others suggest that it probably represents a *primordial cyst* that formed in a supernumerary tooth bud. Still others champion the possibility that it is in reality a *lateral periodontal cyst* developing on the medial aspect of the central incisors. Soskolne and Shteyer (1977) discuss these possibilities in more detail.

Research techniques have not yet been sufficiently refined to demonstrate the genesis of this cyst in all cases. Certainly, though, if the central incisors adjacent to a median mandibular cyst are nonvital, a reasonable conclusion would be that the particular example is a radicular cyst. Conversely, if the teeth are vital a radicular cyst can be ruled out.

EARLY STAGE OF CEMENTIFYING AND OSSIFYING FIBROMAS (BENIGN FIBRO-OSSEOUS LESIONS OF PERIODONTAL LIGAMENT ORIGIN)

Cementifying and ossifying fibromas as well as cemento-ossifying fibromas are considered by most pathologists to be variants of the same basic entity.

These lesions are classified as neoplastic fibro-osseous lesions that arise from elements of the periodontal ligament (Hamner et al., 1968; Waldron and Giansanti, 1973a and b). They differ from the much more common periapical cementomas by the fact that they are seen in younger patients, occur most often in the premolar-molar region of the mandible instead of the incisor region, and if left untreated will attain a much larger size, frequently causing expansion of the jaws. The lesion may be labeled as ossifying or cementifying depending on which tissue is present. A mixture of bone and cementum may be seen in some lesions, and such would be identified as a "cemento-ossifying fibroma." Despite the foregoing it is important to be aware of the fact that a significant number of oral pathologists believe it is not often possible to differentiate between cementum and bone. Hence such pathologists prefer to use the term "fibrocalcific lesions of periodontal ligament origin" (Cornyn, 1975). The majority of cementifying and ossifying fibromas will occur in the periapex because they originate from elements in the periodontal ligament. Occasionally, however, they will not be in contact with the roots of teeth but will occur in the body of the maxilla or mandible in edentulous areas or, when teeth are present, not be associated with the teeth.

The early stage is osteolytic, in which the surrounding bone is resorbed and replaced by a fibrovascular type of soft tissue containing osteoblasts or cementoblasts or both. Cementifying cementomas and ossifying fibromas at this stage may appear as solitary cystlike radiolucencies that are not in contact with teeth (Fig. 18-21).

FEATURES

Cementifying and ossifying fibromas when small are asymptomatic but frequently may grow

A

B

Fig. 18-21. Immature fibro-osseous lesions (PDLO). The biopsy report indicated ossifying fibroma in both cases. (**A** courtesy S. Atsaves, D.D.S., Chicago. **B** courtesy R. Goepp, D.D.S., Zoller Clinic, University of Chicago.)

sufficiently large to expand the jawbone; 70% occur in the mandible and are primarily found in the premolar-molar region. The average age of patients with ossifying fibroma is 26.4 years, and the sexes are approximately equally affected. The age range in the study by Hamner and co-workers (1968) was 7 to 58 years. In contrast to the periapical cementomas these lesions classically occur as solitary entities.

The initial radiolucent stage usually changes progressively from a predominantly fibroblastic lesion to an increasingly calcified structure. During maturation, microscopic examination discloses a number of small droplets of cementum, spicules of bone, cementoblasts, and osteoblasts in a fibrous vascular stroma (Fig. 16-20, C). As these entities continue to mature, the calcified components become larger, coalesce, and are then apparent on radiographs as radiopaque foci

within a well-described radiolucency. Still later, in the mature stage, most of the lesion will consist of calcified tissue and will appear on radiographs as a well-defined radiopacity generally surrounded by a uniform radiolucent zone that represents a noncalcified area of fibrous tissue at the periphery.

DIFFERENTIAL DIAGNOSIS

At least 6 years are required for the lesion to pass from the radiolucent to the radiopaque stage. Usually this pathosis will show varying degrees of soft tissue density with a few small radiopaque foci present; and accordingly it would generally be included in the differential diagnosis of radiolucent areas with radiopaque foci discussed in Chapter 23. When the lesion (infrequently) is found to be completely radiolucent and not in contact with teeth, however, it is assigned a low ranking in the differential discussion of such cystlike radiolucencies.

MANAGEMENT

To make the correct diagnosis, a surgical approach is necessary to obtain biopsy material. Excision and curettement of the lesion are all that is required since this lesion does not have a tendency to recur.

BENIGN NONODONTOGENIC TUMORS

Specific benign nonodontogenic tumors are rarely observed within the jawbones. If they are considered as a group, however, their composite incidence is high enough to warrant their exemption from the category of rarities. The following tumors have occurred with some frequency within the jaws as cystlike radiolucencies not necessarily in contact with teeth: lipoma, salivary gland adenoma, amputation neuroma, neurofibroma, schwannoma, fibroma, and myxoma. Because their growth is slow, they demonstrate well-defined radiolucencies of varying shape (Fig. 18-22).

FEATURES

The majority of these lesions are asymptomatic, except for the peripheral nerve tumors that develop in conjunction with major sensory nerves. The patient will then usually complain of pain, paresthesia, or anesthesia in a region. The patient with an amputation neuroma will almost invariably describe a previous traumatic incident: a tooth extraction, a jaw fracture, or major jaw surgery.

If benign tumors of the jaw go untreated, they

Fig. 18-22. Neurilemoma. Note the cystlike radiolucency between the mandibular canine and premolar. (From Morgan, G., and Morgan, P.: Oral Surg. **25:**182-189, 1968.)

slowly grow and expand the cortical plates—which because of the slow growth of the tumor frequently remain intact. Aspiration will be nonproductive for the benign nonodontogenic tumors just discussed.

DIFFERENTIAL DIAGNOSIS

Benign nonodontogenic tumors of the jawbone should be assigned a low ranking in the differential diagnosis of solitary cystlike radiolucencies.

A *neurofibroma* involving the mandibular canal is sometimes found as an elongated broadening of the canal. When this picture is observed, therefore, the possibility that it represents a peripheral nervous tissue tumor should be considered. *Arteriovenous pathology,* however, also must be considered in such a case.

When the patient gives a history of major surgery or fracture in a region that has a painful cystlike radiolucency, an *amputation neuroma* must be considered as a possibility.

If the patient has neurofibromatosis, the likelihood that a cystlike radiolucency of the jawbones is a peripheral nerve tumor would be much greater than for the general population.

MANAGEMENT

Conservative excision—after a presurgical aspiration test has proved to be nonproductive—is the treatment of choice for these lesions. If the tumor involves the mandibular canal and its contents, the patient should be forewarned of the likelihood that he will experience a postoperative paresthesia or anesthesia of the lip. Also, if the radiolucency is large, the possibility of jaw fracture during surgery should be mentioned.

RARITIES

The following entities, which may appear as cystlike radiolucencies not necessarily in contact with teeth, represent either rare pathoses or else are more common lesions that rarely occur in the jaws (Fig. 18-23):

Adenomatoid odontogenic tumor
Ameloblastic variants
Aneurysmal bone cyst (Fig. 18-23, *D*)
Aneurysms in bone
Calcifying epithelial odontogenic tumor
Cementoma
Central hemangioma of bone
Central squamous cell carcinoma in cyst lining

Fig. 18-23. Rarities. **A,** Cystlike metastatic bronchogenic carcinoma (arrow). **B,** A pericoronal radiolucency involving an impacted canine proved to be a myxoma. **C,** Myxoma between the canine and lateral incisor. **D,** Cystlike aneurysmal bone cyst. **E,** Eosinophilic granuloma (arrow). (**B** and **E** courtesy N. Barakat, D.D.S., Beirut, Lebanon. **C** and **D** courtesy R. Kallal, D.D.S., Chicago.)

Table 18-1. Solitary cystlike radiolucencies

Entity	Predominant sex	Usual age (years)	Predominant jaw	Predominant region	Other radiographic appearances	Additional features
Marrow spaces	M = F	All	Mandible	Molar	Routine Multilocular Multiple cystlike	Asymptomatic Similar patterns contralaterally
Postextraction sockets	M = F	Over 20	Mandible	Molar	Osteosclerosis	Radiolucency does not enlarge History of extraction Asymptomatic
Residual cysts	$\frac{M}{F} = \frac{3}{2}$	Over 20 (avg. 52)	Maxilla—57%		Multilocular	Asymptomatic Preextraction radiograph showing tooth with associated cyst
Traumatic bone cysts	M > F Slight	Under 30	Uncommon in maxilla	Premolar-molar Incisor	Periapical radiolucency	Teeth vital Asymptomatic Possible history of trauma Usually no aspirate
Primordial cysts	M ~ F*	10-30	Mandible	Third molar	Multilocular	Permanent tooth fails to develop
Odontogenic keratocysts	M = 56.9%	Peak—10-30 (avg. 28)	Mandible—65%	Third molar	Scalloped borders Multilocular	Occasionally radiolucency appears hazy High recurrence rate
Ameloblastomas	M ~ F	20-50 (avg. 40)	Mandible—80%	Posterior—70%	Ill-defined ragged borders Multilocular	Erode cortical plates May cause paresthesia
Surgical defects	M = F	Over 10	Equal	Anterior	Ragged irregularly shaped borders	History of previous surgery Radiolucency does not enlarge
Central giant cell granulomas	$\frac{F}{M} = \frac{2.4}{1}$	Under 30 (avg. 26)	Mandible—70%	Anterior to second molars	Multilocular	Previous history of trauma Serum chemistries normal
Giant cell lesions (secondary hyperparathyroidism)	$\frac{F}{M} = \frac{2}{1}$	50-80	Mandible	None	Multilocular Indistinct borders	History of kidney disease Serum calcium normal to↓ Serum phosphate↑ Serum alkaline phosphatase↑
Giant cell lesions (primary hyperparathyroidism)	$\frac{F}{M} = \frac{7}{1}$	30-60	Mandible	None	Multilocular Indistinct borders	Polydipsia Polyuria Serum calcium↑ Serum phosphate↓ Serum alkaline phosphatase↑

*~ Approximately equal.

Continued.

Table 18-1. Solitary cystlike radiolucencies—cont'd

Entity	Predominant sex	Usual age (years)	Predominant jaw	Predominant region	Other radiographic appearances	Additional features
Incisive canal cysts	$\frac{M}{F} = \frac{3}{1}$		Maxilla only	Incisive canal	Heart shaped	Teeth vital Salty taste
Globulomaxillary cysts			Maxilla only	Between lateral incisor and canine	Tear shaped	Teeth vital
Midpalatal cysts			Maxilla only	Palatal midline Posterior to papilla	None	Uncommon
Median mandibular cysts			Mandible only	Midline	Multilocular	Rare lesions Teeth vital
Developmental bone defects	F > M	All ages	Mandible only	Third molar	Semicircular Oval	Teeth vital
Early cementifying/ossifying fibromas	M ~ F	Avg. 26.4	Mandible— 70%	Premolar-molar	Radiolucent-radiopaque Radiopaque	Teeth vital
Benign nonodontogenic tumors			Mandible	Molar Ramus	Elongated	Teeth vital

Desmoplastic fibroma
Histiocytosis X (Fig. 18-23, *E*)
Lateral periodontal cyst
Low-grade metastatic carcinoma
Minor salivary gland tumor in bone
Myxoma (Fig. 18-23, *B* and *C*)
Odontogenic fibroma
Odontoma (early stage)
Osteoblastoma (early stage)
Plasmacytoma
Squamous odontogenic tumor

SPECIFIC REFERENCES

Azaz, B., and Lustmann, J.: Anatomic configurations in dry mandibles, Br. J. Oral Surg. **11**:1-9, 1973.

Brannon, R. B.: The odontogenic keratocyst: a clinicopathologic study of 312 cases. I. Clinical features, Oral Surg. **42**:54-72, 1976.

Brannon, R. B.: The odontogenic keratocyst: a clinicopathologic study of 312 cases. II. Histologic features, Oral Surg. **43**:233-255, 1977.

Cabrini, R. L., Barros, R. E., and Albano, H.: Cysts of the jaws: a statistical analysis, J. Oral Surg. **28**:485-489, 1970.

Christ, T. F.: The globulomaxillary cyst: an embryonic misconception, Oral Surg. **30**:515-526, 1970.

Cornyn, J.: Fibro-calcific lesions to the jaws. Presentation to American Academy of Dental Radiology, Chicago, October 24, 1975.

Cunat, J. J., and Collard, J.: Late developing premolars: report of two cases, J. Am. Dent. Assoc. **87**:183-185, 1973.

Forssell, K., Sorvari, T. E., and Oksala, E.: An analysis of the recurrence of odontogenic keratocysts, Proc. Finn. Dent. Soc. **70**:135-140, 1974a.

Forssell, K., Sorvari, T. E., and Oksala, E.: A clinical and radiographic study of odontogenic keratocysts in jaws, Proc. Finn. Dent. Soc. **70**:121-134, 1974b.

Hamner, J. E., Scofield, H. H., and Cornyn, J.: Benign fibro-osseous jaw lesions of periodontal membrane origin, Cancer **22**:861-878, 1968.

Hansson, L.: Development of a lingual mandibular bone cavity in an 11-year-old boy, Oral Surg. **49**:376-378, 1980.

Little, J. W., and Jakobsen, J.: Origin of the globulomaxillary cyst, J. Oral Surg. **31**:188-195, 1973.

Lurie, A. G., Puri, S., James, R. B., and Jensen, T. W.: Radionuclide bone imaging in the surgical treatment planning of odontogenic keratocysts, Oral Surg. **42**:726-730, 1976.

Marciani, R. D., Trodahl, J. N., Suckiel, M. J., and Dubick, M. N.: Cryotherapy in the treatment of ameloblastoma of the mandible: report of cases, J. Oral Surg. **35**:289-295, 1977.

Mehlisch, R. D., Dahlin, D. C., and Masson, J. K.: Ameloblastoma: a clinicopathologic report, J. Oral Surg. **30**:9-22, 1972.

Minderjahn, A.: Incidence and clinical differentiation of odontogenic tumors, J. Maxillofac. Surg. **7**:142-150, 1979.

Payne, T. F.: An analysis of the clinical and histopathologic parameters of the odontogenic keratocyst, Oral Surg. **33**:538-546, 1972.

Raibley, S. O., and Shafer, W. G.: Unpublished data, 1979.

Rao, P., Solomon, M., Auramides, A., et al.: Brown giant cell tumors associated with second hyperparathyroidism of chronic renal failure, J. Oral Surg. **36**:154-159, 1978.

Regezi, J. A., Kerr, D. A., and Courtney, R. M.: Odontogenic tumors: analysis of 706 cases, J. Oral Surg. **36**:771-778, 1978.

Shafer, W. G.: Presentation to American College of Stomatologic Surgeons, Maywood, Ill., 1978.

Soskolne, W. A., and Shteyer, A.: Median mandibular cyst, Oral Surg. **44**:84-88, 1977.

Struthers, P., and Shear, M.: Root resorption by ameloblastomas and cysts of the jaws, Int. J. Oral Surg. **5**:128-132, 1976.

Taicher, S., and Azaz, B.: Lesions resembling globulomaxillary cysts, Oral Surg. **44**:25-29, 1977.

Waldron, C. A., and Giansanti, J. S.: Benign fibro-osseous lesions of the jaws: a clinical-radiologic-histologic review of sixty-five cases. I. Fibrous dysplasia of the jaws, Oral Surg. **35**:190-201, 1973a.

Waldron, C. A., and Giansanti, J. S.: Benign fibro-osseous lesions of the jaws: a clinical-radiologic-histologic review of sixty-five cases. II. Benign fibro-osseous lesions of periodontal ligament origin, Oral Surg. **35**:340-350, 1973b.

Wilson, D. F., and Ross, A. S.: Ultrastructure of odontogenic keratocysts, Oral Surg. **45**:887-893, 1978.

Winer, R. A., and Doku, H. C.: Traumatic bone cyst in the maxilla, Oral Surg. **46**:367-370, 1978.

Zegarelli, D. J., and Zegarelli, E. V.: Radiolucent lesions in the globulomaxillary region, J. Oral Surg. **31**:767-771, 1973.

GENERAL REFERENCES

Ahlstrom, U., Johnson, C. C., and Lantz, B.: Radicular and residual cysts of the jaws: a long term roentgenographic study following cystectomies. Odontol. Rev. **20**:11-117, 1969.

Albers, D. D.: Median mandibular cyst partially lined with pseudostratified columnar epithelium, Oral Surg. **36**:11-15, 1973.

Arwill, T., and Kahnberg, K-E.: Odontogenic keratocyst associated with an intramandibular chondroma, J. Oral Surg. **35**:64-67, 1977.

Biedeman, R. W.: Pitfalls in interpreting radiographs of developing third molars, J. Am. Dent. Assoc. **86**:870-871, 1973.

Biewald, H. F.: A variation in the management of hemorrhagic, traumatic or simple bone cyst, J. Oral Surg. **25**:627-638, 1967.

Blair, A. E., and Wadsworth, W.: Median mandibular developmental cyst, J. Oral Surg. **26**:735-738, 1968.

Boerger, W. G.: Idiopathic bone cavities of the mandible: a review of literature and report of case, J. Oral Surg. **30**:506-509, 1972.

Borg, G., Persson, G., and Thilander, H.: A study of odontogenic cysts with special reference to comparisons between keratinizing and non-keratinizing cysts, Swed. Dent. J. **67**:311-325, 1974.

Buchner, A., and Ramon, Y.: Median mandibular cyst—a rare lesion of debatable origin, Oral Surg. **37**:431-437, 1974.

Budal, J.: The surgical removal of large osteofibromas, Oral Surg. **30**:303-308, 1970.

Campbell, J. J., Baden, E., and Williams, A. C.: Nasopalatine cyst of unusual size: report of case, J. Oral Surg. **31**:776-779, 1973.

Choukas, N. C.: Developmental submandibular gland defect of the mandible, J. Oral Surg. **31**:209-211, 1973.

Ciola, B., and Catena, D. L.: Midline, maxillary cyst, complicated by unerupted mesiodens, Oral Surg. **34**:978-983, 1972.

Crawford, B. E., and Weathers, D. R.: Osteoporotic marrow defects of the jaws, J. Oral Surg. **28**:600-603, 1970.

Curry, J. T., and Zallen, R. D.: Ossifying fibroma of the maxilla occurring with hyperthyroidism, Oral Surg. **35**:28-34, 1973.

Curtis, M. L., Hatfield, C. G., and Pierce, J. M.: A destructive giant cell lesion of the mandible, J. Oral Surg. **31**:705-709, 1973.

Daugherty, J. W., and Eversole, L. R.: Aneurysmal bone cyst of the mandible, J. Oral Surg. **29**:737-741, 1971.

Davis, R. B., Baker, R. D., and Alling, C. C.: Odontogenic myxoma. Clinical-pathologic conference. Case 24. I, J. Oral Surg. **36:**534-538, 1978.

Davis, R. B., Baker, R. D., and Alling, C. C.: Odontogenic myxoma. Clinical-pathologic conference. Case 24. II, J. Oral Surg. **36:**610-615, 1978.

Davis, W. M., Buchs, A. V., and Davis, W. M.: Extravasation cyst diagnostic curettement: a treatment. Report of 15 cases and suggested treatment, Oral Surg. **47:**2-7, 1979.

Donoff, R. B., Guralnick, W. C., and Clayman, L.: Keratocysts of the jaw, J. Oral Surg. **30:**800-804, 1972.

Doyle, J. L., Grodjesk, J. E., Dolinski, H. B., and Rafel, S. S.: Squamous odontogenic tumor: report of three cases, J. Oral Surg. **35:**994-996, 1977.

Duell, R. C., and Montgomery, J. C.: Concurrent management of a central giant cell granuloma, J. Am. Dent. Assoc. **81:** 148-150, 1970.

Eversole, L. R., Sabes, W. R., Brandebura, J., and Massey, G. B.: Medulloblastoma: extradural metastasis to the jaw, Oral Surg. **34:**634-640, 1972.

Eversole, L. R., Sabes, W. R., and Rovin, S.: Aggressive growth and neoplastic potentials of odontogenic cysts, with special reference to central epidermoid and central mucoepidermoid carcinoma, Cancer **35:**270-282, 1975.

Fantasia, J. E.: Lateral periodontal cyst, Oral Surg. **48:**237-243, 1979.

Farman, A. G., Nortje, C. J., Grotepass, F. W., et al.: Myxofibroma of the jaws, Br. J. Oral Surg. **15:**3-18, 1977.

Freedman, P. D., Cardo, V. A., and Kerpel, S. M.: Desmoplastic fibroma (fibromatosis) of the jaw bones, Oral Surg. **46:**386-395, 1978.

Goldblatt, L. I., and Edesess, R. B.: Central leiomyoma of the mandible. Report of a case with ultrastructural confirmation, Oral Surg. **43:**591-597, 1977.

Hansen, L. S., Sapone, J., and Sproat, R. C.: Traumatic bone cysts of jaws: report of sixty-six cases, Oral Surg. **37:**899-910, 1974.

Harris, W. E.: Unusual response to treatment of traumatic bone cyst: report of a case, J. Am. Dent. Assoc. **84:**632-635, 1972.

Hylton, R. P., McKean, T. W., and Albright, J. E.: Simple ameloblastoma: report of case, J. Oral Surg. **30:**59-62, 1972.

Kennett, S., and Pollick, H.: Jaw lesions in familial hyperparathyroidism, Oral Surg. **31:**502-510, 1971.

Leban, S. G., Lepow, H., Stratigos, G. T., and Chu, F.: The giant cell lesion of the jaws: neoplastic or reparative? J. Oral Surg. **29:**398-404, 1971.

Lorson, E. L., DeLong, P. E., Osbon, D. B., and Dolan, K. D.: Neurofibromatosis with central neurofibroma of the mandible: review of the literature and report of case, J. Oral Surg. **35:**733-738, 1977.

Martinelli, C., Melhado, R. M., and Callestini, E. A.: Squamous cell carcinoma in a residual mandibular cyst, Oral Surg. **44:** 274-278, 1977.

Miller, C. E., Goltry, R. R., and Shenasky, J. H.: Multiple myeloma involving the mandible, Oral Surg. **28:**603-609, 1969.

Morgan, G. A., and Morgan, P. R.: Neurilemmoma-neurofibroma, Oral Surg. **25:**182-189, 1968.

Moss, M., and Levey, A. C.: The traumatic bone cyst: report of three cases, J. Am. Dent. Assoc. **72:**397-402, 1966.

Oikarinen, V. J., Wolf, J., and Julku, M.: A stereosialographic study of developmental mandibular bone defects (Stafne's idiopathic bone cavities), Int. J. Oral Surg. **4:**51-54, 1975.

Palladino, V. S., and Danziger, A. E.: Hemangioma of the maxilla, J. Am. Dent. Assoc. **70:**636-641, 1965.

Payne, T. F.: An analysis of the clinical and histopathologic parameters of the odontogenic keratocyst, Oral Surg. **33:** 538-546, 1972.

Pedersen, G. W.: Central giant cell lesion of the maxilla: enucleation and immediate reconstruction, Oral Surg. **36:**790-799, 1973.

Poyton, H. G., Mustard, R. A., and Sim, J.: Cirsoid aneurysm secondary to an arteriovenous fistula of the facial artery and vein, Oral Surg. **37:**474-479, 1974.

Prescott, G. H., and White, R. E.: Solitary, central neurofibroma of the mandible: report of case and review of the literature, J. Oral Surg. **28:**305-309, 1970.

Pullon, P. A., Shafer, W. G., Elzay, R. P., et al.: Squamous odontogenic tumor: report of six cases of a previously undescribed lesion, Oral Surg. **40:**616-630, 1975.

Reyneke, J. P.: Aneurysmal bone cyst of the maxilla, Oral Surg. **45:**441-447, 1978.

Richter, K. G., Grammer, F. C., and Boies, L.: Central giant cell lesion in the angle of the mandible: review of the literature and report of case, J. Oral Surg. **31:**26-30, 1973.

Rittersma, J., and Westerink, P.: Neurofibromatosis with mandibular deformities, Oral Surg. **33:**718-727, 1972.

Robinson, M., and Slaukin, H. C.: Dental amputation neuromas, J. Am. Dent. Assoc. **70:**662-675, 1965.

Roser, S. M., and Davee, J. S.: An infiltrating odontogenic keratocyst: a clinical pathological correlation, J. Oral Med. **33:**28-30, 1978.

Rud, J., and Pindborg, J. J.: Odontogenic keratocysts: a follow-up study of 21 cases, J. Oral Surg. **27:**323-330, 1969.

Samartano, J. G., and Haar, J. G.: A large keratinizing dentigerous cyst: report of case, J. Oral Surg. **29:**60-62, 1971.

Samules, H. S.: Marsupialization: effective management of large maxillary cysts, Oral Surg. **20:**676-683, 1965.

Schiff, B. A., Kringstein, G., and Stoopack, J. C.: An extremely large and facially distorting nasopalatine duct cyst, Oral Surg. **27:**590-594, 1969.

Schneider, L. C., Mesa, M., Weisinger, E., and Weiner, P.: Solitary intramandibular neurofibroma: report of a case, J. Oral Med. **34:**37-39, 1979.

Shensa, D. R., and Nasseri, S.: Central giant cell reparative granuloma of the mandibular condyle, J. Oral Surg. **36:**642-643, 1978.

Shimura, K., Allen, E. C., Kinoshita, Y., and Takaesu, T.: Central neurilemoma of the mandible: report of case and review of the literature, J. Oral Surg. **31:**363-367, 1973.

Shira, R. B.: Treatment planning, J. Oral Surg. **28:**70-73, 1970.

Shklar, G., and Meyer, I.: Neurogenic tumors of the mouth and jaws, Oral Surg. **16:**1075-1093, 1963.

Singer, C. F., Gienger, G. L., and Kullbom, T. L.: Solitary intraosseous neurofibroma involving the mandibular canal: report of case, J. Oral Surg. **31:**127-129, 1973.

Smith, G. A., and Ward, P. H.: Giant-cell lesions of the facial skeleton, Arch. Otolaryngol. **104:**186-196, 1978.

Snyder, S. R., Merkow, L. P., and White, N. S.: Eosinophilic granuloma of bone: report of case, J. Oral Surg. **31:**712-715, 1973.

Stene, T., and Pedersen, K. N.: Aberrant salivary gland tissue in the anterior mandible, Oral Surg. **44:**72-75, 1977.

Stewart, S., Sherman, P., and Stoopack, J. C.: Large bilateral traumatic bone cysts of the mandible: report of case, J. Oral Surg. **31:**865-868, 1973.

Taintor, J. F., and Fahid, A.: Case report: median palatine cyst, Dent. Survey **53:**33-36, 1977.

Tasanen, A., Konow, L., and Nordling, S.: Central giant cell lesion in the mandibular condyle, Oral Surg. **45:**532-539, 1978.

Thornton, W. E., Allen, J. W., and Byrd, L. D.: Median palatal cyst: report of case, J. Oral Surg. **30:**661-663, 1972.

Tilson, H. B., and Bauerle, J. E.: Median mandibular cyst: report of case, J. Oral Surg. **28:**519-522, 1970.

Torres, J. S., and Higa, T. T.: Epidermoid cysts in the oral cavity, Oral Surg. **30:**592-600, 1970.

Waldron, C. A., and Shafer, W. G.: Central giant repara-tive granuloma of the jaws, Am. J. Clin. Pathol. **45:**437-447, 1966.

Wesley, R. K., Horan, M., Helfrick, J. F., et al.: Central giant cell granuloma of the mandible. Clinical-pathological confer-ence. Case 25. I, J. Oral Surg. **36:**713-715, 1978.

19

Multilocular radiolucencies

Norman K. Wood
Paul W. Goaz
Roger H. Kallal

"Soap bubble"   "Honeycomb"   "Tennis racket"

Multilocular radiolucencies of the oral cavity include the following:

Anatomic patterns
Multilocular cyst
Ameloblastoma
Central giant cell granuloma
Giant cell lesion of hyperparathyroidism
Cherubism
Odontogenic myxoma
Aneurysmal bone cyst
Metastatic tumors to the jaws
Central hemangioma of bone
Rarities
    Ameloblastic variants
    Arteriovenous malformations
    Burkitt's lymphoma
    Calcifying epithelial odontogenic tumor
    Cementifying and ossifying fibroma
    Central mucoepidermoid tumor
    Central odontogenic and nonodontogenic fibromas
    Chondroma
    Eosinophilic granuloma
    Fibrous dysplasia
    Immature odontoma
    Neurilemoma
    Neuroectodermal tumor of infancy
    Odontogenic keratocyst
    Osteomyelitis
    Pseudotumor of hemophilia
    Squamous odontogenic tumor

Multilocular radiolucencies are produced by multiple, adjacent, frequently coalescing, and overlapping pathologic compartments in bone. They may occur in the maxilla but are found much more commonly in the mandible.

Whereas all the entities that are included in this chapter appear as multilocular lesions, they may also occur as a single sharp cystlike radiolucency or even as a poorly defined radiolucency.

The presentation of these lesions in the outline at the beginning of this chapter and in Chapter 18 is according to incidence (to whatever extent such order is known or ordering is possible).

It is important to note that unilocular lesions that have perforated the cortical plate in one or more areas may cause radiographic images that resemble those from multilocular entities (Fig. 19-1). The true multilocular lesion will contain two or more pathologic chambers partially separated by usually radiographically discernible septae of bone. On occasion, the septae may be so thin and their images so indistinct as to cause the multilocular lesion to appear unilocular radiographically.

The terms "soap bubble," "honeycomb," and "tennis racket" are frequently used to describe the various radiographic images of multilocular lesions. "Soap bubble" is reserved for lesions consisting of several *circular* compartments that vary in size and usually appear to overlap somewhat. "Honeycomb" applies to lesions whose compartments are *small* and tend to be quite *uniform*. The "tennis racket" designation is descriptive of lesions composed of *angular* rather than rounded compartments that result from the development of more or less straight septae. Thus these compartments tend to be triangular, rectangular, or square. (Refer to the introductory figure for this chapter.)

To amplify the connotation of the term "multilocular lesion" as used in this chapter, we shall merely remind the reader that multilocular is used only as a *radiographic*, not a microscopic, description. Many lesions demonstrate micro-

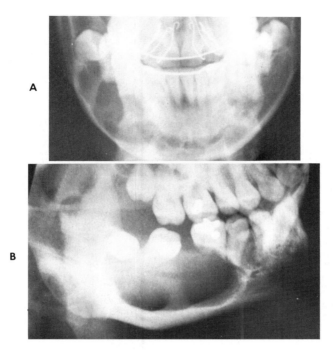

Fig. 19-1. Pseudomultilocular radiolucencies. Both lesions proved at surgery to be unilocular. **A,** Traumatic bone cyst. **B,** Ameloblastoma. (Courtesy M. Kaminski, D.D.S., and S. Atsaves, D.D.S., Chicago.)

scopic projections, but these tiny bosses are usually not large enough to be radiographically evident. When studying radiographs of the lesions described in this chapter, the clinician should be cognizant that the radiolucent areas making up the images are not empty spaces, as they appear, but rather are compartments filled usually with neoplastic tissue or at least with cystic fluid or blood.

The following presentation includes, in addition to descriptions of the primary and distinctive features of each lesions, illustrations of the development of a differential diagnosis and the contributing circumstances and considerations that support a suggested course of treatment.

ANATOMIC PATTERNS

To preclude their being mistaken for multilocular lesions, two normal radiolucent structures of the perioral regions and their radiographic variations are noted and described in this section: the maxillary sinus and bone marrow spaces.

The *maxillary sinus* usually has several compartments that project into the surrounding maxilla and zygoma and give the radiographic appearance of septa dividing the sinus into lobes.

When many such lobes or compartments are present, the resultant image may be of soap bubbles (Fig. 19-2). The anatomic location of the variable extensions of the sinus and the relative movement of adjacent structures on radiographs taken from different angles, coupled with the absence of symptoms, are usually sufficient to identify these areas as pouches from the maxillary sinus.

Bone marrow spaces and trabecular patterns appear frequently as multilocular radiolucencies, especially in the mandible (Fig. 19-3). Usually when these spaces and patterns resemble pathologic multilocular radiolucencies, a comparison with the pattern of trabeculation in the remainder of the jawbone will show a similar image so the examiner can conclude with reasonable certainty that the suspicious-looking region is a normal variation.

When a trabecular pattern appears only as an isolated area, the correct diagnosis is more difficult to make. In the absence of additional manifestations of disease, however, a satisfactory technique is to observe the area semiannually with radiographs to be certain that no growth occurs and that it is an innocent variation of the normal trabecular pattern.

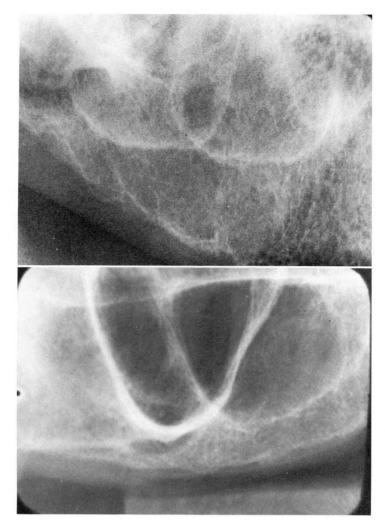

Fig. 19-2. Maxillary sinus. Note the multilocular patterns.

Fig. 19-3. Marrow spaces. Note the soap bubble patterns.

MULTILOCULAR CYST

The multilocular cyst is the most frequently encountered pathologic multilocular radiolucency in the jaws. It is always of the soap bubble variety, occurs most frequently in the mandible (usually in the premolar-molar region), and varies greatly in size (Fig. 19-4).

Theoretically any of the cysts occurring in the jaws could develop multiple compartments; but particularly the odontogenic keratocyst, the primordial cyst, the follicular cyst, and the residual cyst occur with some frequency as multilocular cysts whereas the radicular and fissural cysts are almost always unilocular lesions.

FEATURES

The multilocular cyst is a true cyst of the jaws and may be found in any age group but is more frequent in persons over 15 years of age. The small cyst is usually asymptomatic and generally noticed on routine radiographic examination (Fig. 19-4). It increases in size slowly and may cause displacement of adjacent teeth and occasionally root resorption; but it rarely give rise to a paresthesia unless secondarily infected. If undetected, the cyst may expand the cortical plates as it enlarges and may become clinically apparent as a smooth bony-hard swelling. If the overlying bone becomes quite thin, a crackling sound

Fig. 19-4. Multilocular cysts. **A,** Residual cyst. **B,** Botryoid cyst. **C,** Radicular cyst. **D** and **E,** Follicular cysts. (**A** courtesy M. Smulson, D.D.S., Maywood, Ill. **C** courtesy R. Kallal, D.D.S., Flossmoor, Ill. **D** and **E** courtesy O. H. Stuteville, D.D.S., M.D., St. Joe, Ark.)

(crepitus) may be produced by palpation. Later, if the covering plate is destroyed, the cyst will appear as a soft to rubbery fluctuant mass with perhaps a bluish color.

Aspiration will generally yield a thin straw-colored fluid unless the mass is a keratocyst, which will yield a thick granular yellow fluid that requires a large-bore needle for successful aspiration. Microscopic study will reveal a lumen lined with epithelium and surrounded by a cyst wall varying in thickness and in fibrous tissue content.

DIFFERENTIAL DIAGNOSIS

All the lesions in this chapter must be considered in the differential diagnosis of multilocular cyst. These are given in the differential diagnosis section at the end of this chapter (p. 417) and in Table 19-1.

MANAGEMENT

The treatment of cysts is presented in detail in Chapters 16 and 17. The four alternate methods are as follows:

1. Total surgical enucleation plus a bone graft if the size of the defect is large
2. Marsupialization
3. Decompression
4. Partial decompression followed by surgical enucleation at a later date

Many factors must be considered before a method of treatment is selected. In general, total removal is the treatment of choice for multilocular cysts because ensuring that all compartments have been eradicated is especially difficult if the more conservative methods are employed. A conservative approach may be preferable in some cases, however.

Fig. 19-5. Ameloblastoma. **A,** Note the facial asymmetry due to the expansion of the left ramus in a 68-year-old man. **B,** Intraoral swelling in the third molar region of the same patient. Note the ulcerated surface caused by trauma from a maxillary molar. **C,** Left lateral oblique radiograph, same patient. **D,** Radiograph of the surgical specimen showing the soap bubble pattern. **E to J,** Radiographs of other ameloblastomas. (Note the honeycomb patterns in **E** and **G,** the soap bubble patterns in **H** and **I,** and the angular multilocular pattern in **J.**) (**E** courtesy P. Akers, D.D.S., Chicago. **F to J** courtesy O. H. Stuteville, D.D.S., M.D., St. Joe, Ark.)

The final diagnosis must await surgery and microscopic examination. If the suspicious-looking lesion is a cyst, the surgeon will usually encounter a thin soft tissue lining and a lumen filled with fluid. Any solid areas of soft tissue should alert him to the probability that he is dealing with a more serious lesion, such as one of those listed at the beginning of this chapter. In addition, he should be alert to the possibility of a mural ameloblastoma. Regardless of the method of treatment chosen, the surgical site must be observed radiographically for several years to ensure that healing is complete or that recurrences are detected.

Inasmuch as the central hemangioma represents such a potential threat of uncontrolled hemorrhage when it is unexpectedly encountered at surgery and since it might be confused with another entity detailed in this chapter, aspiration of any lesion is in order. This test is best employed just prior to initiating the surgical procedure because of the possibility of contaminating the lesion during aspiration.

AMELOBLASTOMA

The ameloblastoma is an odontogenic tumor usually described as locally malignant. It may cast a unilocular cystlike radiolucency or a multilocular image. The multilocular image may be of either the soap bubble or the honeycomb variety (Fig. 19-5). Most frequently ameloblastomas of the maxilla are unilocular whereas those of the mandible are more equally divided between unilocular and multilocular lesions. The frequency of multilocular ameloblastomas of the maxilla must be low since a thorough search of literature

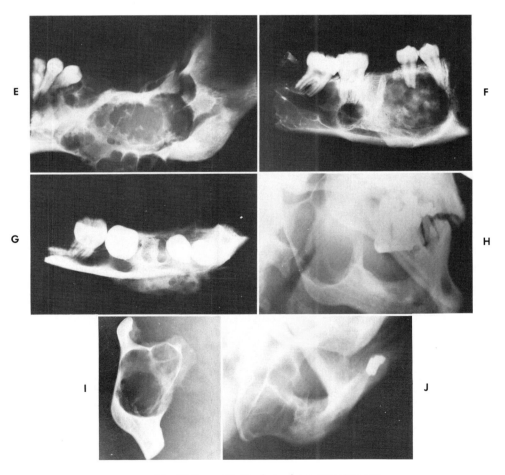

Fig. 19-5, cont'd. For legend see opposite page.

has failed to reveal an example. The ameloblastoma is discussed in detail in Chapter 18.

DIFFERENTIAL DIAGNOSIS

For a discussion of the differential diagnosis of ameloblastoma, refer to the differential diagnosis section at the end of this chapter (p. 417) and to Table 19-1 as well as to the differential diagnosis section for ameloblastoma in Chapter 18 (p. 377).

CENTRAL GIANT CELL (REPARATIVE) GRANULOMA

The central giant cell granuloma may occur initially as a solitary cystlike radiolucency; but as it grows larger, it frequently develops an architecture that causes a soap bubble type of multilocular radiolucency (Fig. 19-6). Although trauma was thought to be the causative factor, now many pathologists believe that this is not true.

Fig. 19-6. Giant cell granuloma. **A,** Arrows indicate the lateral limits of the soap bubble lesion. **B,** Large soap bubble lesion producing marked expansion in the mandible of a 5-year-old boy. **C,** Divergence of the lateral incisor and canine roots produced by giant cell granuloma. For the histopathology see Fig. 18-15. **D,** Lesion in a middle-aged white woman. (**A** to **C** courtesy R. Goepp, D.D.S., Zoller Clinic, University of Chicago. **D** courtesy V. Barresi, D.D.S., DeKalb, Ill.)

At present the cause is still in doubt. The lesion is discussed in detail in Chapter 18.

DIFFERENTIAL DIAGNOSIS

For a discussion of the differential diagnosis of central giant cell granuloma, refer to the differential diagnosis section at the end of this chapter (p. 417) and to Table 19-1 as well as to the differential diagnosis section for giant cell granuloma in Chapter 18 (p. 383).

GIANT CELL LESION OF HYPERPARATHYROIDISM

The clinical, radiographic, and histologic characteristics of the giant cell lesion of hyperparathyroidism are identical with those of the giant cell granuloma. It occurs as a unilocular or a multilocular radiolucency (Fig. 19-7) and is found in patients with primary, secondary, or tertiary hyperparathyroidism. The establishment of its true identity is dependent on demonstrating the concomitant parathyroid hormone or kidney disorder. This giant cell lesion is discussed in detail in Chapter 18.

DIFFERENTIAL DIAGNOSIS

For a discussion of the differential diagnosis of the giant cell lesion of hyperparathyroidism, refer to the differential diagnosis section at the end of the chapter (p. 417) and to Table 19-1 as well as to the differential diagnosis section of this giant cell lesion in Chapter 18 (p. 384).

CHERUBISM (FAMILIAL INTRAOSSEOUS SWELLING OF THE JAWS)

Although cases have been reported without familial involvement, cherubism is usually inherited as an autosomal dominant trait. Expressivity and penetrance are more pronounced in males. The disease occurs as two or more separate multilocular-appearing lesions (Fig. 19-8). Sometimes the interlocular bone will become so indistinct that the multilocular appearance is lost.

FEATURES

Cherubism occurs between the ages of 2 and 20 years. It usually commences bilaterally in the rami of the mandible and becomes apparent as painless swellings of the face in these areas. Occasionally the whole mandible is involved. Other bones (e.g., the walls of the maxillary sinus, orbital floor, and tuberosity regions) may also be affected; and the resultant enlargement in these areas produces the cherublike expression by tilting the eyeballs superiorly (Fig. 19-8). The lesion grows slowly, expanding but not perforating the cortex. Paresthesia is not a feature.

At about 8 or 9 years of age, growth of the pathologic region may plateau—until puberty, when the lesion may begin to regress. Usually the bony architecture will return to normal by age 30, except for a few instances in which the involved bone of the ramus will retain a somewhat ground-glass radiographic appearance.

Fig. 19-7. Brown giant cell lesion of hyperparathyroidism. Note the soap bubble pattern. (From Rotblat, S., and Laskin, D.: J. Oral Surg. **27:**820-825, 1969. Copyright by the American Dental Association. Reprinted by permission.)

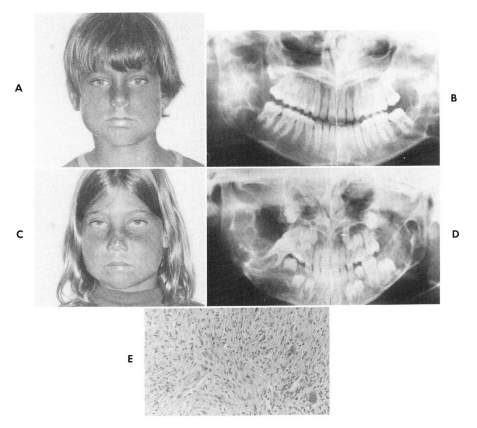

Fig. 19-8. Cherubism. **A,** Clinical appearance of bilateral expansion of the rami in a 12-year-old boy. **B,** Panograph reveals the bilateral soap bubble expansions of the rami. The maxilla was not involved in this case. **C** and **D,** Seven-year-old sister of this patient. Both the maxilla and the mandible are involved. Note the superior tilt of the eyeballs, which gives the cherub appearance. **E,** Microscopy of cherubism. (**A** to **D** courtesy J. Hebert, D.D.S., Houston.)

Some patients may demonstrate a persistent swelling for years.

A few posterior teeth may be missing in this disease because of the early-developing expanding masses; these expansions destroy the buds and the incipient follicles.

On posteroanterior views the teeth associated with the lesion often seem to be hanging in air. Microscopically the lesion is composed of mature fibroblasts in a surprisingly pale edematous background that contains little collagen. Multinucleated giant cells are few and occur in clusters (Fig. 19-8).

DIFFERENTIAL DIAGNOSIS

The multiple lesions occurring bilaterally in the ramus—coupled with the cherub appearance, the specific age group, and a history of kindred involvement—should readily guide the clinician to the correct impression. This disease entity is the only one in the present chapter with characteristics specific enough to enable the clinician to feel confident of his working diagnosis. Nevertheless, because nonfamilial cases as well as unilateral lesions have been reported, he should also consider a list of possible diagnoses. For more differential information the reader is referred to Table 19-1 and to the differential diagnosis section at the end of the chapter (p. 417).

MANAGEMENT

The correct identification of the condition and periodic clinical and radiographic examinations are required. An incisional biopsy will provide the correct diagnosis if the clinical picture is confusing.

Orthodontic care may be needed to ensure proper alignment of the teeth; and occasionally surgical contouring of the lesion will be necessary to improve esthetics and also in cases of active growth (Kuepper and Harrigan, 1978). Usually by the fourth decade, most evidence of the disease has disappeared although unusual cases will show activity through age 60 (Waldron, 1976).

ODONTOGENIC MYXOMA

The odontogenic myxoma is a benign tumor of bone that apparently occurs exclusively in the jaws and is usually classified as an odontogenic tumor. The myxomatous tissue, of which this tumor is composed, is thought to originate by one of three mechanisms:

1. As a direct outgrowth of the dental papilla of a tooth
2. As an inductive effect of nests of odontogenic epithelium on mesenchymal tissue
3. As a direct myxomatous change in fibrous tissue

The myxoma is rarely seen in other bones of the skeleton, and this fact strengthens the theory of odontogenic origin. Although it has been previously believed that the odontogenic myxoma frequently occurs in the region of a missing tooth a recent extensive review of the literature failed to substantiate this opinion (Farman et al., 1977). There is also a malignant variant of this tumor.

Radiographically the odontogenic myxoma may be found as a unilocular cystlike radiolucency, a pericoronal radiolucency, and a mixed radiolucent-radiopaque image. More frequently it occurs as a multilocular radiolucency, however (Fig. 19-9).

The tennis racket appearance is the most common. The individual compartments may appear radiographically in the form of triangles, rectangles, or squares, depending on the random arrangement of the bony septae. Very fine trabeculation is often seen distributed within the individual compartments. The radiographic margins of the tumor may be either well defined or poorly defined. Myxomas may also occur with soap bubble and honeycomb patterns.

FEATURES

The myxoma accounts for 3% to 6% of all odontogenic tumors (Minderjahn, 1979; Regezi et al., 1978). Farman and co-workers (1977) reviewed the literature and found that the approximate ratio of maxillary to mandibular lesions is 3:4. Many of the maxillary lesions involved the maxillary sinus, and very few cases crossed the midline. Farman reported that most of the mandibular lesions occurred in the premolar-molar region. Only a few lesions involved the non-tooth-bearing areas of the jaw. Only a slight predilection for females was found by Farman and co-workers. The average age for various categories ranged between 25 and 35 years. These reviewers found that root resorption was very rare. Harder (1978) reported that myxomas rarely occur before age 10 or after age 50.

The chief complaint of a patient with an odontogenic myxoma may be a slowly enlarging painless expansion of the jaw with possible spreading, loosening, and migration of teeth in the involved area. Rarely there may be numbness of the lip and occasionally pain. The earlier asymptomatic stage, before cortical expansion occurs, may be detected only by a routine radiographic survey.

If the tumor is not detected and treated in the early stage, it will cause facial asymmetry as it expands the cortical plates and effects a smooth enlargement of the alveolus of the jaw (Fig. 19-9). Sometimes it will perforate the cortical plates in several places, thus producing a bosselated surface (several small nodules on the surface). The mucosa or skin over the tumor will appear normal unless continually traumatized.

Histologically the tumor consists of tissue resembling that of the dental papillae. Thin triangular cells with fibers streaming from the corners are seen scattered throughout a pale myxomatous background (Fig. 19-9). Small cords or nests of odontogenic epithelium may be present. Mature collagen fibers are scarce. The loosely arranged fibrillar pale-staining microscopic picture of this lesion confirms the fact that if the cortical plates are perforated the expanding mass will be soft to palpation and will give the impression of fluctuance because of the high water content of the tissue. Aspiration will be nonproductive.

DIFFERENTIAL DIAGNOSIS

Again, even though a lesion of this type may be suspected when the clinician encounters a typical multilocular radiolucency, all the lesions discussed in the present chapter should be included in the differential diagnosis.

If there is a honeycomb or tennis racket picture, however, the myxoma must be considered along with the *ameloblastoma* and the *intrabony hemangioma*. The honeycomb variant of the myxoma generally shows very fine trabeculations within the small lobules, which are not present in the ameloblastoma.

Fig. 19-9. Odontogenic myxoma. **A,** Orthopantomograph and, **B,** radiograph of a surgical specimen. **C,** Lateral oblique radiograph of another patient and, **D,** radiograph of the surgical specimen. **E,** Myxoma producing a smoothly contoured oral swelling. **F** and **G,** Radiographs of the lesion shown in **E. H,** Photomicrograph of a myxoma. (**A** and **B** courtesy N. Barakat, D.D.S., Beirut, Lebanon. **C** and **D** courtesy O. H. Stuteville, D.D.S., M.D., St. Joe, Ark. **F** courtesy R. Kallal, D.D.S., Flossmoor, Ill. **G** courtesy D. Bonomo, D.D.S., Flossmoor, Ill.)

The fact that the myxoma occurs as a solitary lesion, usually in a slightly older age group, should obviate confusing this lesion with the multiple lesions of *cherubism*.

The *giant cell granuloma* occurs most commonly in the anterior regions of the jaws, whereas the myxoma is seen most frequently in the ramus and molar-premolar areas of the mandible.

MANAGEMENT

Recurrences of the odontogenic myxoma are quite common and have been reported in 25% of the treated patients. Apparently this behavior is due to the fact that the tumor tends to spill into the surrounding marrow spaces. As a result normal resection of the tumor with a generous amount of surrounding bone is necessary in extensive lesions to minimize recurrences. Teeth in the region often must be included in the sec-

tion. Many cases are successfully managed, however, with enucleation and cautery. The tumor does not respond to radiation.

Occasionally an odontogenic myxoma will extend into the mandibular canal; and in these cases the neurovascular bundle is usually sacrificed. Recurrences may, on occasion, be observed years after treatment when the involved regions of the jaws have appeared radiographically to be completely healed. A more extensive resection is then required; but the inferior border of the mandible should be retained if possible.

ANEURYSMAL BONE CYST

The aneurysmal bone cyst is characterized as a false cyst because it does not have an epithelial lining. It occurs as a unilocular or multilocular radiolucency (Fig. 19-10) that frequently balloons out the cortex. It has been reported most

Fig. 19-10. Aneurysmal bone cyst. **A,** Arrow indicates the faint soap bubble pattern in the premolar region. **B** and **C,** Posteroanterior and lateral oblique radiographs and, **D,** radiograph of the surgical specimen from the 12-year-old girl shown in **B** and **C. E,** Panograph and, **F,** occlusal radiograph of a large lesion found in a 20-year-old woman. The soap bubble pattern and retention of a thin cortex are characteristic of this benign condition. **G,** Photomicrograph showing a large vascular space. Multinucleated giant cells are frequently present. (**A** courtesy R. Goepp, D.D.S., Zoller Clinic, University of Chicago. **B** to **D** from Hoppe, W.: Oral Surg. **25**:1-5, 1968. **E** and **F** from Oliver, L. P.: Oral Surg. **35**:67-76, 1973.) *Continued.*

Fig. 19-10, cont'd. For legend see p. 411.

frequently in the long bones, the vertebrae, and occasionally the jaws. Its cause, although unproved, is thought to be trauma. Some pathologists believe that it forms a continuum with the traumatic bone cyst and the central giant cell granuloma.

FEATURES

The aneurysmal bone cyst is a slow-growing lesion that affects the mandible much more often than the maxilla (3:1) but is seldom encountered in the perioral regions. It most frequently involves persons under 20 years of age. As it grows slowly, it may expand the cortical plates; but it usually does not destroy them. It may be slightly tender and teeth may be missing or displaced, but root resorption is seldom seen. The lesion does not appear to show a predilection for either sex (Reyneke, 1978; Steidler et al., 1979). Paresthesia is not a feature.

Grossly the lesion is soft reddish brown because of its rich blood supply and it resembles a sponge filled with blood. Microscopically it contains giant cells scattered through a fibrous stroma that contains cavernous thin-walled blood spaces. Bone spicules and osteoid may be present (Fig. 19-10).

Some pathologists are of the opinion that the aneurysmal bone cyst is actually a response to an alteration in the vasculature of the area involved (e.g., trauma and subsequent intrabony bleeding). Such a response, an exaggerated proliferative reaction, is thought to be similar to the central and peripheral giant cell reparative granulomas, which it resembles in many respects; however, the developing aneurysmal bone cyst is apparently continually effused with circulating blood from the injured vessels whereas the granulomas are not.

In light of the suggested similarity in pathogenesis between the aneurysmal bone cyst and the two giant cell lesions, it is of interest to contemplate that all three of these entities usually develop in younger patients (i.e., less than 30 years of age), at which time the repair response is more vigorous.

DIFFERENTIAL DIAGNOSIS

For a discussion of the differential diagnosis of aneurysmal bone cyst, refer to the differential diagnosis section at the end of this chapter (p. 417) and to Table 19-1.

MANAGEMENT

As he must with the other lesions detailed in this chapter, the surgeon should organize a differential diagnosis since the clinical and radiographic pictures of the aneurysmal bone cyst are similar to those of several other entities included in the group. Aspiration of the involved area of the bone is recommended to obviate the dangerous unexpected entrance into an intrabony hemangioma or arteriovenous shunt.

Usually a copious amount of blood can be aspirated from an aneurysmal bone cyst—but not the syringe fulls of blood that are readily obtained from hemangiomas or shunts. Surgical curettement is the treatment of choice. Hemorrhage is usually moderate, and its arrest is not difficult. Recurrences are rare.

METASTATIC TUMORS TO THE JAWS

The most common malignant tumors that metastasize to the jaws are carcinomas of the lung, breast, gastrointestinal tract, kidney, prostate gland, testis, and thyroid gland. Metastatic jaw tumors have been reported to arise from parent tumors in other organs and sites, but these are rare occurrences.

Malignant cells from distant sites usually are carried via arterial blood. Some pathologists, however, believe that malignant cells travel from their primary site to the jaws via the prevertebral veins of Batson.

The mandible is much more frequently the site of secondary tumors than is the maxilla, and the premolar-molar area is the most commonly affected region.

Although metastatic jaw tumors are included in this chapter, which is devoted to multilocular lesions, a multilocular pattern is not the only radiographic picture produced by a secondary tumor.

Intrabony metastatic jaw tumors may cause several other radiographic appearances:

1. *A solitary well-defined cystlike radiolucency.* Tumors giving this picture are usually of the slow-growing, well-differentiated type or else the patient is being successfully treated with cytotoxic drugs.
2. *A solitary poorly defined radiolucency.* This picture is usually caused by a localized, rapidly growing tumor.
3. *Multiple, separate, poorly defined radiolucencies.* This picture usually occurs where several foci of malignant nests are present and growing separately from each other.
4. *Multiple punched-out radiolucencies (multiple myeloma–like).* This picture is characteristic when several nests of slow-growing tumor cells are located close to each other in the bone.

Fig. 19-11. Metastatic renal adenocarcinoma.

5. *Radiopaque patterns with any of the foregoing radiolucent pictures.* The tumors in these cases have either induced osteoblastic activity or produced osteosclerosis in the bone.
6. *An irregular salt-and-pepper appearance.* This picture usually involves a large segment of the jaws and indicates that the tumor is widely disseminated in multiple nests in the bone. These nests appear as small radiolucencies (pepper). They induce sclerotic areas about themselves and thus sprinkle the overall picture with small radiopaque foci (salt).
7. *A relatively dense solitary radiopaque area.* Sometimes a prostatic or a mammary tumor demonstrates osteoblastic activity; the bone thus produced shows as a rather radiopaque area and may resemble condensing osteitis.

When a metastatic tumor of bone produces a multilocular radiographic lesion, it is almost always of the honeycomb or tennis racket structure (Fig. 19-11).

FEATURES

The patient with a secondary tumor of the jaw may seek treatment for pain resulting from a local jaw metastasis or from the parent tumor itself (if it has not been successfully treated). Symptoms induced by the parent tumor will usually reflect the altered physiology of the affected organ.

For example, a large bronchogenic carcinoma in the lung may produce symptoms that include chronic cough, hemoptysis, dyspnea, orthopnea, tachycardia, and an overall cachectic appearance. Thus, if a bony lesion is found in the jaws of such a patient, the clinician should consider the increased possibility that it is a metastatic tumor. He must be aware, however, that in certain cases the metastatic lesion will be the first discovered. In such cases the primary tumor is said to be occult; and if the secondary tumor is poorly differentiated histologically, the primary tumor may be difficult to locate.

The local symptoms produced by a metastatic tumor of the jaws are similar to those produced by a primary malignant jaw tumor. Thus a spectrum of manifestations may be expected, ranging from nonexistent in an early lesion to marked in an advanced lesion that has caused substantial bone destruction. Advanced tumors often involve the inferior dental canal and cause a paresthesia or anesthesia of the lower lip on the affected side. As the lesion becomes more extensive, pathologic fractures are a distinct possibility.

An enlarging lesion may erode rapidly through the cortical plates, usually without expanding them, and then invade the surrounding soft tissues, which thus become fixed to the jawbone. The phenomenon of normally movable soft tissue fixed to bone is an ominous sign and indicates either a sclerosing fibrosis or a malignant invasion. If fibrosis or invasion or both occur in a region where muscles are present, function will be impaired. For example, a tumor that has perforated the bone and invaded one of the muscles of mastication will cause restriction of mandibular opening or perhaps deviation to the affected side. Similarly, if the tongue is fixed in one region by the tumor, its movements may be curtailed and speech may also be affected.

Pain is not a frequent complaint, but occasionally it is present later in the course of growth of the tumor when sensory nerves within the bone are encroached on. It is usually of short duration, however, because the tumor rapidly destroys the affected nerve.

The tumor usually erodes rather than expands the adjacent cortical plates. Thus detectable expansion is not bony hard to palpation but firm. This firmness is due to the nests, cords, and sheets of closely packed tumor cells that are surrounded by a relatively broad and dense boundary of fibrous tissue. The exophytic mass will frequently be nodular and smoothly contoured with a normal-appearing mucosal surface.

The microscopic picture of a metastatic tumor may vary greatly from that of the parent tumor, or both tumors may have an identical microstructure. In addition, a secondary tumor may appear to be more or less malignant than the primary tumor. When a tumor of the jaws is very anaplastic (poorly differentiated) and very aggressive and when a primary lesion has not been detected, a positive diagnosis may be difficult if not impossible to make. Such a nondescript lesion could actually be a primary anaplastic tumor of the jaws.

DIFFERENTIAL DIAGNOSIS

Although the clinician must consider all the multilocular lesions, if the patient has a history of a primary malignancy elsewhere in the body, the possibility of metastatic tumor must be assigned a high rank in the differential diagnosis. For additional features, refer to Table 19-1.

MANAGEMENT

Once the diagnosis of a metastatic tumor has been made and the primary tumor identified, the case should be managed by a tumor board. The course of action of the tumor board will be dictated by several factors:

1. If the primary tumor was successfully treated some time previously and the present jaw lesion is the only detectable metastatic tumor after a complete examination (including a radiographic skeletal survey) and if the patient's general medical condition permits, then the metastatic lesion should be *treated aggressively.*

2. Depending on the type and location of the jaw lesion and how the primary tumor responded to treatment, *surgery, radiation, antitumor medication,* or combinations of these techniques might be used. Despite this statement, however, the clinician must realize that the secondary tumor may react differently to similar treatment from the way the primary tumor reacted.

3. If the primary tumor has shown gross recurrence and there is wide metastasis, then the jaw lesion should be *managed conservatively. Palliative measures* may be instituted to provide as much comfort as possible (e.g., an alcohol nerve block to arrest pain).

CENTRAL HEMANGIOMA OF BONE

The central hemangioma of bone is a benign tumor that rarely occurs in the jaws. It is more frequent in the skull and the vertebrae. It may be congenital or traumatic in origin.

The central hemangioma of bone has been referred to as "the great imitator" because it can produce so many different radiographic images. Worth and Stoneman (1979) have prepared an excellent and unusually thorough review of the various radiographic appearances of this tumor. In about 50% of cases a multilocular appearance can be detected (Fig. 19-12).

Another form this lesion can take reveals coarse

Fig. 19-12. Intrabony hemangioma. **A,** Panograph showing multilocular expansion of the right ramus. Note the malposition of the developing right mandibular molars. **B,** Multilocular lesion in the frontal bone. **C,** Histology showing many vascular spaces between the radiating spicules of bone. (**A** from Gamez-Araujo, J. J., et al.: Oral Surg. **37:**230-238, 1974. **B** courtesy E. Palacios, M.D., Maywood, Ill.)

linear trabeculae that appear to radiate from an approximate center of the lesion. Small angular locules of varying shape are seen; however, the general outline is round.

A third appearance that may be observed is a cystlike radiolucency with an empty cavity and sometimes a hyperostotic border.

The radiographic margins of these images may be either well defined or poorly defined. Resorption of roots of the involved teeth occurs with some frequency; and calcifications (phleboliths) appearing as radiopaque rings are occasionally seen.

FEATURES

The usual complaint of a patient with an intrabony hemangioma is of a slow-growing asymmetry of the jaw or of localized gingival bleeding. Numbness and tenderness or pain may also be described. This solitary tumor is found approximately twice as often in females, and about 65% occur in the mandible. Although the tumors affect all ages, the majority have been discovered between the ages of 10 and 20 years. Some tumors demonstrate pulsation and bruits. Paresthesia is occasionally a feature.

As the slow-growing tumor expands the cortical plates, the examiner may observe that the swelling has become bony hard and possesses a smooth or bosselated surface covered with a normal-appearing mucosa. Microscopic study will reveal that the tumor comprises many thin-walled vascular spaces, some of which are quite cavernous, separated by bony septae (Fig. 19-12).

Local hemorrhage may be evident about the cervices of the teeth encountered by the enlarging lesion. These teeth may also demonstrate a pumping action; that is, if the examiner depresses the crown of the tooth in an apical direction, the tooth will rapidly assume its former position when the pressure is removed.

Aspiration of an intrabony hemangioma will readily yield a copious amount of blood and demands caution. A recommended approach is to introduce the needle through the mucosa some distance from the point where the bone is to be perforated. The bleeding that results from this method will usually be more easily arrested since the mucosa over the point where the bone was penetrated is still intact and the channel through the mucosa can be more effectively compressed.

DIFFERENTIAL DIAGNOSIS

The intrabony hemangioma is a dangerous jaw tumor because of the probability that rapid exsanguination will follow tooth extraction or jaw fracture.

Because of this lethal potential, when a bony

radiolucent lesion is encountered in the jaws, a central hemangioma or arteriovenous aneurysm must always be considered—especially since such a tumor will often demonstrate a variety of radiographic appearances. Because the multilocular appearance is not pathognomonic for an intrabony hemangioma, however, the features listed in Table 19-1 must also be considered in the development of a differential diagnosis.

Specifically the clinician should form a strong impression of intrabony hemangioma when he encounters a pumping tooth or localized gingival bleeding around a loose tooth coupled with radiographic evidence of bony change in the region. This impression may be further strengthened when large quantities of blood are easily aspirated from the area.

MANAGEMENT

Once the surgeon has reached a working diagnosis of intrabony hemangioma, it is incumbent on him to urge a complete examination of the patient and the institution of immediate treatment because death may accompany a traumatic incident to the jaws. Angiograms will aid greatly in identifying a hemangioma or arteriovenous aneurysm.

Courses of radiation have successfully eliminated manifestations of the tumor and have even induced regression of the bony defects. If surgery is the treatment selected, a block resection of the lesion (including a good margin of uninvolved bone) must be performed. Prior to surgery the external carotid artery must be ligated; but even this may not control the bleeding during surgery

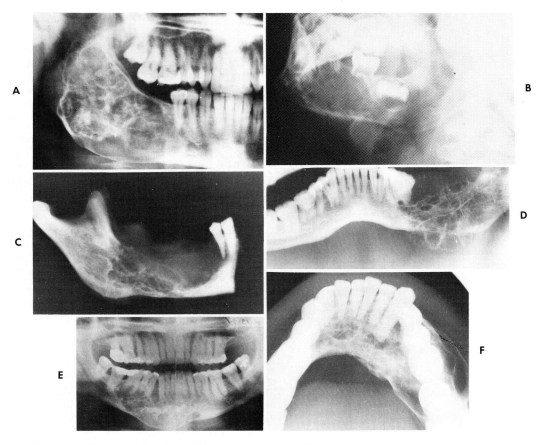

Fig. 19-13. Rare multilocular radiolucencies. **A,** Ameloblastic odontoma. **B,** Intrabony fibroma. **C,** Malignant ameloblastoma. **D,** Intrabony fibroma. **E and F,** Panograph and occlusal view, respectively, of intrabony central mucoepidermoid carcinoma of the mandible. (**A** and **C** courtesy O. H. Stuteville, D.D.S., M.D., St. Joe, Ark. **B** courtesy N. Barakat, D.D.S., Beirut, Lebanon. **D** from Martis, C., and Karakasis, D.: J. Oral Surg. **30:**758-759, 1972. Copyright by the American Dental Association. Reprinted by permission. **E** and **F** courtesy A. Moroff, D.D.S., and W. Schoenheider, D.D.S., Maywood, Ill.)

since unusual vessel aberrations sometimes accompany these tumors.

A promising new surgical approach involves ligating the external carotid artery and utilizing muscle fragments, Gelfoam, and metallic pellets (which lodge in the hemangioma) to reduce the size of the vascular channels.

RARITIES

Several other lesions in bone can cause multilocular radiolucencies. Although less than complete, a list of these entities would include the following (Figs. 19-13 to 19-17):

Ameloblastic variants
Arteriovenous malformation (Fig. 19-16)
Burkitt's lymphoma (Fig. 19-17)
Calcifying epithelial odontogenic tumor
Cementifying and ossifying fibroma (Fig. 19-18)
Central mucoepidermoid tumor
Central odontogenic and nonodontogenic fibromas
Chondroma
Eosinophilic granuloma
Fibrous dysplasia (Fig. 20-6, *B*)
Immature odontoma

Neurilemoma (Fig. 19-16)
Neuroectodermal tumor of infancy
Odontogenic keratocyst
Osteomyelitis
Pseudotumor of hemophilia (Fig. 19-15)
Squamous odontogenic tumor

DIFFERENTIAL DIAGNOSIS OF MULTILOCULAR RADIOLUCENCIES

As can be determined from the previous discussions of multilocular radiolucencies, it is fruitless to attempt to diagnose these lesions using radiographs alone. The clinician can, however, develop a sound differential diagnosis when confronted by a multilocular radiolucency.

If the suspicious-looking region is in the maxillary molar segment of the jaw, a *multilobed maxillary sinus* must be considered as the most likely diagnosis—especially if the pattern is bilateral and the region asymptomatic.

If the multilocular region is in the mandible, the diagnosis most likely will be a soap bubble type of *marrow pattern*—especially if such a pattern is prominent throughout the mandible.

If the multilocular lesion is situated anteriorly in the jaws of a patient under 30 years of age, it

Fig. 19-14. Calcifying epithelial odontogenic tumor of the left mandible. Various views of the same case showing a multilocular pattern. **A** and **B,** Periapical radiographs. **C,** Occlusal radiograph. (Courtesy D. Waite, D.D.S., Minneapolis.)

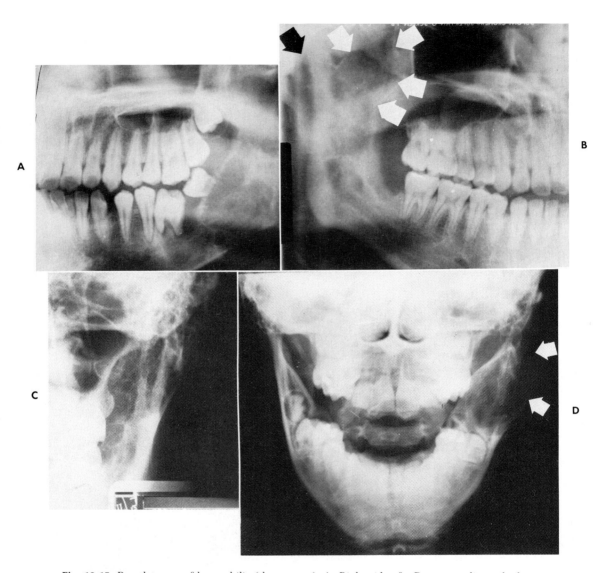

Fig. 19-15. Pseudotumor of hemophilia (three cases). **A,** Right side of a Panorex radiograph showing the multilocular lesion in a 16-year-old Oriental boy with severe hemophilia. **B** and **C,** Another case of pseudotumor in the left ramus of a 23-year-old hemophiliac. **B,** Panorex radiograph showing the multilocular expansion of the ramus, coronoid process, and condyle. **C,** Cropped posteroanterior radiograph of the affected ramus showing the mediolateral dimension of the multilocular expansion. **D,** Another case in an 11-year-old white boy with severe hemophilia. (**A** from Mulkey, T. F.: J. Oral Surg. **35:**561-568, 1977. Copyright by the American Dental Association. Reprinted by permission. **B** and **C** courtesy T. Mulkey, D.D.S., Inglewood, Calif. **D** courtesy G. Blozis, D.D.S., Columbus, Ohio.)

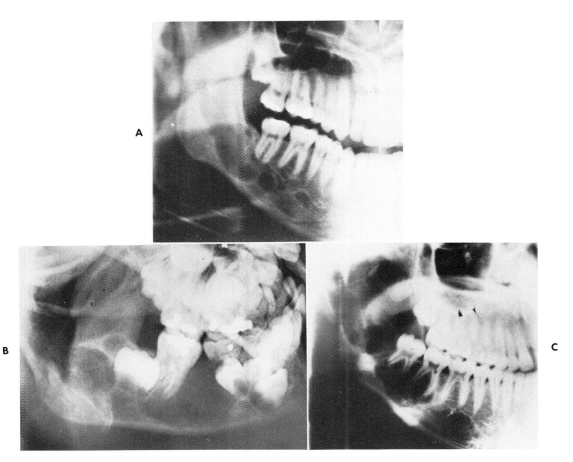

Fig. 19-16. A, Arteriovenous malformation in a 25-year-old white man. B, Arteriovenous malformation in a 10-year-old patient. C, Intrabony neurilemoma. (A from Kelly, D. E., Terry, B. C., and Small, E. W.: J. Oral Surg. **35:**387-393, 1977. Copyright by the American Dental Association. Reprinted by permission. B and C courtesy J. Lehnert, D.D.S., Minneapolis.)

Fig. 19-17. Unilateral case of Burkitt's lymphoma in a young girl. Lateral oblique radiographs showing a rarefied and multilocular pattern of bone loss. (Courtesy D. R. Sawyer, D.D.S., and A. L. Nwoka, M.D., D.M.D., Lagos, Nigeria.)

Table 19-1. Features of lesions producing multilocular radiolucencies

Lesion	Predominant sex	Usual age (years)	Predominant jaw	Predominant region	Predominant multilocular type	Other radiographic appearances	Additional features
Multilocular cysts	M = F	Over 16	Mandible Maxilla—rare	Posterior	Soap bubble	Unilocular cystlike	
Ameloblastomas	M ~ F*	20-50 (avg. 40)	Mandible—80%	Posterior—70%	Soap bubble or honeycomb Maxilla—unilocular	Unilocular a. Ragged b. Ill defined	Paresthesia in some cases
Central giant cell granulomas	$\frac{F}{M} = \frac{2.4}{1}$	Under 30 (avg. 26)	Mandible—70%	Anterior to second molars	Soap bubble	Unilocular a. Cystlike b. Borders indistinct	Serum chemistries normal; 20% cross midline
Giant cell lesions of hyperparathyroidism (secondary)	$\frac{F}{M} = \frac{2}{1}$	50-80	Mandible	None	Soap bubble	Unilocular a. Cystlike b. Borders indistinct	Occasionally multiple Kidney disease Serum calcium↓ Serum phosphorus↑ Serum alkaline phosphatase↑
Giant cell lesions of hyperparathyroidism (primary)	$\frac{F}{M} = \frac{7}{1}$	30-60	Mandible	None	Soap bubble	Unilocular a. Cystlike b. Borders indistinct	Occasionally multiple Polydipsia Polyuria Serum calcium↑ Serum phosphorus↓ Serum alkaline phosphatase↑
Cherubism	M > F	2-20	Mandible Maxilla and zygoma	Ramus and molar Sinus and orbital floor	Soap bubble	Unilocular	Multiple Familial history of lesion
Odontogenic myxomas	M = F	10-50 (avg. 25-35)	Maxilla/mandible — ¾	Ramus, premolar-molar	Soap bubble Honeycomb Tennis racket	Unilocular a. Cystlike b. Borders indistinct	Congenitally missing tooth Pain and paresthesia occasionally
Aneurysmal bone cysts	M ~ F	70% under 20	Maxilla/mandible — ⅓	Ramus and molar	Soap bubble	Unilocular	Tender
Metastatic tumors to jaws	M = F	50-80	Mandible—95%	Premolar-molar	Honeycomb	Many (see discussion in chapter)	History and symptoms of primary tumor in addition to local lesion
Central hemangiomas of bone	$\frac{F}{M} = \frac{2}{1}$	10-20	Mandible—65%	Body and ramus	Honeycomb	Tennis racket Unilocular a. Cystlike b. Borders indistinct	Local gingival bleeding Pumping action of tooth

*~ Approximately equal.

Fig. 19-18. Ossifying and cementifying fibroma. **A,** Multilocular-appearing lesion in premolar–first molar region of the mandible in a 13-year-old white boy. **B,** Another multilocular-appearing lesion in the premolar-molar region of a 28-year-old white woman. (**A** courtesy W. Heaton, D.D.S., Chicago.)

is much more likely to be a *giant cell granuloma* than an ameloblastoma.

If the lesion is situated in the posterior of the mandible in a patient over 30 years of age, it is more likely to be an *ameloblastoma*—especially if there is an accompanying paresthesia of the lip. If there is no paresthesia present, the lesion is more likely to be a *multilocular cyst*.

If the patient complains of polydipsia and polyuria or has a history of kidney disease along with abnormal serum calcium, phosphorus, and alkaline phosphatase levels, then the lesion is most likely a *giant cell lesion of hyperparathyroidism*.

If the lesions occur in a child and are multiple and if there is a family history of such lesions, then the diagnosis is almost certainly *cherubism*.

A history of primary malignant tumor elsewhere would give *metastatic carcinoma* a high rank.

Myxoma and *intrabony hemangioma* show several features in common: both frequently have either a honeycomb or a tennis racket appearance; both are usually found in patients between 10 and 30 years of age; and both are usually found in the ramus and premolar-molar regions. A history of a missing tooth of developmental origin might prompt the clinician to favor a diagnosis of myxoma whereas copious amounts of blood obtained by aspiration or the pumping tooth syndrome or cervical hemorrhage will be highly suggestive of intrabony hemangioma.

Finally, the clinician must be cognizant of the various rarities and be ready to elevate one of these within his list of possibilities when the peculiar circumstances so dictate.

SPECIFIC REFERENCES

Farman, A. G., Nortje, C. J., Grotepass, F. W., et al.: Myxofibroma of the jaws, Br. J. Oral Surg. **15:**3-18, 1977.

Kelly, D. E., Terry, B. C., and Small, E. W.: Arteriovenous malformation of the mandible: report of case, J. Oral Surg. **35:**387-393, 1977.

Kuepper, R. C., and Harrigan, W. F.: Treatment of mandibular cherubism, J. Oral Surg. **36:**638-642, 1978.

Harder, F.: Myxomas of the jaws, Int. J. Oral Surg. **7:**148-155, 1978.

Minderjahn, A.: Incidence and clinical differentiation of odontogenic tumors, J. Maxillofac. Surg. **7:**142-150, 1979.

Mulkey, T. F.: Hemophilic pseudotumors of the mandible, J. Oral Surg. **35:**561-568, 1977.

Regezi, J. A., Kerr, D. A., and Courtney, R. M.: Odontogenic tumors: analysis of 706 cases, J. Oral Surg. **36:**771-778, 1978.

Reyneke, J. P.: Aneurysmal bone cyst of the maxilla, Oral Surg. **45:**441-447, 1978.

Steidler, N. E., Cook, R. M., and Reade, P. C.: Aneurysmal bone cysts of the jaws: a case report and review of the literature, Br. J. Oral Surg. **16:**254-261, 1979.

Waldron, C. A.: Personal communication, 1976.

Worth, H. M., and Stoneman, D. W.: Radiology of vascular abnormalities in and about the jaws, Dent. Radiogr. Photog. **52:**1-23, 1979.

GENERAL REFERENCES

Abaza, N. A., El-Khashab, M., and Kreutner, A.: Central myxoma of the mandible, Oral Surg. **31:**465-471, 1971.

Balogh, G., and Inovoy, J.: Recurrent mandibular myxoma: report of case, J. Oral Surg. **30:**121-124, 1972.

Baum, S. M., Pochaczeusky, R., Sussman, R., and Stoopack, J. C.: Central hemangioma of the maxilla, J. Oral Surg. **30:**885-892, 1972.

Biesecker, J. L., Marcove, R. C., Huros, A. G., and Mike, V.: Aneurysmal bone cysts: a clinicopathologic study of 66 cases, Cancer **26:**615-627, 1970.

Boyd, R. C.: Aneurysmal bone cysts of the jaws, Br. J. Oral Surg. **16:**248-253, 1979.

Brown, D. G., Hilal, S. K., and Robinson, M.: Arteriovenous malformations of the mandible, maxilla, orbit, and cerebrum:

report of case with 20-year follow-up, J. Oral Surg. **31**:553-555, 1973.

Byrd, D. L., Kindrick, R. D., and Dunsworth, A. R.: Myxoma of the maxilla: report of case, J. Oral Surg. **31**:123-126, 1973.

Carlotti, A. E., Camitta, F. D., and Connor, T. B.: Primary hyperparathyroidism with giant cell tumors of the maxilla: report of case, J. Oral Surg. **27**:722-727, 1969.

Cohen, P. B., and Gamble, J. W.: Maxillary resection for odontogenic myxoma: report of case, J. Oral Surg. **35**:573-577, 1977.

Curtis, M. L., Hatfield, C. G., and Pierce, J. M.: A destructive giant cell lesion of the mandible, J. Oral Surg. **31**:705-709, 1973.

Daramola, J. O., Ajagbe, H. A., Oluwasanmi, J. O., et al.: Ameloblastic sarcoma of the mandible: report of case, J. Oral Surg. **37**:432-436, 1979.

Duell, R. C., and Montgomery, J. C.: Concurrent management of a central giant cell reparative granuloma, J. Am. Dent. Assoc. **81**:148-150, 1970.

Ebling, H., and Goldenberg, N.: Central angioma, Oral Surg. **21,** 9-14, 1966.

Ellis, D. J., and Walters, P. J.: Aneurysmal bone cyst of the mandible, J. Oral Surg. **34**:26-32, 1972.

Fisher, A. V., and Philipsen, H. P.: Desmoplastic fibroma of the jawbones, Int. J. Oral Surg. **5**:285-291, 1976.

Franklin, C. D., and Hindle, M. O.: The calcifying epithelial odontogenic tumor—report of four cases: two with long-term follow-up, Br. J. Oral Surg. **13**:230-238, 1976.

Franklin, C. D., and Pindborg, J. J.: The calcifying epithelial odontogenic tumor, Oral Surg. **42**:753-765, 1976.

Fredrickson, C., and Cherrick, H. M.: Central mucoepidermoid carcinoma of the jaws, J. Oral Med. **33**:80-85, 1978.

Gamez-Araujo, J. J., Toth, B. B., and Luna, A.: Central hemangioma of the mandible and maxilla: review of a vascular lesion, Oral Surg. **37**:230-238, 1974.

Goldblatt, L. I.: Ultrastructural study of an odontogenic myxoma, Oral Surg. **42**:206-220, 1976.

Gorlin, R. J., and Goldman, H. M.: Thoma's oral pathology, ed. 6, St. Louis, 1970, The C. V. Mosby Co.

Greer, R. O., and Richardson, J. F.: Clear-cell calcifying odontogenic tumor viewed relative to the Pindborg tumor, Oral Surg. **42**:775-779, 1976.

Grunebaum, M.: Nonfamilial cherubism: report of two cases, J. Oral Surg. **31**:632-635, 1973.

Gruskin, S. E., and Dahlin, D. C.: Aneurysmal bone cysts of the jaws, J. Oral Surg. **26**:523-528, 1968.

Hartley, J. H., and Shatten, W. E.: Cavernous hemangioma of the mandible, Plast. Reconstr. Surg. **50**:287-290, 1972.

Hebert, J. M., Fraire, A. E., and Reid, R.: Cherubism: report of case, J. Oral Surg. **30**:827-831, 1972.

Hindler, B. H., Abaza, N. A., and Quinn, P.: Odontogenic myxoma, surgical management and an ultrastructural study, Oral Surg. **47**:203-217, 1979.

Hoey, M. F., Courage, G. R., Newton, T. H., and Hoyt, W. F.: Management of vascular malformations of the mandible and maxilla, J. Oral Surg. **28**:696-706, 1970.

Hoppe, W.: An aneurysmal bone cyst of the mandible, Oral Surg. **25**:1-5, 1968.

Hylton, R. P., McKean, T. W., and Albright, J. E.: Simple ameloblastoma: report of case, J. Oral Surg. **30**:59-62, 1972.

Leban, S. G., Lepow, H., Straligus, G. T., and Chu, F.: The giant cell lesion of jaws: neoplastic or reparative? J. Oral Surg. **29**:398-404, 1971.

Leider, A. S., Nelson, J. B., and Trodahl, J. N.: Ameloblastic fibrosarcoma of the jaws, Oral Surg. **33**:559-569, 1972.

Loscalzo, L. J., and Marcotullio, R. G.: The multilocular cyst: a surgical approach, Oral Surg. **24**:559-562, 1967.

Lund, B. A.: Hemangiomas of the mandible and maxilla, J. Oral Surg. **22**:234-242, 1972.

Macansh, J. D., and Owen, M. D.: Central cavernous hemangioma of the mandible: report of cases, J. Oral Surg. **30**:293-297, 1972.

Martis, C., and Karakasis, D.: Central fibroma of the mandible: report of case, J. Oral Surg. **30**:758-760, 1972.

Martis, C., and Karakasis, D.: Central hemangioma of the mandible: report of case, J. Oral Surg. **31**:613-616, 1973.

Martis, C., and Karakasis, D.: Central fibroma of the mandible: report of case, J. Oral Surg. **31**:613-616, 1973.

Mehlisch, D. R., Dahlin, D. C., and Masson, J. K.: Ameloblastoma: a clinicopathologic report, J. Oral Surg. **30**:9-22, 1972.

Oikarinen, V. J., Calonius, P. E. B., and Meretoja, J.: Calcifying epithelial odontogenic tumor (Pindborg tumor) case report, Int. J. Oral Surg. **5**:187-191, 1976.

Oliver, L. P.: Aneurysmal bone cyst, Oral Surg. **35**:67-76, 1973.

Palladino, V. S., and Danziger, A. E.: Hemangioma of the maxilla, J. Am. Dent. Assoc. **70**:636-641, 1965.

Peeples, G., and Sanders, B.: Mandibular ramal odontogenic keratocysts involving the coronoid and condyle, J. Oral Med. **34**:90-91, 1979.

Pendya, N. J., and Stuteville, O. H.: Treatment of ameloblastoma, Plast. Reconstr. Surg. **50**:242-248, 1972.

Perrige, M. L., and Finkleman, A.: Myxoma of the left mandible, Oral Surg. **28**:797-799, 1969.

Richter, K. J., Grammer, F. C., and Boies, L.: Central giant cell lesion in the angle of the mandible: review of the literature and report of a case, J. Oral Surg. **31**:26-30, 1973.

Rotblat, N., and Laskin, D. M.: Radiolucent lesions of the mandible: differential diagnosis and report of case, J. Oral Surg. **27**:820-826, 1969.

Sachs, S. A., and Eisenbud, L.: Tuberculosis osteomyelitis of the mandible, Oral Surg. **44**:425-429, 1977.

Shira, R. B., and Guernsey, L. H.: Central cavernous hemangioma of the mandible: report of case, J. Oral Surg. **23**:636-642, 1965.

Steidler, N. E., Cook, R. M., and Reade, P. C.: Aneurysmal bone cysts of the jaws: a case report and review of the literature, Br. J. Oral Surg. **16**:254-261, 1979.

Stewart, S. S., Baum, S. M., Arlen, M., and Elquezabal, A.: Myxoma of the lower jaw, Oral Surg. **26**:800-808, 1973.

Struthers, P., and Shear, M.: Root resorption by ameloblastomas and cysts of the jaws, Int. J. Oral Surg. **5**:128-132, 1976.

Weathers, D. R., and Waldron, C. A.: Unusual multilocular cysts of the jaws (botryoid odontogenic cysts), Oral Surg. **36**:235-241, 1973.

Wysocki, G. P., and Sapp, J. P.: Scanning and transmission electron microscopy of odontogenic keratocysts, Oral Surg. **40**:494-501, 1975.

20

Solitary radiolucencies with ragged and poorly defined borders

Norman K. Wood
Paul W. Goaz
Orion H. Stuteville

Solitary radiolucencies of the jaws with ragged and poorly defined borders include the following:

Chronic osteitis
Chronic osteomyelitis
Squamous cell carcinoma
Fibrous dysplasia—early lesion
Metastatic tumors to the jaws
Malignant minor salivary gland tumors
Osteogenic sarcoma—osteolytic type
Chondrosarcoma
Rarities
    Ameloblastic carcinoma
    Ameloblastoma
    Angiosarcoma
    Benign tumor in the rarefied jaw
    Burkitt's tumor
    Desmoplastic fibroma
    Eosinophilic granuloma
    Ewing's sarcoma
    Fibromatosis
    Fibrosarcoma
    Intrabony hemangioma
    Liposarcoma
    Lymphosarcoma
    Malignant ameloblastoma
    Medulloblastoma
    Melanoma
    Myeloma (solitary; plasmacytoma)
    Myosarcoma
    Neuroectodermal tumor of infancy
    Neurosarcoma
    Odontogenic fibroma
    Odontogenic sarcoma
    Osteoblastoma
    Reticulum cell sarcoma
    Spindle cell carcinoma
    Surgical defect
    Wilms' tumor

Central

Peripheral

The vast majority of solitary radiolucencies with ragged and indistinct borders* are produced by three basic types of pathologic processes: inflammation and/or infection of bone, fibrous dysplasia (early stage), and osteolytic malignancy of bone. Because of the potentially serious nature of the lesion, every ill-defined radiolucency should be considered as possibly malignant until proved otherwise.

Some clinicians depend too heavily on blood chemistry values (e.g., concentration of plasma calcium, phosphorus, and alkaline phosphatase) for the differentiation of osteolytic lesions. It should be understood, however, that a substantial

---

*The term "ragged" or "moth eaten" is also used to connote destructive lesions without smoothly contoured borders. The descriptive phrase "poorly defined" conveys the notion that the borders are fuzzy, indistinct, or difficult to delineate.

amount of bony activity, either mineral absorption or mineral deposition, would have to be induced by these lesions before significant changes in the blood chemistry values could occur. In addition, since pathologic bony activity does not progress at a constant rate, the biochemical values would fluctuate with shifts in activity of the pathologic processes. Thus specific altered values of blood chemistry would be pathognomonic only periodically and in only a few diseases.

Such instances will be identified where they complement the discussion of a particular entity.

CHRONIC OSTEITIS (CHRONIC ALVEOLAR ABSCESS)

Chronic osteitis is a local mild inflammation or infection in bone* that usually occurs around the roots of a tooth. It is quite frequently a sequela of pulpitis and is perhaps identical with the chronic alveolar abscess that is discussed as a periapical radiolucency in Chapter 16. It is included in this chapter because it often has ragged poorly defined borders (Fig. 20-1). As described in Chapter 16, where the features of the chronic alveolar abscess are discussed, the inciting tooth is pulpless and usually tender to percussion. A sinus may be present and may pass through the alveolar bone to open onto the mucosa generally near the level of the apex.

DIFFERENTIAL DIAGNOSIS

The presence of an intra-alveolar draining sinus is not conclusive evidence that a radiolucent area is a *chronic osteitis, abscess,* or *osteomyelitis.*

Such a lesion could represent an *infected malignant tumor* in the periapical area. Because of the low incidence of such tumors, however, and also because a small malignant lesion would not likely become infected, this entity would be assigned a low rank in the differential diagnosis of a draining periapical radiolucent lesion.

MANAGEMENT

Although the management of the chronic alveolar abscess has been detailed in Chapter 16, it is is important to reiterate at least three precepts pertaining to the treatment of radiolucent lesions of the jaws. Compliance with these rules either will enable the clinician to initially establish a valid diagnosis or at least will provide him the op-

---

*The dry socket is a type of chronic or acute osteitis, but it is excluded from the present discussion because it seldom if ever is a diagnostic problem.

Fig. 20-1. Chronic alveolar abscess at the apex of a lateral incisor preceded the root canal filling, which was recently completed.

portunity to reevaluate his initial impression and treatment. Such confirmation may well obviate the disastrous delay that could result if a small periapical malignancy were misdiagnosed as a periapical sequela of pulpitis, treated as such, and then neglected. The three circumstances and the attending considerations are as follows:

1. If the clinician chooses to treat a periapical radiolucency nonsurgically by only obliterating the root canal(s) of the associated tooth, he must substantiate his initial impression by *follow-up radiographs* that the bony lesion was the result of inflammation.
2. If he believes that curettage with or without root resection is needed to complement the canal obliteration, he must not fail to subject the periapical tissue to *microscopic examination.*
3. If he chooses to extract the tooth, the *periapical lesion should also be removed and studied microscopically.* Since small malignancies in the area of the roots are uncommon, however, surgical removal and biopsy of every periapical radiolucency is not justified *except* in extraction cases.

The foregoing philosophy would appear to be the best regarding the management of benign-appearing periapical radiolucencies, which include chronic osteitis (chronic alveolar abscess).

CHRONIC OSTEOMYELITIS

In its usual context the term "osteomyelitis" conveys the notion of an inflammatory reaction of bone marrow that produces clinically apparent pus. An effort to classify the inflammatory diseases of bone, however, according to whether the process is completely confined to the periosteum (periostitis), cortical bone, or marrow is more an academic exercise than a useful diagnostic procedure. In reality, there is seldom if ever such a sharp demarcation among these entities. For our purposes here, if the infection is restricted to the alveolar process we will refer to it as an alveolar abscess. If the basal bone is involved then this will be considered an osteomyelitis.

The inflammation may involve any of the soft parts of the bone, the marrow, the Haversian canals, and the periosteum—separately or in combination—depending on the initiating circumstances and the duration of the process. For example, an infection of local or hematogenous origin may be initiated in any area of the interstitial connective tissues of the bone and be confined to the area where the infectious agents were deposited; or it may subsequently spread to involve the other layers of the bone.

Another consideration that helps keep the concept of a bone infection in the proper perspective is that the calcified portion of the bone does not play an active role in the disease. The calcified portion is affected secondarily by the loss of blood supply, and a greater or lesser portion may die and be resorbed or sequestered. In contrast, however, some areas may become sclerotic as the result of a mild inflammation and/or infectious process stimulating adjacent bone production.

Osteomyelitis of the jaws is a rare disease in normal healthy persons; and the practitioner can readily appreciate this fact by noting the high incidence of odontogenic infections as well as the vast number of successful intraoral surgeries performed in contaminated fields without the development of an osteomyelitis.

A predisposing condition must be present for an osteomyelitis to develop. Uncontrolled and/or undiagnosed debilitating systemic diseases (e.g., diabetes, leukemia, alcoholic states, various anemias and neutropenias, uremias, previous ionizing radiation to the bone, trauma, complications after jaw fracture) are common predisposing conditions. Furthermore, certain diseases (e.g., Paget's, osteopetrosis, sclerosing cemental masses) produce a very dense avascular type of bone, which is prone to the development of osteomyelitis.

Whereas staphylococci and streptococci are the most frequent causative microorganisms in osteomyelitis of the jaws, other microorganisms may also be the infecting agent (Gallo et al., 1976; Igo et al., 1978; Rosenquist and Beskow, 1977). For example, *Actinomyces israelii*, one of the etiologic organisms in cervicofacial actinomycosis (considered to be primarily a soft tissue infection, often situated at the angle of the mandible) may also cause an osteomyelitis of the bone (Fig. 20-2, *F*) (Musser et al., 1977; Yakata et al., 1978).

The acute type of osteomyelitis of the jaws will not be discussed in the present chapter since this form does not produce radiolucent lesions because of its rapid onset, especially in an initial infection. Furthermore, because of the widespread use of antibiotics for the treatment of odontogenic infections and traumatic injuries to the jaws, acute osteomyelitis of the jaws is not common today in the United States.

Chronic osteomyelitis may produce at least four different radiographic images:
1. A radiolucency with ragged borders
2. A radiolucency containing one or more radiopaque foci
3. A dense radiopacity
4. A salt-and-pepper appearance

The patient history, the clinical and laboratory features, and the processes fundamental to the development of all four types of bony change are the same.

Examples of osteomyelitis that may appear as radiolucencies containing radiopaque foci are discussed in Chapter 24. The salt-and-pepper lesions are also discussed in Chapter 24, whereas the completely radiopaque lesions are discussed in Chapter 27. The discussion in this chapter will focus on the conditions that attend the radiolucent type of lesion.

The completely radiolucent type of bony lesion that results from a chronic osteomyelitis usually has irregular shapes with ragged and poorly defined borders (Fig. 20-2).

The infection may originate in a recent extraction site or in a fracture line. When a fracture line is the site, the infection often appears as a more or less linear radiolucency having ragged poorly defined borders and possibly varying in width as it follows the fracture line through the bone (Fig. 20-2).

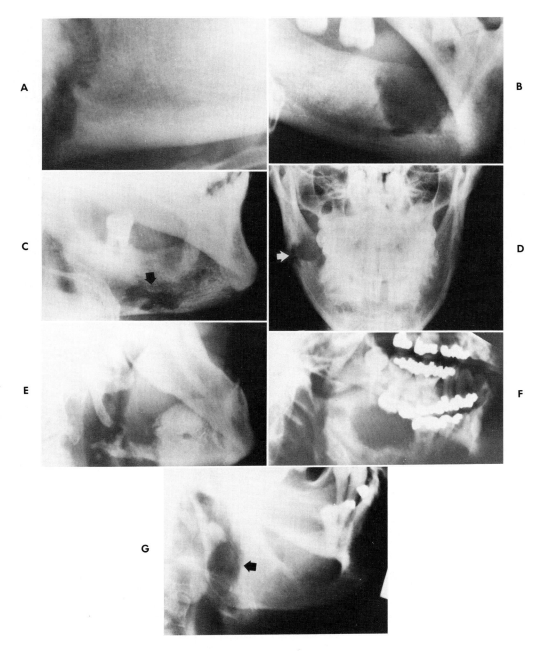

Fig. 20-2. Chronic osteomyelitis. **A,** In a fracture line. **B,** In an extraction site in a diabetic patient. (Refer to Fig. 16-18, *B,* for an illustration of a draining sinus; and to Fig. 16-18, *C,* for the histopathology of chronic osteomyelitis.) **C** to **E,** Additional examples of osteomyelitis. **F,** Actinomycotic osteomyelitis. **G,** Airway shadow (arrow) simulating a radiolucent pathosis with ragged borders. (**C, D,** and **E** courtesy O. H. Stuteville, D.D.S., M.D., St. Joe, Ark. **F** courtesy E. Palacios, M.D., Maywood, Ill.)

Often the surrounding bony borders are denser than the adjacent normal bone, reflecting a degree of sclerosis induced by the chronic infection.

Osteoradionecrosis seldom occurs as a completely radiolucent lesion. Usually there is a radiolucency with large radiopaque foci (sequestra) or perhaps a salt-and-pepper appearance.

Microscopically the radiolucent lesions of chronic osteomyelitis are characterized by small spicules of dead bone with empty lacunae scattered throughout necrotic tissue. The radiolucent areas contain varying numbers of lymphocytes, plasma cells, macrophages, and polymorphonuclear leukocytes (Fig. 16-18). The small sequestra of bone that are microscopically apparent are not large enough to be seen on the radiographs.

FEATURES

In an interview with a patient who either has or is suspected of having a chronic osteomyelitis of the jaws, the questioning should be especially directed to disclose symptoms that may be related to a contributing systemic disease.

For example, the patient may reveal that he experiences polydipsia or polyuria or both, symptoms suggesting diabetes. He may divulge that he is taking antitumor drugs*; and immediately the possibility would occur that his leukocyte count had been reduced to a level which would predispose him to infection. He may indicate that he has received radiation therapy directed to or about the oral cavity. He may report a history of facial trauma or a difficult extraction—followed by a suspected or confirmed jaw fracture.

If the examiner is aware of the spectrum of conditions that may contribute to the initiation of an osteomyelitis, appropriate questioning will often lead to the discovery of such pertinent states as Paget's disease or osteopetrosis. In addition, the clinician should always be alert to the possibility that the patient may have a primary infection elsewhere (particularly in the skin or urinary tract).

Usually the patient's first complaint related to the local problem is tenderness or pain and swelling over the affected region of the bone. If a muscle of mastication is involved, he will experience trismus during mandibular excursions. Regional lymph nodes may be inflamed and painful. A

sinus from the abscess sometimes develops and discharges a purulent material onto the overlying skin or mucosa (Fig. 16-18); but the drainage in chronic osteomyelitis is characteristically intermittent and of small volume.

Unlike a sinus that opens onto the face and is a frequent source of complaint, an osteomyelitic sinus that communicates with the oral cavity will many times be unnoticed. The patient may complain of a fetid breath, however; and if teeth are involved in an area of osteomyelitis, he may complain that they are loose and painful. If there is a nonunited jaw fracture, he may describe crepitus or abnormal jaw mobility. He may complain of intermittent fever as the chronic condition flares into an acute phase because of occlusion of the sinus, a decrease in his resistance, the introduction of a more virulent type of organism, or the interruption of therapy.

Osteomyelitis may occur at any age. In the absence of predisposing systemic disease, however, it is not common in the first three decades of life—except for the proliferative periostitis type, which is discussed in Chapter 27.

The incidence of osteomyelitis slowly increases from the third decade on, which parallels the increase in systemic disease and the decreased resistance of bone to infection in later life. This decreased resistance of bone is thought to result from the increased density combined with a decreased vascularity.

Osteomyelitis is found more frequently in men, probably because men are more commonly involved with traumatic events and their bones are usually denser.

The mandible is involved more often than the maxilla, which is rarely the site of an osteomyelitis, since the mandibular bone is much less vascular than the maxilla. Also spontaneous drainage is more readily initiated from an alveolar abscess within the spongiosa of the maxilla because the cortical plates are thinner in this jaw. Such drainage often prevents the development of an osteomyelitis. Conversely, spontaneous drainage is not so readily established in the body of the mandible because the thicker and denser mandibular cortical plates tend to contain the purulent process within the bone and thus promote the development of a more serious lesion.

This difference in the incidence of osteomyelitis between the two jaws also parallels the nature and frequency of fractures of these bones:

1. Fractures of the mandible are more common than fractures of the maxilla.
2. Fractures of the mandible anterior to the

---

*The cytotoxic drugs commercially available for prescription by the medical profession are listed in the *Physicians' Desk Reference* (Medical Economics Co.) under the classification of antineoplastics. In general, they produce a marked depression of the bone marrow and may produce anemia, leukopenia, and thrombocytopenia.

last tooth are the most common; and these, in turn, involve the largest bulk of the more easily infected dense cortical bone.

3. Fractures of the maxilla usually follow lines of low mechanical resistance that do not involve areas of dense cortical bone.

Osteomyelitis of the mandible most frequently occurs in the body because compound fractures occur more in this segment.

Intraoral contamination of the fracture site, as quite often will happen in compound fractures, greatly increases the likelihood of the development of an osteomyelitis. Thus fractures of the ramus, condyle, and coronoid process seldom become infected since they are rarely compounded intraorally because of the thick coverage of these segments of the lower jaw by muscles and other tissues. Furthermore, odontogenic infection does not commonly reach these areas because such abscesses occur primarily in the tooth-bearing areas of the jaws.

In a chronic osteomyelitis a sinus will frequently open onto the skin or the mucosal surface. There will usually be a firm swelling of the bone* and of the soft tissue covering the infected region. This swelling will often have a reddish surface and will be tender or painful on palpation. Pressure on the swelling may cause the expression of some purulent material from a sinus opening. Teeth in the radiolucent region may be somewhat sensitive when percussed. They may be loose and malposed and may show root resorption.

If the osteomyelitis has occurred in a fracture line, there may be a nonunion—which can be demonstrated by grasping both segments of the fractured bone in two hands and causing mobility about the fracture line.

When the mandible is involved at the angle or in the premolar-molar region, paresthesia of the lip may be a feature if the mandibular canal and its contents are compromised.

Occasionally before the sinus becomes patent or when it is later obliterated, a space abscess will develop in the soft tissue over the segment of involved bone. This mass will be fluctuant, nonemptiable, hot, and painful and will yield pus on aspiration.

Laboratory tests will be helpful in establishing a diagnosis of osteomyelitis. Not only will the picture of chronic bacterial infection be reflected by

---

*This swelling is produced by the formation of pus (or edema fluid) under considerable tension beneath the periosteum. The pus lifts the membrane from the bone, causing a firm enlargement. Inflammation of the adjacent soft tissues as well as fibrosis contributes increased firmness.

the blood counts (total leukocyte count increased with a lymphocytosis), but abnormal values consistent with a predisposing underlying systemic disease may also be evident.

DIFFERENTIAL DIAGNOSIS

For a discussion of the differential diagnosis of osteomyelitis, refer to the differential diagnosis section at the end of this chapter (p. 441).

MANAGEMENT

Although because of the availability of many effective antibiotic preparations osteomyelitis is not as serious today as it was a few decades ago, it is still a difficult disease to eradicate.

There are several reasons for this:

1. The blood supply to the involved bone was probably initially poor, and the decreased supply after the loss of tissue viability adds to the bone's susceptibility.

2. The greatly diminished blood supply terminates at the periphery of the infected bony segment; thus the body's defenses and any systemically administered medication (e.g., antibiotics) can advance only to the perimeters of the disease process.

3. There is frequently an open wound communicating with the oral cavity, which permits the continual contamination of the osteomyelitic area by the oral flora and juices and indeed constitutes a serious problem to manage.

The clinician must first determine whether an underlying debilitating systemic disease is present. If so and it is not being effectively treated, it must be brought under control as soon as possible with the cooperation of the patient's physician. Specimens must be obtained from the purulent drainage for culture and sensitivity tests. As soon as these results are available, the proper antibiotic therapy should be initiated in adequate doses and for a suitable length of time.

If space abscesses are present, they must be incised and drained using a through-and-through rubber drain technique. The drains should be irrigated copiously several times a day with a solution of 3% hydrogen peroxide and normal saline (1:1).

If oral wounds are present, these must likewise be frequently and adequately irrigated. Excellent oral hygiene must be maintained. Recently it has been reported that the use of hyperbaric oxygen appears to speed recovery from osteomyelitis (Goupil et al., 1978; Hart and Mainous, 1976; Mainous et al., 1973).

Infected teeth in the area must usually be extracted since to try to conserve some of them through endodontic treatment at the risk of losing a large section of the jaw is unwarranted. An attempt, nevertheless, should be made to close any oral wound that may be present if the lesion is draining extraorally and especially after the initiation of antibiotic therapy. If bone is protruding through the wound, it should be adequately contoured to permit mucosal closure. If the osteomyelitis is complicating a nonunited fracture, the fragments should be reduced and immobilized as soon as possible.

If drainage continues through the sinus, surgical saucerization may be necessary (Nakajima et al., 1977). Such a procedure requires removing all dead bone along with the granulation and necrotic tissue and recontouring the remaining bone to eliminate sharp edges. If too much bone is lost, a bone graft may be needed to approximate the two ends.

Sanders (1978) reviewed the current concepts in the management of osteomyelitis of the mandible.

In view of the very difficult management problem posed by the treatment of patients with osteomyelitis, prevention is very important. Detailing complete histories before surgery will aid in revealing systemic disease—which can then be regulated before the surgical procedure is undertaken.

Patients undergoing surgical mandibular extractions may be given 500 mg of penicillin or erythromycin 1 hour before surgery and four times per day for 5 days thereafter, or until all the postoperative symptoms have subsided. When a tooth lies in the fracture line of a mandibular fracture and the oral hygiene is poor, some clinicians recommend that the tooth be removed prior to or at the time of reduction and fixation of the fracture.

SQUAMOUS CELL CARCINOMA (EPIDERMOID CARCINOMA)

Squamous cell carcinoma of the oral cavity is discussed in Chapter 5 as a white lesion, in Chapter 6 as a type of mucosal ulcer, in Chapter 7 as an exophytic or verrucous type of lesion, and in Chapter 10 as a red lesion. The present discussion will attend primarily to its bone-destroying aspects.

Since squamous cell carcinoma is the most common malignant lesion to appear in the oral cavity, it is also the most common malignancy to produce radiolucent lesions in the jawbones. All intraoral squamous cell carcinomas do not invade and destroy bone, however. Squamous cell carcinomas of the tongue, floor of the mouth, buccal mucosa, lips, soft palate, and oropharynx do not invade bone unless they are permitted to reach a large size and develop unusual extensions. This is true because the mucosa in these sites is not close to bone. The carcinomas that originate on or near the crest of the mandibular ridge, the maxillary molar ridges, or the posterior hard palate are the tumors most likely to cause bony destruction. Not all types of squamous cell carcinoma seem to possess the same ability to invade bone. For example, the ulcerative variety seems to be more apt than the exophytic and verrucous types to invade and destroy bone.

Basically squamous cell carcinomas that destroy bone can be divided into two types according to origin: the peripheral or mucosal type, which is the more common, and the central type (within bone), which is rare. Since clinicians and pathologists have become increasingly aware of the central type, however, more of these tumors are being recognized and reported; they are thought to originate in nests of epithelium either within the jawbone or within the epithelial lining of cysts.

FEATURES

If the squamous cell carcinoma is of the peripheral type, the patient may complain of a worsening oral ulcer or mass that bleeds easily, may be somewhat tender, and is situated over bone of the alveolus or jaw or on the hard palate (Fig. 20-3). The patient usually has poor oral hygiene and admits to the heavy use of tobacco or alcohol or both. Recently the question has been raised concerning the carcinogenic potential of mouthwashes (Weaver et al., 1979). Other frequent complaints are foul odor and taste, paresthesia or anesthesia of the lip, and, if a pathologic jaw fracture is present, crepitus and pain on moving the jaw. However, it is surprising that frequently overt symptoms are not present with pathologic fracture (Ciola, 1978). Fig. 20-4 illustrates cases with advanced bone loss and fracture.

If the lesion is of the central type, the patient will frequently complain of pain, paresthesia, and swelling of the jaw—the last in the more advanced stages of the disease (Fig. 20-5, *E*).

Radiographs of bone invaded by the peripheral type of squamous cell carcinoma show lytic defects with either of two forms:

1. A roughly semicircular or saucer-shaped erosion into the bony surface with ragged ill-defined borders that illustrate the varying, uneven osteolytic invasion (Fig. 20-3).
2. A mandibular lesion with advanced hori-

Fig. 20-3. Squamous cell carcinoma. **A,** Expansion of the face over the left molar region in a 58-year-old man. **B,** Intraoral ulcer in the same patient. **C,** Lateral oblique radiograph showing a craterlike radiolucency with ragged ill-defined borders. **D,** Radiograph of the surgical specimen. **E,** Histopathology of the tumor showing features of a moderately well-differentiated squamous cell carcinoma.

zontal resorption of the ridge and basal bone in the involved area and only a thin fairly well-defined inferior border of the mandible remaining (Fig. 20-5).

Small sequestra of bone may be present as ragged radiopacities in either type of radiolucent lesion (Fig. 24-2).

Teeth involved with either type of lesion become loose, migrate, and/or have some root resorption.

If the advancing tumor has originated in the maxillary sinus, destroyed the sinus floor, and infiltrated the posterior maxillary ridge, its ragged and poorly defined borders will be toward the

Fig. 20-4. A and **B,** Pathologic fractures of the mandible through areas of gross bone destruction caused by invasive squamous cell carcinomas. **C,** Ragged ill-defined radiolucency lying between the maxillary canine and central incisor tooth. Although this appearance resembles malignancy the missing bone represents an anterior cleft palate. (**A** and **B** courtesy W. Heaton, D.D.S., Chicago.)

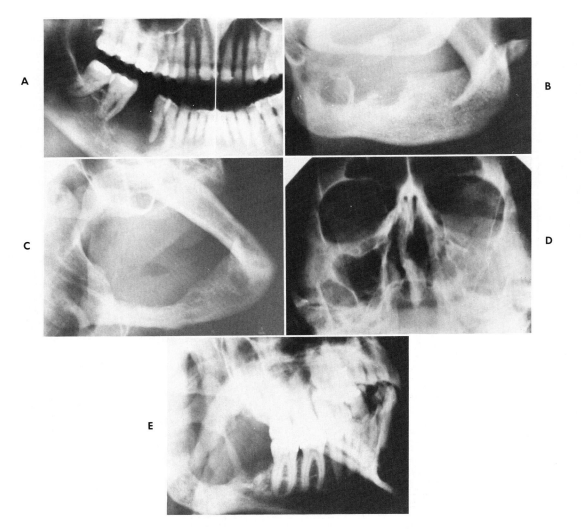

Fig. 20-5. Squamous cell carcinoma. **A** to **C,** Peripheral lesions in the mandible. **D,** In the maxillary sinus. Note the clouding of the left sinus with partial destruction of its walls. **E,** Central lesion in the ramus. (**A** to **C** courtesy O. H. Stuteville, D.D.S., M.D., St. Joe, Ark. **E** courtesy R. Nolan, D.D.S., Waukegan, Ill.)

ridge away from the sinus. This then is a useful feature for differentiating between a tumor that has originated in the maxillary sinus and one that has developed on the ridge.

The bony destruction will usually delineate the path of the advancing lesion. If the maxillary sinus has been involved with a malignant tumor, the sinus walls will be less well defined and perhaps one or more will be destroyed. The sinus itself will show increased density (clouding) where it is filled with tumor (Fig. 20-5).

Enlarged regional lymph nodes are a frequent finding in oral squamous cell carcinoma and may represent either a benign lymphadenitis (caused by infection of the lesion by the oral flora) or metastatic spread. Usually inflamed nodes can be differentiated from nodes involved with metastatic tumor by the fact that the former tend to be enlarged, painful, firm, freely movable, and discrete whereas the latter are enlarged, painless, very firm, immovable, and frequently matted together. In advanced cases the lymph nodes are bound to adjacent structures by the infiltrating tumor and are not freely movable.

Central squamous cell carcinoma is quite rare and frequently appears radiographically as a more or less rounded radiolucency that is completely surrounded by bone (Fig. 20-5) (Coonar, 1979;

Fig. 20-6. Fibrous dysplasia. **A** and **B,** In a 16-year-old boy. Note the ill-defined margins of the radiolucency. **C,** Advanced ossification at the periphery in this patient. Note the dense radiopaque appearance, which gives the illusion of well-defined borders. Periapical films of this peripheral region showed a ground-glass pattern. **D,** Note the Chinese-character spicules of woven osteoid tissue among the active fibrous stroma. Osteoblastic rimming was not a feature.

Martinelli et al., 1977). When its early appearance suggests that it originated in the wall of a cyst, the radiographic borders are evenly contoured and well defined. Later, when the malignancy has infiltrated the cyst wall and destroyed the bone, its borders become ragged and lose their sharp definition (Nolan and Wood, 1976; Sirsat et al., 1973).

Central squamous cell carcinoma predominantly is seen in patients in the fourth through seventh decades of life. Males are affected two to three times as frequently as females. The mandible is involved almost four times as often as the maxilla (Shear, 1969). Conversely, peripheral squamous cell carcinoma affects an older age group and shows a steady increase in incidence from the fourth decade on. No age group is completely immune to either type, however.

The histologic picture of either the central or the peripheral type may be quite variable, ranging from a well-differentiated to a very anaplastic squamous cell carcinoma (Fig. 20-3).

DIFFERENTIAL DIAGNOSIS

The problems attending a differential diagnosis of squamous cell carcinoma are discussed in the differential diagnosis section at the end of this chapter (p. 441).

MANAGEMENT

The management of patients with squamous cell carcinoma is discussed in Chapter 6.

FIBROUS DYSPLASIA—EARLY LESION

Fibrous dysplasia (benign fibro-osseous lesion not of periodontal ligament origin) is a lesion of bone that arises as a result of an abnormal proliferation of fibrous tissue. As the lesion matures and enlarges, destroying trabeculae and expanding cortices, peculiar trabecular shapes resembling Chinese characters are formed in the fibrous stroma (Fig. 20-6).

There is considerable variation in the proportion of fibrous to osseous tissue among lesions, depending on the stage of development of the lesion. The radiographic features of fibrous dysplasia will therefore vary, depending on its state of maturity. An early fibrous (osteolytic) stage will appear as a radiolucent lesion whereas an intermediate stage may be recognized by a smoky, mottled, or hazy pattern produced by the poorly defined intense aggregations of small spicules randomly distributed throughout the radiolucent area (Chapter 24). Finally, a mature stage may be variously described as having a salt-and-pepper, ground-glass, or orange peel appearance, which varies in radiopaqueness depending on the number, size, and degree of calcification of the trabeculae. (Fibrous dysplasia is discussed as a solitary radiopacity in Chapter 27).

When a lesion is discovered in the early osteolytic stage, its border will usually be diffuse in character and will appear to blend with the adjacent normal bony pattern without distinct demarcation (Fig. 20-6). Thus the early stage of fibrous dysplasia is included in this chapter, which encompasses the lesions having ill-defined borders.

FEATURES

Although its cause is unknown, fibrous dysplasia primarily affects adolescents and young adults, showing no predilection for either sex. It may produce asymmetry of the jaws but usually no pain. If teeth are situated in an involved section of jawbone, malocclusion, spreading, or migration may be noted but not mobility. Growth is slow and usually ceases in the early 20s or before. The molar, premolar, and canine areas, the ramus and symphysis of the mandible, and the premolar-molar regions of the maxilla as well as the zygoma and maxillary sinus are the most frequent maxillofacial sites involved.

Radiographically the early lesion of fibrous dysplasia is radiolucent with poorly defined borders (Fig. 20-6). It is usually situated deep within the bone rather than superficially in the alveolus. The maturing changes that produce the ground-glass appearance frequently commence at the periphery of the lesion and are a clue to its correct identity (Fig. 20-6). Other features are discussed in detail in Chapter 24.

DIFFERENTIAL DIAGNOSIS

The differential diagnosis of fibrous dysplasia is discussed in the differential diagnosis section at the end of this chapter (p. 441).

MANAGEMENT

The management of fibrous dysplasia is discussed in Chapter 24.

METASTATIC TUMORS TO THE JAWS

Metastatic tumors to the jaws are second only to primary squamous cell carcinoma as the most common group of malignant tumors in the jawbones. This group is discussed in Chapter 19, where it is stated that the secondary jaw tumor may produce some six different radiographic images. One possible image is a solitary radiolucency with ragged poorly defined borders, which is the feature of metastatic tumors that explains their inclusion in the present chapter.

FEATURES

The more common primary tumors that metastasize to the jaws are from the breast, lung, gastrointestinal tract, prostate gland, kidney, and thyroid gland. Although the majority of secondary jaw tumors are found in the fifth decade and later, a few (e.g., neuroblastoma, retinoblastoma) have a high incidence in children and metastasize to bone in some cases; thus the possibility of metastatic tumors to the jaws in the lower age groups must not be completely excluded.

Although it may occur at the periphery and expand into the oral cavity, the secondary jaw tumor is usually situated deep in the bone. When it produces an expansion the exophytic lesion is usually dome shaped and covered with normal-appearing mucosa. Later because it increases in size and there is concomitant masticatory trauma, its surface will frequently develop a mucositis; and if the trauma continues, the surface will ulcerate and become necrotic (Fig. 20-7).

Fig. 20-7. Metastatic bronchogenic carcinoma to the maxillary molar–premolar region. Note the smoothly contoured expanded alveolar process in this region. The surface ulceration recently occurred as a result of masticatory trauma. (Courtesy W. Heaton, D.D.S., Chicago.)

Although metastatic tumors have been reported in different regions of the jaws, most occur in the premolar-molar area of the mandible; the incidence of secondary tumors in the maxilla is quite low.

A radiolucent area that may vary greatly in size with ragged poorly defined borders is one of the radiographic pictures produced by metastatic tumors in the jaws (Fig. 20-8). Pain and numbness are frequent complaints. If there are teeth in the affected section of bone, any combination of loss of lamina dura, root resorption, and loosening and spreading of teeth is a common finding.

DIFFERENTIAL DIAGNOSIS

For a discussion of the differential diagnosis of metastatic tumors to the jaws refer to the differential diagnosis section at the end of this chapter (p. 441).

MANAGEMENT

The management of metastatic tumors is discussed in Chapter 19.

MALIGNANT MINOR SALIVARY GLAND TUMORS

Malignant salivary gland tumors are discussed in Chapter 6 as mucosal ulcers and in Chapter 7 as exophytic lesions. In the present chapter the features produced by these tumors when they infiltrate and destroy jawbone are emphasized. The more commonly occurring varieties are the pleomorphic and monomorphic adenocarcinoma, adenoid cystic carcinoma, mucoepidermoid tumor, and unclassified adenocarcinoma.

Although their incidence is much lower than that of the squamous cell carcinoma, malignant salivary gland tumors may occur as peripheral or central lesions; and, like the squamous cell carcinoma, those originating within the jawbones are rare. Peripheral malignant salivary gland tumors may occur anywhere in the soft tissue lining of the oral cavity, but seldom in the gingiva or on the anterior hard palate because the minor salivary glands are not usually found in these sites.

The posterior hard palate, the upper lip and anterior vestibule, the retromolar regions, and the base of the tongue are the most common peripheral sites affected. The glandular tissue is most proximal to bone on the hard palate and in the retromolar areas so these are the main sites where malignant minor salivary gland tumors invade the bone relatively early and produce poorly defined radiolucencies with ragged borders.

The central variety occurs so seldom that it will not be discussed further—other than to indicate that its features are similar to those produced by a central squamous cell carcinoma or any malignancy originating in the jawbones. An example that produced a multilocular radiolucency of the mandible is illustrated in Fig. 19-13.

FEATURES

The malignant minor salivary gland tumor usually occurs in patients between 40 and 70 years of age and is more common in women. It usually grows slowly but may demonstrate alternate rates of growth. It frequently is found on routine examination, or sometimes the patient will complain of a painful swelling. Because it develops as an increasing mass of tumor cells beneath and separate from the epithelial surface, it is most frequently somewhat dome shaped with a smooth surface and quite firm to palpation.

A mucus-producing adenocarcinoma and a mucoepidermoid tumor may have areas that are fluctuant because of pooling of the mucus pro-

A   **B**

Fig. 20-8. Metastatic tumors. **A,** Metastatic bronchogenic carcinoma. **B,** Metastatic squamous cell carcinoma from the lower lip. (**A** courtesy R. Latronica, D.D.S., Albany, N.Y. **B** courtesy O. H. Stuteville, D.D.S., M.D., St. Joe, Ark.)

Fig. 20-9. Peripheral malignant salivary gland tumors. **A,** Mucoepidermoid tumor in the retromolar region destroying the alveolar bone (arrow). **B,** Mucoepidermoid tumor (arrows), which originated in the floor of the mouth and infiltrated the lingual alveolar plate in the premolar-molar region. **C,** Radiograph of a surgical specimen of an adenocystic carcinoma. **D,** Adenocarcinoma of minor salivary gland origin. (**A** and **B** courtesy R. Kallal, D.D.S., Chicago. **C** courtesy O. H. Stuteville, D.D.S., M.D., St. Joe, Ark. **D** courtesy R. Goepp, D.D.S., Zoller Clinic, University of Chicago.)

duced by these special types of tumors. Aspiration will yield mucus that is clear, viscous, and sticky. When mucus pools near the surface of a mucus-producing tumor, the tumor may clinically mimic a mucocele. Furthermore, if it has cystic areas of mucus retention, the areas may rupture and produce a persistent ulcerated surface.

Early in its development the malignant salivary tumor is usually covered with a smooth normal-appearing mucosa. Later if it is chronically traumatized, its surface will demonstrate a mucositis. If the trauma is severe or if a biopsy of the mass is done, the surface will ulcerate and remain ulcerated; and this frequently leads to the production of a necrotic surface.

When a malignant salivary gland tumor infiltrates bone, it produces a radiolucency identical with that produced by a peripheral squamous cell carcinoma (i.e., a semicircular radiolucency with poorly defined ragged advancing borders eroding from the surface into the bone; Fig. 20-9). An undetected lesion on the posterolateral hard palate will often destroy the floor of the maxillary sinus and invade the air-filled cavity. Although the radiographic appearances of both tumors may be similar, the fact that the malignant salivary gland tumor seldom originates on the crest of the alveolar ridge will be useful in distinguishing this lesion from squamous cell carcinoma.

DIFFERENTIAL DIAGNOSIS

For a discussion of the management of malignant minor salivary gland tumors, refer to the section on differential diagnosis at the end of this chapter (p. 441).

MANAGEMENT

The management of malignant minor salivary gland tumors is discussed in Chapter 7.

Fig. 20-10. A, Osteogenic sarcoma (osteolytic variety) (arrows). **B,** Microscopy of the lesion showing scanty osteoid and malignant osteoblasts. (**A** courtesy R. Goepp, D.D.S., Zoller Clinic, University of Chicago.)

OSTEOGENIC SARCOMA— OSTEOLYTIC TYPE

Osteogenic sarcoma is second only to multiple myeloma as the most frequently encountered *primary* tumor of the jawbones. It is thought to arise from primitive undifferentiated cells and from malignant transformation of osteoblasts. Radiographically it may present three basic appearances; completely radiolucent, radiolucent with radiopaque areas, and predominantly radiopaque. The classic sunburst effect may be seen in the latter two types. Discussion in this chapter stresses the radiolucent variety.

Like other malignant tumors the osteogenic sarcoma is of unknown cause. Bones that have been previously radiated and bones affected with Pagent's disease, however, show an increased incidence. Osteogenic sarcoma of the jaws differs from that found in other bones as follows:

1. The peak age of incidence is about 27 years, an average 10 years above the incidence observed in other bones.
2. The jaw lesions have less tendency to metastasize.
3. The prognosis is better for jaw lesions.

Osteogenic sarcoma metastasizes almost exclusively by hematogenous spread. Pulmonary metastasis is the most common, being frequently found at autopsy. Examples of lymph node involvement are rare.

FEATURES

A patient with an osteogenic sarcoma may complain of intermittent local pain, swelling, paresthesia or anesthesia, perhaps tooth mobility, intraoral bleeding, asymmetry of the jaws, and in some cases a mass on the ridge or gingivae. Garrington and co-workers (1967) reported that of their series, 40% had pain, 14% had paresthesia, and 25% experienced dental symptoms. There may be a history of recent tooth extraction with a nodular or polypoid, somewhat reddish, granulomatous-appearing mass growing from the tooth socket.

Approximately 60% of osteogenic sarcomas occur in men. The majority of patients affected are in the second to fifth decade, and incidence peaks at about 27 years of age. Investigators differ as to which jaw is more frequently involved, but most favor the mandible. In the series reported by Garrington and co-workers (1967) the mandible was affected two times as often as the maxilla.

As the tumor grows, eroding the cortical plates, the expansion is very firm because of the dense fibrous tumor tissue produced. Initially the swelling is smoothly contoured and covered with normal-appearing mucosa. Later, when the expansion becomes chronically traumatized, the surface develops a mucositis; and still later it ulcerates and a necrotic surface that is whitish gray results. This surface can be removed with a tongue blade.

The bony lesion is radiolucent with poorly defined ragged borders; and early in the course of the disease, it is usually located centrally in the jaws (Fig. 20-10). Sometimes it will be discovered as a radiolucency in the periapex or more toward the periphery of the ridge or cortical plates. It may originate adjacent to or seemingly in the periodontal ligament space, and in such cases it will be encountered radiographically as a bandlike widening involving the complete length of the periodontal ligament space on one side of the root (Gardner and Mills, 1976). This particular picture

Fig. 20-11. Bandlike widening of the periodontal ligament. **A,** Chondrosarcoma of the anterior of the mandible in a young woman. **B,** Osteosarcoma of the anterior of the mandible. Note the presence of both symmetric and asymmetric bandlike widening of the periodontal ligament in **A** and **B. C,** Asymmetric widening of the periodontal ligament on the mesial aspect of the canine tooth, which is due to the presence of calculus. **D,** Asymmetric widening of the periodontal ligament on mesial aspect of upper lateral incisor tooth, which has been produced by recent orthodontic movement. (**A** courtesy R. Goepp, D.D.S., Zoller Dental Clinic, University of Chicago. **B** courtesy O. H. Stuteville, D.D.S., M.D., St. Joe, Ark.)

is not pathognomonic for osteogenic sarcoma, however, but may also be seen with other types of mesenchymal malignancies as well as in patients undergoing orthodontic therapy and also unusual unilateral bone resorption in periodontal disease (Fig. 20-11). In addition, Shafer (1980) illustrated a case of osteoblastoma that produced a unilateral bandlike widening of the periodontal ligament.

Microscopically the radiolucent type of osteogenic sarcoma will be basically fibroblastic in nature—showing malignant changes, good vascularity, and a few areas of osteoid tissue. It may also form some cartilage. A tumor composed primarily of osteoid or cartilage may rapidly calcify in these areas and become evident as a mixed radiolucent-radiopaque area or as a predominantly radiopaque lesion. The latter two types are discussed in Chapter 24.

DIFFERENTIAL DIAGNOSIS

The differentiation of radiolucent lesions such as osteogenic sarcoma is discussed in the differential diagnosis section at the end of this chapter (p. 441).

MANAGEMENT

Although a diagnosis of osteogenic sarcoma of the jaws is grave (approximately 25% of the patients survive 5 years), the prognosis is better than for osteogenic sarcoma of other bones of the skeleton (Garrington et al., 1967). Lesions in the symphysial region of the mandible have the best outlook, and those in the maxillary sinus have the poorest.

As with all malignant tumors, the management of a case of osteogenic sarcoma should be determined by the tumor board. Once a positive diagnosis of osteogenic sarcoma has been made by the pathologist, a thorough examination of the patient must be conducted in an attempt to determine whether secondary lesions are present. If extensive secondary lesions are found, palliative radiation is usually decided on. If no secondary lesions are discovered, the tumor board usually decides on radical resection if possible. Regional lymph node dissection is rarely indicated or necessary since spread to such nodes is infrequent. Presurgical radiation has been advised by some authors on the basis that it reduces the threat of metastasis imposed by the surgical procedure. Recent studies have indicated that radiation or chemotherapy may yield as good results as radical surgery. High and Glass (1978) reported achieving a complete remission in a recurrent case of osteosarcoma of the mandible.

The osteolytic type is the least differentiated and carries the poorest prognosis.

CHONDROSARCOMA

Chondrosarcoma follows multiple myeloma and osteogenic sarcoma as the third most common primary malignant tumor of the jawbones. It is, however, an uncommon jaw tumor, osteogenic sarcoma being at least three times more common. Although its exact origin is obscure, the chondrosarcoma may be found developing in normal cartilage, chondromas, or osteochondromas. It may originate centrally or on the periphery of the bone.

Radiographically the chondrosarcoma may present two images: a frank radiolucency (usually in an early stage) or a radiolucency containing various shapes and sizes of radiopaque shadows. These radiopaque shadows are the result of calcification and/or ossification in areas of cartilage formation and are a feature of relatively long-standing tumors; they are found in the older parts of the tumors.

There is also a comparatively rare primitive type of chondrosarcoma, the mesenchymal chondrosarcoma, that is apparently derived from cartilage-forming mesenchyme. Some authors believe this lesion is more aptly described as a mesenchymal sarcoma showing some chondroid differentiation.

In keeping with the subject of this chapter, only the completely radiolucent type will be discussed.

FEATURES

The chondrosarcoma is a tumor primarily of adulthood and old age—the majority of jaw tumors occurring in patients between the ages of 20 and 60 years, with an average age of approximately 40 years (Sato et al., 1977). Over 60% of chondrosarcomas are found in men, and the maxilla is involved more often than the mandible. Some of the maxillary tumors represent lesions that have originated in the cartilages of the nasal cavity and have invaded the maxillary bone. The premolar-molar regions, the symphysis, and coronoid and condyloid processes are the most frequent mandibular sites (Martis, 1978).

Unlike the osteogenic sarcoma, the chondrosarcoma metastasizes relatively rarely, especially in its early stages. As with osteogenic sarcoma, however, metastatic spread is almost entirely by vascular channels. Malignant cells may erode through the walls of a venule and extend along inside the venule without adhering to the vessel walls but still attached at their site of entry. When metastasis does occur, the lung is the organ most frequently involved.

Recurrence happens when resection has been inadequate, usually only after many years. A patient whose tumor has not been adequately excised will experience several recurrences and finally die because the tumor has invaded or metastasized to a surgically inaccessible site.

Although the common type of chondrosarcoma occurs more frequently throughout the body than does the mesenchymal type, a greater portion of the mesenchymal type occurs in the jaws. The mesenchymal chondrosarcoma represents a more malignant variety and demonstrates more rapid growth as well as earlier and more frequent metastasis; as a result it carries a much poorer prognosis.

Except for the mesenchymal variety, the chondrosarcoma behaves in a much less aggressive fashion than does the osteosarcoma. The patient frequently complains of a painful slowly enlarging swelling in the affected region of the bone, often of several years' duration. The pain is strongly suggestive of an actively growing central type of bony tumor. Paresthesia is experienced in many cases. Occasionally when there is malignant transformation in a previously benign carti-

laginous tumor, the patient will experience a rapid growth in an existing mass of long standing.

Before the chondrosarcoma has caused expansion of the bone, pain alone may be the only clinical indications of the developing tumor. If it has eroded through the cortical plates, a tender or painful smoothly contoured mass can be palpated over the bone. The mass will be very firm if the particular tumor or region contains substantial amounts of cartilage or fibrous tissue. If, however, much myxomatous-type tissue is present near its periphery, the tumor will feel soft. The mucosal covering will appear normal in the early stage but later may ulcerate and develop a necrotic surface if chronically traumatized. Teeth in the affected region may demonstrate spreading, migration, increased mobility, and root resorption. Sato and co-workers (1977) found that in maxillary tumors the most common symptoms were nasal.

The earlier lesion in bone is usually radiolucent because the neoplastic cartilage has not yet become calcified (Figs. 20-11, *B,* and 20-12).

Microscopically the lesion shows varying degrees of myxomatous-type tissue, atypical cartilage, endochondral bone, and nests of malignant chondrocytes (Fig. 20-12, *B*). A low-grade chon-

Fig. 20-12. Chondrosarcoma. **A,** Radiograph of surgical specimen of a mandibular lesion. **B,** Photomicrograph of a chondrosarcoma. (**A** courtesy O. H. Stuteville, D.D.S., M.D., St. Joe, Ark.)

drosarcoma is difficult to differentiate microscopically from an aggressive chondroma.

Radiographically the central tumor is bordered by a ragged poorly defined perimeter of bone. Conversely, the peripheral type may show only one border in bone and the rest of the tumor may be a vague hazy mass peripheral to the uneven area of bony erosion. The peripheral lesion generally tends to be more circumscribed. A lesion involving the teeth may appear as a periapical radiolucency or as an asymmetric broadening of the periodontal ligament space (Fig. 20-11, B).

DIFFERENTIAL DIAGNOSIS

The discussion of the differential diagnosis of the chondrosarcoma is included in the differential diagnosis section that begins at the bottom of this page.

MANAGEMENT

As with other oral malignant tumors, the treatment of a chondrosarcoma should be directed by a tumor board. Adequate surgical resection of the diseased bone is the only treatment offering any real chance of a cure; and the surgeon should assume that the initial procedure is the only opportunity he will have to effect the cure. Consequently the treatment must be radical and the excision should include as wide a margin of adjacent normal bone as is practical.

The surgeon should be prepared for a radical procedure if the clinical appearance of the lesion causes him to suspect it is malignant. If this precaution is observed, he will be able to resect as soon as a frozen section is evaluated. Such preparedness will reduce the time interval between the initial biopsy and the resection—when the potential for vascular dissemination of tumor cells is high because of the surgical manipulation.

The chondrosarcoma is quite radioinsensitive, and radiation therapy is used only as a palliative procedure with large inoperable tumors. Local more conservative block resection, not including the full thickness of the bone, may be the treatment of choice in some early peripheral chondrosarcomas.

There is a good long-term survival rate in 50% of the patients who have received early surgical treatment if wide margins of adjacent normal bone have also been excised. The prognosis for a jaw chondrosarcoma is not generally considered to be as good as for a chondrosarcoma of another bone since a greater portion of jaw chondrosarcomas are of the more aggressive mesenchymal variety. A tumor involving the symphysial region has the most favorable prognosis.

RARITIES

There are considerable number and variety of rare lesions of the jaws that may appear as solitary radiolucencies with ragged poorly defined borders. Following is a partial list of such lesions—considered as rarities because they either seldom occur in the United States or do not usually cause a solitary radiolucent lesion with poorly defined borders characteristic of the others in this group (Figs. 20-13 to 20-15):

Ameloblastic carcinoma (Fig. 20-13, G)
Ameloblastoma (Fig. 20-13, A and H)
Angiosarcoma
Benign tumor in the rarefied jaw
Burkitt's tumor
Desmoplastic fibroma
Eosinophilic granuloma (Figs. 20-13, E, and 20-14, D)
Ewing's sarcoma (Fig. 20-15)
Fibromatosis
Fibrosarcoma (Fig. 20-13, D)
Intrabony hemangioma
Liposarcoma
Lymphosarcoma
Malignant ameloblastoma
Medulloblastoma
Melanoma
Myeloma (solitary; plasmacytoma) (Fig. 20-14)
Myosarcoma
Neuroectodermal tumor of infancy
Neurosarcoma
Odontogenic fibroma
Odontogenic sarcoma
Osteoblastoma
Reticulum cell sarcoma (Fig. 20-13, B and C)
Spindle cell carcinoma
Surgical defect
Wilms' tumor

Furthermore, benign lesions in rarefied jaws may appear to have ill-defined borders. For example, a giant cell lesion situated in a jaw that is rarefied by osteitis generalisata of hyperparathyroidism will appear as an ill-defined lesion because of the overall radiolucent appearance of the bone (Fig. 18-16).

DIFFERENTIAL DIAGNOSIS OF SOLITARY RADIOLUCENCIES WITH RAGGED POORLY DEFINED BORDERS

The finding of a radiolucency with ill-defined ragged borders must be regarded as an ominous

Fig. 20-13. Rare ill-defined ragged radiolucencies. **A,** Ameloblastoma. **B,** Lateral oblique and, **C,** periapical radiographs of a reticulum cell sarcoma. **D,** Surgical specimen of a fibrosarcoma of the mandible. **E,** Eosinophilic granuloma in the mandibular molar region. **F,** Central squamous cell carcinoma. **G,** Ameloblastic carcinoma. **H,** Simple ameloblastoma. (**A** courtesy D. Skuble, D.D.S., Hinsdale, Ill. **B** and **C** courtesy R. Goepp, D.D.S., Zoller Clinic, University of Chicago. **D** courtesy R. Oglesby, D.D.S., Chicago. **E** courtesy N. Barakat, D.D.S., Beirut, Lebanon. **F** courtesy O. H. Stuteville, D.D.S., M.D., St. Joe, Ark. **G** courtesy R. Latronica, D.D.S., Albany, N.Y. **H** courtesy R. Newman, D.D.S., Chicago.)

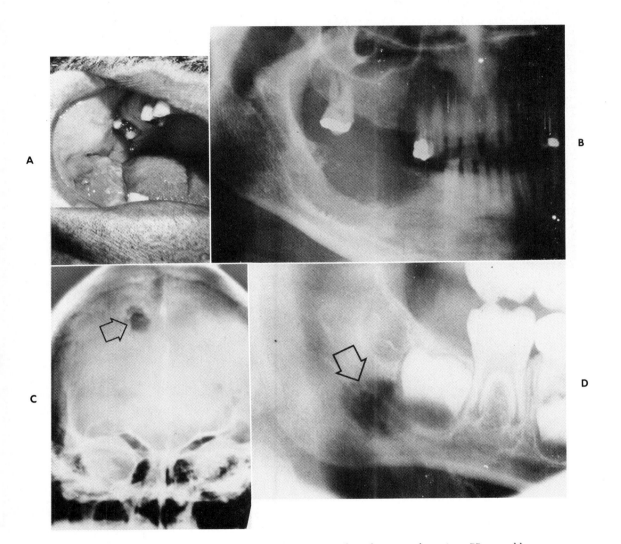

Fig. 20-14. A and **B,** Clinical and radiographic picture of a solitary myeloma in a 55-year-old man. **C,** Radiograph of a solitary myeloma in the frontal bone. **D,** Eosinophilic granuloma in a 9-year-old child. (**A** and **B** courtesy N. Barakat, D.D.S., Beirut, Lebanon. **C** courtesy W. Heaton, Chicago. **D** courtesy R. Warpeha, D.D.S., M.D., Maywood, Ill.)

Fig. 20-15. Ewing's sarcoma in a 13-year-old girl. **A,** Full-face view showing asymmetry caused by a swelling in left mandible. **B,** Intraoral view showing smoothly contoured bony expansion in the premolar–first molar region. **C,** Lateral oblique radiograph showing ill-defined radiolucency and malposition of the premolar tooth. **D,** Occlusal view showing some central bone loss and also some destruction of the buccal plate (arrow). Some bony spicules could be seen radiating out from the bone at this location in the original radiograph. The posteroanterior view of the mandible (see Fig. 27-12, *A*) showed periosteal bone growth at the inferior border of the mandible with an onionskin appearance. (Courtesy N. Barakat, Beirut, Lebanon.)

sign. When such a picture is observed on good diagnostic films, it is recommended practice to obtain additional radiographs of the suspected area from various angles to determine the following:

1. Whether the radiolucency actually has ill-defined borders or whether by happenstance the angle at which the original film was exposed combined with an unusual variation in anatomic structure to produce the mistaken impression
2. The exact size, extent, and location of the lesion

The differential diagnosis of lesions included in the present chapter is relatively difficult since the clinical characteristics of most of the entities are so similar—an enlarging tender or painful swelling of the jawbone accompanied by paresthesia or numbness. Likewise the radiographic appearances of these lesions are not uniquely characteristic during the radiolucent stage. As a result of this local clinical similarity, the diagnostician must be alert to the more subtle features of each lesion: the relative frequency of occurrence, sexual predilection, age range of patients affected, incidence peaks, jaw regions usually involved, and accompanying systemic signs or symptoms.

An inflamed surface of an expanding jaw lesion, or even the presence of purulent drainage from a sinus, will not positively establish whether the suspicious pathosis is a chronic infection, however, since any of the tumors listed in this chapter may be complicated by the superimposition of an osteomyelitis.

Because the differential diagnosis of solitary poorly defined ragged radiolucencies in children will be quite different from that of lesions having the same appearance in adults, this aspect will be discussed separately for the two age groups.

Solitary lesion in an adult
PERIPHERALLY LOCATED

A 59-year-old white man complained of a tender swelling on the right side of the lower jaw in the molar area (Fig. 20-16). He also described a paresthesia of the lower lip on that side. He had first noticed the swelling about 1 month previously. He smoked and drank excessively and had poor oral hygiene. On examination the clinician found an ulcer on the mucosa over the edentulous mandibular alveolar ridge in the right molar region (Fig. 20-16). The opposing posterior maxillary arch was also edentulous.

The ulcer had firm borders and was 2 cm in

Fig. 20-16. Peripheral squamous cell carcinoma. **A,** Note the bony destruction (arrows). **B,** Radiograph of the surgical specimen. (Courtesy E. Palacios, M.D., Maywood, Ill.)

diameter. There was a firm nontender expansion of soft tissue on the buccal and lingual surfaces of the ridge in the area of the ulcer. This soft tissue mass was tightly bound to the alveolar bone beneath. Several firm, nontender, enlarged, and matted nodes were present in the right submandibular space. The hematologic examination revealed that, although the patient was anemic, the total leukocyte count and differential were within normal limits.

A broad roughly semicircular destructive lesion on the alveolar crest of the right mandibular molar region was apparent on a lateral oblique radiograph. The margin of this saucer-shaped erosion was ragged and poorly defined (Fig. 20-16).

In evaluating this lesion the clinician can initially rule out *fibrous dysplasia* because its early (radiolucent) stage would seldom if ever be seen at age 59 years. Also fibrous dysplasia almost never causes pain or paresthesia, and enlarged lymph nodes are not a feature of the disease.

The more common metastatic tumors of childhood, *neuroblastoma* and *retinoblastoma*, may be assigned a low rank on the basis of the patient's age. Also *osteogenic sarcoma* usually occurs in a younger age group. Other metastatic tumors more common to this age would be assigned a low priority because of the absence of symptoms that would suggest the presence of a distant primary tumor.

Chronic osteomyelitis and *chronic osteitis* are not prime suspects for consideration because there are no manifestations of infection (e.g., local pain, cervical lymphadenitis, leukocytosis).

The age of the patient would not contraindicate *chondrosarcoma,* but a chondrosarcoma that had reached this size would usually show some calcified foci within the radiolucency. Furthermore, a chondrosarcoma would seldom involve the regional lymph nodes. Also chondrosarcomas are more common in the maxilla.

Squamous cell carcinoma, malignant minor salivary gland tumor, and *reticulum cell carcinoma* (see Table 20-1) must be considered as possible diagnoses on the basis of the patient's age and the fact that they may involve lymph nodes. On the basis of incidence, these entities would be ranked in the following order in the working diagnosis:

1. Squamous cell carcinoma
2. Malignant minor salivary gland tumor
3. Reticulum cell sarcoma

Peripheral squamous cell carcinoma is the most likely diagnosis for this lesion since minor salivary gland tissue is unlikely to be found on the crest of the alveolar ridge. Also the radiographic appearance of the tumor suggests that it originated in the soft tissue and was invading the bone from the periphery, which would be atypical of the usual initial manifestation of a localized reticulum cell sarcoma (a rare lesion). Finally, the diagnosis of peripheral squamous cell carcinoma is strongly supported by the fact that this oral lesion is frequently associated with poor oral hygiene, excessive smoking, and heavy alcohol consumption.

CENTRALLY LOCATED

A 30-year-old white man described appreciable pain of about 1 month's duration in the right body of his lower jaw. Shortly before this time, he had noticed a tingling in his lower lip on the right side. There was no history of trauma to the area.

During the examination the clinician noticed a slight swelling on the buccal aspect of the alveolus between and beneath the first molar and second premolar. These two teeth were found to be abnormally mobile, but they were not sensitive to percussion and they tested vital. The examination of the remainder of the oral cavity did not disclose additional significant abnormal conditions, and no cervical masses were found. A medical examination failed to disclose any systemic problems, and a skeletal radiographic survey revealed no other bony lesions. Likewise the results from all the appropriate laboratory tests[*] were within normal ranges.

Periapical radiographs of the right mandible revealed a solitary radiolucency at the junction of the molar and premolar areas. It was approximately round with irregular poorly defined borders. The first molar and second premolar were found to have advanced and uneven root resorption although the crowns of both appeared to be free of caries and there were no restorations. The lower borders of the radiolucency appeared to be encroaching on the mandibular canal.

Chronic osteitis and *osteomyelitis* can be excluded as likely causes of this man's discomfort since there were no local signs of infection and no apparent evidence of predisposing conditions, fractures, or teeth with probable pulpitis.

Fibrous dysplasia can be eliminated from further consideration on the basis of the patient's pain, lip paresthesia, and root resorption—which point to the probability of a malignancy.

Peripheral squamous cell carcinoma may be dismissed as an unlikely choice since there is no mucosal involvement; and the possibility that the lesion is a *central squamous cell carcinoma* can be assigned a low rank since this tumor is rare. Also the peripheral and central squamous cell carcinomas are usually seen in an older age group.

Because of the patient's age, *Ewing's sarcoma,* which occurs most commonly at a younger age, *lymphosarcoma,* which is seldom seen between the ages of 20 and 30 years, and *metastatic lesions of childhood* should be assigned a low ranking in the differential diagnosis.

Chondrosarcoma is more commonly seen in an older age group, and it affects the maxilla more frequently than the lower jaw.

The patient is too young for *adult metastatic disease* to be strongly suspected, and there were no systemic symptoms to suggest a primary tumor elsewhere (although there could have been an occult primary lesion).

Central malignant minor salivary gland tu-

---

[*]Erythrocyte and leukocyte counts (complete and differential), serum calcium, alkaline and acid phosphatase, urine calcium, and Bence Jones protein are usually determined.

mors are rare and are usually found in older individuals.

Reticulum cell sarcoma of bone is a possibility, but it is also usually found in older people and occurs much less frequently than osteogenic sarcoma.

Finally, the location, signs and symptoms, age of the patient, and incidence prompt the clinician to assign a top ranking to *osteogenic sarcoma (osteolytic type).*

Solitary lesion in a child

A mother described the chief complaint of her 5-year-old daughter as a rapidly growing painful swelling in the molar region of the right mandible. The mother reported that she had first noticed the swelling about 1 month before and that pain had initially been intermittent but soon became constant. The child had recently experienced a tingling sensation on the right side of the lower lip; a history of recent trauma could not be established; and vital signs, including temperature, were normal. Examination of the child's neck failed to reveal any abnormalities such as lymph node involvement or tender areas.

The intraoral swelling, which was clinically apparent to the examiner, was tender and firm to palpation; and the jaw was somewhat expanded both buccally and lingually. The smoothly contoured swelling was covered with normal-appearing mucosa, and there was no draining sinus present. The two deciduous molars in the area of the swelling were mobile, and there was some bleeding from their gingival sulci.

A complete radiographic survey of the skeleton disclosed only a solitary radiolucent lesion in the right mandible. It was completely surrounded by bone measuring about 2 cm in diameter, and its ragged borders were poorly defined. An occlusal radiograph showed that, although there was minimal evidence of destruction of both lingual and buccal cortical plates, multiple layers of subperiosteal new bone were faintly evident. The first and second right deciduous molars were not carious and had not been restored, but their roots were almost entirely resorbed. The lamina dura surrounding the root and crypt of the developing first permanent molar was missing.

A detailed medical examination, including complete blood and urine tests, failed to provide any pathognomonic results.

An early (osteolytic) lesion of *fibrous dysplasia* can immediately be eliminated as a possible diagnosis for this child's condition since pain is not a feature of fibrous dysplasia and the lesion does not enlarge rapidly, does not cause root resorption or paresthesia, and infrequently develops in children as young as 5 years of age.

Chronic osteitis or *osteomyelitis,* with the exception of Garré's type, may be assigned a low rank because there was no obvious precipitating injury or predisposing systemic disease and the occurrence of osteomyelitis would be very rare under such circumstances. Also the local and systemic pictures did not show an infection since there was an absence of local inflammation, there were no tender regional lymph nodes, and the patient's temperature and leukocyte count and differential were within normal limits.

The *neuroectodermal tumor* of infancy can be rejected as a possible diagnosis not only because this entity is rare but also because it almost always occurs in the anterior maxilla and is seldom if ever seen in children who have reached 5 years of age.

The patient's lesion is not likely to be an *intrabony hemangioma* since pain is seldom a feature of the central hemangioma and such rapid expansion is not characteristic. Also its superior border is usually contoured around the roots of the adjacent teeth. Furthermore, once the cortical plates were eroded, this vascular tumor would be relatively soft to palpation. If doubt still remained, judicious aspiration of the mass would provide convincing evidence of its vascular nature.

The foregoing considerations point to a conclusion of *malignant tumor* in bone. On the basis of age alone, however, this 5-year-old girl would not be likely to have a *squamous cell carcinoma, malignant minor salivary gland tumor,* or *chondrosarcoma.* Furthermore, a diagnosis of *peripheral squamous cell carcinoma* or *peripheral malignant minor salivary gland tumor* would be precluded by the radiographic appearance of the lesion—which indicated an origin in bone (central lesion)—and by the fact that there was no peripheral soft tissue mass or ulceration of the mucosa. Then, too, the *central varieties of squamous cell carcinoma* and *minor salivary gland tumor* would be rare.

Although the foregoing speculations do not permit specific identification of the lesion, they do emphasize the important fact that the malignant tumors prone to involve this age group are quite different from those that usually occur in adults. Also malignant tumors in children are far less common than in adults and must be considered rare. Consequently, in identifying this child's pathosis, the clinician would be compelled to consider the entities listed as rarities.

The history, physical examination, and laboratory tests in this case provide presumptive evidence of a bone tumor; but there are no definite features that would permit the conclusion of either a primary or a metastatic lesion. To establish a working diagnosis, the clinician must consider a catalogue of the most frequent childhood tumors of bone.

The primary tumors are fortunately few in number and include osteogenic sarcoma, Ewing's sarcoma, lymphosarcoma, and chondrosarcoma. The most common metastatic bone tumors in children include Ewing's sarcoma (a primary osseous tumor that regularly metastasizes to other bones), neuroblastoma, and retinoblastoma. (Wilms' tumor might also be placed in this working diagnosis since it occurs with some frequency in children; but it rarely metastasizes to bone.)

Two of the metastatic tumors, *retinoblastoma* and *neuroblastoma*, should be assigned a very low ranking. Retinoblastoma seems quite unlikely since, on the one hand, the tumor is most uncommon in this group of possibilities and, on the other hand, the physical examination failed to reveal any ocular symptoms. Similarly neuroblastoma almost always effects multiple metastases, and the clinical examination of the patient did not suggest either the presence of a primary tumor of this type or that such a primary tumor had spread. Neither did the laboratory examination of the urine disclose high levels of catecholamines, which are almost always raised in neuroblastoma.

A diagnosis of *lymphosarcoma* seems less probable than one of osteogenic sarcoma or Ewing's sarcoma since a lymphosarcoma is less common than either an osteogenic or a Ewing's sarcoma and, in contrast, does not form bone. Furthermore, its peak incidence occurs at a considerably older age.

Although *osteogenic sarcoma* is more common than *Ewing's sarcoma,* the age distribution of the latter is more skewed toward the younger ages. Osteogenic sarcoma also produces a more extensive erosion of the cortex than does Ewing's sarcoma (not a feature of this case). The concentric layers of laminated subperiosteal new bone (onionskin) observed in the patient may be produced by both tumors but are a more frequent characteristic of Ewing's sarcoma. (Such a pattern of laminated subperiosteal bone is also seen with Garré's osteomyelitis, but this diagnosis is

Table 20-1. Solitary ill-defined radiolucencies

Lesion	Predominant sex	Usual age (years)	Predominant jaw	Predominant region	Additional features	Other radiographic appearances
Chronic osteitis	$M > F$	50-80 and 5-15			Usually associated with root of pulpless tooth Slow course	Cystlike radiolucency Radiopacity
Chronic osteomyelitis	$\frac{M}{F} = \frac{5}{1}$	30-80	Mandible/maxilla = 7/1	Premolar-molar Angle Symphysis	History of debilitating systemic disease and/or fracture Slow course	Radiolucency with radiopaque foci Radiopacity
Peripheral squamous cell carcinomas	$\frac{M}{F} = \frac{2-4}{1}$	40-80 (peak 65)	Mandible/maxilla = 3/1	Mandibular molar	Tobacco, alcohol, poor hygiene Metastasizes—frequently early to regional lymph nodes Rapid growth	Radiolucency with radiopaque foci (sequestra)
Fibrous dysplasia (early stage)*	M ~ F†	10-20 (peak 17)	Maxilla/mandible = 4/3	Rare in anterior maxilla and symphysis	No pain No paresthesia No root resorption Slow expansion	Mottled or smoky Ground-glass

Lesion	Sex	Age	Jaw	Region	Course	Radiographic features
Metastatic tumors to jaws						
Adults	$\frac{F}{M} = \frac{3}{2}$	40-60	Mandible/maxilla = 7/1	Premolar-molar	Signs and symptoms from primary tumor / Unpredictable course	Solitary cystlike radiolucency / Multiple cystlike radiolucencies
Children	M ~ F	0-10	Mandible > maxilla	Premolar-molar	Signs and symptoms from primary tumor / Usually rapid course	Generalized rarefaction / Salt and pepper / Radiopacity / Radiolucency with smooth well-defined borders
Malignant minor salivary gland tumors	$\frac{F}{M} = \frac{2}{1}$	40-70	Mandible ~ maxilla	Posterior hard palate / Retromolar	Metastasizes to regional lymph nodes / Local extension by perineural space / Moderately slow but unpredictable course	
Osteogenic sarcomas	M > F	10-40 (peak 27)	Mandible/maxilla = 2/1	Mandibular body	Metastasizes by vascular route to lungs and other organs / Variable course	Radiolucency with radiopaque foci / Sunburst
Chondrosarcomas	M > F	20-60 (avg. 40)	Maxilla > mandible		Metastasizes late by vascular route to lungs and other organs / Usually slow course	Radiopacity / Asymmetric broadening of periodontal ligament
Mesenchymal type	M > F	30-60 (peak 50s)			Metastasizes early by vascular route to lungs and other organs / Unpredictable course	Onionskin growth of periosteal bone / Codman's triangle / Cumulus cloud formation
Reticulum cell sarcomas	$\frac{M}{F} = \frac{2}{1}$	10-60 (avg. 37)	Rare in maxilla	Molar / Angle / Ramus	Metastasizes to bone or lymph nodes / Moderately slow course	RL and RO
Ewing's sarcomas	$\frac{M}{F} = \frac{2}{1}$	5-24 (peak 14-18)	Rare in maxilla		Metastasizes to lymph nodes, lungs, and other bones / Rapid course	Onionskin growth of periosteal bone / Sunburst
Central squamous cell carcinomas	$\frac{M}{F} = \frac{2}{1}$	30-70 (peak 57)	Mandible/maxilla = 4-2/1	No predilection	Metastasizes to regional lymph nodes / Perhaps slow growth initially, then rapid growth	Cystlike radiolucency

*Pain, paresthesia, and root resorption are common features of all these lesions except fibrous dysplasia, although pain is not characteristically present in early lesions of peripheral squamous cell carcinoma and minor salivary gland tumors.

†~ Approximately equal.

unlikely because there are no signs or symptoms of infection present.)

In view of this correlation of the patient's symptoms with the features of those bone tumors under suspicion, the following working diagnosis seems to provide the best compromise:

1. Ewing's sarcoma
2. Osteogenic sarcoma
3. Lymphosarcoma
4. Metastatic tumor

Although a working diagnosis of malignant tumor may be appropriate for this case, only the microscopic examination of representative excised tissue will identify the specific type of tumor and prove whether the lesion is really malignant.

SPECIFIC REFERENCES

Ciola, B.: Pathologic fractures of the mandible following invasive oral carcinomas, Oral Surg. **46:**725-731, 1978.

Coonar, H.: Primary intraosseous carcinoma of maxilla, Br. Dent. J. **147:**47-48, 1979.

Gallo, W. J., Shapiro, D. N., and Moss, M.: Suppurative candidiasis: review of the literature and report of case, J. Am. Dent. Assoc. **92:**936-939, 1976.

Gardner, D. G., and Mills, D. M.: The widened periodontal ligament of osteosarcoma of the jaws, Oral Surg. **41:**652-656, 1976.

Garrington, G. E., Scofield, H. H., Cornyn, J., and Hooker, S. P.: Osteosarcoma of the jaws, Cancer **20:**377-391, 1967.

Goupil, M. T., Steed, D. L., and Kolodny, S. C.: Hyperbaric oxygen in the adjunctive treatment of chronic osteomyelitis of the mandible: report of case, J. Oral Surg. **36:**138-140, 1978.

Hart, G. B., and Mainous, E. G.: The treatment of radiation necrosis with hyperbaric oxygen, Cancer **37:**2580-2585, 1976.

High, C. L., and Glass, R. T.: Osteosarcoma of the mandible, Oral Surg. **45:**678-684, 1978.

Igo, R. M., Taylor, C. G., Scott, A. S., and Jacoby, J. K.: Coccidioidomycosis involving the mandible: report of case, J. Oral Surg. **36:**72-75, 1978.

Mainous, E. G., Boyne, P. J., and Hart, G. B.: Hyperbaric oxygen treatment of mandibular osteomyelitis: report of three cases, J. Am. Dent. Assoc. **87:**1426-1430, 1973.

Martinelli, C., Melhado, R. M., and Callestini, E. A.: Squamous cell carcinoma in a residual mandibular cyst, Oral Surg. **44:**274-278, 1977.

Martis, C.: Chondrosarcoma of the mandible: report of case, J. Oral Surg. **36:**227-230, 1978.

Musser, L. M., Tulumello, T. N., and Hiatt, W. R.: Actinomycosis of the anterior maxilla, Oral Surg. **44:**21-24, 1977.

Nakajima, T., Yagata, H., Kato, H., and Tokiwa, N.: Surgical treatment of chronic osteomyelitis of the mandible resistant to intraarterial infusion of antibiotics: report of case, J. Oral Surg. **35:**823-827, 1977.

Nolan, R., and Wood, N. K.: Central squamous cell carcinoma of the mandible: report of case, J. Oral Surg. **34:**260-264, 1976.

Rosenquist, J. B., and Beskow, R.: Tuberculosis of the maxilla, J. Oral Surg. **35:**309-310, 1977.

Sanders, B.: Current concepts in the management of osteomyelitis of the mandible, J. Oral Med. **33:**40-43, 1978.

Sato, K., Nukaga, H., and Horikoshi, T.: Chondrosarcoma of the jaws and facial skeleton: a review of the Japanese literature, J. Oral Surg. **35:**892-897, 1977.

Shafer, W. G.: Personal communication, 1980.

Shear, M.: Primary intra-alveolar epidermoid carcinoma of the jaw, J. Pathol. **97:**645-651, 1969.

Sirsat, M. V., Sampat, M. B., and Shrikhande, S. E.: Primary intra-alveolar squamous cell carcinoma of the mandible, Oral Surg. **35:**366-371, 1973.

Weaver, A., Fleming, S. M., and Smith, D. B.: Mouthwash and oral cancer: carcinogenic or coincidence? J. Oral Surg. **37:**250-253, 1979.

Yakata, H., Nakajima, T., Yamada, H., and Tokiwa, N.: Actinomycotic osteomyelitis of the mandible, J. Oral Surg. **36:**720-724, 1978.

GENERAL REFERENCES

Adler, C. I., Sotereanos, G. C., and Valdivieso, J. G.: Metastatic bronchogenic carcinoma to the maxilla: report of case, J. Oral Surg. **31:**543-546, 1973.

Al-Ani, S.: Metastatic tumors to the mouth: report of two cases, J. Oral Surg. **31:**120-122, 1973.

Angelopoulas, A. P., Tilson, H. B., and Stewart, F. W.: Metastatic neuroblastoma of the mandible: review of literature and report of case, J. Oral Surg. **30:**93-106, 1972.

Appenzeller, J., Weitzner, S., and Long, G. W.: Hepatocellular carcinoma metastatic to the mandible: report of case and review of literature, J. Oral Surg. **29:**660-671, 1971.

Batsakis, J., and McBurney, T.: Metastatic neoplasms to the head and neck, Surg. Gynecol. Obstet. **133:**673-677, 1971.

Bhaskar, S. N.: Synopsis of oral pathology, ed. 5, St. Louis, 1977, The C. V. Mosby Co.

Binnie, W. H., De Lathoower, C., Broncheriou, C., and Panders, A. K.: Symposium on maxillofacial bone pathology, Int. J. Oral Surg. **4:**80-92, 1975.

Borghelli, R. F., Barros, R. E., and Zampieri, J.: Ewing sarcoma of the mandible. Report of case, J. Oral Surg. **36:**473-475, 1978.

Browne, R. M.: Metaplasia and degeneration in odontogenic cysts in man, J. Oral Pathol. **1:**145-158, 1972.

Cangiano, R., Stratigos, G. T., and Williams, F. A.: Clinical and radiographic manifestations of fibro-osseous lesions of the jaws: report of five cases, J. Oral Surg. **29:**872-881, 1971.

Carl, W., Schaaf, N. G., Gaeta, J., and Sinks, L. F.: Ewing's sarcoma, J. Oral Surg. **31:**472-478, 1971.

Caron, A. S.: Osteogenic sarcoma of the facial and cranial bones: a review of 43 cases, Am. J. Surg. **122:**719-725, 1971.

Carter, D. G., Anderson, E. E., and Currie, D. P.: Renal cell carcinoma metastatic to the mandible, J. Oral Surg. **35:**992-993, 1977.

Cherrick, H. M., and Demkee, D.: Metastatic carcinoma of the jaws, J. Am. Dent. Assoc. **87:**180-181, 1973.

Cherry, C. Q., and Glass, R. T.: Large-cell carcinoma metastatic to the jaws, Oral Surg. **44:**358-361, 1977.

Ciola, B., and Yesner, R.: Radiographic manifestations of a lung carcinoma with metastases to the anterior maxilla, Oral Surg. **44:**811-816, 1977.

Dahlin, D. C.: Bone tumors, ed. 2, Springfield, Ill., 1973, Charles C Thomas, Publisher.

Draper, B. W., Precious, D. S., and Priddy, R. W.: Follicular thyroid carcinoma metastatic to the mandible. Clinical-pathological conference. Case 29. I, J. Oral Surg. **37:**657-658, 1979.

Draper, B. W., Precious, D. S., and Priddy, R. W.: Follicular thyroid carcinoma metastatic to the mandible. Clinical-pathologic conference. Case 29. II, J. Oral Surg. **37:**736-739, 1979.

Eversole, L. R., Sabes, W. R., and Rovin, S.: Fibrous dysplasia, a nosologic problem in the diagnosis of fibro-osseous lesions of the jaws, J. Oral Pathol. **1:**189-220, 1972.

Forman, G., and Garrett, J.: Ameloblastic sarcoma: report of case, J. Oral Surg. **30:**50-54, 1972.

Gardner, A. F.: The odontogenic cyst as a potential carcinoma, a clinicopathologic appraisal, J. Am. Dent. Assoc. **78:**746-755, 1969.

Garrington, G. E., Scofield, H. H., Cornyn, J., and Hooker, S. P.: Osteosarcoma of the jaws. Analysis of 56 cases, Cancer **20:**377-391, 1967.

Goveia, G., and Bahn, S.: Asymptomatic hepatocellular carcinoma metastatic to the mandible, Oral Surg. **45:**424-430, 1978.

Griboff, S. I., Herrmann, J. B., Smelin, A., and Moss, J.: Hypercalcemia secondary to bone metastases from carcinoma of the breast, J. Clin. Endocrinol. **14:**378-388, 1954.

Hampl, P. F., and Harrigan, W. F.: Squamous cell carcinoma possibly arising from an odontogenic cyst: report of case, J. Oral Surg. **31:**359-362, 1973.

Hartman, G. L., Robertson, G. R., Sugg, W. E., and Hiatt, W. R.: Metastatic carcinoma of the mandibular condyle: report of case, J. Oral Surg. **31:**716-717, 1973.

Henefer, E. P., Bishop, H. C., and Brown, A.: Juvenile fibromatosis with invasion of the mandible: report of two cases, J. Oral Surg. **36:**965-970, 1978.

Higashi, T., Sugimoto, K., Shimura, A., et al.: Technetium 99m bone imaging in the evaluation of cancer of the maxillofacial region, J. Oral Surg. **37:**254-258, 1979.

Lapin, R., Garfinkle, A. V., Catinia, A. F., and Kane, A. A.: Squamous cell carcinoma arising in a dentigerous cyst, J. Oral Surg. **31:**354-358, 1973.

Lewis, J. S., and Castro, E. B.: Cancer of the nasal cavity and paranasal sinuses, J. Laryngol. Otol. **86:**255-262, 1972.

Lichtenstein, L.: Bone tumors, ed. 5, St. Louis, 1977, The C. V. Mosby Co.

Mainous, E. G., Boyne, P. J., and Hart, G. B.: Hyperbaric oxygen treatment of mandibular osteomyelitis: report of three cases, J. Am. Dent. Assoc. **87:**1426-1430, 1973.

Mainous, E. G., Boyne, P. J., Hart, G. B., and Terry, B. C.: Restoration of resected mandible by grafting with combination of mandible homograft and autogenous iliac marrow, and postoperative treatment with hyperbaric oxygenation, Oral Surg. **35:**13-20, 1973.

Martis, C.: Chondrosarcoma of the mandible: report of case, Oral Surg. **36:**227-230, 1978.

Martis, C., Karakasis, D., and Lazaridia, N.: Metastatic adenocarcinoma to the mandible: report of case, J. Am. Dent. Assoc. **94:**1163-1168, 1977.

Moss, M., and Shapiro, D. N.: Mandibular metastasis of breast cancer, J. Am. Dent. Assoc. **78:**756-757, 1969.

Newman, G. W., and Burdick, F. A.: Rare cause of osteomyelitis of the mandible: report of case, J. Am. Dent. Assoc. **87:**189-191, 1973.

Peede, L. F., and Epker, B. N.: Aggressive juvenile fibromatosis involving the mandible: surgical excision with immediate reconstruction, Oral Surg. **43:**651-657, 1977.

Perriman, A. O., and Figures, K. H.: Metastatic retinoblastoma of the mandible, Oral Surg. **45:**741-748, 1978.

Rapoport, A., Sobrinho, J. D., Carvalho, J. M., et al.: Ewing's sarcoma of the mandible, Oral Surg. **44:**89-94, 1977.

Richardson, J. F., Fine, M. A., and Goldman, H. M.: Fibrosarcoma of the mandible: a clinico-pathologic controversy: report of case, J. Oral Surg. **30:**664-667, 1972.

Roistacher, S. L.: Numbness—a significant finding, Oral Surg. **36:**22-27, 1973.

Samit, A., Falk, H. J., Ohanian, M., et al.: Malignant melanoma metastatic to the mandible, J. Oral Surg. **36:**816-821, 1978.

Saud, A.: Metastatic tumors of the mouth: report of two cases, J. Oral Surg. **31:**120-122, 1973.

Saw, D.: Fibrosarcoma of maxilla, Oral Surg. **47:**164-168, 1979.

Schultz, W., and Whitten, J. B.: Mucoepidermoid carcinoma in the mandible: report of case, J. Oral Surg. **27:**337-340, 1969.

Seldin, E. B.: New hope for patients with Ewing sarcoma (letter), J. Oral Surg. **36:**583, 1978.

Shafer, W. G., Hine, M. K., and Levy, B. M.: A textbook of oral pathology, ed. 3, Philadelphia, 1974, W. B. Saunders Co.

Silbermann, M., Maloney, P. L., and Doku, C. H.: Spontaneous healing of a large osteomyelitic defect in the mandible: report of case, J. Oral Surg. **30:**821-823, 1972.

Skiba, T. J., Williams, R. A., Dixon, R. A., and Mercuri, L. G.: Eosinophilic granuloma. Clinical-pathological conference. Case 26. I, J. Oral Surg. **36:**887-889, 1978.

Skiba, T. J., Williams, R. A., Dixon, R. A., and Mercuri, L. G.: Eosinophilic granuloma. Clinical-pathological conference. Case 26. II, J. Oral Surg. **36:**960-962, 1978.

Uhler, I. V., Fahs, G. R., and Dolan, L. A.: Metastasis of cervical carcinoma to the mandible: report of case, J. Am. Dent. Assoc. **85:**363-364, 1972.

Upton, L. G., Hayward, J. R., and Kerr, D. A.: Neurofibrosarcoma of the mandible, J. Oral Surg. **35:**504-506, 1977.

Van der Kwast, W. A. M., and van der Waal, I.: Jaw metastases, Oral Surg. **37:**850-857, 1974.

Waldron, C. A., and Giansanti, J. S.: Benign fibro-osseous lesions of the jaws: a clinical-radiologic-histologic review of sixty-five cases. I. Fibrous dysplasia of the jaws, Oral Surg. **35:**190-201, 1973.

Walker, R. D., and Schenck, K. L.: Infarct of the mandible in sickle cell anemia: report of case, J. Am. Dent. Assoc. **87:**661-664, 1973.

Wilcox, J. W., Dukart, R. C., Kolodny, S. C., and Jacoby, J. K.: Osteogenic sarcoma of the mandible: review of the literature and report of case, J. Oral Surg. **31:**49-52, 1973.

Wright, J. A., and Kuehn, P. G.: Fibrosarcoma of the mandible, Oral Surg. **36:**16-20, 1973.

Yacabucci, J. E. Mainous, E. G., and Kramer, H. S.: Hepatocellular carcinoma diagnosed following metastasis to the mandible, Oral Surg. **33:**880-893, 1972.

21

Multiple separate well-defined radiolucencies

Norman K. Wood
Paul W. Goaz

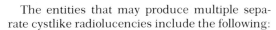

The entities that may produce multiple separate cystlike radiolucencies include the following:

Anatomic variations
Multiple cysts or granulomas
Basal cell nevus syndrome
Multiple myeloma
Metastatic carcinoma
Histiocytosis X
Rarities
    Ameloblastomas
    Cherubism
    Craniofacial dysostosis
    Gaucher's disease
    Hunter's or Hurler's syndrome
    Hyperparathyroidism with multiple distinct osteolytic lesions
    Leukemia
    Lymphosarcoma
    Multiple dental cysts in arachnodactyly
    Neimann-Pick disease
    Sclerosing cemental masses (early stage)
    Oxycephaly
    Pseudotumors of hemophilia
    Scleroderma
    Traumatic bone cysts

The multiple separate cystlike radiolucencies must be distinguished from the multilocular type of radiolucency (which is not made up of numerous distinctly separate lesions but appears to be a single lesion formed of contiguous and coalescent cystic spaces).

ANATOMIC VARIATIONS

As is true of other radiolucent anatomic structures, those that cause multiple separate cystlike radiolucencies may be mistaken for pathoses.

Marrow spaces are an anatomic structure discussed in Chapter 18 that may produce the radio-graphic image of a cystlike radiolucency. Occasionally several such separate marrow spaces will be observed on radiographs of a patient's jaw (Fig. 21-1), and the clinician is then faced with the dilemma of deciding whether they are marrow spaces or one of the pathologic conditions listed in the left-hand column of this page.

If previous radiographs of the jaws are available, the clinician can compare the areas in question to determine whether there has been a change in the pattern. If he finds that the radiolucencies were apparent on earlier radiographs, are of the same relative proportions and appearance, and are obviously only casually associated with the crown or root of a tooth (and in the absence of other signs and symptoms), then a reasonable assumption would be that they are multiple separate cystlike marrow spaces. If a change in the trabecular pattern of an area in a jaw is evident on a sequence of radiographs, the clinician would do well to determine whether this change is related to a change in function. It is unusual to find such multiple cystlike marrow spaces in the maxilla. Thus, if suspicious images are found there and also in the mandible, they very likely represent a pathologic condition.

Multiple postextraction sockets will sometimes appear as separate cystlike radiolucencies and be misdiagnosed as pathoses by the unwary examiner. Although such images are to be expected on radiographs of a jaw after recent tooth extractions, they may persist for years. Radiolucencies representing multiple extraction wounds would, of course, be found in the alveolar portion of the jawbone in edentulous regions (Fig. 21-2). Man-

Fig. 21-1. Multiple marrow spaces at the apices of the molar and premolar.

Fig. 21-2. Multiple sockets.

dibular sockets are usually much more prominent and better defined than are their maxillary counterparts because the finer architecture of the bone in the upper jaw is less likely to silhouette the sockets so clearly.

If the extractions are recent, the clinician will be able to identify them readily from the patient's history and by the telltale condition of the alveolar ridge (which will clinically show the depressions on the surface mucosa each surrounded by an elevation over the crest of the bony socket walls). If, however, the extractions were done months or years before, only a persistent stable pattern in the alveolar bone apparent on periodic radiographs will indicate their identity.

MULTIPLE CYSTS OR GRANULOMAS (CONVENTIONAL TYPE*)

From time to time, multiple conventional cysts or granulomas will occur in otherwise normal patients who do not have any recognizable syndrome. Reports indicate that these cysts may be follicular cysts, radicular cysts, primordial cysts, and/or keratocysts (Fig. 21-3). There seems to be a familial tendency for multiple odontogenic cysts.

Instances of multiple periapical granulomas have been noted, but they are usually identifiable as sequelae of pulpitis since they are associated with untreated carious teeth (Fig. 21-3). Solitary examples of these individual entities are discussed in Chapters 16, 17, and 18, so they will not be discussed further in this chapter.

---

*In the context of this discussion, the term "conventional" refers to those multiple jaw cysts whose initiation can apparently be attributed to strictly local factors.

DIFFERENTIAL DIAGNOSIS

Uncomplicated multiple cysts must be distinguished from those of the less frequently occurring *basal cell nevus syndrome*. This differentiation is developed in the differential diagnosis section under the basal cell nevus syndrome (p. 455).

MANAGEMENT

The treatment of cysts is discussed in detail in Chapters 16 and 17.

BASAL CELL NEVUS SYNDROME

The basal cell nevus syndrome is a hereditary complex of abnormalities transmitted as an autosomal dominant trait with a poor degree of penetrance and variable expressivity. The feature that prompts its inclusion in this chapter is the multiple jaw cysts—which may be of the follicular, primordial, or radicular variety. The majority of these cysts prove to be keratocysts on microscopic examination.

FEATURES

Characteristic features of the basal cell nevus syndrome embrace varying manifestations of cutaneous and skeletal abnormalities and frequently ectopic calcifications.

Fig. 21-3. Multiple conventional granulomas or cysts (no syndrome). **A,** Multiple periapical granulomas. **B,** Bilateral cysts. **C,** Orthopanograph showing multiple cysts. *1,* Follicular; *2* and *4,* radicular; *3,* residual. (**B** courtesy D. Skuble, D.D.S., Hinsdale, Ill. **C** courtesy N. Barakat, Beirut, Lebanon.)

The syndrome occurs with equal frequency in males and females (autosomal dominant trait) and usually becomes apparent between 5 and 30 years of age. The most notable and characteristic cutaneous manifestation is the nevoid basal cell carcinomas; these are present as flesh-colored or brownish papules, predominantly on the skin of the face, neck, and trunk but occurring anywhere on the skin surface (Fig. 21-4). The papules frequently appear early in childhood, but additional lesions may occur during the second and third decades.

The majority of these papular basal cell carcinomas are less aggressive than the usual solitary basal cell carcinoma, which characteristically produces a rodent ulcer.

Fig. 21-4. Basal cell nevus syndrome. **A,** Multiple nevoid basal cell carcinomas on the face. **B,** Panograph showing four dentigerous cysts associated with impacted third molars. **C,** Anteroposterior radiograph of the chest depicting a bifid rib. (**A** courtesy D. Bonomo, D.D.S., Flossmoor, Ill. **B** and **C** courtesy J. Ireland, D.D.S., and J. Dolce, D.D.S., Mundelein, Ill.)

In some cases pits and/or dyskeratosis is present on the palmar and plantar surfaces.

Skeletal abnormalities may include multiple cysts of the jaws, bifid ribs, synostosis of the ribs, kyphoscoliosis, vertebral fusion, polydactyly, frontal and temporoparietal bossing, a mild ocular hypertelorism, and a mild prognathism (Fig. 21-4).

The ectopic calcifications observed most frequently occur in the falx cerebri, the skin, and the jaw cysts. The jaw cysts generally develop at an earlier age than do the basal cell carcinomas. Thus the dental clinician may be the first to encounter and identify this syndrome when he discovers the multiple cystlike radiolucencies on radiographs of the jaws.

The jaw cysts, which vary in size from a millimeter or less to several centimeters in diameter, occur more frequently in the mandible and in the premolar-molar region. They may be of follicular, primordial, or radicular types, Histologically all types and variations of epithelial linings may occur, but there is a preponderance of the keratocystic type. Frequently microcysts develop in the cyst wall, and a peculiar budding of the basal epithelial cells into the deeper layers of the wall may be a feature.

The Elsworth-Howard test is utilized to differentiate the basal cell nevus syndrome from other disease states that may manifest some of the same clinical characteristics. It evaluates kidney tubular function after parathyroid hormone injection. An absence of significant phosphorus diuresis after an intravenous injection of the hormone is observed in this syndrome.

DIFFERENTIAL DIAGNOSIS

When most of the features associated with the basal cell nevus syndrome are manifested and apparent, the syndrome does not present a problem in differential diagnosis. Sometimes only two or three features are present, however; and the clinician must then be cognizant of the fact that early in childhood only the jaw cysts may be apparent—which can cause a diagnostic problem.

In developing a working diagnosis, the clinician should furthermore remember that *multiple conventional jaw cysts* occur more frequently than do those that are a feature of the basal cell nevus syndrome. Consequently, if no other expressions of the disease are present, he may have to proceed with a working diagnosis of multiple conventional jaw cysts while maintaining close posttreatment surveillance to ensure that the additional characteristics of the syndrome do not develop at a later date.

Such an occurrence would, of course, be convincing evidence that the case was indeed a basal cell nevus syndrome. The examiner must therefore make the distinction between multiple conventional jaw cysts and the jaw cysts of the basal cell nevus syndrome because the management of the latter condition is much more complex and difficult.

Usually multiple conventional jaw cysts are well defined and relatively large so they cannot be confused with *multiple cystlike marrow spaces* or *multiple postextraction wounds* or *scars*, which are more uniform in shape and arrangement. Should the suspicious lesion be associated with an expansion of the buccal plates, however, the diagnosis of either marrow spaces or postextraction sockets would be ruled out.

The multiple radiolucent lesions of *multiple myeloma, metastatic carcinoma,* and *histiocytosis X* can generally be distinguished from multiple conventional jaw cysts and cysts of the basal cell nevus syndrome. The two former lesions are usually smaller and more numerous, and they affect other bones of the skull and skeleton in addition to the jaws. Lesions of histiocytosis X usually have ragged vague margins and so are not cystlike.

Multiple radiolucent lesions of *cherubism* may be scattered throughout the jaws of a patient in the first or second decade of life. Contrary to multiple cysts of the syndrome, however, these radiolucencies frequently have a multilocular appearance. Although they may be unilocular, they will show a more elliptic expansion of the jaws without well-circumscribed or hyperostotic borders.

The abnormal response of a patient with the basal cell nevus syndrome to injections of parathyroid hormone—plus the ectopic calcifications (some of which involve the jaw cysts) and the other skeletal abnormalities—may be confused with such entities as *idiopathic hypoparathyroidism, pseudohypoparathyroidism, pseudo-pseudo-hypoparathyroidism, basal ganglion calcification syndrome, Turner's syndrome,* and *Gardner's syndrome.* Witkop (1968) has reviewed the differential diagnosis of these entities in considerable detail.

MANAGEMENT

It is important for the clinician to identify and differentiate the basal cell nevus syndrome from multiple conventional jaw cysts since the management of the former is so much more difficult and complex than that of the latter.

The jaw cysts associated with the basal cell nevus syndrome show a much higher recurrence rate (36.4% in Brannon's series [1976]), possibly because of the microcyst and/or budding phenomena in the keratocysts. Thus a more vigorous enucleation and more vigilant postoperative surveillance are in order.

The other systemic manifestations and complications (i.e., the basal cell carcinomas, the spinal problems, the increased risk of medulloblastoma in the probands and siblings) require careful evaluation and management by a physician.

MULTIPLE MYELOMA

Multiple myeloma is the most common primary malignant tumor of bone and usually involves a number of bones in the same individual. Although in advanced cases it may appear radiographically as a generalized rarefaction of the skeleton or as numerous radiolucencies with ill-defined ragged borders, it most frequently occurs as small circular multiple but separate well-defined (punched-out) radiolucencies; and this latter appearance explains the inclusion of the lesion in the present chapter.

FEATURES

Multiple myeloma is a malignant plasma cell tumor that is thought to originate from reticulum cells within the bone marrow. It appears with equal frequency in men and women, most commonly affecting the age group between 40 and 70 years. The bones usually involved are the skull, clavicle, vertebrae, ribs, pelvis, femurs, and jaws (all of which play a prominent role in hematopoiesis); however, any part of the skeleton may be involved. In approximately 30% of the cases, the jawbones are affected—especially the premolar region and coronoid process.

The patient may complain of pain in the involved bones, which is aggravated by exercise and relieved by rest. When the mandible is involved, paresthesia or numbness of the lip may be a complaint as may looseness and migration of the teeth. Sometimes the myeloma will erode through the buccal plates and produce a rubbery expansion of the jaws. At first the expansion is covered with normal mucosa; but chronic trauma produces an inflamed and eventually an ulcerated necrotic surface.

Sedimentation rates in multiple myeloma are markedly elevated, and pancytopenias are present. The increased serum gamma globulin produces a reverse in the albumin/globulin ratio as well as an elevation in the total plasma protein. Plasma cells are usually found in peripheral blood smears.

As in most lytic bone diseases that apparently demonstrate alternate active and quiescent phases, the serum calcium values in multiple myeloma may be normal. Hypercalcemia, however, is detected in 20% to 40% of the cases; but since the bone resorption is generally not rapid enough to cause a rise in plasma calcium if the filtration rate is normal, the hypercalcemia is believed to result from an increase in the bone resorption combined with a reduction in the glomerular filtration rate.

Although the plasma phosphate in multiple myeloma is usually normal, a hypophosphatemia is sometimes observed. The serum chemistry levels may resemble those seen in primary hyperparathyroidism, but the serum alkaline phosphatase level is usually normal. In approximately half the cases Bence Jones proteins* are produced by the abnormal plasma cells making up the multiple tumors.

Complications of multiple myeloma include pathologic fracture, secondary anemia, increased susceptibility to infection, a bleeding tendency, kidney failure, and amyloidosis. Such symptoms as nausea, lethargy caused by the anemia, and vomiting caused in part by the increased serum calcium level are also observed.

The pathologic fractures, which are more frequent than in metastatic carcinoma, result from the myeloma tissue's advancing on adjacent bone, thinning the cortex, and reducing the trabeculae in thickness and number (Moseley, 1963, p. 137).

---

*This protein precipitates when the patient's urine is heated to 50 or 60 C, but the precipitate disappears on boiling and then reappears when the urine is cooled to 60 or 70 C.

The secondary anemia, increased susceptibility to infection, and bleeding tendency result from the overgrowth of myeloma cells in the bone marrow; these cells replace the normal centers of erythrocyte, granulocyte, and megakarocyte formation.

The kidney failure, which (after pneumonia) is the second most common cause of death in multiple myeloma, is due in part to the hypercalcemia, amyloidosis, and blockage of the renal tubules with casts of Bence Jones protein (Nordin, 1973, p. 17).

As mentioned previously, multiple myeloma may occur with three different radiographic appearances.* The multiple and scattered small round well-defined radiolucencies without sclerotic borders, involving several bones of the skeleton, will be stressed in this chapter (Fig. 21-5).

---

*Although certain features and locations of radiographic lesions are strongly suggestive of multiple myeloma, none of the bone changes that might be observed in this disease are pathognomonic. At one time, punched-out areas of bone destruction were considered the most common appearance of multiple myeloma. Now there is general agreement that the usual tendency is for the skeleton to be involved by a combination of types of lesions. Also the degree and extent of bone involvement are directly related to the duration of the disease. The involvement of the skull, coupled with other skeletal lesions, was once considered unequivocal evidence of multiple myeloma; but now authorities recognize that the skull is not always involved (Moseley, 1963, p. 137).

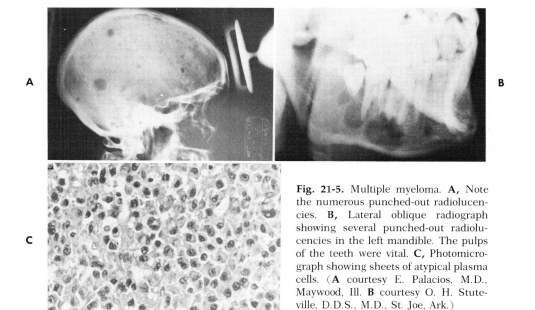

Fig. 21-5. Multiple myeloma. **A,** Note the numerous punched-out radiolucencies. **B,** Lateral oblique radiograph showing several punched-out radiolucencies in the left mandible. The pulps of the teeth were vital. **C,** Photomicrograph showing sheets of atypical plasma cells. (**A** courtesy E. Palacios, M.D., Maywood, Ill. **B** courtesy O. H. Stuteville, D.D.S., M.D., St. Joe, Ark.)

The definitive diagnosis is made from a smear of bone marrow aspirate, from a biopsy of an affected region of bone, or from plasma electrophoresis.

The tumors vary greatly in degree of malignancy. They are composed of solid sheets of plasma cells with few or no connective tissue septa (Fig. 21-5). Because of the frequent accumulation of plasma cells in chronic inflammatory proliferations in the oral cavity, differentiation of such lesions from those of solitary myeloma sometimes presents a problem for the pathologist. Solitary myeloma lesions of bone are invariably followed by multiple myeloma although in some cases it may take as long as 20 years for the disseminated disease to become manifest.

DIFFERENTIAL DIAGNOSIS

The differential diagnosis of multiple myeloma and similar-appearing lesions is discussed under the differential diagnosis section of histiocytosis X (p. 461).

MANAGEMENT

Multiple myeloma is a rapidly fatal disease. About half the patients die within 2 years of the onset of symptoms. The 5-year survival rate is approximately 10%. The primary disease is treated usually by systemic administration of cytotoxic drugs (e.g., melphalan, urethan, cyclophosphamide) as well as by steroids and radiation. Palliative measures are used to control the accompanying pain, bleeding, anemia, and kidney problem.

Inorganic fluoride and phosphate supplements have been utilized in attempts to relieve the bone pain to reverse some of the abnormal serum electrolyte patterns. Early reports on fluoride therapy were promising; but studies by Harley and coworkers (1972) and other investigators revealed that fluoride therapy, while effecting some relief of pain, is not as beneficial for resolving bone lesions as it was first considered and may even be harmful.

The immune and other defense mechanisms are seriously impaired, so the patient is highly susceptible to infection. Hence any surgical procedure that cannot be postponed should be accompanied by an antibiotic effective against both gram-positive and gram-negative microorganisms.

METASTATIC CARCINOMA

The spread from a primary carcinoma may result in the development of multiple metastases in the skeleton. When this happens, the metastatic bone lesions may assume a variety of radiographic appearances, one of which is multiple small rounded and well-defined (punched-out) radiolucencies (Fig. 21-6). Consequently metastatic carcinoma is included in the present chapter.

FEATURES

Metastatic carcinoma is discussed in Chapter 20, so its characteristics will not be detailed further here except to indicate that a patient with such a disseminated malignant disease is obviously very ill and may manifest some of the symptoms and problems described for multiple myeloma: fatigue, pancytopenia, bleeding, and abnormal serum calcium, phosphorus, and alkaline phosphatase levels.

DIFFERENTIAL DIAGNOSIS

The differential diagnosis for metastatic carcinoma and similar-appearing lesions is discussed under the differential diagnosis section for histiocytosis X (p. 461).

MANAGEMENT

The major considerations determining the management of patients with metastatic carcinoma are enumerated in Chapter 20. Since a patient with multiple metastases would be considered terminal, palliative procedures are usually all that can rationally be prescribed.

HISTIOCYTOSIS X

Histiocytosis X is a group of reticuloendothelial diseases that are not well understood. Although there is not complete agreement, many authors believe that the three entities making up this group (Letterer-Siwe disease, Hand-Schüller-Christian disease, and eosinophilic granuloma) represent interrelated manifestations of the same basic pathologic process. Histiocytosis X is classified as a nonlipid reticuloendotheliosis and differs from the lipid reticuloendothelioses (e.g., Gaucher's disease, Niemann-Pick disease), which are the result of inborn errors of metabolism and in which the reticulum cells produce and store abnormal lipids. Histiocytosis X affects the reticuloendothelial organs such as the spleen, liver, lymph nodes, and bone marrow and may infiltrate mucosa, skin, or viscera.

Two of the entities making up histiocytosis X, Letterer-Siwe disease and Hand-Schüller-Christian disease, may produce multiple lytic lesions in bone that affect several bones simultaneously; and the lesion may appear as multiple small regular well-defined radiolucencies. Thus these two

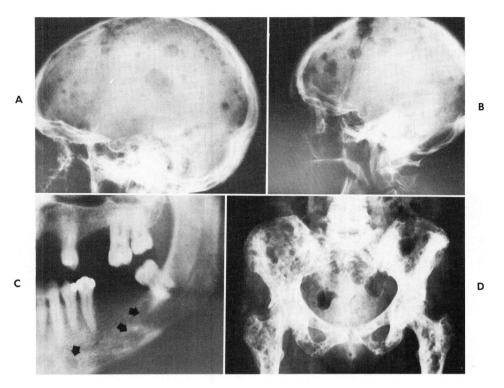

Fig. 21-6. A and **B,** Two patients with multiple metastatic carcinomas. **C,** Three distinct mandibular lesions (arrows) of metastatic bronchogenic carcinoma in a 58-year-old man. **D,** Another example of metastatic carcinoma. The multiple punched-out lesions in the pelvic bones and femurs are from a renal carcinoma. (**A** and **B** courtesy E. Palacios, M.D., Maywood, Ill.)

entities are included in the present chapter. Eosinophilic granuloma usually occurs as a solitary radiolucency; however, a significant number of cases have been reported with bilateral involvement (Ragab and Rake, 1975).

FEATURES

Letterer-Siwe disease. Letterer-Siwe disease is the acute widely disseminated form of histiocytosis X; it is generally fatal and occurs almost exclusively in infants under 1 year of age. Numerous enlargements of organs and other swellings caused by accumulations of histiocytes are seen. The patient appears cachectic and frequently has petechiae and necrotic ulcers on the skin and mucous membranes. When there are extensive bony lesions, a severe pancytopenia is produced because of the masses of proliferating histiocytes that displace the hematopoietic marrow. When the skeleton is involved, lesions are usually present in several bones and may appear as multiple small rounded radiolucencies with well-defined borders (Fig. 21-7). If teeth are present in the

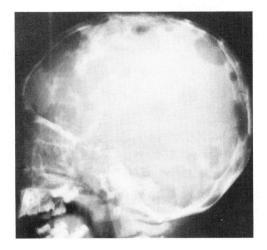

Fig. 21-7. Letterer-Siwe disease in a 15-month-old child. (Courtesy E. Palacios, M.D., Maywood, Ill.)

affected region, they are frequently mobile and there is associated gingival bleeding.

Hand-Schüller-Christian disease. In its classic form Hand-Schüller-Christian disease affects children and young adults with three principal manifestations:

1. Bony lesions
2. Exophthalmos
3. Diabetes insipidus

It represents a chronic disseminated form of histiocytosis X and carries a much more favorable prognosis than does the Letterer-Siwe variety. The triad of symptoms listed above are not always present in the same patient, however, nor does the presence of additional manifestations rule out the disease. The nature of the symptoms depends on the locations of the histiocytic proliferations.

Frequently the lymph nodes, spleen, and liver will be enlarged and there may be petechial and/or papular eruptions on the skin and oral mucosa. Ulcerations in the mouth with necrotic lesions and edematous gingivae as well as loosened teeth

Fig. 21-8. Hand-Schüller-Christian disease. **A,** Note the multiple punched-out radiolucencies. **B,** Mandibular lesion in the same patient. **C,** Ramus of a 14-year-old boy with Hand-Schüller-Christian disease. Note the multiple punched-out radiolucencies. **D,** Multiple radiolucent jaw lesions in a patient with histiocytosis X. **E,** Several punched-out radiolucencies in another patient with histiocytosis X. (**A, B,** and **E** courtesy E. Palacios, M.D., Maywood, Ill. **D** courtesy N. Barakat, D.D.S., Beirut, Lebanon.)

are sometimes seen. Although the most common complaint is a chronic otitis media, loose teeth will frequently be one of the initial complaints. Patients with the classical triad of symptoms will complain of polydipsia and polyuria due to the diabetes insipidus. When there is disseminated bony involvement, a pancytopenia will likely be present. The bony lesions may appear ragged and patchy and may tend to coalesce, giving a geographic appearance on radiographs of the skull (Fig. 21-8, *A* and *B*); but the multiple punched-out lesions are also fairly frequent on radiographs of the jaws (Figs. 21-8 and 21-9).

The histologic appearances are basically similar in Letterer-Siwe disease and Hand-Schüller-Christian disease. Sheets of histiocytes make up the bulk of the enlargements. Scattered accumulations of eosinophils may be seen around areas of necrosis. The histiocytes in Letterer-Siwe disease usually appear more atypical.

DIFFERENTIAL DIAGNOSIS

When developing the differential diagnosis for the multiple separate well-defined radiolucencies of histiocytosis X, the clinician should divide the pathoses into two groups: large cystlike lesions of the jaws and multiple smaller punched-out radiolucencies that may occur in the jaws and in several other bones simultaneously.

The large cystlike lesions are usually characterized by two or more radiolucent areas in the jaws without involvement of other bones. Post-extraction sockets, multiple conventional cysts or granulomas, the basal cell nevus syndrome, and cherubism are in this group.

The multiple smaller lesions occurring simultaneously in other bones of the skeleton may be confused with marrow spaces, multiple myeloma, multiple metastatic lesions, and histiocytosis X.

Since the differential diagnosis for the first group is discussed earlier in this chapter (p. 455), only the differentiation for the second group will be described here.

Children. When multiple punched-out bony lesions are found in children, *histiocytosis X* or *metastatic carcinoma* is the most likely diagnosis. Both diseases would be expected to cause a cachectic condition with many similar systemic manifestations; but the higher incidence of the former in children should lead the watchful clinician to suspect histiocytosis X, as should likewise an inconclusive biopsy report. A history of primary tumor, however, such as medulloblastoma or Wilms' tumor (which usually occur in children), should promote metastatic carcinoma to a higher ranking in the list of possible entities.

Adults. Multiple punched-out lesions in several bones of the skeleton in adults should prompt

Fig. 21-9. Adult patient with multiple jaw lesions of histiocytosis X. (Courtesy W. Heaton, D.D.S., Chicago.)

the clinician to rank *multiple myeloma* or *metastatic carcinoma* high in the working diagnosis. Many of the signs and symptoms of these two entities are similar, however; and thus the clinical manifestations are not often beneficial in helping to differentiate between multiple myeloma and metastatic carcinoma. The comparative incidence, however, should lead to the assigning of a higher rank to multiple myeloma than to multiple metastatic carcinoma. Furthermore, if the albumin/globulin ratio is reversed and Bence Jones proteins are present in the urine, this is almost conclusive proof that the disease in question is multiple myeloma; but, in the absence of definitive serum characteristics, a history of treatment for an earlier primary tumor would improve the possibility that the disease is a metastatic tumor. The final decision will depend on the microscopic examination of excised tissue or aspirated sample.

Suspicious asymptomatic multiple and usually relatively small radiolucencies in the jaw of an apparently healthy adult patient in whom no abnormalities have been disclosed by a general systemic and/or radiographic examination most likely represent multiple distinct *marrow spaces*.

MANAGEMENT

Letterer-Siwe disease is the more serious variant of histiocytosis X but is no longer considered invariably fatal; for with good clinical management some infants and children can live for years in a more chronic phase.

Hand-Schüller-Christian disease, the chronic form of histiocytosis X, carries a better prognosis.

There may be a potential for one form of the

Fig. 21-10. Ameloblastoma showing multiple punched-out radiolucencies in the right ramus. (Courtesy O. H. Stuteville, D.D.S., M.D., St. Joe, Ark.)

Fig. 21-11. Multiple brown giant cell lesions in the maxilla and mandible in a patient with primary hyperparathyroidism exacerbated by pregnancy. Note also generalized loss of lamina dura and root resorption of lower left first molar tooth. Radiograph has been printed lighter to show detail in rarefied jawbone. (From Pellegrino, S. V.: J. Oral Surg. **37:**915-917, 1977. Copyright by the American Dental Association. Reprinted by permission.)

disease to be transformed into the other, however, and carry with it the coincident prognosis. Radiation frequently proves helpful and often palliative. Corrective therapy is necessary to regulate the altered physiology.

RARITIES

In unusual cases multiple separate cystlike radiolucencies may prove to be ameloblastomas (Fig. 21-10).

Following is a list of the entities that rarely produce multiple separate well-defined radiolucencies:

Ameloblastomas
Cherubism
Craniofacial dysostosis
Gaucher's disease
Hunter's or Hurler's syndrome
Hyperparathyroidism with multiple distinct osteolytic lesions (Fig. 21-11)
Leukemia
Lymphosarcoma
Multiple dental cysts in arachnodactyly
Neimann-Pick disease
Nodular cemental masses (early stage; Fig. 21-12)
Oxycephaly
Pseudotumors of hemophilia
Scleroderma
Traumatic bone cysts

The lipid reticuloendothelioses (e.g., Niemann-Pick disease, Gaucher's disease) may produce bony lesions that are multiple, well defined, and somewhat round; and there may be a generalized rarefaction.

Cherubism frequently produces multiple radiolucent lesions of the jawbones, but the pattern is usually multilocular. In some instances, however, the pattern is unilocular and the outlines of the radiolucencies may be well defined or poorly defined.

Sometimes multiple well-defined osteolytic lesions (brown giant cell lesions) will be seen in hyperparathyroidism (Fig. 21-11), although generalized rarefaction of the skeleton is more commonly produced (Fig. 22-1).

Multiple cystic areas are also seen in the jaws of patients with Hunter's or Hurler's syndrome.

Leukemias, especially the acute varieties, may be seen with multiple punched-out radiolucent lesions in the skull and other bones, but seldom are the jawbones thus affected.

Lymphosarcoma rarely also may give the same appearance.

Multiple dental cysts have been reported in arachnodactyly.

Radiographs of the skull in craniofacial dysostosis or oxycephaly often reveal multiple radiolucencies (Fig. 21-13); but such radiolucencies are not seen in radiographs of the jaws.

Fig. 21-12. Multiple radiolucent jaw lesions in a 26-year-old woman with sclerosing cemental masses. Some of the lesions are completely radiolucent while some are in the more radiopaque stage.

Fig. 21-13. Note the cranial convolutions in this patient who experienced early closure of the sutures of the skull. (Courtesy A. C. W. Hutchinson collection, Northwestern University Dental School Library, Chicago.)

SPECIFIC REFERENCES

Brannon, R. B.: The odontogenic keratocyst, a clinicopathologic study of 312 cases. I. Clinical features, Oral Surg. **42:** 54-72, 1976.

Harley, J. B., Schilling, A., and Glidewell, O.: Ineffectiveness of fluoride therapy in multiple myeloma, N. Engl. J. Med. **286:**1283-1288, 1972.

Moseley, J. E.: Bone changes in hematologic disorders, New York, 1963, Grune & Stratton.

Nordin, B. E. C.: Metabolic bone and stone disease, Baltimore, 1973, The Williams & Wilkins Co.

Ragab, R. R., and Rake, O.: Eosinophilic granuloma with bilateral involvement of both jaws, Int. J. Oral Surg. **4:**73-79, 1975.

Witkop, C. J.: Gardner's syndrome and other osteognathodermal disorders with defects in parathyroid functions, J. Oral Surg. **26:**639-642, 1968.

GENERAL REFERENCES

Bhaskar, S. N.: Synopsis of oral pathology, ed. 5, St. Louis, 1977, The C. V. Mosby Co.

Carbone, P. P., Zipkin, I., Sokoloff, L., et al.: Fluoride effect on bone in plasma cell myeloma, Arch. Intern. Med. **121:** 130-140, 1968.

Dahlin, D. C.: Bone tumors, ed. 2, Springfield, Ill., 1973, Charles C Thomas, Publisher.

Ellis, D. J., Akin, R. K., and Bernhard, R.: Nevoid basal cell carcinoma syndrome: report of case, J. Oral Surg. **30:**851-856, 1972.

Giansanti, J. S., and Baker, G. O.: Nevoid basal cell carcinoma syndrome in Negroes: report of five cases, J. Oral Surg. **32:** 138-144, 1974.

Goldsmith, R. S., Bartos, H., Halley, S. B., et al.: Phosphate supplementation as adjunction in therapy of multiple myeloma, Arch. Intern. Med. **122:**128-133, 1968.

Gorlin, R. J., and Goldman, H. M.: Thoma's oral pathology, ed. 6, St. Louis, 1970, The C. V. Mosby Co.

Halpern, K. L., and Calhoun, N. R.: Pathological fracture of mandibular condyloid process associated with multiple myeloma: report of case, J. Oral Surg. **36:**560-561, 1978.

Jagger, R. G., Helkimo, M., and Carlsson, G. E.: Multiple myeloma involving the temporomandibular joint: report of case, J. Oral Surg. **36:**557-559, 1978.

Koutnik, A. W., Kolodny, S. C., Hooker, S. P., and Roche, W. C.: Multiple nevoid basal cell epithelioma, cysts of the jaws, and bifid rib syndrome: report of case, J. Oral Surg. **33:**686-689, 1975.

Laurian, N., Zoahar, Y., and Kende, L.: Solitary myeloma with multiple mandibular lesions: report of case, J. Oral Surg. **30:** 841-844, 1972.

Lichtenstein, L.: Bone tumors, ed. 5, St. Louis, 1977, The C. V. Mosby Co.

Markus, A. F.: Bilateral hemorrhagic bone cysts of the mandible: a case report, Br. J. Oral Surg. **16:**270-273, 1979.

Maw, R. B., and McKean, T. W.: Hand-Schüller-Christian disease: report of case, J. Am. Dent. Assoc. **85:**1353-1357, 1972.

Miller, A. S., Leifer, C., Pullon, P. A., and Bowser, M. W.: Nevoid basal cell carcinoma syndrome, Oral Surg. **36:**533-543, 1973.

Miller, A. S., and Pullon, P. A.: Mobile teeth and ulcerated soft tissue lesions, Dent. Survey **55:**71, 1979.

Pellegrino, S. V.: Primary hyperparathyroidism exacerbated by pregnancy, J. Oral Surg. **35:**915-917, 1977.

Raibley, S. O., Beckett, R. P., and Nowakowski, A.: Multiple traumatic bone cysts of the mandible, J. Oral Surg. **37:**335-337, 1979.

Rapidis, A. D., Langdon, J. D., Harvey, P. W., and Patel, M. F.: Histiocytosis X, Int. J. Oral Surg. **7:**76-84, 1978.

Ryan, D. E., and Burkes, E. J.: The multiple basal cell nevus syndrome in a Negro family, Oral Surg. **36:**831-840, 1973.

Scott, J., and Finch, L. D.: Histiocytosis X with oral lesions: report of case, J. Oral Surg. **30:**748-753, 1972.

Sigala, J. I., Silverman, S., Brody, H. A., and Kushner, J. H.: Dental involvement in histiocytosis, Oral Surg. **33:**42-48, 1972.

Soskolne, W. A., Lustmann, J., and Azaz, B.: Histiocytosis X: report of six cases initially in the jaws, J. Oral Surg. **35:**30-33, 1977.

Stoelinga, P. J. W., Cohen, M., and Morgan, A. F.: The origin of keratocysts in the basal cell nevus syndrome, J. Oral Surg. **33:**659-663, 1975.

Tabachnick, T. T., and Levine, B.: Multiple myeloma involving the jaws and oral soft tissue, J. Oral Surg. **34:**931-933, 1976.

White, S. C., Frey, N. W., Blaschke, D. D., et al.: Oral radiographic changes in patients with progressive systemic sclerosis (scleroderma), J. Am. Dent. Assoc. **94:**1178-1182, 1977.

22

Generalized rarefactions of the jawbones

Norman K. Wood
Paul W. Goaz

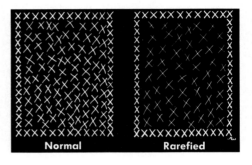

Normal | **Rarefied**

Following is a list of the generalized rarefactions of the jawbones:

Hyperparathyroidism
    Primary
    Secondary
    Tertiary
Osteoporosis
    Postmenopausal and senile
    Cushing's syndrome
    Drug-induced
    Malnutritional states
    Thyrotoxic
Osteomalacia
Hereditary hemolytic anemia
    Thalassemia
    Sickle cell
Leukemia
Histiocytosis X
Paget's disease
Multiple myeloma
Rarities
    Acromegaly (pseudo-osteoporosis)
    Agranulocytosis
    Burkitt's lymphoma
    Central cavernous hemangioma
    Congenital heart disease
    Cyclic neutropenia
    Diabetes
    Down's syndrome
    Erythroblastosis fetalis
    Gaucher's disease
    Hypervitaminosis D
    Hypogonadism
    Hypoparathyroidism
    Hypophosphatasia
    Hypovitaminosis C
    Lymphosarcoma
    Massive osteolysis (phantom bone disease)
    Multiple metastatic carcinomas
    Multiple sclerosis
    Osteogenesis imperfecta

    Other diffuse malignant tumors
    Oxalosis
    Polycythemia
    Postradiation rarefaction
    Pregnancy—late stages
    Progeria
    Protein-deficiency states
    Rickets
    Sarcoidosis
    Spherocytosis
    Urticaria pigmentosa
    XO syndrome
    XXY syndrome

HOMEOSTASIS OF BONE

Bones are complex organs consisting of a dense outer cortex covered with a specialized connective tissue of varying thickness, the periosteum. The inner medullary portion comprises small communicating cavities, or marrow spaces, filled with red (hematopoietic) and/or yellow (adipose) marrow. These marrow spaces and the inner surface of the cortex are lined with a delicate connective tissue, the endosteum.

Osteoblasts, which proliferate from undifferentiated cells, are responsible for the formation of the organic bone matrix (osteoid). The osteoid soon becomes mineralized under normal conditions.

Osteoclasts actively resorb bone and are thought to form from the coalescence of macrophages and from undifferentiated cells (Little, 1973b).

466

Maintenance of normal bone density or mass requires normal (mechanical) function along with the interaction of a number of intricate and delicate systems: osseous, endocrine, renal, gastrointestinal, nutritional, hematopoietic, and neurocirculatory.

The endocrine glands play important and often antagonistic roles in maintaining normal bone mass. Hormones such as the following, in physiologic amounts, usually promote the formation of bone: growth hormone, testosterone and other androgens, estrogens, and calcitonin. Hormones such as parathyroid hormone, cortisol, and thyroxine usually promote the resorption of bone.

All the rarefying diseases included in this chapter represent a disruption of bone homeostasis that may result from either an imbalance between the factors just noted or the direct influence of a disease process on the bone itself.

NORMAL VARIATIONS IN THE RADIODENSITY OF BONE

Radiographs reveal a considerable variation in the density of normal jawbones. Men frequently have heavier bones than women because of the more powerful anabolic effects of testosterone. Heavy vigorous men usually have more osseous tissue, which in turn produces a denser radiographic image. The bones of thin delicate people (men and women) usually cast a less dense, more fragile-appearing radiographic shadow. This normal variation in radiodensity is in part caused by differences in the size and shape of the marrow spaces and the number and prominence of the trabeculae.

Although differences in radiodensity are apparent on radiographs from several persons, variations in radiodensity are also apparent in the jaws of the same person. For example, bone is frequently denser in the anterior region of the mandible than in the more posterior regions, and the mandible is more radiolucent inferior than superior to the external oblique and mylohyoid ridges, partly because of the salivary gland depression, which thins the bone in this region. Furthermore, the thickness of soft tissue overlying the bone, the patient's complexion, the variations due to equipment, and the exposure and developing factors all contribute to the apparent differences in the radiodensities of bone.

Functional stress is also closely related to the bony architecture. Usually, within physiologic limits, the greater the mechanical forces applied the more radiopaque will be the image of the bone. This relationship between structure and function is illustrated by the frequent observation that when teeth are lost the alveolar bone in the edentulous area becomes relatively radiolucent.

When all the modifying factors are considered, it is not surprising that images which mimic changes seen in rarefying disease are frequently found in radiographs of normal jaws.

HYPERPARATHYROIDISM

Parathyroid hormone plays an important role in maintaining calcium homeostasis. A decrease in the plasma calcium level below the normal level stimulates the parathyroid gland to secrete additional parathyroid hormone, which in turn causes the plasma calcium to rise until it has been restored to the normal level. When the plasma calcium reaches the normal concentration, the secretion of hormone is reduced.

Although the manner in which parathyroid hormone elevates plasma calcium is the subject of active research (and some controversy), the following sequence of events is well established and serves to provide a useful outline of the reactions promoted by this hormone:

1. The bone and kidneys are the target organs of parathyroid hormone, which mediates the coalescence of macrophages to form mobile-type osteoclasts; and these osteoclasts actively resorb bone (Little, 1973b).
2. When bone is resorbed, calcium is released to the extracellular fluid and the serum calcium level may be elevated.
3. The level of serum phosphorus, unlike that of serum calcium, is not elevated because parathyroid hormone acts on the epithelium of the kidney tubules and causes a phosphorus diuresis while concomitantly inducing an increased calcium reabsorption from the glomerular filtrate.
4. Parathyroid hormone may also increase the absorption of calcium from the intestine, but this has not been definitely established (Jaworski, 1972).

Hence in the healthy person injections of parathyroid hormone produce an elevated plasma calcium level, a decreased plasma phosphorus level, and an increased alkaline phosphatase level. An increase in this serum enzyme is observed whenever there is increased bone activity.

Hyperparathyroidism is a disease in which there may be a complex of biochemical, anatomic, and clinical abnormalities resulting from the increased secretion of parathyroid hormone. It may occur in primary, secondary, and tertiary forms. It is included in the present chapter because all three types may produce a generalized rarefaction of the jawbones as well as several other changes. Worth (1963, p. 356) stated that this entity is the most common cause of a generalized rarefaction of the jaws.

Since it has become traditional to consider hyperparathyroidism as classically producing marked and predictable changes in the serum chemistry values as well as loss of the lamina dura, it is important for the clinician to know that such changes do not always occur and indeed have proved to be the exception rather than the rule. This is especially true regarding changes in the lamina dura that have been traditionally described and reputed to be specific for the disease.

With the development of immunoassay techniques for measuring plasma levels of parathyroid hormone, it has been shown that approximately 50% of the cases of primary hyperparathyroidism now detectable do not show radiologic, clinical, or biochemical changes other than increased parathyroid hormone levels (Bartter, 1973). Such cases are termed "normocalcemic" hyperparathyroidism. It is evident that in mild or early cases abnormalities will not usually be detected whereas in more advanced cases symptoms may be mild, marked, or variable. Radiographic changes in bone are now considered to develop and become apparent only in the more advanced stages of the disorder; and changes in the jawbones are often late manifestations of the radiographically demonstrable bony disease (Silverman et al., 1968).

To emphasize the fact that the following features are characteristic of all three types of hyperparathyroidism, we shall undertake the discussion of the disorder itself before the three forms of the disease are described.

FEATURES

Hyperparathyroidism is a relatively common disease. Jackson and Frame (1972) estimated that one of every 1000 patients examined at a general diagnostic clinic will have some form of hyperparathyroidism; however, a significant percentage of these patients will be symptomless. These authors aptly described the features of the advanced disease as a composite of "bones, stones, abdominal groans, and psychic moans with fatigue overtones." Such patients complain of weakness, anorexia, nausea, vomiting, constipation, abdominal pains, muscular and joint pains, polyuria, polydipsia, and emotional instability.

In addition, a variety of osseous changes, including the following, may be present: metastatic calcification, subperiosteal erosion, osteitis fibrosa generalisata, disturbances in the jawbones, brown giant cell lesion, and rarely osteosclerosis.

Metastatic calcification. Ectopic calcification in soft tissue is the most common feature of hyperparathyroidism. A reported 45% to 80% of the patients have nephrolithiasis and/or nephrocalcinosis. Other soft tissues involved are the subcutaneous tissues, walls of blood vessels, articular cartilages, and joint capsules. The pancreas and the salivary glands frequently develop lithiasis.

Subperiosteal erosion. Subperiosteal erosion of bone, especially of the middle phalanges, is considered to be the radiographic hallmark of hyperparathyroidism (Fig. 22-1). It is also frequently seen in other sites (e.g., outer third of the clavicle, distal end of the femur, medial surface of the neck of the femur, upper end of the tibia). Walsh and Karmiol (1969) considered the loss of lamina dura as a type of subperiosteal erosion, likening the periodontal ligament to periosteum. Subperiosteal resorption of bone is the most characteristic radiographic feature of osteitis fibrosa; and when present, it is almost always pathognomonic for some variety of parathyroid dysfunction (Jackson and Frame, 1972).

Osteitis fibrosa generalisata (cystica). The older term "osteitis fibrosa cystica" was adopted because osteitis fibrosa lesions often appeared cystlike on radiographs. These areas were later found to be made up of fibrous tissue, however, so the term "cystica" was not appropriate and its use was discontinued. The term "osteitis fibrosa generalisata" refers to the pattern of generalized rarefaction seen in the skeleton as a late change in primary, secondary, or tertiary hyperparathyroidism and occasionally in pseudohypoparathyroidism* (Fig. 22-1). It occurs in approximately 13% of patients with hyperparathyroidism (Bartter, 1973). Early symptoms include vague aches and pains, which may be quite disseminated; later symptoms are severe bone pain and tenderness followed by fractures and the development of deformities.

Radiographically the bones may appear quite radiolucent with thin cortices and hazy indistinct trabeculae. Some bones may be less homogenous, presenting a moth-eaten image. Regions

---

*Pseudohypoparathyroidism with osteitis fibrosa is a rare condition. It is characterized by the serum changes typical of hypoparathyroidism (hypocalcemia, hyperphosphatemia, and normophosphatasia), by increased levels of circulating parathyroid hormone, and by the skeletal changes of hyperparathyroidism.

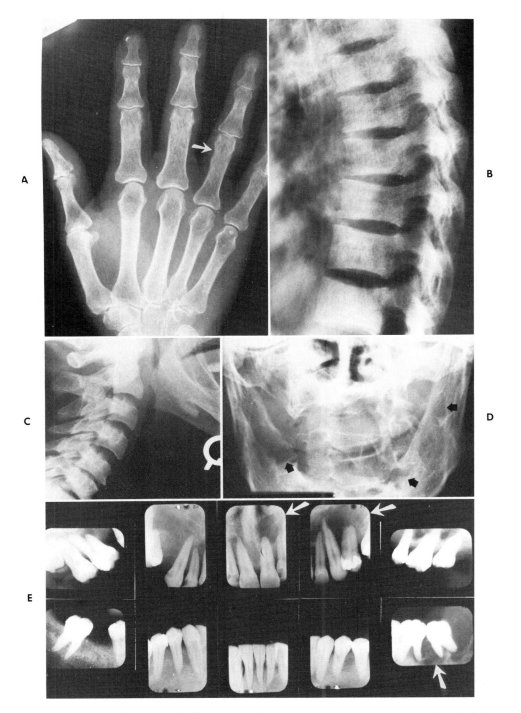

Fig. 22-1. Hyperparathyroidism. **A,** The arrow indicates early subperiosteal erosion on the third phalanx. **B,** Note the generalized rarefaction and loss of cortical margins in the thoracic vertebrae. **C,** Similar findings in the cervical vertebrae and mandible. **D,** Generalized rarefaction of the maxilla and mandible with thinning or loss of the cortical plates. Note the three brown giant cell lesions (arrows). **E,** Note the generalized rarefaction, the loss of lamina dura, and the two brown giant cell lesions (arrows). Most of these pictures have been printed lighter than normal to elucidate detail in the rarefied bones. (**A** to **C** courtesy E. Palacios, M.D., and J. Adamski, Maywood, Ill. **D** and **E** courtesy O. H. Stuteville, D.D.S., M.D., St. Joe, Ark.)

in which the trabeculae are completely missing will have a cystlike appearance on radiographs.

On histologic examination the radiolucent areas are found to contain sparse narrow trabeculae scattered throughout a fibrous stroma. A few osteoclasts may be present in Howship's lacunae. Watson (1973) referred to brown giant cell lesions as localized regions of osteitis fibrosa—which prompts us to question whether indeed histologic studies of areas of osteitis fibrosa generalisata in their earlier, more active stages might yield a picture similar to that seen in brown giant cell lesions. Certainly the examiner would expect to see a more vascular and cellular stroma, with an abundance of osteoclasts, in the early stages.

Jawbone changes. The bone changes of hyperparathyroidism do not occur so frequently in the jawbones as in the long bones and the skull; but hyperparathyroidism is the most common cause of generalized rarefaction of the jaws (Worth, 1963, p. 356).

Generalized rarefaction of the skeleton is not specific for hyperparathyroidism since identical radiographic changes may be seen in several of the other conditions detailed in this chapter. If the jaws are affected, the complete maxilla and mandible will usually be involved. The rarefaction may be of a homogenous nature in which the normal trabecular pattern is lost and replaced by a granular or ground-glass appearance (Fig. 22-1). Sometimes the rarefaction will have a mottled or moth-eaten appearance, showing variation in density. If the alveolus is severely affected, the teeth may be mobile and may migrate (Worth, 1963, p. 357). The radiopaque cortical plates outlining the bones and anatomic regions and features (e.g., nasal fossa, maxillary sinus, mandibular canal, mental foramen, alveolar crest, crypts of unerupted teeth, lamina dura) may be thinned or lost entirely (Fig. 22-1). Likewise, the oblique and mylohyoid ridges may be less prominent or may not show at all.

The lamina dura is diminished or completely absent in only about 10% of the cases. Silverman and co-workers (1968) stated that the loss of lamina dura is the most overrated characteristic of hyperparathyroidism. The degree of loss depends on the severity and/or duration of the disease. The teeth are not affected but appear relatively more radiopaque because of the contrast resulting from the loss of the lamina dura and the decrease in density of the surrounding bone (Fig. 22-1).

The clinician should realize that, even though reduced radiopacity of the jaws is a late manifestation of the disease, in some cases the jawbones may be the first to show such a change. Also, since the jawbones are examined radiographically more frequently than any other bones of the skeleton, bone changes in the jaws may be the first indication of the disease.

Brown giant cell lesion. The brown giant cell lesion of hyperparathyroidism is discussed as a cystlike radiolucency in Chapter 18 and as a multilocular radiolucency in Chapter 19. Although described by some authors as a localized area of osteitis fibrosa, these two conditions are generally considered to be separate entities.

Giant cell lesions occur slightly less often than osteitis fibrosa generalisata, developing in less than 10% of the patients with hypercalcemia. Although they may occur in the pelvis, ribs, and femurs, they are most common in the jaws—where they may cause radiolucencies that are either peripheral or central and unilocular or multilocular. Their margins will not be well defined if they arise in the osteoporotic jaw (Fig. 22-1). Worth (1963, p. 360) maintained that giant cell lesions are not so common in secondary hyperparathyroidism, but other authorities do not mention this distinction. Giant cell lesions may be the only sign of hyperparathyroidism; and when a giant cell lesion recurs after excision, hyperparathyroidism should be suspected.

The gross specimen is moderately soft and reddish brown, and it bleeds readily. Histologically it has giant cells scattered throughout a fibrovascular stroma in which foci of hemosiderin are present (Fig. 18-13, *F*). It cannot be distinguished on a histologic basis from the giant cell granuloma. Giant cell granulomas are more common in younger individuals, however; so if the patient is over 30 years of age, he is more likely to have a brown giant cell lesion than if he were younger.

Surgical excision of the giant cell lesion is generally considered unnecessary since the lesion resolves after the hyperparathyroidism is controlled. Nevertheless, a biopsy is advised for identification.

PRIMARY HYPERPARATHYROIDISM

Primary hyperparathyroidism is the result of a primary hyperplasia or a benign or malignant tumor of the parathyroid glands. Bartter (1973) reported that 50% of the patients with hyperparathyroidism have a mild form of the disease and do not show clinical, radiographic, or biochemical changes. He referred to this variety as "normocalcemic" hyperparathyroidism. Depending on the level of parathyroid hormone production, any or all of the changes described for hyperparathyroidism will be apparent. In advanced cases the classic serum changes of increased calcium, alkaline phosphatase, and decreased phorphorus will usually be present.

SECONDARY HYPERPARATHYROIDISM

Secondary hyperparathyroidism is a condition that results when the parathyroid glands are stimulated to produce increased amounts of parathyroid hormone to correct abnormally low serum calcium levels. Chronic renal disease and osteomalacia (delayed mineralization of new bone stemming from a lack of or an inability to utilize dietary calcium) are the most common conditions in which the hypocalcemic state is a feature. The low serum calcium levels stimulate increased production and secretion of parathyroid hormone, which then induce bone resorption with the liberation of calcium and phosphate ions. Contrary to the situation in primary hyperparathyroidism, however, there is an inverse relationship in secondary hyperparathyroidism between the levels of serum parathyroid hormone and serum calcium. The increased parathyroid activity and calcium mobilization are reflected not by an increase but by a decrease in the serum calcium level (Rasmussen and Bordier, 1974, p. 150).

In osteomalacia the most common cause of hypocalcemia is an impaired absorption of calcium from the intestine caused by a deficiency of vitamin D.

The cause of hypocalcemia in secondary hyperparathyroidism resulting from kidney disease is more obscure. Although phosphorus excretion is known to be impaired, with a resultant hyperphosphatemia in certain types of chronic kidney disease, what produces the hypocalcemia is not known. Several theories have been proposed; but on the basis of some contradictory evidence or observation, none are free of question. The resultant demand on the parathyroid glands usually produces a hyperplasia of all four glands, and the increased parathyroid hormone secretion causes an increased resorption of bone—which becomes radiographically evident in advanced cases. The classic serum chemistry changes in secondary hyperparathyroidism are hypocalcemia, hyperphosphatemia, and an increased serum alkaline phosphatase.

With the increased number of patients being managed by dialysis, it is likely that an increased incidence of secondary hyperparathyroidism will be seen. Fletcher and co-workers (1977) discussed the oral manifestations of secondary hyperparathyroidism related to long-term hemodialysis therapy.

TERTIARY HYPERPARATHYROIDISM

Occasionally parathyroid tumors develop after a long-standing secondary hyperparathyroidism, and this condition is known as "tertiary hyperparathyroidism." In effect, a secondary hyperparathyroidism has developed into a type of primary hyperparathyroidism. The increased parathyroid hormone levels produce increased bone resorption and a resultant hypercalcemia. All the skeletal manifestations of the other types of hyperparathyroidism may be seen in this rather rare variation of the disease.

DIFFERENTIAL DIAGNOSIS

See the differential diagnosis section at the end of the chapter (p. 486) for comments relative to the basic clinical and biochemical features that will aid in distinguishing the disorders that are the subject of this chapter.

MANAGEMENT

Early detection of hyperparathyroidism is necessary since the advanced disease may cause irreversible kidney damage, hypertension, and death (not to mention the discomfort, pain, fractures, and emotional problems that attend the condition).

Treatment of the primary and tertiary types requires excision of the parathyroid tumors. Patients usually are relieved of back pain within 48 hours after the excision, but radiographic improvement may not appear for about 1 month (Watson, 1973).

In the secondary type complete restoration of kidney function is usually not possible, but a subtotal parathyroidectomy is frequently beneficial. Watson (1973) reported that in secondary hyperparathyroidism the oral administration of adjusted doses of vitamin D will restore a normocalcemia by enhancing the absorption of calcium from the intestine. The ingestion of 1 g of calcium daily (equivalent to 1 quart of milk) can prevent skeletal demineralization in most cases of severe hyperparathyroidism (Walsh and Karmiol, 1969); and the skeletal changes will return to normal when the hyperparathyroidism is brought under control.

If the fibrosis is not too severe in advanced cases of osteitis fibrosa generalisata, the radiographic appearance of the bones will usually return to normal 6 months after treatment. If fibrosis is extensive, fibrotic bone may be replaced by sclerotic bone (Stafne, 1969, p. 264).

OSTEOPOROSIS

Osteoporosis of the skeleton is the most common form of metabolic bone disease. It is not a specific disease entity but represents a nonspecific reaction of the skeleton to several predisposing factors or diseases. It is a generalized rarefaction of the bones resulting from a deficiency of bone matrix rather than a deficit of mineral. The bone is normal in composition, but deficient in amount; in other words, there is a reduced volume of bone tissue relative to the volume of anatomic bone.

Osteoporosis develops in disease states in which there is an imbalance between bone formation (anabolism) and bone resorption (catabolism). Such disturbances develop in one of three ways:

1. A slight increase in bone resorption with a slight decrease in formation
2. A severe increase in bone resorption with a normal rate of formation
3. Normal bone resorption with a severe decrease in formation

Osteoporosis may be acquired or congenital, regional or generalized. In the present context the regional (isolated) examples will not be considered.

FEATURES

The majority of patients with osteoporosis show no symptoms. In advanced cases the clinical onset is frequently heralded by an attack of severe pain that is aggravated by movement and occurs after trauma or strenuous muscular effort. Osteoporosis is probably the most common cause of backache in elderly persons (Watson, 1973).

The pathologic bone changes in osteoporosis tend to involve the central axial part of the skeleton (spine, long bones, pelvis, skull, feet) in contrast to the bone changes in osteomalacia, which more frequently involve the peripheral skeleton. A gradual loss of height may be noticed by the osteoporotic patient because of shortening of the trunk.

Radiographic changes. Whatever the factor predisposing a patient to the development of an osteoporosis, the radiographic changes are quite similar. Since there must be at least a 30% to possibly a 50% or 60% loss of calcium content from a bone before the loss can be detected on radiographs, much bone tissue is lost before the

change becomes radiographically apparent. Although radiographic changes in osteoporosis can be described generally as a decrease in the density of the bone, specifically there is a loss of the normal trabecular pattern and a thinning of the cortex. The skull shows a diffuse decrease in density and assumes a spotty appearance.

Jaws. Although the maxilla and the mandible may become osteoporotic from a number of causes, there is a greater tendency for osteoporosis to develop in certain disease conditions than in others. For example, patients with Cushing's syndrome and patients receiving cortisone therapy more frequently develop bone changes in the jaws; and although thyrotoxicosis and postmenopausal or senile osteoporosis do not usually involve the jaws (Worth, 1963, p. 360), jaw changes may occur in advanced stages of these diseases.

If osteoporosis is present in the jaws, a generalized rarefaction of the maxilla and the mandible will be evident. Individual trabeculae will be fine and indistinct, and many will be completely obliterated. The overall picture will be of diffuse granularity. The cortical borders of the bone and anatomic chambers, such as the nose and maxillary sinus, will be thinner and less distinct (Fig. 22-2). The lamina dura characteristically will persist longer than in hyperparathyroidism, but it may be indistinct in advanced and severe cases and sometimes may be completely obliterated.

This description notwithstanding, the jaws have not been adequately studied in most series of osteoporosis that have been reported.

Biochemical changes. The serum calcium, phosphorus, and alkaline phosphatase levels are within normal limits in osteoporosis unless fractures are present.

Histopathology. If a section of osteoporotic bone is studied under low-power magnification, a thinned cortex will be apparent and the trabecular pattern will be irregular. Many of the trabeculae will have disappeared, and most of those remaining will be extremely thin. Otherwise the bone will appear normal.

Types of osteoporosis

There are numerous predisposing conditions or disease states that may induce an osteoporosis: postmenopausal and senile states, Cushing's syndrome, drug therapy, malnutrition, thyrotoxicosis. Regardless of the cause, the histologic changes are similar.

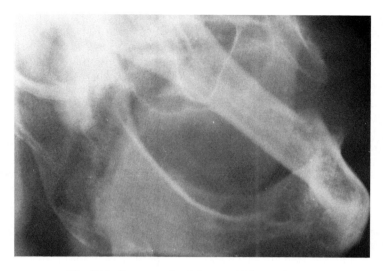

Fig. 22-2. Osteoporosis of the mandible, senile type.

POSTMENOPAUSAL AND SENILE OSTEOPOROSIS

Although precise etiologies have not been identified, the normal aging process in the skeleton of an adult human is known to begin soon after 20 years of age and to progress slowly with the advancing years. This aging process is part of a more generalized condition that affects all the tissues of the body. In some older persons additional contributing factors may accelerate the process and as a result frank osteoporosis develops.

An overall decrease in the anabolic hormones (particularly estrogen) in postmenopausal women may cause a lag in the formation of bone; and since bone resorption continues at about the normal rate, a progressive and extensive resorption of bone results. This condition is referred to as postmenopausal osteoporosis, and the loss of bone substance is limited to the spine, pelvis, and ribs. The skull and extremities remain intact (Snapper, 1957, pp. 201-202).

The imbalance between the formation and resorption of bone continues for about 10 years after the climacteric or menopause. Then the rarefying process levels off. At about the age of 60, a generalized atrophy of the bone—senile osteoporosis—becomes apparent. This atrophy occurs much more frequently and is more marked in women; and it probably represents a summation of postmenopausal and senile osteoporotic damage.

In senile osteoporosis the rarefaction involves mainly the spine, ribs, and vertebrae; but a minor amount of rarefaction also involves the peripheral skeleton. Whereas this slight amount in women is the result of senile osteoporosis, the rarefaction of the spine, ribs, and vertebrae is a combination of postmenopausal and senile osteoporoses.

Senile osteoporosis is thought to be caused by a number of factors operating together, but sometimes one factor is dominant and identifiable. For example, a decline in calcium absorption is not uncommon in elderly men and women partly because of a decrease in absorption and/or metabolism of vitamin D with increasing age. Also in aging, less bone is formed because of a decrease in the anabolic hormones. There is, furthermore, a decrease in muscle protein, which in turn results in less muscular activity; and less muscular activity results in a decreased flow of blood to the bone. Thus the oxygen supply to the bones is decreased and the resulting hypoxic condition favors bone resorption.

In elderly persons the altered hormonal spectrum, which is part of the aging process, predisposes them to the formation of (usually) small thrombi; these thrombi plug small vessels in the bone and cause a loss of bone vitality and hence resorption (osteoporosis). The poor nutritional habits of the elderly also add to this problem.

When the cause cannot be determined, the osteoporosis is termed "idiopathic." Since there is no specific agent yet available to stimulate bone formation, the current treatment for osteoporosis consists mainly of palliative procedures. To this end analgesics are prescribed as well as dietary counseling to ensure a good protein diet with general supplements of calcium and vitamins C and D. The use of intermittent calcium infusions, thyrocalcitonin, and diphosphonates is currently under investigation (Watson, 1973).

CUSHING'S SYNDROME

Cushing's syndrome is a complex of symptoms, including buffalo torso (adiposity about the upper portion of the trunk and a bump at the base of the neck), moon face (puffiness of the face), altered hair distribution (masculinizing effects in females and in male children), hypertension, elevated blood glucose levels, increased excretion of 17-ketosteroids in the urine, and osteoporosis. These are evoked by an increased output of glucocorticoids, especially cortisol.

In children this condition results from hyperplasia or tumors of the adrenal cortex, and in adults most frequently from a pituitary adenoma. The excess cortisol acts to produce osteoporosis in at least two ways:

1. As a catabolic* hormone it contributes to the degradation of protein and severely limits the formation of bone matrix by reducing the amount that each osteoblast synthesizes.
2. It promotes the formation of osteoclasts from the osteogenic undifferentiated cells and thus enhances bone resorption.

Osteoporosis is seen in 64% of the women and 75% of the men afflicted with Cushing's syndrome. The pelvis, ribs, vertebrae, long bones, and skull are most commonly involved. The jaws may show changes in advanced cases, with the density or the lamina dura diminished or even completely missing. After the adrenocortical problem is corrected, the osteoporosis will usually disappear in young growing individuals; but the rarefaction appears to be irreversible in adults (Reynolds and Karo, 1972).

DRUG-INDUCED OSTEOPOROSIS

Cortisol/cortisone. Prolonged administration of glucocorticoid drugs will often produce a cushingoid syndrome with the accompanying osteoporosis occasioned by the same mechanisms described for Cushing's syndrome. Concurrent administration of androgens, estrogens, calcitonin, and fluorides fails to protect the bone from the adverse effects of the corticoids (Duncan, 1972). It has been determined, however, that the

---

*In this chapter the nature of the hormones' effects is described in general terms without distinguishing whether indeed the hormones are acting—for example, as catabolic or antianabolic agents in a particular event.

endocrine imbalance resulting from the continuous use of cortisol can be minimized if the daily dose is synchronized with the physiologic cortisol peak in the normal diurnal cycle between 6:00 A.M. and 8:00 A.M.

Contraceptive drugs. There is an interaction between the progestational compounds used as contraceptive agents and the increased levels of cortisol that are occasioned by stress. In addition to the usual effect of cortisol on the hematopoietic tissue (i.e., causing an increase in the number of megakarocytes formed), the combination of the two compounds causes the production of abnormal megakaryocytes, which in turn form abnormal sticky platelets. These platelets immediately fuse and give rise to multiple small thrombi.

The thrombi occlude small vessels in the tissues; and when the process occurs in osseous tissues, small foci of bone supplied by these occluded vessels die and the dead bone is subsequently resorbed (Little, 1973b). When sufficient bone has been removed, radiographic changes become evident. The levels of cortisol required for thrombus formation vary with each progestational steroid, but they are the lowest with the efficient contraceptive agents (Little, 1973a).

MALNUTRITIONAL STATES

Sufficient protein must be absorbed from the intestine to supply the constant need for matrix formation. A deficiency in protein can cause osteoporosis and may result from a protein-poor diet or from gastrointestinal disturbances such as gastric resection (the patient usually eats less), colitis, regional enteritis, and malabsorption syndromes.

A vitamin C deficiency will produce an osteoporosis by (1) causing a defective matrix to be formed by the osteoblasts and (2) weakening the sinusoidal vessel walls in medullary bone. The sinusoidal vessels tend to dilate and rupture, resulting in the pooling of blood and hypoxia, which subsequently leads to loss of vitality and the removal of bone by phagocytic osteoclasts.

THYROTOXIC OSTEOPOROSIS

A hyperthyroid patient may have an increased basal metabolic rate, increased temperature, flushing, weight loss, emotional instability, overalertness, tremors, and exophthalmos.

The hyperthyroid state leads to osteoporosis if it remains untreated for several years. Since most patients receive definitive treatment at a relatively early stage of their disease, radiographic bone changes are not a usual feature of the condition. This consideration may help to explain the variation in frequency with which osteoporosis has been reported to occur in hyperthyroidism (Koutras et al., 1973).

There is not unanimous agreement concerning the mechanism(s) responsible for the production of osteoporosis in hyperthyroidism; nevertheless, one theory holds that thyroxine mediates the action of cortisol on bone and an excess of thyroxine results in a more efficient utilization of this steroid. Thus there is increased bone resorption. Although the thyroxine appears to increase both the formation and the resorption of bone, the balance of bone activity favors resorption (Rasmussen and Bordier, 1974, p. 192). There is a tendency toward hypercalcemia; but the serum calcium level is generally within normal range and the alkaline phosphatase level is increased—the latter correlating well with the increased bone activity.

Osteoporosis is more often seen in children with hyperthyroidism, and the radiographic picture is similar to that of osteoporosis produced by other causes. The jaws may be involved as a late change, and both the maxilla and the mandible will show uniform involvement.

In young patients the treatment of thyrotoxicosis usually results in a restoration of the bone mass. In older patients the osteoporosis generally persists after treatment (Koutras et al., 1973).

DIFFERENTIAL DIAGNOSIS

For a discussion of the differential diagnosis of osteoporosis, see the differential diagnosis section at the end of the chapter (p. 486).

MANAGEMENT

If a dental clinician observes osteoporosis on radiographs of the jaws, he should consult with an internist. Treatment and prognosis of osteoporosis are discussed under the individual types.

OSTEOMALACIA

The terms "rickets" in children and "osteomalacia" in adults embrace a group of disorders characterized by a rarefaction of the skeleton and caused by a deficiency of calcium for the mineralization of normal osteoid. The calcium deficiency responsible for the rachitic or osteomalacic state may be the result of one or a combination of the following: vitamin D deficiency, calcium malabsorption, liver and renal disorders, prolonged anticonvulsive drug therapy, and hypophosphatemic rickets.

Vitamin D acts to promote the absorption of calcium from the intestine and also induces the rapid calcification of osteoid (Bartter, 1973). Thus a deficiency of this vitamin can readily lead to rarefaction of the skeleton.

Calcium-deficient diets, as well as malabsorption states such as those encountered after gastric resection (probably due to deficient intake of calcium and vitamin D since these patients tend to eat less) and in chronic pancreatitis, small bowel ischemia, and gluten enteropathy, may be the cause of the calcium deficiency even if adequate amounts of vitamin D are present. Biliary obstruction may also produce a calcium deficiency by preventing bile salts from reaching the intestine; the presence of bile salts in the intestine is necessary for fat absorption. The resulting impairment of fat absorption causes a deficiency in vitamin D absorption (vitamin D is fat soluble) and hence the decreased absorption of calcium.

Prolonged administration of anticonvulsant drugs (e.g., phenobarbital, primidone) can result in calcium deficiency because these drugs enhance liver enzyme activity, which leads to an increased breakdown of vitamin D to biologically inert products (Conacher, 1973).

A variety of renal diseases, which may be congenital or may result from a chronic nephritis, are associated with an imbalance of serum calcium and/or phosphorus; and as a result an osteomalacia is produced. Such cases are often complicated by a secondary hyperparathyroidism that is consequent to a low serum calcium, so both an osteomalacia and an osteitis fibrosa generalisata may be present.

Except that serum calcium level tends to be normal, hypophosphatemic rickets seems to be a specific disease entity showing the features of vitamin D deficiency. These patients require much larger doses of vitamin D to correct the deficiency than would normally suffice to correct an avitaminosis D. Generally there is a familial background, but not invariably. Although the pathogenesis is not clear, the main problem may be due to reduced phosphorus absorption and/or reduced tubular reabsorption of phosphorus (Nordin, 1973, pp. 78-80).

FEATURES

The clinical features of osteomalacia include weakness and generalized bone pain. The pain is localized in the bones rather than in the joints, and back pain is not so common as in osteoporosis. Approximately one third of the patients suffer spontaneous fractures (Conacher, 1973).

Characteristic radiographic features are not apparent in many osteomalacic patients. When a change is evidenced, however, it is often a non-specific generalized demineralization of the skeleton such as that seen in osteoporosis. Pseudofractures (or Milkman's fractures) and greenstick fractures are practically pathognomonic for osteomalacia in adults.

Pseudofractures in osteomalacia appear as radiolucent bands extending into the bones from the cortex, usually at right angles to the periosteal margins. These are partial or complete fractures without displacement, in which callus has been deposited but has failed to calcify. The pseudofractures are at sites of entry of the nutrient arteries. In cases of advanced osteomalacia, there will be complete fractures and bowing.

Radiographic changes do occur in the jaws of osteomalacic patients and are identical with those found in osteoporosis: a generalized rarefaction, a cortical thinning, and a homogeneous granular appearance throughout the maxilla and mandible. The lamina dura may be less prominent or completely absent.

In osteomalacia caused by a vitamin D deficiency, the serum calcium level is initially decreased. This prompts an increased parathyroid activity, which causes a decrease in serum phosphorus levels by inducing a phosphorus diuresis. Although the parathyroid hormone causes a resorption of bone and the alkaline phosphatase level is concurrently elevated with the increased bone activity,* insufficient calcium is mobilized to maintain calcium homeostasis (Rasmussen and Brodier, 1974, p. 150).

Overly wide osteoid seams may be observed microscopically surrounding thinned cortices and trabeculae.

DIFFERENTIAL DIAGNOSIS

For a discussion of the differential diagnoses of osteomalacia, see the differential diagnosis section at the end of the chapter (p. 486).

MANAGEMENT

Management of osteomalacia is directed toward correcting the basic defect, whether a dietary deficiency of calcium or vitamin D or a gastrointestinal or renal problem.

---

*The elevation of bone serum alkaline phosphatase in osteomalacia, rickets, and certain other bone disease is generally attributed to increased osteoblastic activity; the osteoblasts are the cells richest in alkaline phosphatase. Whether this is the correct explanation, however, is uncertain. Sometimes serum alkaline phosphatase appears to correlate better with the resorption than with the formation of bone (Nordin, 1973, p. 68).

HEREDITARY HEMOLYTIC ANEMIAS

Hemolytic anemias are discussed in this chapter because they produce a somewhat characteristic type of rarefaction of the bones. The rarefaction is caused by the development of larger than usual marrow spaces as well as, in some instances, a greater ratio of medullary bone to cortical bone. These changes are the result of a marked hyperplasia of the hematopoietic tissue induced by the increased demand for effective erythrocytes in the anemias.

Since there is a potential to replace fatty marrow with red marrow when a need for more erythrocytes arises, the hyperplastic changes in the hemolytic anemias are not restricted to bones that normally show erythropoiesis.* (The changes are often more pronounced in these bones, however.) Accordingly the fatty marrow of the adult mandible and maxilla may revert to the hyperplastic hematopoietic variety in response to stress imposed by the anemias. The skeletal changes are directly proportional to the severity of the disease. Although prominent changes may be observed in severe untreated cases, in mild cases no radiographic changes will be evident.

Thalassemia (Mediterranean or Cooley's anemia)

Thalassemia (Greek, *thalasso*, sea) was once considered to be found almost exclusively in people of Mediterranean origin, but it is now recognized to be a relatively common disorder of wide distribution (Moseley, 1963, pp. 26-27). It occurs in a number of different genetic forms with similar hematologic and clinical features. Although there are several classifications of the thalassemias, the most widely accepted consists of two main categories: major and minor.†

There is a type of thalassemia between these two that has a rather hazy clinical picture and is sometimes designated as intermediate thalassemia. This entity is not well defined but includes some features of the more severe thalassemia minors and the less severe thalassemia majors.

The basic anomaly in thalassemia is a defective erythrocyte with the individual having a markedly shortened life span.

---

*In the embryo and neonate the cavities of all the bones contain only red marrow. With advancing age the red marrow is gradually replaced by yellow or fatty marrow. In the normal adult the red marrow is found only in the vertebrae, ribs, sternum, diploë, and proximal epiphyses of the femur and humerus.

†Thalassemia major occurs in persons who are homozygous for the autosomal dominant trait. Thalassemia minor occurs in persons who are heterozygous for the condition.

FEATURES

Thalassemia major is a severe disorder of infants and children that usually becomes evident within the first year or two of life. Its clinical picture is of pallor, weakness, severe anemia, irritability, lethargy, and in some cases hepatosplenomegaly. The patient seldom survives beyond adolescence.

Patients with the intermediate type of thalassemia have similar but less severe symptoms.

Patients with the minor type of thalassemia are asymptomatic or have barely perceptible symptoms and show mild changes in the hemogram.

Radiographically the skull in thalassemia major is enlarged because of an increase in the width of the diploë. Sometimes numerous white hairlike shadows arising from the inner table of the cranial vault appear to protrude from the surface of the bone and produce the hair-on-end effect. The outer plate is displaced externally and may be less prominent or missing completely (Fig. 22-3). In severe cases the maxilla, mandible, and zygoma are markedly increased in size and the paranasal sinuses reduced.

Although a range of changes may be apparent in the jaws of patients with thalassemia, not all the changes will be evident in a particular patient. The cortices may be thinned, and the tooth roots short and spike shaped (Fig. 22-4). In general, there will be a blurring of the trabeculae—but with large circular bone marrow spaces delineated by pronounced trabeculae. The lamina dura about the tooth roots and the opaque lamina around the crypts of developing teeth may be thin. There will be a generalized rarefaction (Poyton and Davey, 1968), and occasionally a honeycombed pattern will be seen throughout the jaws (Fig. 22-4).

Aspiration biopsy of the bone marrow will reveal a very active immature hematopoietic tissue.

DIFFERENTIAL DIAGNOSIS

The radiographic picture of the thalassemias is distinct from that produced by *osteoporosis*,

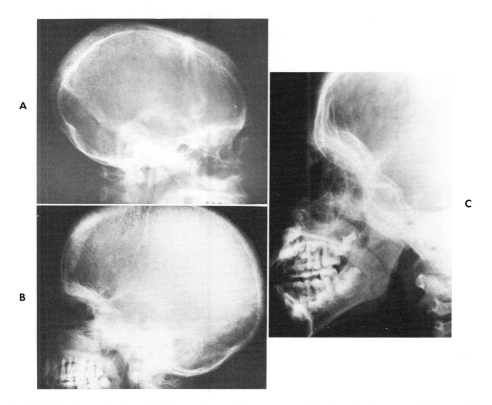

Fig. 22-3. Thalassemia. **A** and **B,** Two patients. Note the generalized rarefaction, the widening of the inner table, and the hair-on-end effect. **C,** Generalized rarefaction of the skull and jaws in another patient. (**A** and **B** courtesy E. Palacios, M.D., Maywood, Ill. **C** courtesy R. Moncada, M.D., Maywood, Ill.)

Fig. 22-4. Thalassemia. **A** and **B,** Note the honeycomb rarefaction in these periapical radiographs. The lamina dura is present. **C,** A similar pattern in a normal person. (**A** and **B** courtesy A. P. Angelopolous, D.D.S., Athens, Greece.)

osteomalacia, and *osteitis fibrosa generalisata* but is similar to what might be seen in other *hemolytic anemias.* The mild changes that may be found in the minor form, however, will not differ greatly from the minor variations expected in normal marrow patterns (Fig. 22-4). The history, clinical features, and blood studies are necessary for identification of the general condition as well as the specific form of the anemia.

MANAGEMENT

Treatment of the thalassemias is limited to administering transfusions and other supportive therapy. The dental clinician must consult the patient's internist before initiating dental procedures because of the potential bleeding and hypoxic problems as well as the increased possibility of infection.

Sickle cell anemia

Sickle cell anemia is a hereditary disease affecting blacks almost exclusively. The clinically apparent disease occurs in homozygotes; heterozygotes for the characteristic possess only the sickle cell trait, which does not (except in rare instances) produce any clinical manifestations. Approximately 10% of American blacks carry the sickle cell trait whereas only 0.5% have the disease. The manifestations usually appear early in childhood.

Fig. 22-5. Sickle cell anemia. **A,** Smear of peripheral blood showing sickle-shaped erythrocytes. **B,** Periapical radiograph showing the stepladder pattern. This pattern is also observed in normal patients. **C,** Spherocytosis. Note the honeycomb radiolucency and the faint lamina dura.

The sickle cell defect lies in the inherited abnormal hemoglobin—which has diminished oxygen-carrying capacity and is less soluble in the reduced state than is normal hemoglobin. The result is that under conditions of low oxygen tension, the reduced abnormal hemoglobin crystallizes from solution within the red cells and causes the cells to take on abnormal shapes (especially crescents or sickles). The episode is termed a "sickle cell crisis"; and during these phases the sickled erythrocytes become physically trapped in small vessels, form thrombi, and cause the development of tiny infarctions. When these infarctions occur in bone, foci of dead bone develop and are then resorbed. Thus the rarefaction related to the anemia-induced erythroblastic hyperplasia is intensified. Repeated infarctions are thought to produce sclerotic regions in the bone.

FEATURES

The patient with sickle cell disease may exhibit pallor, fatigue, weakness, dyspnea, retardation of growth, acute abdominal pain, and joint and muscle pains. A child with sickle cell disease will be quite susceptible to infection. Most patients die before reaching 40 years of age.

The sickle cell patient often has relatively long gangling extremities, which are particularly striking when contrasted with his short often rotund torso (Chernoff, 1967, p. 1046).

Oral ulcers may be present, particularly on the gingivae, and represent infarcts that have become secondarily infected (Fig. 6-11, *A*).

Splenomegaly is present in about 30% of adolescents with sickle cell anemia; but by adulthood the spleen has become fibrosed and small. The hemogram shows a mild to severe anemia, increased reticulocyte count, and marked poikilocytosis. A special sickle cell preparation applied to a drop of blood on a glass slide will demonstrate the sickling phenomenon (Fig. 22-5).

Electrophoretic analysis of the hemoglobin is also utilized in establishing the diagnosis.

Although Robinson and Sarnat (1952) reported that 18 out of 22 patients with sickle cell disease showed generalized rarefaction of the skeleton, most authors believe that bone changes are not found so frequently and are not so pronounced as those in thalassemia. The skull may show the hair-on-end appearance, which again is usually not so marked as in thalassemia. The following radiographic changes in the jaws, either singly or in combination, have been reported to be indicative of sickle cell anemia (Sanger et al., 1977):

1. The trabeculae may be reduced in number.
2. The remaining trabeculae appear coarsened and sharply defined.
3. Occasionally prominent horizontal trabeculae between the teeth have a stepladder appearance (Figs. 22-5 and 22-6).
4. Although the lamina dura and other cortices are usually normal, a thinning of the inferior border of the mandible and the alveolar crestal cortex may be observed.

Fig. 22-6. A and **B,** Periapical films of a young black with sickle cell anemia. Note the rarefied appearance of the bone, the generalized decrease in number of trabeculae, and also the sketchy traces of thick opaque trabeculae. **C,** Periapical radiograph of a normal patient showing a similar appearance.

5. There may be sclerotic areas in the bone that represent healed infarcts.
6. Changes are more remarkable in children (Sanger and Bystrum, 1977).

In contrast to the classic radiographic appearances just described, Mourshed and Tuckson (1974), in the most extensive study of the radiographic features of the jaws in sickle cell anemia to date, reported that similar radiographic appearances may be observed in normal patients (Fig. 22-6). Furthermore, these authors did not observe cortical thinning of the inferior border of the mandible or sclerotic areas in their series of sickle cell patients.

They stressed rather that radiographic features of the jaws should not be regarded as reliable diagnostic criteria for sickle cell disease. They strongly recommended, however, that if any of these radiographic features are present the clinician should resort to the appropriate laboratory procedures to determine whether the patient has sickle cell disease.

DIFFERENTIAL DIAGNOSIS

When the radiographic changes described for sickle cell disease are present, they are suggestive of *hemolytic anemia* but may also be frequently found in radiographs of a normal individual. If the patient is a black and has a family history of sickle cell anemia, this will prompt a high ranking of sickle cell anemia in the differential diagnosis. If the patient displays suggestive symptoms, the working diagnosis must be sickle cell anemia. The final diagnosis, of course, will depend on a hemoglobin analysis by electrophoresis, hemogram, and a special erythrocyte sickle cell preparation.

MANAGEMENT

The dental clinician must closely consult with the patient's internist before dental work is undertaken on a person with sickle cell disease. This is necessary because of the increased possibility of infection and the precipitation of a sickle cell crisis by the stressful situations frequently associated with dental procedures. Girasole and Lyon (1977) reported three cases of sickle cell osteomyelitis of the mandible

LEUKEMIA

Leukemia is a malignancy of the hematopoietic tissue involving one of the leukocytic cell types. Marrow replacement by proliferating cells of the myeloid series causes general rarefactions of bone, so the disease is included in this

chapter. The more aggressive is the disease, or the younger the patient, the more likely are gross bone changes to develop (Van Slyck, 1972).

The radiographic appearance of leukemia may vary from multiple punched-out defects to solitary moderately well-defined areas of osteolysis to generalized rarefaction. Occasionally osteosclerosis is observed. The fact that the maxilla and the mandible in growing persons possess active hematopoietic marrow prompts the clinician to anticipate that these bones will be involved with a leukemic infiltrate and develop osteolytic lesions.

FEATURES

The onset of leukemia may be insidious or abrupt; and the symptoms will be related to the resulting anemia, thrombocytopenia, and tissues that may be infiltrated and/or infected by the proliferating leukemic cells. The patient may exhibit pallor and weakness as well as petechiae or ecchymoses in the mucous membrane or skin. Michaud and co-workers (1977) detailed a thorough description of oral manifestations of leukemia in children.

The pallor will be noticeable on the oral mucosa, which will usually be normal in other respects, except in monocytic leukemia. This type of leukemia frequently causes the development of ulcers on the oral mucosa, gingival enlargements, bleeding, and/or gangrenous stomatitis. The ulcers are often covered with a yellow-gray fibrinous pseudomembrane that bleeds readily (Williamson, 1970, pp. 943-944).

Occasionally oral changes are observed in other types of leukemia also. Leukemic infiltration of the oral soft tissues may produce swelling of the palate and other regions of the jaws. Lymph nodes are frequently enlarged (Michaud et al., 1977), and there may be a slight hepatosplenomegaly. Fever is a common symptom, as are abdominal and bone pains. Leukocyte counts in active stages may range from 20,000 to 100,000 per milliliter. In chronic leukemias or in remission phases of acute types, the signs and symptoms are more moderate.

Radiographically discernible osteolytic changes are present in over 60% of the acute childhood leukemias. Demonstrable bone lesions, however, are not so common in acute adult leukemias[*];

---

[*]In adults very little hematopoietic tissue remains in the skeleton, so there is much greater reserve space in the fatty marrow cavities for the expansion of the proliferating leukemic cells before they eventually encroach on the bone itself.

and only about 12% of the lymphosarcomas* involve bone (Van Slyck, 1972). The rarefaction may be quite pronounced—with the trabecular architecture of the jawbone almost completely destroyed, the cortices thinned, and the lamina dura missing.

Worth (1966) described the following radiographic changes observed in the jaws of patients with leukemia or lymphosarcoma:

1. The formation of the tooth crowns may be incomplete and delayed.
2. The cortices of the tooth crypts may be partially or completely destroyed.
3. There may be enlargement of the crypts with failure of bone formation about the apical portion of erupting or developing teeth (Fig. 22-7).
4. The developing tooth may assume an asymmetric position within the crypt with or

---

*Lymphosarcoma is mentioned here because although it arises in aggregates of lymphoid tissue it does occasionally infiltrate and replace bone marrow and may be associated with a blood picture of lymphatic leukemia.

without destruction of some or part of the crypt cortex.

5. Incompletely formed crowns may be situated entirely above the alveolar crest, being completely elevated out of the bone.
6. Partially formed teeth, especially those having incomplete root formation, may be found to have excessively rapid eruption.

In a study of 214 children with acute leukemia, Curtis (1971) reported finding jawbone changes in 65% of the acute lymphatic leukemias and 55% of the acute myelogenous leukemias. He observed that osteoporosis usually commenced with the destruction of the apical portion of the cortex about the most distal developing mandibular molar crypt and progressed forward. He indicated that this was the most frequently found abnormality in the jaws. Some patients developed unilateral changes in the jaws, others developed bilateral changes, some in only one jaw, and others in both jaws. The alveolar crests were not usually involved; but when changes in the crest were

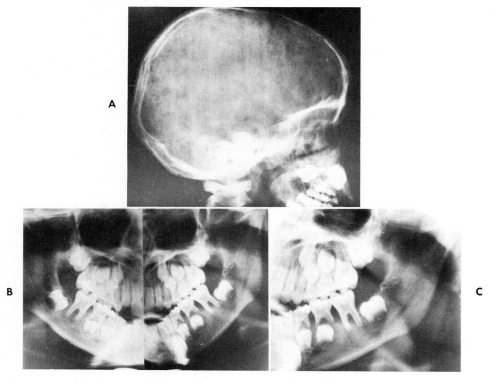

Fig. 22-7. Acute leukemia. **A,** Note the generalized rarefaction of the skull and ramus. **B,** Generalized rarefaction and diminution or loss of the lamina dura around roots and crypts. Note that the left mandible is more severely affected than the right. **C,** Enlarged view of the left mandible in **B.** Radiographs have been printed lighter than normal to elucidate detail in the rarefied bone. (**A** courtesy R. Moncada, M.D., Maywood, Ill. **B** and **C** courtesy T. Emmering, D.D.S., Maywood, Ill.)

present, they were the result of an extension of a medullary lesion rather than of the disease process's commencing at the crest. Changes in the lymphatic and myelogenous types were indistinguishable. Remissions were reflected by improvement in the radiographic picture.

In addition to the osseous defects of leukemia, there may be discernible periosteal new bone apposition, developing as a reaction to the penetration by the leukemic cells between the cortex and the periosteum (Lichtenstein, 1977, p. 325).

Contrary to the lytic changes, osteosclerosis is an occasional finding and is more common in myelogenous leukemia than in the other types (Worth, 1963, p. 371).

DIFFERENTIAL DIAGNOSIS

For a discussion of the differential diagnosis of leukemia, see the differential diagnosis section at the end of this chapter (p. 486).

MANAGEMENT

Antitumor drugs (e.g., methotrexate, prednisone) are used for the induction and maintenance of remissions of the leukemias. Palliative measures to counteract anemia, bleeding problems, and infection are necessary, especially in the acute phase of the disease. Acute childhood leukemias carry the poorest prognosis.

HISTIOCYTOSIS X

Histiocytosis X is a reticuloendothelial disease that may cause a generalized rarefaction of the jaws, especially in the Letterer-Siwe and Hand-Schüller-Christian varieties. This reticuloendotheliosis is discussed in Chapter 21 as a disease producing multiple separate radiolucencies that are well defined but without a cortical margin.

FEATURES

The rarefied appearance of the jawbone produced by Letterer-Siwe or Hand-Schüller-Christian disease may closely mimic the leukemic changes. In most cases, however, the bone destruction in histiocytosis X commences at the alveolar crest instead of in the medullary region of the bone, which is more typical of leukemia. Extrusion of the teeth, thinning of the cortices and lamina dura, and crypt and tooth involvement (all changes seen in leukemia) may be present in histiocytosis X (Fig. 22-8). New bone formation is not characteristic of the latter disease, however.

DIFFERENTIAL DIAGNOSIS

See the differential diagnosis section at the end of this chapter (p. 486) for comments relative to the basic clinical and biochemical features that will aid in distinguishing the disorders that are the subject of the chapter.

MANAGEMENT

Although the acute disseminated form, Letterer-Siwe, is the more serious variant of this disease, it is no longer considered invariably fatal; for with good clinical management some infants and children can be carried for years into a more chronic phase (Lichtenstein, 1977, p. 418).

Hand-Schüller-Christian disease, being a chronic form of histiocytosis X, carries a better prognosis. Radiation therapy frequently proves helpful. Often palliative and corrective measures are also necessary to regulate the altered physiol-

Fig. 22-8. Histiocytosis X. **A,** Generalized rarefaction and a discrete lesion. **B,** Diffuse radiolucency of bone in another patient. (**A** courtesy R. Goepp, D.D.S., Zoller Clinic, University of Chicago.)

Fig. 22-9. Paget's disease, early stage. **A,** Osteoporosis circumscripta of the skull. **B,** Two stages of Paget's disease: intermediate stage in the skull and early osteolytic stage in the maxilla (which is almost completely radiolucent). **C,** Same patient as in **B.** Note the generalized rarefaction of the maxilla, the loss of lamina dura, and the relative increase in radiopacity of the teeth. The mandible was unaffected. **D,** Photomicrograph of early Paget's disease. Note the increased amount of fibrous tissue and the numerous osteoclasts resorbing thinned bony trabeculae. (**A** courtesy R. Moncada, M.D., Maywood, Ill.)

ogy (diabetes insipidus) and control potentially serious secondary infections. Allard and co-workers (1978) reported satisfactory results from marrow-cancellous bone grafting of the defects in the alveolar bone.

PAGET'S DISEASE (OSTEITIS DEFORMANS)

The intermediate stage of Paget's disease is discussed in detail in Chapter 24, which emphasizes the mixed radiolucent and radiopaque appearance of the disease. The late stage, with its dense cotton-wool appearance, is stressed in Chapter 29. The early stage, characterized by a radiographic picture of rarefaction, is discussed in this chapter.

FEATURES

Inclusive features of Paget's disease will not be reviewed here since they are presented in detail in Chapters 24 and 29.

In general, the clinician will not be as well ac-

quainted with the radiolucent stage of Paget's disease as he is with the cotton-wool (late) stage. Osteitis deformans circumscripta of the skull is an example of this disease in its osteolytic phase (Fig. 22-9) (Anderson and Dehner, 1976). Furthermore, Paget's disease may initially cause a general homogenous rarefaction of the jawbone and a fine ground-glass appearance identical with that seen in hyperparathyroidism. The entire jawbone may be involved, with the cortices thinned and the lamina dura missing (Fig. 22-9, C).

Whereas both jaws may be affected, it is not characteristic for the same stage of the disease to be manifested in both simultaneously. (There is a progressive development of the disease from one bone to another.) The maxilla is more frequently involved than the mandible and is practically always affected first (Fig. 22-9).

Paget's disease may also involve the pelvis, vertebrae, and femurs; but the rarefaction stage is less common in these bones. The serum alkaline phosphatase levels are markedly elevated, as high as or higher than in any other disease (Goldsmith, 1972).

Histopathology of the early stage will show active resorption, with osteoclasts present in Howship's lacunae. The trabeculae will be small, disorganized, and scattered throughout a fibrous stroma (Fig. 22-9). Bone with the mosaic pattern will usually not be present at this stage, being characteristic of a more advanced phase of the disease.

DIFFERENTIAL DIAGNOSIS

For a discussion of the differential diagnosis of Paget's disease, see the differential diagnosis section at the end of the chapter (p. 486).

MANAGEMENT

Palliative measures are necessary to alleviate symptoms of the disease (e.g., early and persistent pain). Various regimens have been used to curb the degenerative advance of Paget's disease; and although some have been effective in relieving the pain, most have been disappointing in their effects on bone lesions.

MULTIPLE MYELOMA

Multiple myeloma is a disease characterized by the development of multiple malignant tumors of plasma cells. It originates in the bone marrow and represents the most common primary malignancy of bone. It is discussed in Chapter 21, where its radiographic appearance of multiple punched-out radiolucencies is emphasized.

FEATURES

In advanced cases the gross destruction of the medullary portions of the bones, coupled with resorption of the cortices from within, is so extensive that a generalized osteoporosis is obvious (Fig. 22-10).

DIFFERENTIAL DIAGNOSIS

For a discussion of the differential diagnosis of multiple myeloma, see the differential diagnosis section at the end of the chapter (p. 486).

MANAGEMENT

Multiple myeloma is a rapidly fatal disease; about half the patients die within 2 years of onset of symptoms. The 5-year survival rate is approximately 10%. The disease is treated with cytotoxic drugs (e.g., melphalan, urethan, steroids) and radiation. Palliative measures are used to alleviate

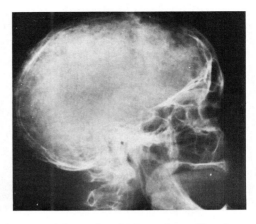

Fig. 22-10. Advanced multiple myeloma. Note the generalized rarefaction of the skull and jaws. Most of the radiopaque appearance of the skull is produced by the brain. (Courtesy E. Palacios, M.D., Maywood, Ill.)

the accompanying pain, bleeding, anemia, and kidney problems.

RARITIES

As shown in the list of rarities at the beginning of this chapter (and below), a varied group of diseases may produce generalized rarefactions of the skeleton, including the jaws (Figs. 22-11 and 22-12).

Either these diseases occur rarely, however, or they seldom produce rarefactions of the bone and/or jaws. Nevertheless, the clinician must be cognizant of them when he is developing a differential diagnosis for a particular case. Hopefully the other symptoms coincidental with the rarefaction will direct him to include the appropriate diseases in his working diagnosis:

The following list includes rare generalized rarefactions:

Acromegaly (pseudo-osteoporosis)
Agranulocytosis
Burkitt's lymphoma (Fig. 22-12)
Central cavernous hemangioma
Congenital heart disease
Cyclic neutropenia
Diabetes
Down's syndrome
Erythroblastosis fetalis
Gaucher's disease
Hypervitaminosis D
Hypogonadism
Hypoparathyroidism
Hypophosphatasia
Hypovitaminosis C

Fig. 22-11. Rarities. **A** to **C,** Lymphosarcoma. (Note the generalized rarefaction and loss of the lamina dura around the roots, **A,** as well as the blurred appearance of bone and loss of lamina dura, **B** and **C**). **D** and **E,** Diffuse squamous cell carcinoma of the anterior mandible. Note the loss of lamina dura and the generalized rarefaction.

Lymphosarcoma (Fig. 22-11)
Massive osteolysis (phantom bone disease)
Multiple metastatic carcinomas (Fig. 22-13)
Multiple sclerosis
Osteogenesis imperfecta
Other diffuse malignant tumors
Oxalosis
Polycythemia
Postradiation rarefaction
Pregnancy—late stages
Progeria
Protein-deficiency states

Rickets
Sarcoidosis
Spherocytosis
Urticaria pigmentosa
XO syndrome
XXY syndrome

DIFFERENTIAL DIAGNOSIS OF RAREFACTIONS OF THE JAWBONE

Because of the wide range of naturally occurring anatomic variations in healthy bone, distinguishing the radiographic appearance of normal

Fig. 22-12. Panorex radiograph of a patient with Burkitt's lymphoma. Note the gross rarefaction and almost complete loss of the bone in the molar and ramus areas bilaterally. (Courtesy N. Palm, D.D.S., Detroit.)

jawbone from changes produced by disease is frequently quite difficult. The jawbones of frail but healthy persons with delicate structures may appear to be more radiolucent than usual. Some persons may normally have relatively large marrow spaces, whereas others normally have a faint lamina dura. As a general rule, if the patient is well and changes are not evident on serial radiographs, then the bone picture is most likely within the range of normal variation.

The ensuing discussion, which pertains to the development of a differential diagnosis and a working diagnosis for the disorders included in the present chapter, requires some initial qualification since it is unique in relation to other similar sections of this text.

All the pathoses discussed herein are systemic diseases; and, needless to say, the differential diagnosis of bone diseases requires a very detailed history and careful physical examination. Therefore to describe all the manifest and subtle differences characterizing these entities is too large an undertaking.

An effort has been made, however, to present sufficient detail that the dental practitioner can appreciate the relationships between the oral and systemic manifestations and thereby be prepared for a consultation with the physician by perhaps first recognizing the need for the consultation, and second providing the most appropriate dental therapy when necessary.

Another consideration that seems important for overall orientation is that, in addition to causing similar rarefactions of the skeleton, the conditions listed herein (except two or three of the rarities) also produce other systemic changes. These features are identified by the general clinical examination and laboratory tests—supplementing the radiographic findings. Thus although there are no pat formulas, the clinical and laboratory examinations are significant in establishing the priorities of the probable entities in the differential diagnosis.

Following are some hints that will be of help in specific instances:

1. *There is a tendency to immediately diagnose a rarefaction of the jawbones accompanied by a loss of lamina dura as hyperparathyroidism.* True, a hyperparathyroidism may be the most common cause of rarefaction; but when one considers the many and varied disease processes that can produce a similar radiographic appearance, it becomes obvious that all the local and systemic features of a case must be carefully evaluated be-

Fig. 22-13. Disseminated metastatic retinoblastoma to the mandible in a 3-year-old girl. **A,** Intraoral view showing the tumorous expansion of the anterior alveolus. **B** and **C,** Right and left lateral oblique radiographs showing the general rarefaction of the mandible with a loss of most of the cortices and disruption of several developing permanent teeth. (From Perriman, A. P., and Figures, K. H.: Oral Surg. **45:**741-748, 1978.)

Table 22-1. Comparison of the serum values in metabolic bone diseases

Disease	Calcium	Phosphorus	Alkaline phosphatase
Hyperparathyroidism			
Primary	Increased	Decreased	Increased
Secondary	Normal to decreased	Increased	Increased
Tertiary	Increased	Normal to increased	Increased
Osteoporosis	Normal	Normal	Normal
Osteomalacia			
Vitamin D deficiency	Decreased	Decreased	Increased
Hypophosphatemia	Normal	Decreased	Increased
Paget's disease	Normal	Normal	Increased
Multiple myeloma	Normal to increased	Normal	Increased

fore an adequate working diagnosis can be developed.

Subperiosteal erosions, especially of the middle phalanges, are almost pathognomonic for hyperparathyroidism, as are the recurrent benign giant cell lesions of the jaws. Another important feature that will point to primary hyperparathyroidism is hypophosphatemia. Except for its occurrence in hyperparathyroidism, hypophosphatemia occurs only in avitaminosis D and hypophosphatemic rickets and in osteomalacia. Contrary to primary hyperparathyroidism, however, hypercalcemia is not found in the other conditions (Table 22-1).

2. *The lamina dura in osteoporosis is more apt to be deficient than in osteomalacia* (Worth, 1963, p. 360). The lamina dura characteristically appears normal in the hemolytic anemias (especially sickle cell anemia).

3. *Pseudofractures in adults are almost pathognomonic for osteomalacia.* The same can be said of greenstick fractures.

4. *Jawbone lesions of histiocytosis X more often commence at the crest of the alveolar ridge.* By contrast, those of leukemia characteristically originate in the deeper medullary portion. Also bone proliferation is foreign to the former condition but may be a feature of leukemia or lymphoma.

5. *Several diseases occur primarily in young persons:*
Thalassemia
Sickle cell anemia
Acute leukemia
Histiocytosis X

Older persons (over 40 years) are affected primarily by the following:
Hyperparathyroidism (especially secondary or tertiary)
Osteoporosis
Osteomalacia
Paget's disease
Multiple myeloma

Laboratory values may be particularly useful in differentiating among the afore-mentioned diseases, but the limitations of these parameters must be kept in mind. The biochemical indices and morphologic characteristics of the diseases may undergo spontaneous and independent variations. Thus a disease that characteristically shows an increased serum calcium may not show an increase during a regression of symptoms. Furthermore, variable factors—including diet, stress, and degree of physical activity—may influence these parameters, not to mention the day-to-day fluctuations due to variable technical factors in the laboratory. Then, too, concomitant systemic conditions may present confusing results if their interactions are not considered.

The serum alkaline phosphatase level is generally elevated during accelerated bone activity (whether resorption or apposition). It may be above normal in obstructive liver disease (jaundice), however, and often in nonjaundiced patients with liver damage and in pregnant women as well. Thus an increase is not always pathognomonic of increased bone activity. Consequently, although a high serum alkaline phosphatase level may suggest perhaps Paget's disease, biliary obstruction, or pregnancy, the history and cursory physical examination should also indicate which circumstance was responsible for this change in the patient's biochemistry.

The characteristic changes in the serum chemistry for some of the diseases discussed in this chapter are listed in Table 22-1.

6. *Fifty percent of the cases of multiple myeloma are positive for urinary Bence Jones protein.*

SPECIFIC REFERENCES

Allard, J. R., Landino, R. J., and Cerami, J. J.: Autogenous marrow-cancellous bone grafting in a patient with Hand-Schüller-Christian disease, J. Oral Surg. **36**:293-296, 1978.

Anderson, J. T., and Dehner, L. P.: Osteolytic form of Paget's disease, J. Bone Joint Surg. [Am.] **58**:994-1000, 1976.

Bartter, F. C.: Bone as a target organ: toward a better definition of osteoporosis, Perspect. Biol. Med. **16**:215-231, 1973.

Chernoff, A. I.: The hemoglobinopathies and thalassemia. In Beeson, P. B., and McDermott, W., editors: Textbook of medicine, ed. 2, Philadelphia, 1967, W. B. Saunders Co.

Conacher, W. D.: Metabolic bone disease in the elderly, Practitioner **210**:351-356, 1973.

Curtis, A. B.: Childhood leukemias: osseous changes in jaws on panoramic dental radiographs, J. Am. Dent. Assoc. **83**:844-847, 1971.

Duncan, H.: Osteoporosis in rheumatoid arthritis and corticosteroid-induced osteoporosis: symposium on metabolic bone disease, Orthop. Clin. North Am. **3**:571-583, 1972.

Fletcher, P. D., Scopp, I. W., and Hersh, R. A.: Oral manifestations of secondary hyperparathyroidism related to long-term hemodialysis therapy, Oral Surg. **43**:218-226, 1977.

Girasole, R. V., and Lyon, E. D.: Sickle cell osteomyelitis of the mandible: report of three cases, J. Oral Surg. **35**:231-234, 1977.

Goldsmith, R. S.: Laboratory aids in the diagnosis of metabolic bone disease, Orthop. Clin. North Am. **3**:545-560, 1972.

Jackson, C. E., and Frame, B.: Diagnosis and management of parathyroid disorders: symposium on metabolic bone disease, Orthop. Clin. North Am. **3**:699-712, 1972.

Jaworski, Z. F. G.: Pathophysiology, diagnosis, and treatment of osteomalacia: symposium on metabolic bone disease, Orthop. Clin. North Am. **3**:623-652, 1972.

Koutras, D. A., Pandros, P. G., Koukoulommati, A. S., and Constantes, J.: Radiological signs of bone loss in hyperthyroidism, Br. J. Radiol. **46**:695-698, 1973.

Lichtenstein, L.: Bone tumors, ed. 5, St. Louis, 1977, The C. V. Mosby Co.

Little, K.: Bone behavior, New York, 1973a, Academic Press.

Little, K.: Osteoporotic mechanisms, J. Int. Med. Res. **1**:509-529, 1973b.

Michaud, M., Baehner, R. L., Bixler, D., and Kafrawy, A. H.: Oral manifestations of acute leukemia in children, J. Am. Dent. Assoc. **95**:1145-1150, 1977.

Moseley, J. E.: Bone changes in hematologic disorders (roentgen aspects), New York, 1963, Grune & Stratton.

Mourshed, F., and Tuckson, C. R.: A study of the radiographic features of the jaws in sickle cell anemia, Oral Surg. **37**:812-819, 1974.

Nordin, B. E. C.: Metabolic bone and stone disease, Baltimore, 1973, The Williams & Wilkins Co.

Perriman, A. O., and Figures, K. H.: Metastatic retinoblastoma of the mandible, Oral Surg. **45**:741-748, 1978.

Poyton, H. G., and Davey, K. W.: Thalassemia: changes visible in radiographs used in dentistry, Oral Surg. **25**:564-576, 1968.

Rasmussen, H., and Brodier, P.: The physiological and cellular basis of metabolic bone disease, Baltimore, 1974, The Williams & Wilkins Co.

Reynolds, W. A., and Karo, J. J.: Radiologic diagnosis of metabolic bone disease: symposium on metabolic bone disease, Orthop. Clin. North Am. **3**:521-543, 1972.

Robinson, I. B., and Sarnat, S. G.: Roentgen studies of the maxilla and mandible in sickle cell anemia, Radiology **58**:517-523, 1952.

Sanger, R. G., and Bystrom, E. B.: Radiographic bone changes in sickle cell anemia, J. Oral Med. **32**:32-37, 1977.

Sanger, R. O., Greer, R. O., and Averbach, R. E.: Differential diagnosis of some simple osseous lesions associated with sickle cell anemia, Oral Surg. **43**:538-545, 1977.

Silverman, S., Ware, W. H., and Gillooly, C.: Dental aspects of hyperparathyroidism, Oral Surg. **26**:184-189, 1968.

Snapper, I.: Bone disease in medical practice, New York, 1957, Grune & Stratton.

Stafne, E. C.: Oral roentgenographic diagnosis, ed. 3, Philadelphia, 1969, W. B. Saunders Co.

Van Slyck, E. J.: The bony changes in malignant hematologic disease: symposium on metabolic bone disease, Orthop. Clin. North Am. **3**:733-744, 1972.

Walsh, R. F., and Karmiol, M.: Oral roentgenographic findings in osteitis fibrosa generalisata associated with chronic renal disease, Oral Surg. **28**:273-281, 1969.

Watson, L.: Endocrine bone disease, Practitioner **210**:376-383, 1973.

Williamson, J. J.: Blood dyscrasias. In Gorlin, R. J., and Goldman, H. M., editors: Thoma's oral pathology, ed. 6, St. Louis, 1970, The C. V. Mosby Co., vol. 2.

Worth, H. M.: Principles and practice of oral radiologic interpretation, Chicago, 1963, Year Book Medical Publishers.

Worth, H. M.: Some significant radiographic appearances in young jaws, Oral Surg. **21**:609-617, 1966.

GENERAL REFERENCES

Adatia, A. K.: Significance of jaw lesions in Burkitt's lymphoma, Br. Dent. J. **145**:263-266, 1978.

Alexander, W. N., and Bechtold, W. A.: Alpha thalassemia minor trait accompanied by clinical oral signs, Oral Surg. **43**:892-897, 1977.

Atkinson, P. J., and Woodhead, C.: The development of osteoporosis: a hypothesis based on a study of human bone structure, Clin. Orthop. **90**:217-228, 1973.

Baylink, D. J., Wergedal, J. E., Yamamoto, K., and Manzke, E.: Systemic factors in alveolar bone loss, J. Prosthet. Dent. **31**:486-505, 1974.

Beumer, J., Trowbridge, H. O., Silverman, S., and Eisenberg, E.: Childhood hypophosphatasia and the premature loss of teeth, Oral Surg. **35**:631-640, 1973.

Bildman, B., Martinez, M., and Robinson, L. H.: Gaucher's disease discovered by mandibular biopsy: report of case, J. Oral Surg. **30**:510-512, 1972.

Cardo, N. A., and Zambito, R. F.: Burkitt's lymphoma: report of case in New York City, J. Oral Surg. **30**:138-142, 1972.

Caudill, R., Saltzman, D., Guam, S., and Granite, E.: Possible relationship of primary hyperparathyroidism and fibrous dysplasia: report of case, J. Oral Surg. **35**:482-490, 1977.

Choremis, C., Liakakos, D., Tsoghi, C., and Moschovakis, C.: Pathogenesis of osseous lesions in thalassemia, J. Pediatr. **66**:962-963, 1965.

Garn, S. M.: The course of bone gain and the phase of bone loss: symposium on metabolic bone disease, Orthop. Clin. North Am. **3**:503-520, 1972.

Goldsmith, R. S.: Laboratory aids in the diagnosis of metabolic bone disease: symposium on metabolic bone disease, Orthop. Clin. North Am. **3**:545-570, 1972.

Hammer, W. S., Soni, N. N., and Fraleigh, C. M.: Quantitative study of bone activity in the diabetic rat mandible: triple fluorochrome study, Oral Surg. **35**:718-729, 1973.

Hays, G. L.: Nuclear characteristics of buccal mucosa cells in sickle-cell anemia, Oral Surg. **43**:554-561, 1977.

Houston, J. B., Dolan, K. D., Appleby, R. C., et al.: Radiography of secondary hyperparathyroidism, Oral Surg. **26**:746-750, 1968.

Joncas, J., and Rioux, E.: Burkitt's lymphoma of the jaw in a Canadian child, Can. Med. Assoc. J. **117**(4):367-368, 1977.

Kalish, S. R.: Hyperthyroid osteoporosis: a case study in differential diagnosis, J. Am. Podiatry Assoc. **64**:35-45, 1974.

Koutras, D. A., Pandos, P. G., Koukoulommati, A. S., and Constantes, J.: Radiological signs of bone loss in hyperthyroidism, Br. J. Radiol. **46**:695-698, 1973.

Macchia, A. F., and Cassalia, P. T.: Primary hyperparathyroidism: report of case, J. Am. Dent. Assoc. **81**:1153-1155, 1970.

Meunier, P. J., Bianchi, G. G. S., Edouard, C. M., et al.: Bony manifestations of thyrotoxicosis: symposium on metabolic bone disease, Orthop. Clin. North Am. **3**:745-774, 1972.

Murphy, J. B., Doku, H. C., and Carter, B. L.: Massive osteolysis: phantom bone disease, J. Oral Surg. **36**(4):318-322, 1978.

Nathan, A. S., Traiger, J., and Berman, S. A.: Secondary hyperparathyroidism as a cause of generalized enlargement of the maxialla and the mandible, Oral Surg. **21**:724-731, 1966.

Phillips, R. M., Bush, O. B., and Hall, D. H.: Massive osteolysis (phantom bone, disappearing bone): report of case with mandibular involvement, Oral Surg. **34**:886-896, 1972.

Sanner, J. R., and Ramin, J. E.: Osteoporotic, hematopoietic mandibular marrow of defect: an osseous manifestation of sickle cell anemia, J. Oral Surg. **35**:986-988, 1977.

Schindel, J., Matz, S., Edlan, A., and Abraham, A.: Central cavernous hemangioma of the jaws, J. Oral Surg. **36**:803-807, 1978.

Scott, J., and Finch, L. D.: Histiocytosis X with oral lesions: report of case, J. Oral Surg. **30**:748-753, 1972.

Sela, M. N., and Pisanti, S.: Early diagnosis and treatment of patients with leukemia, a dental problem, J. Oral Med. **32**:46-50, 1977.

Shepherd, J. P.: The management of the oral complications of leukemia, Oral Surg. **45**:543-548, 1978.

Sidhu, S. S., Sukhija, D. S., and Parkash, H.: Burkitt's lymphoma, Oral Surg. **39**:463-468, 1975.

Sippel, H. W., and Samartano, J. G.: Leukemia manifested as lymphosarcoma of the mandible: report of case, J. Oral Surg. **29**:363-366, 1971.

Stern, M. H., and Cole, W. L.: Radiographic changes in the mandible associated with leukemic infiltration in a case of acute myelogenous leukemia, Oral Surg. **36**:343-346, 1973.

Terezhalmy, G. T., Fletman, R., and Bottomly, W. T.: Initial evidence of primary hyperparathyroidism presenting in the mouth: a case report, J. Oral Med. **33**:4-8, 1978.

Terril, D. G., Lee, A., Le Donne, M. A., and Nusbaum, T. G.: American Burkitt's lymphoma in Pittsburgh, Pennsylvania, Oral Surg. **44**:411-418, 1977.

Warren, R.: Osteoporosis, J. Oral Med. **32**:113-119, 1977.

Section B · **Radiolucent lesions with radiopaque foci or mixed radiolucent and radiopaque lesions**

The normal anatomic structures and disease states that produce mixed radiolucent-radiopaque images on radiographs are especially challenging since there is such a wide variety of normal and pathologic conditions that can produce them.

It is especially instructive to note that several of the radiolucent-radiopaque lesions in this group represent intermediate stages in the development or maturation of more opaque lesions—that is to say, a particular pathologic entity may commence as an osteolytic lesion, which shows as a radiolucency on the radiograph; during its development, foci of calcified material may form within the osteolytic area; and when these foci become large enough and sufficiently mineralized, they will become radiographically apparent. Thus the mixed radiolucent-radiopaque condition frequently represents an intermediate stage in the development of the lesion.

Often maturation or mineralization will continue until most of the lesion, with the possible exception of a thin radiolucent rim, becomes opaque.

The outstanding feature that makes this group especially interesting is the close correlation between the radiographic appearance and the microstructure of the individual lesions.

Histologically all the lesions in the radiolucent-radiopaque stage contain calcified areas of either hard tooth tissue (or bone) or nondescript mineralized material. In a few instances the radiopacities will be hazy and poorly defined and microscopic examination will show that they are not produced by calcified material but by dense composites of fibrous tissue. This effect will be even more pronounced when the lesion is large and causes a buccolingual expansion of the mandible (see Fig. 23-14).

The response of bone to some extrinsic state or to frank bone disease may, however, cause a sclerosis without an initial radiographically apparent osteolytic stage. The influence of the disease state on the bone will then be mild and the primary effect will be stimulation of osteoblastic activity, resulting in a bony sclerosis. These sclerosed regions usually appear as radiopacities within (and not sharply demarcated from) normal-appearing bone.

23

Mixed radiolucent-radiopaque lesions associated with teeth

Norman K. Wood
Paul W. Goaz

The following are mixed radiolucent-radiopaque lesions associated with teeth:

Periapical mixed lesions
Calcifying crown of developing tooth
Tooth root with rarefying osteitis
Rarefying and condensing osteitis
Periapical cementoma (intermediate)
Cementifying and/or ossifying fibroma
Rarities
    Calcifying and keratinizing odontogenic cyst
    Cementoblastoma (intermediate)
    Foreign bodies
    Generalized (nodular cemental masses; Paget's disease)
    Odontoma (intermediate)

Pericoronal mixed lesions
Odontoma (intermediate)
Adenomatoid odontogenic tumor
Keratinizing and calcifying odontogenic cyst
Ameloblastic fibro-odontoma
Calcifying epithelial odontogenic tumor
Odontogenic fibroma
Rarities
    Ameloblastic fibrodentinoma
    Cystic odontoma

Periapical mixed lesions

CALCIFYING CROWN OF DEVELOPING TOOTH

The radiographic appearance of crypts containing tooth germs in early stages of development is discussed in Chapter 18, where it is stated that they appear as cystlike radiolucencies. The cusp tips are the first part of the developing tooth to calcify; and as soon as sufficient mineral is deposited in the matrix of the cusp tips to make them radiographically apparent, the developing tooth can be recognized as a radiolucency with radiopaque foci (Fig. 23-1). Thus the intermedi-

ate stage of tooth formation may be imprudently mistaken for a mixed radiolucent-radiopaque lesion.

Presumably the clinician trained to interpret radiographs of the jaws would not make this error since he would expect to encounter such normal structures in the radiographs of patients under 20 years of age. In unusual cases, however, third molar tooth buds may develop later than 20 years of age and the development of the maxillary second premolar buds may be delayed until about the eleventh year.

Prior to calcification, permanent tooth buds may appear in the periapical regions of deciduous teeth and in a few months undergo sufficient mineralization to appear as periapical radiolucencies with radiopaque foci. The clinician should therefore be familiar with the normal positions, chronologies, and radiographic appearances of the tooth buds of calcifying crowns. If there is a question, he can compare the appearances of the developing contralateral teeth to confirm the identity of these calcifying crowns.

493

Fig. 23-1. Calcifying crowns of developing teeth. **A,** Mandibular right second premolar. **B,** Mandibular left third molar.

Fig. 23-2. Root tip with accompanying rarefying osteitis.

The radiographic appearance in an isolated case may not be definite enough to allow the clinician to make a firm diagnosis of calcifying crown (e.g., when the developing tooth's formation or calcification is delayed, when the tooth is not in its normal position, or when the tooth is supernumerary and not immediately identifiable). Periodic radiographs will then reveal the true nature of the suspicious-looking region as the form of the calcifying crown becomes more typical on subsequent radiographs.

TOOTH ROOT WITH RAREFYING OSTEITIS

Retained roots and root tips are the most common abnormal radiopacities found in edentulous regions of the jaws. Retained roots may be present in the jaws of one of every four edentulous persons; 80% of these retained roots will be in the posterior region of the jaws, and 6% of all retained root tips will be associated with radiolucent areas. (This latter statistic is a corollary to the observation that the root canal of a retained root is frequently continuous with the oral cavity at its coronal end. Thus the root canal may become the channel for infection, with a resulting

rarefying osteitis in the periapex and the production of a radiolucent-radiopaque jaw lesion. Such root tips are surrounded by granulation tissue; and they may be totally asymptomatic, or the patient may complain of intermittent slight pain or swelling. When the patient's resistance becomes depressed, an acute infection may ensue and produce a fluctuant painful smooth-surfaced mass (abscess).

Microscopically a section of the lesion will show chronic granulation tissue about a cross section of the tooth root with perhaps a purulent root canal.

Identification of the retained root will be relatively easy when the shape of the root has persisted along with the linear radiolucent shadow of the root canal, a portion of the periodontal membrane space, and the surrounding lamina dura. In other instances, however, when the root fragment has been resorbed to some extent, the root canal is not discernible, the lamina dura is no longer present, and chronic inflammation has produced a rarefaction of the surrounding bone (Fig. 23-2), the clinician's diagnostic problem will be more difficult.

DIFFERENTIAL DIAGNOSIS

Root tips that are atypical in appearance (partially resorbed with the root canal and lamina dura obscured) and surrounded by rarefying osteitis may be confused with an intermediate-stage cementoma or odontoma, a chronic osteomyelitis, an ossifying fibroma, an osteogenic sarcoma, a chondrosarcoma, or a metastatic osteoblastic carcinoma. If recent preextraction radiographs are available, however, they will usually aid in identifying the lesion as a root tip.

The *metastatic osteoblastic carcinoma, chon-*

drosarcoma, and *osteogenic sarcoma* may share two common characteristics with a retained root tip whose identity is obscured by rarefying osteitis: local discomfort and a radiolucency with usually ill-defined ragged margins. The malignant tumors will all show moderate to rapid growth, as evidenced by an enlargement of the region that becomes evident within a few weeks. An acute abscess originating from an infected root tip, however, will usually increase rapidly in size within a few days and become quite painful, inflamed, and perhaps fluctuant. If the infection is chronic, a draining sinus will probably develop. A medical history indicating that the patient has a primary malignancy elsewhere or has symptoms suggesting such a tumor will, of course, prompt the examiner to suspect a metastatic osteoblastic tumor.

If the patient has no predisposing systemic disease and no history of trauma to the area and if the lesion is in the maxilla, then *osteomyelitis* may be assigned a low rank in the differential diagnosis. Also an absence of pain, swelling, or drainage will further deemphasize osteomyelitis.

If the patient is over 20 years of age, the radiolucent-radiopaque lesion is not likely to be an *odontoma* that has yet to develop beyond the intermediate stage.

The radiopacities in fibro-osseous lesions of periodontal ligament origin (PDLO) (e.g., a *cementoma*) are frequently multiple and have a more uneven density and a less well-defined outline than do those of root tips. Thus the clinician would be influenced to assign a low rank to this entity in the list of possible diagnoses. Also, if the lesion is single, asymptomatic, and situated in the maxilla or the molar region of a white man, it is unlikely to be a cementoma. Furthermore, in contrast to the margins of the radiolucency surrounding an infected root tip, which are usually poorly defined and somewhat ragged, the radiolucent margins about a cementoma will be well defined and smoothly contoured.

On the basis of incidence alone, the working diagnosis for a relatively small well-defined smoothly outlined homogeneously dense radiopaque image surrounded by an ill-defined ragged radiolucency in a tooth-bearing area of the jaws would be a root tip surrounded by rarefying osteitis.

MANAGEMENT

Retained root tips that are infected should be removed. If an acute abscess is present, it should be incised, drained, cultured, and irrigated at least twice daily and the patient should be given suitable antibiotic therapy. After the infection has subsided, the root tip and surrounding soft tissue should be removed, the bone defect curetted, and the tissue microscopically examined.

RAREFYING AND CONDENSING OSTEITIS

Frequently a chronic infection in the jawbone, precipitated by a nonvital tooth or a retained root, will induce both a rarefying and a condensing osteitis (Fig. 23-3). The chronic infection thus acts as an irritating factor (causing resorption of bone) and as a stimulating factor (producing denser bone)—perhaps as a defense mechanism to contain the local problem.

Bone resorption occurs where the irritating products of the chronic infection are most concentrated (i.e., about the apex), whereas bone apposition occurs some distance from this point (at the periphery of the rarefying lesion). The diffusion of the irritating products of the infection through the tissues results in their alteration or dilution, and they then induce osteoblastic activity and sclerosis at the periphery of the osteolytic area.

When the chronic infection has run a steady course, a reasonably well-defined somewhat homogeneous radiopacity is seen more or less circumscribing the radiolucency around the root end (Fig. 26-3). When the course of the chronic infection is punctuated by acute exacerbations, however, the radiographic picture will be less orderly and the sclerosis more diffuse and less homogeneous.

FEATURES, DIFFERENTIAL DIAGNOSIS, AND MANAGEMENT

Features, differential diagnosis, and management of rarefying and condensing osteitis are similar to those discussed for a root tip with rarefying osteitis. Further discussion of the differential diagnosis may be found in the differential diagnosis sections under benign fibro-osseous lesions of periodontal ligament origin (p. 498) and the intermediate stage of odontoma (p. 504).

PERIAPICAL CEMENTOMA— INTERMEDIATE STAGE

The periapical cementoma is thought to be a reactive phenomenon that arises from elements within the periodontal ligament (Hamner et al., 1968; Waldron and Giansanti, 1973a and b).

The cementoma or periapical cemental dysplasia is discussed in Chapter 16 as a periapical

Fig. 23-3. Combined periapical rarefying and condensing osteitis. The teeth in the three cases were nonvital. Note that the rarefying osteitis contacts the root end and that the condensing osteitis (radiopaque halo) is located around the periphery of the rarefied area.

radiolucency, in Chapter 18 as a cystlike radiolucency, and in Chapter 26 as a periapical radiopacity. In this chapter the emphasis will be on its intermediate radiolucent-radiopaque stage, which embraces a spectrum of radiographic appearances between the totally radiolucent and the mature radiopaque stage (Figs. 23-4 and 23-5).

FEATURES

Cementomas most often occur in the periapices of vital teeth; but they may also be found elsewhere in either jaw, as a solitary lesion and as multiple lesions. Approximately 90% occur in the mandible, usually in the anterior region. They are seldom if ever found in the anterior maxilla. They have a higher predilection for women (approximately 80%) and for blacks. They may vary in size from a few millimeters to several centimeters in diameter; and they seldom occur before 30 years of age. They will ordinarily be asymptomatic; and the usual periapical lesion seldom grows large enough to expand the jaw, but in rare cases some may.

The initial lesion of the cementoma is osteo-

lytic; and as it matures, particles or spicules of calcified material develop in the cystlike radiolucency (Figs. 23-4 and 23-5). When these foci of calcification become radiographically apparent, the lesion is considered to be in its intermediate stage of maturation. The size, shape, number, and discreteness of the contained radiopacities vary greatly from lesion to lesion and from patient to patient as the calcified components become larger and coalesce and the lesion becomes more radiopaque.

Regardless of its stage of development, the cementoma will usually have well-defined, smoothly contoured, radiolucent borders (Figs. 23-4 and 23-5). Sometimes sclerosis will be induced in the bone at the periphery of the radiolucent border and will show on the radiograph as a hyperostotic margin.

The microscopic picture reflects what is seen on the radiograph. At the intermediate stage a cementoma is made up of a fibroblastic-type matrix that is moderately vascular and contains a varied number of calcified zones of cementum or bone, or cementum and bone in varying com-

Fig. 23-4. Intermediate-stage fibro-osseous lesions (PDLO). **A** to **C,** Cementomas in periapices of teeth with vital pulps.

Fig. 23-5. Intermediate-stage fibro-osseous lesions (PDLO). **A,** Cementoma. **B,** Microscopy showing the small separate masses of acellular cementum characteristic of cementomas. (**A** courtesy M. Smulson, D.D.S., Maywood, Ill.)

binations (Fig. 23-5). The cementum may be distinguished from bone by the differences in width and pattern of the intrinsic collagenous bundles under polarized light (Waldron and Giansanti, 1973a).

DIFFERENTIAL DIAGNOSIS

The following entities should be included in the differential diagnosis of the intermediate stage of cementoma: rarefying osteitis in combination with condensing osteitis, chronic osteomyelitis, fibrous dysplasia, calcifying crowns, ossifying and cementifying fibroma, postsurgical calcifying bone defect, odontoma (intermediate stage), juxtaposed pericoronal mixed lesions, osteogenic sarcoma, chondrosarcoma, and metastatic osteoblastic carcinoma.

The cementomas are slow growing, which distinguishes them from the more rapidly growing malignant *metastatic osteoblastic carcinoma, chondrosarcoma,* and *osteogenic sarcoma.* Like the cementomas these malignancies may appear as mixed radiolucent-radiopaque lesions; but unlike the smooth well-defined fibro-osseous lesions, they are usually irregular and ill-defined. Furthermore, these malignancies (together with the chondroma) frequently cause root resorption whereas the cementomas characteristically do not.

The mass or masses of calcified material within an *intermediate-stage odontoma,* especially the compound variety, will frequently show a somewhat orderly relationship of the radiodense enamel to the dentin and pulp spaces. The *complex odontoma,* on the other hand, will be more difficult to recognize because the hard dental tissues may be so disorganized that they appear as irregular masses of calcified material. Even in these lesions, however, the more radiopaque enamel component may be discernible and will frequently provide a clue to the true identity of the lesion. In addition, the odontoma is usually located above the crown of an unerupted tooth, sometimes between teeth but seldom in the periapex.

The scattered calcifying foci in a *healing postsurgical bone defect* may be identified by a history of a recent enucleation.

Calcifying crowns, which are present in the jaws of patients in the first and second decades, are easily identified by their anticipated location in the jaw, the radiographically distinguishable tissues of the tooth, and usually the presence of a similar picture in the contralateral jaw.

After these considerations the working diagnosis will be narrowed to periapical cementoma, cementifying and ossifying fibroma, rarefying osteitis combined with condensing osteitis, chronic osteomyelitis, and fibrous dysplasia.

The current generally accepted concept of *fibrous dysplasia* of the jaws poses several glaring dissimilarities between this entity and the fibro-osseous lesions originating from the periodontal ligament (the cementoma and the cementifying and ossifying fibroma; PDLO):

1. Fibrous dysplasia is slightly more common in the maxilla, whereas 90% of fibro-osseous lesions (PDLO) are found in the mandible.
2. Fibrous dysplasia has a definite tendency to develop during the first and second decades of life, whereas the periapical cementoma is seldom observed in people who are under 30 years of age.
3. Fibrous dysplasia affects men and women equally whereas the cementoma has a high predilection for women.
4. Jaw expansion caused by lesions of fibrous dysplasia is usually of the elongated fusiform type, whereas jaw expansion caused by fibro-osseous lesions (PDLO) is less common and is usually more nodular or dome shaped.
5. The radiographic borders of the lesions of fibrous dysplasia are characteristically poorly defined (i.e., merge imperceptibly with normal bone), whereas the radiographic borders of fibro-osseous lesions (PDLO) are well defined (Waldon and Giansanti, 1973b).

Application of these characteristics should enable the clinician to distinguish between most of the lesions of fibrous dysplasia and lesions of PDLO he will encounter.

Fibrous dysplasia containing only mottled areas of calcification will be more difficult to differentiate; but the fact that this mottled appearance represents an immature stage seldom seen in persons older than 20 years will be helpful to the differentiation.

Of course, if the patient is a young girl with a known case of Albright's syndrome and has jaw lesions, the clinician would have to rank fibrous dysplasia as a likely diagnosis.

If the lesions are periapical and the tooth is vital, then the possibility that a pathosis has resulted from an infection of a root canal, such as might produce the combination of *rarefying* and condensing *osteitis* and *chronic osteomyelitis,* will be minimized. The absence of pain, drainage, inflammation, and tenderness to palpation plus no regional lymphadenitis will further prompt the examiner to assign a lower ranking to these entities, which are a direct result of infection. In addition, it is helpful to consider that in cases of combined periapical rarefying and condensing osteitis, the radiolucent zone always lies next to the root end while the radiopaque zone (condensing) forms a halo outside the radiolucency.

It may be difficult to differentiate between a periapical cementoma and a cementifying and/or ossifying fibroma because both lesions occur at the apices of vital teeth, are basically round in shape with well-defined borders, and mature through the three stages. It is necessary to differentiate between the two lesions because the cementifying and/or ossifying fibroma is a potentially troublesome lesion requiring excision while the periapical cementoma seldom requires removal.

The following clues are helpful: the periapical cementoma (1) is a common lesion, (2) has a predilection for the lower incisor teeth, (3) has a marked predilection for females, (4) almost invariably affects patients over 30 years of age, (5) seldom attains a diameter of over 1 cm, (6) seldom produces clinically discernible expansion, and (7) often occurs as multiple lesions. In contrast, the ossifying fibroma (1) is an uncommon lesion, (2) has a predilection for the premolar-molar area of the mandible, (3) affects males and females equally, (4) occurs in patients who on the average are less than 30 years of age (26.4 years), (5) frequently attains a diameter of 2 to 4 cm (Fig. 23-6), (6) frequently produces a clinically discernible expansion, and (7) occurs as a single lesion.

Occasionally unerupted malposed teeth with a mixed radiolucent-radiopaque lesion will be positioned in such a fashion that the mixed image contacts the periapex of neighboring teeth (Fig. 23-10). The diagnostician then faces the dilemma of whether the lesion was primarily a periapical lesion or a pericoronal lesion. The correct decision in such a case often greatly facilitates the differential diagnosis process. Additional radiographic views frequently will separate the lesion from either the periapex or from the crown of the unerupted tooth.

CEMENTIFYING AND/OR OSSIFYING FIBROMA

The cementifying and/or ossifying fibromas are thought to be uncommon neoplastic processes that originate from elements in the periodontal ligament (Waldron and Giansanti, 1973a and b). Hamner and co-workers (1968) explained that under a variety of stimuli, cells of the periodontal ligament are capable of producing lesions comprised of cementum, lamellar bone, fibrous tissue, or any combination of these tissues. Traditionally if a certain lesion contained only bony spicules and fibrous elements it would be recog-

Fig. 23-6. Ossifying fibroma. Large well-marginated radiolucent lesion with radiopaque foci involving the roots of the mandibular second molar tooth. (Courtesy W. Schoenheider, D.D.S., Oak Lawn, Ill.)

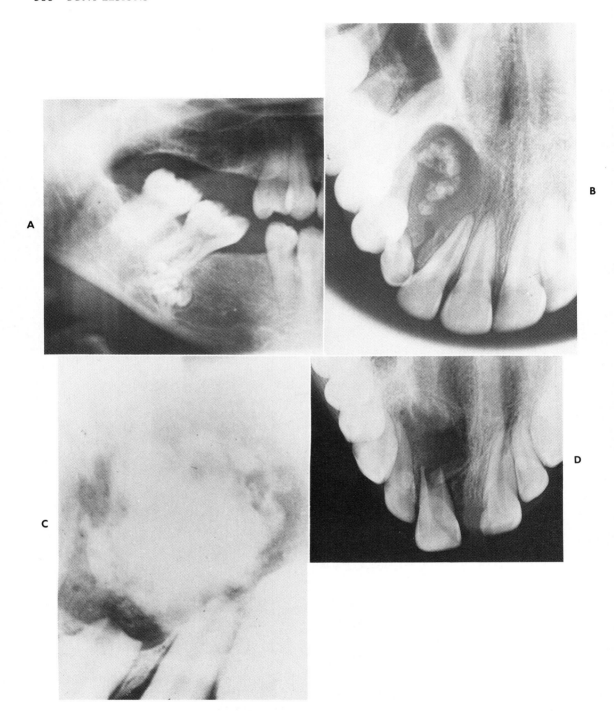

Fig. 23-7. Rare periapical mixed lesions. **A,** Compound odontoma at the apices of a second molar tooth—a most unusual location. **B** and **C,** Calcifying odontogenic cysts. **B,** In the canine region of a 14-year-old girl. **C,** In the maxillary incisor region the unusually radiopaque lesion has caused root resorption. **D,** A mixed radiolucent-radiopaque lesion at the apex of the nonvital central incisor. The lesion was basically a pulpoperiapical lesion and the rectangular radiopaque image was the mesial segment of the crown of the other central incisor, which had been broken off in a traumatic incident and driven up into the tissue.

Fig. 23-7, cont'd. E, Several radiopaque foci (root canal–filling material) within a periapical radiolucency. (**B** from Seeliger, J. E., and Regneke, J. P.: J. Oral Surg. **36:**469-472, 1978. Copyright by the American Dental Association. Reprinted by permission. **C** courtesy K. Kennedy, D.D.S., Chicago. **E** courtesy M. Smulsen, D.D.S., Maywood, Ill.)

nized as an ossifying fibroma. Conversely if the lesion contained only cemental and fibrous tissue it would be called a cementifying fibroma. If the lesion contained a mixture of cementum and bone in a fibrous tissue stroma it would be recognized as a cemento-ossifying fibroma. It is understood that these are three subclassifications of otherwise identical lesions.

FEATURES

The cementifying and ossifying fibromas usually occur as periapical lesions that are basically round and well marginated (Fig. 23-6). Seventy percent occur in the mandible primarily in the premolar-molar region. The average age of patients with ossifying fibroma is 26.4 years, and the sexes are approximately equally affected (Hamner et al., 1968). These authors stated that the age range was from 7 to 58 years. These lesions usually occur as solitary entities, go unnoticed when small, and frequently reach a size of 2 to 4 cm, expanding the jaws as they grow.

DIFFERENTIAL DIAGNOSIS

The differential diagnosis of cementifying and ossifying fibromas is discussed under the differential diagnosis section of periapical cementomas.

MANAGEMENT

The usual periapical cementoma that is not large enough to produce an expansion of the jawbone does not require treatment. Nevertheless, the clinician should periodically examine such lesions radiographically to be certain that the mixed radiolucent-radiopaque area is not enlarging. If a good portion of a lesion has become calcified, this is an indication that the lesion is mature and is not likely to increase in size.

Few fibro-osseous lesions (PDLO) become large enough to produce an expansion of the cortical plate. These should be conservatively enucleated, and the tissue microscopically examined to establish the final diagnosis. Attempts should be made to conserve teeth in the region. If an unusually large lesion is permitted to grow, pathologic fracture may become a threat. Sometimes, when the lesion has been permitted to grow and expand peripherally until subjected to trauma, the overlying mucosa has become ulcerated and a secondary osteomyelitis developed in the fibro-osseous lesion.

RARE PERIAPICAL MIXED LESIONS

There is a vast array of rare lesions and also lesions that are common but rarely appear to be primarily associated with the periapex. For instance, a mixed periapical lesion seen at the root end of a tooth in a periapical film could represent a generalized condition such as sclerosing cemental masses or Paget's disease. Fig. 23-7 illustrates some of the rare mixed periapical lesions.

Pericoronal mixed lesions

ODONTOMA—INTERMEDIATE STAGE

The odontoma is a benign tumor containing all the various component tissues of teeth. It is the most common odontogenic tumor, representing 67% of all odontogenic tumors in the series reported by Regezi and co-workers (1978). They seem to result from a budding of extra odontogenic epithelial cells from the dental lamina. This cluster of cells forms a large mass of tooth tissue that may be deposited in an abnormal arrangement but consists of normal enamel, dentin, cementum, and pulp.

The compound odontoma comprises odontogenic tissues laid down in a normal relationship, and the resulting structure bears considerable morphologic resemblance to teeth. When the tooth components are less well organized and toothlike structures are not formed, however, the lesion is termed a "complex" odontoma. Some tumors are a combination of both types (i.e., they contain not only multiple toothlike structures but also calcified masses of dental tissue in haphazard arrangement). Such lesions are called "compound-complex" odontomas. Another type, the ameloblastic odontoma, is an uncommon tumor and basically represents what the name implies.

In its development the odontoma passes through the same stages as does a developing tooth. Thus, as the odontogenic tissues are laid down and proliferate, there is a resorption of bone so the lesion is radiolucent. An intermediate stage then follows that, because of the partial calcification of the odontogenic tissues, is characterized by a radiolucent-radiopaque image. This process continues to the most radiopaque stage, in which the calcification of the dental tissues is completed.

The early or intermediate stages of the developing odontoma are usually not seen or recognized as often as is the late stage presumably because the earlier lesions are not clinically apparent. Also the formation of odontomas begins in children when the natural dentition is developing, and routine radiographs are rarely done of patients at this age. The intermediate or mixed radiolucent-radiopaque stage in the development of the odontoma is stressed in the present chapter (Figs. 23-8 and 23-9).

FEATURES

The most common complaint of a patient with an odontoma relates to the delayed eruption of a permanent tooth. Some odontomas, however, produce no accompanying symptoms and are discovered on routine radiographic examination.

The compound variety is more common than is

Fig. 23-8. Intermediate-stage odontoma. **A** and **C,** Compound. Note the washer effect produced by partial calcification of the teeth in **A. B,** Compound-complex causing impaction of the molar. (**A** courtesy M. Dettmer, D.D.S., Wheaton, Ill. **B** courtesy R. Latronica, D.D.S., Albany, N.Y.)

the complex, and 62% occur in the maxilla, having a predilection for the incisor-canine region but no sex bias (Minderjahn, 1979). The complex odontoma, on the other hand, is more common in the mandible, and approximately 70% of these tumors are located in the first and second molar areas. About 68% of complex odontomas occur in females (Minderjahn, 1979).

The majority of lesions are almost completely radiopaque when discovered in the second and

third decades of life, which has led to the conclusion that the early and intermediate stages appear at a younger age. The lesions are nonaggressive; and although most measure between 1 and 3 cm in diameter, occasionally one will reach a much larger size and cause extensive asymmetry of the jaw.

A complex odontoma is frequently situated between the crown of an unerupted tooth and the crest of the ridge, thus effectively blocking the

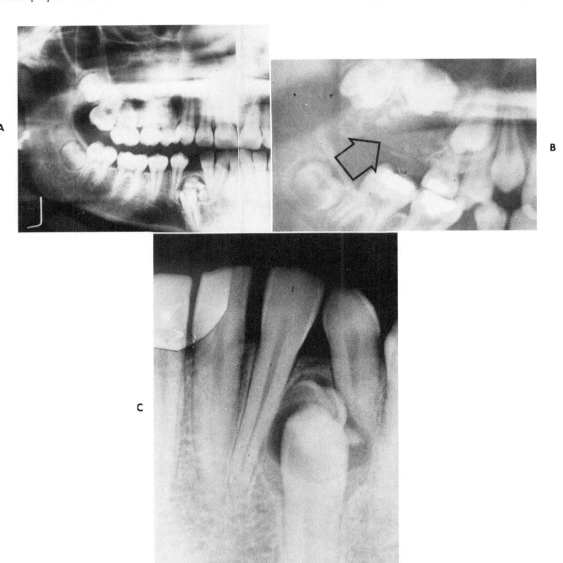

Fig. 23-9. A to **C,** Pericoronal, intermediate-stage odontomas associated with an impacted mandibular canine. **B,** Minimal calcification has occurred in this odontoma located pericoronally in the maxillary first and second molar region. (**A** courtesy J. Ireland and J. Dolce, Chicago. **B** courtesy W. Schoenheider, D.D.S., Oak Lawn, Ill.)

tooth's eruption. For this reason the clinician should secure radiographs of the area when a tooth's eruption has been delayed. In the intermediate stage it may be seen as a mixed pericoronal lesion (Figs. 23-8 and 23-9).

Radiographically the intermediate-stage compound odontoma will show as a well-defined radiolucent lesion containing varying numbers of radiopaque (washerlike) cross sections of developing teeth and longitudinal hollow radiopaque shadows of developing teeth (Figs. 23-8 and 23-9). The degree of calcification and opacity will vary from stage to stage and from lesion to lesion. The complex odontoma will be seen as a well-defined radiolucency with many radiopaque foci that vary greatly in size, shape, and prominence (Figs. 23-8 and 23-9).

Microscopically the compound odontoma will correspond to the histologic structure of normal teeth, whereas the intermediate stage of a complex odontoma will reveal deposits of dentin, enamel, enamel matrix, cementum, and pulp tissue arranged in a completely haphazard relationship.

DIFFERENTIAL DIAGNOSIS

The *compound odontoma* seldom presents a problem in differential diagnosis, even in the intermediate stage, because of its characteristic radiographic appearance. Despite this statement, however, on microscopic examination a particular tumor may show areas of ameloblastic proliferation and thus prove to be an *ameloblastic odontoma*. It is impossible to distinguish these two lesions clinically, radiographically, or on the basis of the history.

On the contrary, the *complex odontoma* in its intermediate stage may mimic several other lesions: fibro-osseous lesions (PDLO), calcifying odontogenic cyst, adenomatoid odontogenic tumor (intermediate stage), calcifying epithelial odontogenic tumor, postsurgical calcifying bone defect, fibrous dysplasia, rarefying osteitis with condensing osteitis, chronic osteomyelitis.

Chronic osteomyelitis and *rarefying osteitis* with *condensing osteitis* may be initially ruled out because of the absence of pain, tenderness, inflammation, drainage, or regional lymphadenopathy. The radiographic margins of these entities are usually poorly defined and roughly contoured whereas the radiolucent borders of the complex odontoma are as well contoured and defined as the margins of a crypt about a developing tooth. Periodic radiographs of untreated infectious lesions will frequently show the lesions to

be increasing in size whereas the complex odontoma will not increase in size after calcification of the odontogenic tissues has commenced.

Even when it appears mottled or has a smoky pattern on the radiograph, *fibrous dysplasia* has poorly defined borders so it can be deemphasized as a possible diagnosis.

These comparisons will narrow the clinician's working diagnosis to include fibro-osseous lesions (PDLO), calcifying odontogenic cyst, adenomatoid odontogenic tumor, calcifying epithelial odontogenic tumor, and postsurgical calcifying bony defect. All these entities will produce well-defined radiolucencies containing radiopaque foci that may be located pericoronally.

The *postsurgical calcifying defect* is easily eliminated if there is not a recent surgical procedure in the patient's history.

The *calcifying epithelial odontogenic tumor (CEOT)* (Pindborg tumor) is the rarest of these conditions. Unlike the odontoma, which develops in the first and second decades of life, the average age for the patient with a CEOT is 40.41 years (Franklin and Pindborg, 1976). Like the complex odontoma the molar region of the mandible is the preferred site and a large percentage are associated with unerupted teeth. In the light of this information a radiolucency with radiopaque foci associated with the crown of an unerupted mandibular molar tooth in a child or adolescent is much more likely to be an intermediate-stage odontoma than a CEOT. After a considerable amount of mineralization has taken place in the odontoma the differentiation would be easier because the CEOT does not often produce large dense masses of calcified tissue.

In its intermediate stage of development, the *adenomatoid odontogenic tumor* is radiographically indistinguishable from the fibro-osseous lesions (PDLO), the calcifying odontogenic cyst, and the complex odontoma; and like the odontoma it occurs most often in the first two decades. Unlike the complex odontoma, however, which is relatively common and is most often found in the molar region of the mandible, the adenomatoid odontogenic tumor is not common and is found usually in the anterior maxilla.

The *calcifying odontogenic cyst*, like the adenomatoid odontogenic tumor, is not a common lesion and 75% occur anterior to the first molars. Also 47% occur in patients below 31 years of age. Like the complex odontoma it has a predilection for the mandible. The aspiration test is often helpful in differentiating the calcifying odontogenic cyst from the odontoma. Whereas aspiration of a calcifying odontogenic cyst may yield a thick granular yellow fluid (keratin), aspiration of an odontoma will be nonproductive.

In the intermediate stage of development, a *fibro-osseous lesion (PDLO)* will share several characteristics with a complex odontoma: both usually develop in the mandible, both are asymptomatic (except in unusual instances when they attain a large size), and both may have a similar radiographic appearance at this stage of development. The fibro-osseous lesion (PDLO), however, is usually situated in a more inferior position in the mandible and frequently appears as a periapical lesion whereas the complex odontoma is usually situated in a more superior position between the crown of a tooth and the crest of the ridge. The fact that the periapical cementoma is seen more in women over 30 years of age and the intermediate-stage complex odontoma is seen in patients under 30 years of age will furnish additional help for the differential diagnosis.

MANAGEMENT

Because of its peripheral fibrous connective tissue capsule, which is really the follicle or periodontal ligament of the abnormal dental structure, the odontoma is easily enucleated. Such treatment is curative, however. Nevertheless, suitable postoperative periodic examination is necessary to ensure that complete healing has taken place. Microscopic examination is especially necessary to ensure the diagnosis.

ADENOMATOID ODONTOGENIC TUMOR

The adenomatoid odontogenic tumor is an uncommon odontogenic tumor that also may undergo different stages of development. Regezi and co-workers (1978) reported that it represented 3% of their series of odontogenic tumors. It may occur as a well-circumscribed radiolucency or it may contain radiopaque foci. The lesion is discussed in detail in Chapter 17, where its pericoronal radiolucent appearance is stressed. The mixed radiolucent-radiopaque stage will be emphasized in this chapter.

FEATURES

The adenomatoid odontogenic tumor is a slow-growing lesion that occurs most often between 10 and 30 years of age. About 95% occur in the anterior regions of the jaws (65% in the maxilla), and 75% are associated with an impacted tooth (most often a canine). Approximately 65% of the lesions occur in females. A delayed eruption of a permanent tooth or a regional swelling of the jaws may be the first symptom. Pain or other neurologic signs are not characteristic.

Radiographically the adenomatoid odontogenic tumor is a pericoronal cystlike radiolucency that mimics the radiographic appearance of a dentigerous cyst. In the maturing stage (which represents 65% of the lesions reviewed by Gargiulo and co-workers, 1974) sharply defined radiopaque foci are seen within the radiolucency (Fig. 23-10).

Microscopically small deposits of calcified material are present and scattered over a background of odontogenic cells that form cords and swirls of ductlike structures and pseudoacinae (Fig. 23-10).

DIFFERENTIAL DIAGNOSIS

The differential diagnosis of the adenomatoid odontogenic tumor is covered under the differential diagnosis section of the odontoma. The lesions most often confused with the adenomatoid odontogenic tumor are the *keratinizing and calcifying odontogenic cyst*, the *intermediate stage odontoma*, and the *calcifying epithelial odontogenic tumor*.

MANAGEMENT

The adenomatoid odontogenic tumor is readily enucleated, and recurrences are very unusual.

KERATINIZING AND CALCIFYING ODONTOGENIC CYST

The keratinizing and calcifying odontogenic cyst is considered to occupy a position between a cyst and an odontogenic tumor—having some characteristics of both. This entity accounted for 2% of all the odontogenic tumors reported by Regezi and co-workers (1978). In its early stages of development, this cystic keratinizing tumor will be completely radiolucent, but later the radiolucency will contain scattered radiopaque foci (Fig. 23-11). When it occurs in a dentigerous cyst position it appears as a pericoronal radiolucency with radiopaque foci.

FEATURES

The keratinizing and calcifying odontogenic cyst is a slow-growing completely benign condition. It occurred with equal frequency in the maxilla and mandible, and 54.2% occurred in females (Freedman et al., 1975). These authors reported that before the age of 41 the calcifying odontogenic cyst was much more common in females while after age 41 it was much more common in

Fig. 23-10. Adenomatoid odontogenic tumors in the intermediate stage seen as pericoronal radiolucencies with radiopaque foci. **A,** In the maxillary canine region. **B,** Another case in the upper premolar region. **C,** Photomicrograph of adenomatoid odontogenic tumor. Note dark foci of calcified material. (**A** courtesy K. Giedt, Aberdeen, S.D. **B** from Abrams, A. M., Melrose, J. R., and Howell, F. V.: Cancer **22:**175-185, 1968.)

males. Their review of cases showed that 47% occurred before 31 years of age, and that 75% of the lesions were situated anterior to the first molar teeth. It may vary in size and enlarge sufficiently to expand the mandible.

Most of the lesions are intrabony, but some occur in the soft tissues and may cause a saucering of the adjacent bone. The lesions are usually cystic, and aspiration may yield a viscous granular yellow fluid.

The radiographic appearance is of a cystlike radiolucency containing quite distinct radiopaque foci (Figs. 23-7 and 23-11).

The microscopic picture is unique for an oral lesion and has some characteristics of the calcifying epithelioma of Malherbe (which occurs in the skin). The basal cells are low cuboidal or columnar with dark large nuclei. The cells above the basal layer are irregular in arrangement and surround nests or sheets of large ghost epithelial

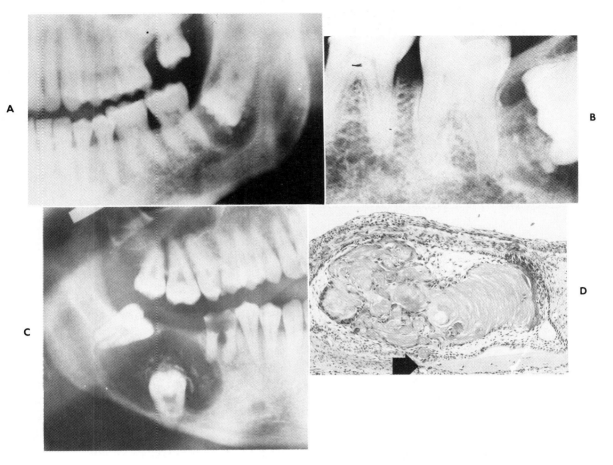

Fig. 23-11. Pericoronal calcifying odontogenic cysts with radiopaque foci within the cystlike radiolucency (**A** and **B** are same case). **C,** Panograph of another calcifying odontogenic cyst. **D,** Photomicrograph of calcifying and keratinizing odontogenic cyst. Note nodular formation of keratin and ghost cells within the epithelium of the cyst wall. Calcified tissue can be observed at the inferior aspect (arrow). (**A** and **B** courtesy R. Latronica, D.D.S., Albany, N.Y. **C** courtesy W. Schoenheider, D.D.S., Oak Lawn, Ill. **D** courtesy S. O. Raibley, D.D.S., Maywood, Ill.)

cells filled with atypical-appearing keratin. Some of these nests of ghost cells calcify (Fig. 23-11); and when they reach a sufficient size, they become recognizable as radiopaque foci in the radiolucent lesion.

DIFFERENTIAL DIAGNOSIS

Because of its radiographic appearance, the keratinizing and calcifying odontogenic cyst is most frequently confused with the partially calcified odontoma, the calcifying epithelial odontogenic tumor, and an adenomatoid odontogenic tumor. The differentiating features of these lesions are discussed under the differential diagnosis section of the odontoma.

MANAGEMENT

Since the keratinizing and calcifying odontogenic cyst has a tendency for continued growth, surgical enucleation is the treatment of choice. Recurrences are very rare.

AMELOBLASTIC FIBRO-ODONTOMA

Ameloblastic fibro-odontomas are benign mixed odontogenic tumors that contain cords and nests of odontogenic epithelium and also some calcified odontogenic tissue in a myxomatous stroma. This tumor represented 2% of the odontogenic tumors reported by Regezi and coworkers (1978).

Fig. 23-12. A and **B,** Case of an ameloblastic fibro-odontoma. **A,** Panorex radiograph. **B,** Periapical view. Note the radiopaque foci within the radiolucency associated with the crown of the impacted first molar. (From Curran, J. B., Owen, D., and Lanoway, J.: J. Can. Dent. Assoc. **46:**314-316, May 1980.)

FEATURES

Minderjahn reviewed statistics of the ameloblastic fibro-odontoma in 1979 and reported the following: the first two decades were the most common age groups affected, with the average age being 12 years; a predponderance of the patients were males (63%); the mandible had a slightly higher incidence, and the most common site affected was the premolar-molar region.

The ameloblastic fibro-odontoma is frequently located in a pericoronal position to an imbedded tooth and is initially completely radiolucent but acquires increasingly prominent radiopaque foci as the hard dental tissues within it become mineralized (Fig. 23-12).

DIFFERENTIAL DIAGNOSIS

The pericoronal variety of ameloblastic fibro-odontoma must be included in the differential diagnosis with such lesions as the intermediate stage odontoma, the calcifying odontogenic cyst, the adenomatoid odontogenic tumor, and the calcifying epithelial odontogenic tumor.

MANAGEMENT

The ameloblastic fibro-odontoma is a benign, well-encapsulated tumor that should be conservatively enucleated. It does not show a tendency to recur but patient follow-up is still necessary.

CALCIFYING EPITHELIAL ODONTOGENIC TUMOR (PINDBORG TUMOR)

The calcifying epithelial odontogenic tumor (CEOT) is considered to be rare and represents about 1% of odontogenic tumors (Franklin and Pindborg, 1976; Regezi et al., 1978). It may have several radiographic appearances: (1) a pericoronal radiolucency, (2) a pericoronal radiolucency with radiopaque foci (Fig. 23-13), (3) a mixed radiolucent-radiopaque lesion not associated with an unerupted tooth, (4) a "driven snow" appearance, and (5) a dense radiopacity (occasionally). In their extensive review Franklin and Pindborg (1976) reported that the most common pictures were that of a pericoronal radiolucency and of diffuse radiopacities within radiolucent areas.

FEATURES

From a review of 113 cases, Franklin and Pindborg (1976) reported the following statistics. All but five of the lesions were intraosseous. The intrabony lesions occurred in patients from 9 to 92, and the mean age at initial diagnosis was 40.41 years. Males and females were equally affected. Sixty-eight percent of the tumors occurred in the mandible, and there was a marked predilection for the molar region of the mandible (Fig. 23-13). The molar region of the maxilla and the premolar region of the mandible were the next most common sites. Fifty-two percent of the cases were undoubtedly associated with an unerupted tooth. The CEOT commonly occurred as a painless, slowly increasing expansion of the jaws. Small lesions were usually entirely asymptomatic.

Microscopically abundant sheets of polyhedral epithelial cells, which usually have prominent intracellular bridges, are seen. There is a variable amount of pleomorphism present but rarely are

Fig. 23-13. Pericoronal calcifying epithelial odontogenic tumor. **A,** An embedded premolar tooth and small radiopaque foci are seen within the radiolucency in this occlusal view of the mandible of a 57-year-old man. **B,** Lateral oblique radiograph of a 77-year-old woman showing a mixed radiolucent-radiopaque image in association with an embedded molar tooth. **C** and **D,** Photomicrographs of calcifying epithelial odontogenic tumor. Notice the pleomorphism of epithelial cells in **C.** **D** shows some clear epithelial cells and calcified material. (**A** and **B** from Franklin, C. D., and Hindle, M. O.: Br. J. Oral Surg. **13:**230-238, 1976. **D** courtesy S. O. Raibley, D.D.S., Maywood, Ill.)

there mitotic figures (Fig. 23-13, *C*). Circular areas within these epithelial cells are filled with a homogeneous eosinophilic material. This eosinophilic material becomes calcified following a pattern of concentric deposition known as Liesegang's rings.

DIFFERENTIAL DIAGNOSIS

The differential diagnosis discussion of the pericoronal radiolucent-radiopaque image of CEOT has been included in the differential diagnosis section of the odontoma.

MANAGEMENT

Surgical excision with a satisfactory border of apparently normal tissue is the recommended treatment for the calcifying epithelial odontogenic tumor. The recurrence rate is considerably lower than that of the ameloblastoma; however, careful patient follow-up is mandatory.

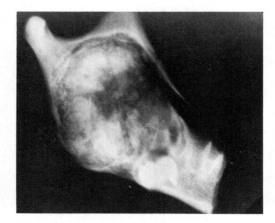

Fig. 23-14. Odontogenic fibroma. Radiograph of a surgical specimen. Note the well-defined borders and the displaced third molar. The radiopacities were due to the density and thickness of the fibrous tumor. Calcifications were not present in this lesion.

Fig. 23-15. Cystic odontomas. **A,** Orthopantomograph showing an odontoma within a large dentigerous cyst. **B,** Cystic odontoma in an intraradicular location between the lateral incisor and canine tooth. (**A** courtesy M. Kaminski, D.D.S., and S. Atsaves, D.D.S., Chicago. **B** courtesy W. Kinsler, D.D.S., Chicago.)

ODONTOGENIC FIBROMA

The central odontogenic fibroma is a rare, poorly understood, benign lesion that is thought to originate from cells of the periodontal ligament or other segments of the odontogenic apparatus. They consist basically of fibrous tissue containing nests of odontogenic epithelium and frequently calcified material that resembles cementum droplets. The hard deposits are apparent as radiopaque foci if they are large enough and adequately mineralized; or the lesion may be completely radiolucent.

Some central lesions have a hazy radiopaque pattern despite the absence of calcification, and this is the result of the dense areas of fibrous tissue in a lesion with considerable buccolingual dimension.

FEATURES

The odontogenic fibroma usually occurs in patients under 40 years of age, shows no sex predilection, and is found more commonly in the mandible. It is a slow-growing lesion and does not cause pain or other neurologic symptoms. It may attain considerable size, producing an expansion and/or destruction of the cortical plate and causing facial asymmetry.

Central odontogenic fibromas will appear as well-defined radiolucencies, perhaps containing radiopaque foci, and may cause spreading and migration of teeth in the region where they occur; but they do not characteristically cause root resorption (Fig. 23-14).

Occasionally a completely radiolucent central odontogenic fibroma will occur as a pericoronal radiolucency and mimic a follicular cyst. One with a combined radiolucent-radiopaque appearance, on the other hand, will resemble a calcifying odontogenic cyst.

The central type of odontogenic fibroma may be confused with a calcifying odontogenic cyst, an intermediate-stage odontoma, an intermediate-stage benign fibro-osseous lesion (PDLO), an adenomatoid odontogenic tumor, a CEOT, or a calcifying postsurgical bone defect.

MANAGEMENT

Complete enucleation and microscopic examination of the surgical specimen is the required treatment for an odontogenic fibroma.

RARITIES

Virtually any mixed radiolucent-radiopaque lesion that occurs in the jaw may contact the crown of an unerupted tooth and so appear as a mixed pericoronal lesion. Because there are many

Table 23-1. Mixed radiolucent-radiopaque periapical lesions

Entity	Predominant sex	Predominant age	Predominant jaw	Predominant region	Distinguishing features
Calcifying crowns	M = F	Under 20	—	Tooth-bearing areas	Compare with appearance in contralateral and opposing arches
Tooth root with rarefying osteitis	M = F	10-60	—	80% posterior	Position of tooth root on preextraction radiograph
Rarefying and condensing osteitis	M = F	20-60	Mandible	Premolar-molar	—
Calcifying postsurgical bone defect	M	—	Mandible	—	History of surgery
Periapical cementoma	F—80%	Over 30	Mandible—90%	Tooth-bearing areas (especially anterior mandible)	Vital teeth Circular Size < 1 cm Well-defined margins with radiolucent rim Often multiple
Cementifying and ossifying fibromas	M ~ F*	Avg. = 26.4†	Mandible—70%	Premolar-molar	Circular 2-5 cm Well marginated Solitary

*Approximately equal.

†For ossifying fibroma.

Table 23-2. Mixed radiolucent-radiopaque pericoronal lesions

Entity	Predominant sex	Predominant age	Predominant jaw	Predominant region	Distinguishing features
Odontoma compound	M ~ F*	5-20	Maxilla—62%	Incisor Canine	Radiolucent, smooth contours with well-defined radiopaque washers within
Odontoma complex	F—68%	5-20	Mandible	Molars—70% First Second Usually supracoronal	Radiolucent, smooth contours with well-defined, patternless radiopacities within Unerupted tooth
Adenomatoid odontogenic tumor	F : M = 2 : 1	Median = 16.5	Maxilla—65%	95% anterior of jaws 65% in canine areas	Pericoronal radiolucency—75% Often small radiopaque foci
Keratinizing and calcifying odontogenic cyst	Overall—M ~ F F—< age 41 M—> age 41	47% before 31 years	Maxilla = mandible	75% anterior to first molar	Viscous yellow aspirate
Ameloblastic fibro-odontoma	M—63%	5-20 Avg. = 12	Mandible ~ maxilla	Premolar-molar	
Calcifying epithelial odontogenic tumor	M ~ F	Avg. = 40.41	Mandible—68%	1. Mandibular molar 2. Maxillary molar; mandibular premolar	At least 52% associated with unerupted tooth
Odontogenic fibroma	M = F	Under 40	Mandible	Tooth-bearing regions	

*Approximately equal.

unerupted teeth in the jaws of patients during the first 15 years of life, one would expect that there would be a greater incidence of such an "accidental" happening during these early years. Fig. 23-15 illustrates two examples of the rare cystic odontoma.

SPECIFIC REFERENCES

Abrams, A. M., Melrose, J. R., and Howell, F. V.: Adenoameloblastoma: a clinical pathological study of 10 new cases, Cancer **22:**175-185, 1968.

Franklin, C. D., and Hindle, M. O.: The calcifying epithelial odontogenic tumor—report of four cases: two with long-term follow-up, Br. J. Oral Surg. **13:**230-238, 1976.

Franklin, C. D., and Pindborg, J. J.: The calcifying epithelial odontogenic tumor, Oral Surg. **42:**753-765, 1976.

Freedman, P. D., Lumerman, H., and Gee, J. K.: Calcifying odontogenic cyst, Oral Surg. **40:**93-106, 1975.

Gargiulo, E. A., Ziter, W. D., Mastrocola, R., and Ballard, B. R.: Odontogenic adenomatoid tumor (adenoameloblastoma): report of case and review of the literature, J. Oral Surg. **32:**286-290, 1974.

Hamner, J. E., Scofield, H. H., and Cornyn, J.: Benign fibro-osseous jaw lesions of periodontal membrane origin, Cancer **22:**861-878, 1968.

Minderjahn, A.: Incidence and clinical differentiation of odontogenic tumors, J. Maxillofac. Surg. **7:**142-150, 1979.

Regezi, J. A., Kerr, D. A., and Courtney, R. M.: Odontogenic tumors: analysis of 706 cases, J. Oral Surg. **36:**771-778, 1978.

Seeliger, J. E., and Reyneke, J. P.: The calcifying odontogenic cyst: report of case, J. Oral Surg. **36:**469-472, 1978.

Waldron, C. A., and Giansanti, J. S.: Benign fibro-osseous lesions of the jaws: a clinical-radiologic-histologic review of sixty-five cases. I. Fibrous dysplasia of the jaws, Oral Surg. **35:**190-201, 1973a.

Waldron, C. A., and Giansanti, J. S.: Benign fibro-osseous lesions of the jaws: a clinical-radiologic-histologic review of sixty-five cases. II. Benign fibro-osseous lesions of periodontal ligament origin, Oral Surg. **35:**340-350, 1973b.

GENERAL REFERENCES

Berk, R. S., Baden, E., Ladov, M., and Williams, A. C.: Adenoameloblastoma (odontogenic adenomatoid tumor): report of a case, J. Oral Surg. **30:**201-208, 1972.

Cangiano, R., Stratigos, G. E., and Williams, F. A.: Clinical and radiographic manifestations of fibro-osseous lesions of the jaws: report of five cases, J. Oral Surg. **29:**872-881, 1971.

Chen, S-Y., and Miller, A. S.: Ultrastructure of the keratinizing and calcifying odontogenic cyst, Oral Surg. **39:**769-780, 1975.

Cherrick, H. M., King, O. H., Lucatorto, F. M., and Suggs, D. M.: Benign cementoblastoma, a clinicopathologic evaluation, Oral Surg. **73:**54-63, 1974.

Eversole, L. R., Sabes, W. R., and Dauchess, V. G.: Benign cementoblastoma, J. Oral Surg. **36:**824-830, 1973.

Eversole, L. R., Sabes, W. R., and Rovin, S.: Fibrous dysplasia: a nosologic problem in the diagnosis of fibro-osseous lesions of the jaws, J. Oral Pathol. **1:**189-220, 1972.

Fahim, M. S., Elmofty, S. K., and El-attar, A. A.: Adenoameloblastoma: report of three cases, J. Oral Surg. **27:**407-414, 1969.

Fejerskov, O., and Krogh, J.: The calcifying ghost cell odontogenic tumor—or the calcifying odontogenic cyst, J. Oral Pathol. **1:**273-287, 1972.

Gould, J. F.: Complex odontoma, three-year follow-up of tooth movement, Oral Surg. **45:**175-177, 1978.

Greer, R. O., and Richardson, J. F.: Clear-cell calcifying odontogenic tumor viewed relative to the Pindborg tumor, Oral Surg. **42:**775-779, 1976.

Hamner, J. E., Gamble, J. W., and Gallegos, G. J.: Odontogenic fibroma: report of two cases, Oral Surg. **21:**111-119, 1966.

Johnson, R. H., and Topazian, R. G.: Calcifying odontogenic cyst, J. Oral Surg. **26:**394-400, 1968.

Kennett, S., and Curran, J. B.: Giant cemento-ossifying fibroma: report of case, J. Oral Surg. **30:**513-516, 1972.

Mallow, R. D., Spatz, S. S., Zubrow, H. J., and Kline, S. N.: Odontogenic fibroma with calcification, Oral Surg. **22:**564-568, 1966.

Marble, H. R., and Topazian, R. G.: Complex odontoma of the maxillary sinus, Oral Surg. **36:**658-662, 1973.

Oikarinen, V. J., Calonius, P. E., and Meretoja, J.: Calcifying epithelial odontogenic tumor (Pindborg tumor). Case report, Int. J. Oral Surg. **5**(4):187-191, 1976.

Sauk, J. J.: Calcifying and keratinizing odontogenic cyst, J. Oral Surg. **30:**893-897, 1972.

Seth, V. K.: Large compound composite odontoma: report of case, J. Oral Surg. **26:**745-748, 1968.

Smith, N. H.: Benign osteoblastoma of the mandible: report of case, J. Oral Surg. **30:**288-292, 1972.

Townes, T. M., Marks, R. B., and Carr, R. F.: Benign (true) cementoblastoma: report of cases, J. Oral Surg. **37:**342-345, 1979.

Ulmansky, M., Azaz, B., and Sela, J.: Calcifying odontogenic cyst: report of cases, J. Oral Surg. **27:**415-419, 1969.

Vegh, T.: Multiple cementomas (periapical cemental dysplasia), Oral Surg. **42:**402-406, 1976.

Wertheimer, F. W., and Sabin, M.: Calcifying odontogenic fibroma: report of case, J. Oral Surg. **30:**367-369, 1972.

Worley, R. D., and McKee, P. E.: Ameloblastic odontoma: report of case, J. Oral Surg. **30:**764-766, 1972.

24

Mixed radiolucent-radiopaque lesions not necessarily contacting teeth

Norman K. Wood
Paul W. Goaz

The following list is composed of mixed radiolucent-radiopaque lesions that are not necessarily associated with teeth:

Ossifying postsurgical bone defect
Chronic osteomyelitis, osteoradionecrosis, and Garré's osteomyelitis
Fibrous dysplasia
Paget's disease
Cementifying and/or ossifying fibroma
Osteogenic sarcoma
Osteoblastic metastatic carcinoma
Chondroma and chondrosarcoma
Ossifying subperiosteal hematoma
Rarities
    Adenomatoid odontogenic tumor
    Ameloblastic fibrodentinoma
    Ameloblastic fibro-odontoma
    Calcifying epithelial odontogenic tumor
    Central hemangioma
    Ewing's sarcoma
    Intrabony hamartoma
    Keratinizing and calcifying odontogenic cyst
    Lymphoma of bone
    Malignant tumors with superimposed osteomyelitis
    Sclerosing cemental masses
    Odontoma (intermediate)
    Osteoblastoma (intermediate)
    Osteoid osteoma

OSSIFYING POSTSURGICAL BONE DEFECT

Frequently, when central benign pathoses have been enucleated and closed, primary healing takes place through the ossification of the surgically produced hematoma, which is then slowly transformed to normal bone under favorable conditions. A radiograph taken shortly after the surgery will show a well-defined homogeneous radiolucency. If the radiograph is made at a later date when some calcification of the hematoma has taken place, the previously well-defined homogeneous radiolucency will contain many poorly defined radiopaque foci (Fig. 24-1).

Sometimes the appearance can be best described as a coarse salt-and-pepper image. Other times the radiopacities seem to concentrate in separate hazy aggregations and may present a puzzling picture if the clinician is not cognizant of the recent surgical procedure (Fig. 24-1, *B*). Later, as the calcification progresses and includes the entire defect, the radiographic image will illustrate the unstructured development of the poorly calcified new bone—in contrast to the regular trabecular pattern of the adjacent normal bone. This unordered picture will usually be remodeled to a normal bony architecture under the influence of internal stresses induced by the masticatory forces.

When bone marrow or chips have been implanted as graft material in a postsurgical defect, many radiopaque images of varying shape and size not unlike those just described for a normally calcifying defect will be seen in the radiolucent wound (Fig. 24-1, *A*).

Fig. 24-1. A, Enucleated cyst cavity grafted with autogenous bone chips (arrow). **B,** Mixed radiolucent-radiopaque appearance of a residual cyst as the cavity begins to ossify after surgical enucleation. (**A** courtesy O. H. Stuteville, D.D.S., M.D., St. Joe, Ark. **B** courtesy W. Heaton, D.D.S., Chicago.)

DIFFERENTIAL DIAGNOSIS AND MANAGEMENT

A recent history of a lesion enucleated in the area in question should establish the identity of postsurgical calcifying defect. Nevertheless, the clinician must always consider the possibility that he is confronting a recurrent pathosis, especially when the initial lesion was aggressive. If there is any question, close periodic clinical and radiographic examinations are in order. This precaution is recommended for all surgical cases but is especially important when the initial lesion was invasive and destructive.

CHRONIC OSTEOMYELITIS, OSTEORADIONECROSIS, AND GARRÉ'S OSTEOMYELITIS

Chronic osteomyelitis is discussed in Chapter 20, where the totally radiolucent type is stressed. In this chapter the mixed radiolucent-radiopaque appearance will be emphasized.

Osteomyelitis rarely afflicts a patient unless such predisposing conditions as the following set the stage for its development: uncontrolled debilitating systemic disease, sclerosing disease of the jawbones in which the vascular supply is compromised (e.g., Paget's disease, osteopetrosis, diffuse cementosis, postirradiation states), and inadequate reduction of jaw fractures or inadequate surgical enucleation of pathoses. The maxilla is rarely affected because of a more fragile bone pattern and richer blood supply.

FEATURES

Clinically the following signs of infection will be present: inflammation, tenderness, possibly pain, swelling, perhaps a draining sinus, regional lymphadenopathy, and likely a leukocytosis and increased sedimentation rate. Nonvital bone fragments or sections of jawbone may protrude from an ulcerated mucosal or cutaneous surface.

Osteoradionecrosis may mimic chronic osteomyelitis in all aspects (Fig. 24-4). The differentiating characteristic is the history of radiation therapy. Also osteoradionecrosis usually involves a larger segment of the jaw. Mizuno and coworkers (1976 and 1978) extensively described the histopathologic and radiographic changes in this condition.

The radiographic appearance of chronic osteomyelitis is most often a mixed radiolucent-radiopaque image. Frequently the borders will be ragged and poorly defined, but other times they may be well defined (Figs. 24-2 to 24-6). The radiolucent areas will usually consist of infected granulation tissue containing areas of necrosis or fibrosis or both. The radiopaque areas represent sclerosed, often nonvital bone or sequestra or both (Fig. 24-3). Garré's osteomyelitis, discussed in Chapter 27, may show an alternating radiolucent-radiopaque laminated appearance (Fig. 24-5).

DIFFERENTIAL DIAGNOSIS

The differential diagnosis of chronic osteomyelitis is covered in the differential diagnosis section under fibrous dysplasia. The lesions most frequently confused with chronic osteomyelitis are fibro-osseous lesions (PDLO), mottled-type lesion of fibrous dysplasia, rarefying and condensing osteitis, Paget's disease, malignant tumors that can produce a ragged radiolucent-radiopaque pattern (osteogenic sarcoma, chondrosarcoma, osteoblastic metastatic carcinoma, lymphoma of bone, Ewing's tumor), and a secondarily infected bone tumor.

A secondarily infected bone tumor and chronic osteomyelitis are indistinguishable clinically or

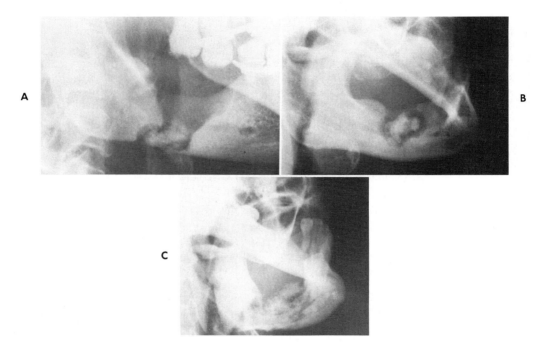

Fig. 24-2. Chronic osteomyelitis. Note the sequestra. The patient in **A** had a compound fracture. The patients in **B** and **C** were uncontrolled diabetics. (**B** courtesy O. H. Stuteville, D.D.S., M.D., St. Joe, Ark. **C** courtesy E. Palacios, M.D., Maywood, Ill.)

Fig. 24-3. Chronic osteomyelitis. **A,** Lesion in the mandible. **B,** Empty lacunae in nonvital trabeculae surrounded by necrotic material. (**A** courtesy the late S. Blackman, B.D.S., Chicago.)

Fig. 24-4. Osteoradionecrosis. Note the characteristically large section of mandible involved with the ill-defined destructive process. Both patients had received radiation for squamous cell carcinoma of the oral cavity. (**A** courtesy R. Kallal, D.D.S., Chicago. **B** courtesy O. H. Stuteville, D.D.S., M.D., St. Joe, Ark.)

Fig. 24-5. Garré's osteomyelitis in an 11-year-old child. Note the rarefaction at the periapices of the first molar. Note also that the periostitis at the inferior border of the mandible has produced alternate light and dark (less calcified) laminations. (Courtesy N. Barakat, D.D.S., Beirut, Lebanon.)

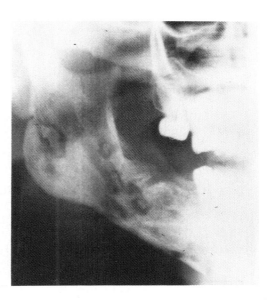

Fig. 24-6. Unusual appearance of the right ramus and body produced by osteomyelitis. (Courtesy A. Indresano, D.D.S., and P. O'Flaherty, D.D.S., Chicago.)

radiographically or by the patient interview. Incidence alone, however, will favor a diagnosis of osteomyelitis.

MANAGEMENT

The management of chronic osteomyelitis is discussed in detail in Chapter 20. Basically it involves controlling the underlying systemic disease (if present), administering the proper antibiotic, and incision, irrigation, saucerization, sequestrectomy (if necessary), and possibly use of hyperbaric oxygen (Mainous et al., 1973).

FIBROUS DYSPLASIA

Fibrous dysplasia is a poorly understood benign disturbance of bone which, although classified as a benign fibro-osseous disease, is currently considered by most oral pathologists to arise from specific bone-forming mesenchyme and to be a separate entity from the benign fibro-osseous lesions of PDLO (Waldon and Giansanti, 1973a and b). Essentially this lesion comprises varying proportions of fibrous tissue and spicules of bone.

There is considerable variation in the radiographic appearance of fibrous dysplasia, and the density of the lesions ranges from relatively radiolucent to quite radiopaque. The lesions are seldom spherical but are usually observed to be elongated or elliptic, especially in the mandible (Fig. 24-7). The shape of the lesions that extend into the maxillary sinus is influenced by the configuration of this chamber.

The lesions may be unilocular or multilocular, and their borders will usually be poorly defined because of the gradual blending of the altered bone with the adjacent normal pattern. This transitional zone may often measure more than 1 cm. The density of the lesion varies with the proportion of fibrous to osseous tissue—which relates to the stage of development of the lesion.

Three basic patterns are usually described:
1. An early primarily osteolytic fibrous stage that may be completely radiolucent
2. An intermediate stage recognizable by its smoky, hazy, or mottled radiolucent-radiopaque pattern (Fig. 24-8), which is pro-

Fig. 24-7. Fibrous dysplasia, intermediate stage. **A,** Note the deformity of the lower left mandible, producing facial asymmetry. **B,** Smoothly contoured expansion of the left mandible, which caused malocclusion. **C,** Occlusal radiograph showing fusiform ground-glass expansion of the left mandible. Note the characteristically indistinct anterior border of the lesion. **D,** Periapical radiograph showing the ground-glass pattern.

duced by poorly defined aggregates of small spicules of bone distributed throughout the radiolucent area (Occasionally radiopaque areas in this pattern will have a ground-glass appearance; or the complete lesion will have a moderately opaque ground-glass pattern, Fig. 24-7).

3. A more mature phase variously described as having a salt-and-pepper, ground-glass, or orange peel appearance, which will vary in opaqueness depending on the number, size, and degree of clacification of the trabeculae

The lesions with the mottled radiolucent-radiopaque appearance will be emphasized in the present chapter, for they are considered to be more immature than those having the uniformly opaque ground-glass appearance.

FEATURES

Fibrous dysplasia of the facial bones appears to show characteristics and behavior patterns that are different from those of fibrous dysplasia involving other bones of the skeleton; consequently it should be considered as a separate entity.

Aside from the lesions accompanying Albright's syndrome, fibrous dysplasia usually occurs as a solitary (monostotic) lesion in the mandible but will frequently involve the maxilla, zygoma, and sphenoid as a unit (Figs. 24-7 and 24-8). The maxilla is involved slightly more often than the mandible. The zygoma and the maxillary sinus are also affected. The anterior maxilla and the mandibular symphysis appear to be immune. Men and women are affected equally.

Clinically the lesion grows very slowly, finally causing a fusiform expansion of the jaw and a nontender facial asymmetry. As a rule the lesion stops growing when skeletal growth ceases. Like most benign conditions originating beneath the surface epithelium, the expansion is smooth and covered with normal-appearing mucosa or skin. Surface ulcerations are uncommon but may be seen when the mass intrudes on the occlusion. Pain or paresthesia is an unusual complaint. Teeth in the involved segment may show minimal migration or displacement but are not characteristically loosened. Serum chemistry levels are within normal limits because of the very slow growth.

The region of hazy radiopaque-radiolucent mottling is often somewhat rectangular in shape and is seen in younger patients (Fig. 24-8). Sometimes the radiopaque foci will be quite dense, but usually they will have a ground-glass

appearance. Minor displacement of teeth or divergence of roots may be present, and occasionally whole segments of teeth will appear to have moved. Root resorption is not a feature.

Microscopically the proportions of fibrous tissue and bone vary from lesion to lesion, as do the size and distribution of the bony aggregations. This accounts for the diverse radiographic appearances. Fibrous tissue predominates in the more radiolucent areas; and if bony trabeculae are present, they will be too small or inadequately mineralized to show as radiopaque foci. The ground-glass areas consist of small trabeculae of bone of approximately equal size, many of which will be radiographically apparent. The dense radiopaque areas are made up of larger trabeculae with less intervening fibrous tissue. The fibrous stroma varies in cellularity and amounts of collagen present. The trabecular margins usually show what appears to be a streaming of collagen fiber bundles from the bone into the stroma.

Fig. 24-8. Fibrous dysplasia, intermediate stage. **A,** Note the smoky or mottled radiopacity within the radiolucency (seen also in **B**). **B,** Note one lesion in the maxilla and one in the mandible. Polyostotic examples in the jaws are unusual without an accompanying Albright's syndrome. The mottled pattern seen in the mandibular lesion in **B** is very similar to the mottled pattern in the skull of Paget's disease shown in Fig. 24-9. (**A** courtesy S. Atsaves, D.D.S., Chicago. **B** courtesy N. Barakat, D.D.S., Beirut, Lebanon.)

The majority of the bony trabeculae are composed of woven bone (not the lamellar type laid down in haversian systems) on which osteoblastic rimming is not usually seen (Waldron and Giansanti, 1973a). As the lesion becomes more mature, spicules of lamellar bone with osteoblastic rimming will be seen.

Albright's syndrome occurs in girls who show the following features:

1. Precocious sexual development
2. Multiple bones affected with lesions of fibrous dysplasia (polyostotic)
3. Café-au-lait spots on the skin and oral mucosa

DIFFERENTIAL DIAGNOSIS

The mottled type of fibrous dysplasia must be differentiated from chronic osteomyelitis, ossifying and cementifying fibromas, Paget's disease, osteosarcoma, osteoblastic metastatic carcinoma, chondrosarcoma, Ewing's sarcoma, and lymphomas of bone. The well-circumscribed entities such as a healing surgical defect, intermediate-stage odontoma, and other odontogenic lesions should not be a differential problem.

Lymphomas of bone are rare and may be seen as poorly defined rarefactions perhaps with a few septa of bone left intact, which give a multilocular appearance. Other lymphomas may exhibit both osteoblastic activity as well as bone resorption and hence produce a mixed radiolucent-radiopaque appearance (Fig. 24-18). The pattern would be much more irregular and bizarre than that seen in the mottled lesion of fibrous dysplasia. Also smooth, well-contoured external bony borders are always maintained in fibrous dysplasia both clinically and radiographically. This is almost never the case in extensive malignancies or osteomyelitis.

Chondrosarcoma is an uncommon malignant tumor of the jaws that usually affects a much older age group (30 to 60) than fibrous dysplasia (5 to 20). In addition, chondrosarcoma frequently produces pain while pain almost never accompanies fibrous dysplasia. Also the typical, rectangular, more-ordered radiographic appearance of fibrous dysplasia frequently differentiates this entity from the chondrosarcoma whose radiolucent-radiopaque image will be completely disorderly, often invading the cortex.

Osteoblastic metastatic carcinoma likewise will seldom be seen with as monotonous a pattern as that seen in the mottled type of fibrous dysplasia. Also a history of either symptoms of or treatment for a primary tumor elsewhere would usually be elicited during the history taking. The majority of osteoblastic metastatic carcinomas are found in an older age group.

Osteosarcoma of the mixed fibroblastic and osteoblastic type will produce a radiolucent-radiopaque image. This tumor has a predilection for a younger age group (average 27 years) and so is more similar in this manner to fibrous dysplasia than most of the other entities in this discussion. Again the radiographic pattern in osteosarcoma will be much more disorderly than that seen with fibrous dysplasia (Figs. 24-11 to 24-13). Generally one of the following radiographic features produced in osteosarcoma will be apparent: (1) sunburst appearance, (2) cumulus cloud, (3) Codman's triangle, (4) asymmetric bandlike widening of the periodontal ligament, or (5) onionskin appearance of redundancy of the cortical plate.

The mottled appearance seen in *Paget's disease* may be identical to that seen in fibrous dysplasia (Figs. 24-8, *B,* and 24-9). Classically Paget's disease simultaneously affects several bones of the skeleton; this feature would enable the clinician to separate such a case from the single isolated lesion of fibrous dysplasia even if it were large and involved almost all of the jaw. However, occasional cases of atypical Paget's disease are seen where only the mandible is involved. Such cases are more difficult to differentiate from fibrous dysplasia. The presence of extensive hypercementosis and an age over 40 years would prompt the clinician to favor Paget's in such a case.

Adding to the difficulty is the possibility of *Albright's syndrome* because two or more of the bones will be affected with fibrous dysplasia.

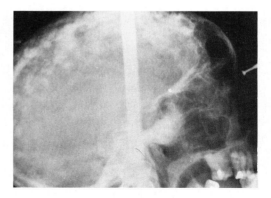

Fig. 24-9. Paget's disease. Note the mottled appearance produced by cotton balls distributed over a generalized radiolucency. The jaws were not involved. (Courtesy R. Goepp, D.D.S., Zoller Clinic, University of Chicago.)

Here the presence of café-au-lait spots on the skin as well as precocious puberty in young girls would identify the case as being Albright's syndrome. The extremely high serum alkaline phosphatase values seen in Paget's disease will direct the diagnostician away from a diagnosis of fibrous dysplasia and permit the establishment of a firm diagnosis of Paget's disease when typical bone changes are present.

Cementifying and ossifying fibroma (fibro-osseous lesions; PDLO) may be seen with a similar mottled appearance (Fig. 24-10) to that seen in fibrous dysplasia. The following differences are now recognized:

1. *Shape.* The cementifying and ossifying fibromas are predominantly round while those of fibrous dysplasia are more rectangular.

2. *Jaw expansion.* Jaw expansion caused by cementifying and ossifying fibroma is usually nodular or dome shaped whereas the jaw expansion of fibrous dysplasia is usually of the elongated fusiform type.

3. *Margins.* The cementifying and ossifying fibroma has sharply defined radiographic margins. In contradistinction, the margins of fibrous dysplasia are indistinct, blending imperceptibly with normal bone.

4. *Predominant jaw.* Approximately 70% of cementifying and ossifying fibromas occur in the mandible. Fibrous dysplasia shows a slight predilection for the maxilla.

5. *Predominant age.* The age range for ossifying fibromas is from 7 to 58 years and the average age is 26.4. The majority of active cases of fibrous dysplasia are found in patients under 20 years of age.

Chronic osteomyelitis in its radiolucent-radiopaque appearance can mimic the mottled appearance of fibrous dysplasia. When pain and purulent drainage are present it is easy to make a diagnosis of osteomyelitis. Likewise, the presence of predisposing conditions in a patient that would render a patient likely to contract osteomyelitis would prompt the clinician to rank this entity higher in the working diagnosis. With the exception of Garré's osteomyelitis, bone infections involve a considerably older age group. Radiographically in osteomyelitis the cortices of the bone are usually irregular at least at one point along the expanded region. This is almost never so in cases of fibrous dysplasia, where the expanded bony periphery, although thinned, will appear smoothly contoured and basically uniform.

MANAGEMENT

The usual course of fibrous dysplasia is for a lesion to appear in a young person, grow slowly for a decade or so, then stabilize, and slowly return to normal. Consequently, occlusion as well as tooth-jaw relation should be observed carefully during the years of bone growth. Occasionally, surgical recontouring is required to improve esthetics or as a preprosthetic preparation.

PAGET'S DISEASE (OSTEITIS DEFORMANS)—INTERMEDIATE STAGE

Paget's disease is also described in Chapter 22, where its generalized osteolytic stage—producing a generalized rarefaction of the involved bones—is emphasized. The dense mature cotton-wool appearance is described in Chapter 29. Like many of the other pathoses discussed in this chapter, Paget's disease may pass through three progressive stages:

1. The initial stage is osteolytic and fibroblastic, causing a generalized radiolucency.

2. The intermediate stage is both osteolytic and osteoblastic, producing some large trabecular clusters, which appear as radiopaque areas within the generalized radiolucency.

3. The mature stage, although still possessing some osteoclastic behavior, is predominantly osteoblastic and shows as a dense cotton-wool pattern on radiographs.

The intermediate stage of this disease is emphasized in the present chapter. The course of

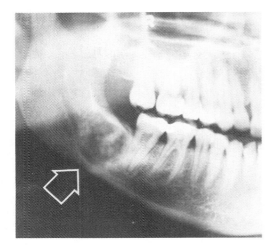

Fig. 24-10. Ossifying fibroma in the third molar region of a 36-year-old black woman.

the disease suggests that it is the result of a disorder in the coordination of osteoblastic and osteoclastic activity.

FEATURES

Paget's disease appears to be a familial disease transmitted as an autosomal dominant trait, seldom becoming evident before 40 years of age. The bones most frequently involved are the skull, vertebrae, pelvis, femurs, and jaws. Clinically the involved bones are thickened and the foramina are often constricted. Thus pressure is induced on the structures that pass through the foramina, causing neurologic signs.

A spectrum of radiographic features characterizes the intermediate stage of this lesion— from the first indication of a developing radiopacity in the osteolytic stage to the appearance of calcified areas (cotton balls) interspersed with radiolucent areas and producing the distinctive cotton-wool appearance (Fig. 24-9).

It is important to point out that frequently the affected bones in the same person are not at the same stage of the disease. The skull frequently becomes involved prior to the maxilla, and the maxilla before the mandible. We have seen patients in whom the skull was in the radiopaque stage (almost completely radiopaque), the maxilla was in the mixed radiolucent-radiopaque stage, and the mandible was either uninvolved or in the radiolucent stage. Teeth in the involved jaw may demonstrate spreading, migration, and (characteristically) hypercementosis.

Microscopically the intermediate stage of Paget's disease shows areas made up chiefly of fibroblastic tissue containing a few trabeculae of bone with osteoclasts often evident in Howship's lacunae at the periphery. Other areas show heavy trabeculae with osteoblasts and osteoclasts both present rimming the bone in closely adjacent areas.

Using low-power examination, the clinician may detect a mosaic pattern within the larger trabeculae. This pattern is produced by the many reversal lines caused by the sequences of destruction and repair repeated again and again in the same spicule.

Although the serum chemistry levels may vary with lapses and progressions of the disease, the alkaline phosphatase levels are usually very high whereas the calcium and phosphorus levels are within normal limits.

DIFFERENTIAL DIAGNOSIS

Paget's disease should be suspected in persons who have generalized mixed radiolucent-radiopaque lesions throughout the jaws. If a radiographic survey demonstrates generalized radiolucent, mixed radiolucent-radiopaque, or cotton-wool changes in other bones, the disturbance is almost certain to be Paget's disease. A high serum alkaline phosphatase level should strengthen this impression.

None of the other mixed radiolucent-radiopaque lesions discussed in the present chapter affect multiple bones and show such complete involvement of the individual bones as does Paget's disease.

Several bones may be involved by *fibrous dysplasia in Albright's sundrome;* but, contrary to Paget's disease, which is a disturbance in adults over 40 years of age, this disorder affects young girls. If the clinician has only one periapical radiograph of the involved jaw, he may easily mistake the radiographic image for many of the other lesions discussed in this chapter. It is inexcusable, however, to attempt to diagnose a case without access to radiographs showing the full extent of the lesions.

MANAGEMENT

Paget's disease is a slowly progressive pathosis with no known cure. Palliative procedures to alleviate the neurologic and locomotive problems are indicated. Edentulous patients may require frequent adjustment or the continued fabrication of new dentures because of the constantly expanding jawbones.

As the disease progresses, the involved bones initially become more fragile and thus subject to pathologic fracture. As apposition exceeds resorption, however, and the mature stage of Paget's disease is reached, the bone becomes condensed and avascular and is then predisposed to develop osteomyelitis. There is a greatly increased incidence of osteogenic sarcoma in patients who have Paget's disease.

CEMENTIFYING AND/OR OSSIFYING FIBROMA

The cementifying and/or ossifying fibromas have been discussed in detail in Chapter 23 where their mixed periapical appearance was stressed. These lesions may also occur separate from teeth. Fig. 24-10 illustrates a mixed spherical radiolucency containing a mottled radiopaque appearance in the edentulous third molar area of a 32-year-old woman. Cementifying and/or ossifying fibromas occur in the teeth-bearing regions of the jaws, particularly the premolar-molar regions of the mandible.

Fig. 24-11. Osteogenic sarcoma. Lateral oblique and occlusal views of the same patient. The gross production of neoplastic bone has produced a cumulus-cloud appearance. Increased width of the periodontal ligament may be seen around the roots of the anterior teeth. In some cases the widening is asymmetric. The marked proliferation of neoplastic bone is evident on both radiographs. (Courtesy R. Goepp, D.D.S., Zoller Clinic, University of Chicago.)

OSTEOGENIC SARCOMA

Osteogenic sarcoma is ranked next to multiple myeloma as the second most common primary malignant tumor of the jawbones. It may display three basically different radiographic images: totally radiolucent, mixed radiolucent-radiopaque, or completely radiopaque. Osteogenic sarcoma is discussed in Chapter 20, where its radiolucent picture is stressed. In the present chapter the mixed radiolucent-radiopaque appearance will be detailed.

FEATURES

Osteogenic sarcoma is usually a rapidly growing tumor of the jaws, which may produce pain, paresthesia, or anesthesia. It occurs more often in the mandible, and the peak age of incidence falls between 25 and 30 years of age. In the early stages, unless the mass is chronically traumatized, its surface will be smoothly contoured and covered with normal mucosa.

The radiolucent-radiopaque lesion usually has ragged ill-defined borders, and its radiographic pattern is the result of areas of excessive bone production intermingled with radiolucent foci of bone destruction (Figs. 24-11 and 24-12). Also in some lesions sequestra are formed, and these usually appear as well-defined dense radiopacities. If the tumor invades the periosteum, many thin irregular spicules of new bone directed outward and perpendicular to the surface of the le-

Fig. 24-12. Osteogenic sarcoma. **A,** Note the ragged borders of the mixed radiolucent-radiopaque lesion. **B,** Bone destruction in the medullary portion of the bone produced by an osteogenic sarcoma in another patient. Note the sunburst effect at the periphery. (**A** courtesy R. Goepp, D.D.S., Zoller Clinic, University of Chicago. **B** courtesy the late S. Blackman, B.D.S., Chicago.)

Fig. 24-13. Osteogenic sarcoma. Radiographs of a surgical specimen. Note the sunburst pattern emanating from the buccal cortex, especially in **A.** (Courtesy O. H. Stuteville, D.D.S., M.D., St. Joe, Ark.)

sion may develop (Figs. 24-12 and 24-13). They produce the so-called sunburst effect, which, although not pathognomonic for osteogenic sarcoma, is highly suggestive of the lesion. Another characteristic appearance is the "cumulus cloud" formation illustrated in Fig. 24-11, *A*.

Sometimes two triangular radiopacities will project from the cortex and mark the lateral extremities of the lesion. These are referred to as Codman's triangles. Rarely osteogenic sarcoma will cause periosteal deposition of bone in an onionskin pattern.

Microscopically fibroblastic tissue occupies the radiolucent areas and contains deposits of osteoid tissue and malignant osteoblasts. The tumor bone in the radiopaque areas is irregular and immature. A transitional type of cartilage may also be present in the tumor.

DIFFERENTIAL DIAGNOSIS

The most frequent lesions to be confused with an osteogenic sarcoma are the chondrosarcoma, osteoblastic metastatic carcinoma, ossifying subperiosteal hematoma, peripheral fibroma with calcification, fibrous dysplasia, and chronic osteomyelitis.

Although the *peripheral fibroma with calcification* may radiographically and clinically resemble the osteogenic sarcoma that has originated in the periodontal ligament, the slow benign growth of the former entity distinguishes it readily from this malignant tumor.

The *ossifying subperiosteal hematoma* may be easily mistaken for an osteogenic sarcoma by the unwary examiner. This particular entity occasionally develops when trauma to the jawbone produces a sizable subperiosteal hematoma. Such hematomas may calcify and produce a disturbing radiographic appearance, often simulating the sunburst effect. A history of recent trauma to the bone should alert the clinician to the possibility that the ill-defined bony margin is a calcifying hematoma.

An *osteoblastic type of metastatic tumor* may also produce a mixed radiographic image similar to that found in osteogenic sarcoma but without the sunburst effect. The absence of a primary tumor or associated symptoms should prompt a low ranking for this entity in the differential diagnosis.

The *chondrosarcoma* can be tentatively distinguished from the osteogenic sarcoma since it usually affects an older age group and more often involves the maxilla. Radiographically and clinically, however, it may closely mimic the osteogenic sarcoma.

Differentiating features of fibrous dysplasia and chronic osteomyelitis are discussed under the differential diagnosis section of fibrous dysplasia.

MANAGEMENT

The recommended treatment for osteogenic sarcoma of the jaws is radical resection as early as possible. The prognosis is grave, although better than for osteogenic sarcoma of other bones.

OSTEOBLASTIC METASTATIC CARCINOMA

Metastatic tumors to the jawbone usually produce poorly defined ragged radiolucencies; they are discussed in Chapter 20. Although as a general rule any osteoblastic metastasis to the jaws is rare, some secondary tumors from primary lesions in the prostate and occasionally from the breast may be of this type (Figs. 24-14 and 24-15).

Metastatic prostatic tumors to bone may develop as entirely radiolucent, entirely radiopaque, or mixed radiolucent-radiopaque lesions.

Whether a metastatic tumor will promote osteoblastic activity in the tissue or organ involved ap-

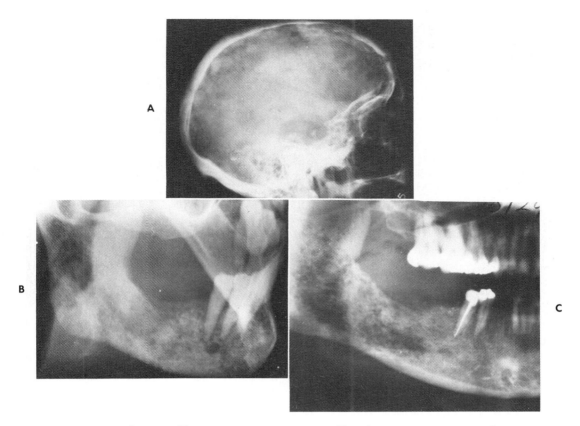

Fig. 24-14. Osteolytic-osteoblastic metastatic carcinoma. **A,** Note the extensive metastasis of a prostatic carcinoma with both osteoblastic and osteolytic activity. **B,** Note the salt-and-pepper appearance of this metastatic breast carcinoma to the mandible. **C,** Another case of metastatic carcinoma from breast producing a coarse, irregular, salt-and-pepper lesion in the right body and ramus. (**A** courtesy E. Palacios, M.D., Maywood, Ill. **B** courtesy R. Goepp, D.D.S., Zoller Clinic, University of Chicago. **C** courtesy D. Cooksey, D.D.S., Los Angeles.)

parently depends primarily on whether there are significant levels of acid and alkaline phosphatase produced by the metastasized tumor cells.

Other metastatic tumors that are usually osteolytic may induce osteoblastic activity in either the tumor or the neighboring bone. Such lesions will also appear as mixed radiolucent-radiopaque lesions on the radiograph with usually vague irregular borders. The dissemination may be so great that the resultant picture mimics Paget's disease (Figs. 24-14 and 24-15).

Whether lesions of this type are well circumscribed or not usually depends on the aggressiveness of the tumor: the less aggressive a lesion behaves, the more circumscribed it will appear on the radiograph.

When multiple small nests of sclerosing or osteoblastic metastatic tumor have become dis-

seminated throughout the jawbone, a coarse salt-and-pepper pattern may be seen on radiographs (Fig. 24-14).

FEATURES

The clinical features of osteoblastic metastatic carcinoma are similar to those described for central malignancies of the jawbones. A history of surgery for or symptoms relatable to a current primary tumor are the factors that usually alert the clinician to the possibility of metastatic disease.

DIFFERENTIAL DIAGNOSIS

The differential diagnosis of osteoblastic metastatic carcinoma is presented in the differential diagnosis section under osteogenic sarcoma (p. 524).

Fig. 24-15. Disseminated osteolytic and osteoblastic metastatic adenoid cystic carcinoma that originated in the oral cavity. **A,** Posteroanterior view of the skull and jaws. Note the cotton-wool appearance in the skull and the large bilateral radiolucent lesions in the mandible. **B,** Lateral radiograph of the skull and jaws showing radiolucent areas as well as radiopaque areas. (**B** courtesy O. H. Stuteville, D.D.S., M.D., St. Joe, Ark.)

MANAGEMENT

The management of patients with metastatic tumors is described in detail in Chapter 19.

CHONDROMA AND CHONDROSARCOMA

Both the chondroma, which is benign, and the chondrosarcoma, which is malignant, originate in cartilage and are uncommon tumors of the jawbones.

FEATURES

The chondroma and chondrosarcoma are considered together in this discussion because, except for the more aggressive behavior and the more irregular clinical and radiographic appearances of a very malignant chondrosarcoma, their features are quite similar. Frequently the differentiation between an aggressive chondroma and a slow-growing chondrosarcoma will be difficult to make since there are few pathognomonic signs or symptoms by which the chondroma can be differentiated from the chondrosarcoma and radiography is of little help.

Both the chondroma and the chondrosarcoma may cause root resorption of the involved teeth,

and both may show as either well-demarcated or ill-defined radiolucencies (the radiolucent type of chondrosarcoma is discussed in Chapter 20). Although the opacities in the chondroma usually appear more orderly than do those in the chondrosarcoma, both tumors may also develop a radiopaque pattern in the osteolytic bone cavity.

The chondroma and chondrosarcoma favor males slightly and occur more frequently in the maxilla; the anterior region is the most common site of involvement (Martis, 1978). When found in the mandible they have a preference for the premolar-molar regions, the symphysis, the condyle, and the coronoid process. Like other central tumors in the early stages, they are covered with a smooth normal-appearing mucosa (Fig. 24-16), which later becomes ulcerated because of trauma.

Pain is a frequent symptoms of both entities.

Sato and co-workers (1977) reviewed the Japanese literature for chondrosarcoma of the jaws and facial skeleton. These authors reported that this tumor affects the maxilla approximately 1.28 times as frequently as the mandible. The age range of patients with chondrosarcoma was from

Fig. 24-16. Chondrosarcoma. **A,** Smoothly contoured nonulcerated swelling in the maxillary premolar region. **B,** Radiograph of the surgical specimen. Note the radiopaque foci in the exophytic mass. **C,** Microscopy of a chondrosarcoma. (**A** and **B** courtesy R. Nolan, D.D.S., Waukegan, Ill.)

3 to 78 years, but most occurred between the ages of 30 and 60. The highest incidence occurred in the fourth decade. Chondrosarcoma of the lower jaw occurred twice as often in men as in women.

Microscopically cartilage as well as chondrocytes and possibly fibrous or myxomatous tissue is seen in the chondrosarcoma. Areas in which the cartilage has calcified may be found, and these are what cause the radiopacities on radiographs. The more aggressive the tumor, the poorer will be the quality of the cartilage formed and the more atypical the chondrocytes will appear.

Considerable variation occurs in the size of the cells of both tumors and many cells are binucleated (Fig. 24-16). Osteoid tissue is not seen in a true chondrosarcoma.

It should be emphasized that these tumors may vary greatly in appearance from area to area, with large intervening masses of normal-appearing hyaline cartilage frequently being present in a particular specimen.

DIFFERENTIAL DIAGNOSIS

The differential diagnosis of the chondroma and the chondrosarcoma is covered in the differential diagnosis section of osteogenic sarcoma (p. 524).

MANAGEMENT

Because of the malignant nature of the chondrosarcoma and the difficulty often encountered in differentiating between an aggressive chondroma and a chondrosarcoma, a wide resection should be done—to ensure the removal of an adequate margin of normal tissue even though the surgeon's working diagnosis is chondroma. Sato and co-workers (1977) reported that the 3-year survival rate was about 50% for chondrosarcoma of the lower jaw but was much lower for tumors of the maxilla.

OSSIFYING SUBPERIOSTEAL HEMATOMA

The ossifying subperiosteal hematoma sometimes occurs when a subperiosteal hematoma is

Fig. 24-17. A, Ameloblastic odontoma of the angle. **B,** Sclerosing cemental masses in a 32-year-old black woman. Note the mixed radiolucent-radiopaque appearance of these cemental masses, which are in the intermediate stage of maturation. (**A** courtesy O. H. Stuteville, D.D.S., St. Joe, Ark. **B** courtesy R. Nolan, D.D.S., Waukegan, Ill.)

induced by trauma to the jawbone. It may also accompany a jaw fracture.

FEATURES

Usually the ossifying subperiosteal hematoma occurs in young people under 15 years of age, in whom the bones are still actively growing. Ossification of the hematoma occurs quite rapidly. The new bone is often formed in perpendicular columns from the cortical plate outward. Such an osseous arrangement gives a sunburst pattern or at times the appearance of an irregularly thickened cortex.

DIFFERENTIAL DIAGNOSIS

Without a recent history of trauma, the clinical and radiographic appearances of ossifying sub-periosteal hematoma may be readily mistaken for such lesions as *osteogenic sarcoma, Ewing's sarcoma, chondrosarcoma,* and *Garré's osteomyelitis.*

These lesions occur predominantly in younger persons except for the chondrosarcoma; and although the clinician cannot differentiate between this calcifying phenomenon in the hematoma and the foregoing lesions, if such a condition is observed soon after a traumatic incident to the jawbone, it is most likely a calcifying subperiosteal hematoma.

MANAGEMENT

A mass such as the calcifying subperiosteal hematoma should be kept under close observation for the following reasons:

Fig. 24-18. Malignant lymphoma of bone in a white man in his 50s. Note the radiolucent and radiopaque appearance. **A,** Panograph. **B,** Periapical film.

Fig. 24-19. Malignant tumors with superimposed osteomyelitis. **A,** Mandibular occlusal film of a squamous cell carcinoma of the symphysis in a 62-year-old man. Note the radiopaque sequestrum within the classic radiolucent lesion with ragged ill-defined borders. **B,** Orthopantograph of osteoradionecrosis and recurrent squamous cell carcinoma in a 68-year-old white man. Note the ragged radiolucent-radiopaque appearance. (**A** courtesy M. Kaminski, D.D.S., and S. Atsaves, D.D.S., Chicago.)

1. The lesion may in reality be a malignant tumor or perhaps Garré's osteomyelitis.
2. The area may have to be surgically excised to improve esthetics and function if the ossified expansion fails to be recontoured by the stresses produced by normal function of the jaws.

RARITIES

The following lesions rarely occur in the jawbones as mixed radiolucent-radiopaque lesions or else are more often associated with teeth:

Adenomatoid odontogenic tumor
Ameloblastic fibrodentinoma
Ameloblastic odontoma (Fig. 24-17, *A*)
Calcifying epithelial odontogenic tumor
Central hemangioma
Ewing's sarcoma
Intrabony hamartoma
Keratinizing and calcifying odontogenic cyst
Lymphoma of bone (Fig. 24-18)
Malignant tumors with superimposed osteomyelitis (Fig. 24-19)
Sclerosing cemental masses (Fig. 24-17, *B*)
Odontoma (intermediate stage)
Osteoblastoma (intermediate stage)
Osteoid osteoma

Table 24-1. Mixed radiolucent-radiopaque lesions not necessarily contacting teeth

Entity	Predominant sex	Predominant age	Predominant jaw	Predominant region	Distinguishing features
Ossifying postsurgical bony defect	M	—	Mandible	—	History of surgery
Chronic osteomyelitis and osteoradionecrosis	M > F	40-80	Rare in maxilla	Body of mandible	Predisposing conditions; i.e., trauma, diabetes, Paget's disease, previous radiation
Fibrous dysplasia	M = F	5-20	Maxilla > mandible (slightly)	Symphysis and anterior maxilla exempt	Noncircular; borders poorly defined; ground-glass, mottled pattern
Paget's disease	M > F (slightly)	Over 40	Maxilla	Generalized	Cotton-wool; multiple bones involved; elevated serum alkaline phosphatase
Cementifying and/or ossifying fibroma	M ~ F*	Avg. = 26.4†	Mandible— 70%	Premolar-molar	Circular, 2-5 cm, well marginated
Osteogenic sarcoma	M > F	10-40; peak = 27	Mandible ~ maxilla	Body of mandible	Sunburst; many radiographic appearances (see Table 20-1); well marginated
Osteoblastic metastatic carcinoma	?	40-80	Mandible	Body of mandible	History of parent tumor in prostate or breast
Chondroma and chondrosarcoma	M > F (slightly)	30-60	Maxilla 1.2 times mandible	Anterior maxilla, mandible; premolar-molar; symphysis; condyle; coronoid	Pain; many radiographic appearances (see Table 20-1)
Ossifying subperiosteal hematoma	M > F	5-20	—	—	Rapid growth after trauma

*Approximately equal.
†For ossifying fibroma.

SPECIFIC REFERENCES

Hamner, J. E., Scofield, H. H., and Cornyn, J.: Benign fibro-osseous jaw lesions of periodontal membrane origin, Cancer **22:**861-878, 1968.

Mainous, E. G., Boyne, P. J., and Hart, G. B.: Elimination of sequestrum and healing of osteoradionecrosis of the mandible after hyperbaric oxygen therapy: report of case, J. Oral Surg. **31:**336-339, 1973.

Martis, C.: Chondrosarcoma of the mandible: report of case, Oral Surg. **36:**227-230, 1978.

Mizuno, A., Sekiyama, S., Seki, S., and Kojima, M.: Clinical observation on osteoradionecrosis of the mandible, Oral Surg. **46:**22-26, 1978.

Mizuno, A., Shimizu, M., and Ueno, T.: Histopathologic and roentgenologic studies on the effects of irradiation on the human mandible, Bull. Tokyo Med. Dent. Univ. **23:**129-201, 1976.

Sato, K., Nukaga, H., and Horikoshi, T.: Chondrosarcoma of the jaws and facial skeleton: a review of the Japanese literature, J. Oral Surg. **35:**892-897, 1977.

Waldron, C. A., and Giansanti, J. S.: Benign fibro-osseous lesions of the jaws: a clinical-radiologic-histologic review of sixty-five cases. I. Fibrous dysplasia of the jaws, Oral Surg. **35:**190-201, 1973a.

Waldron, C. A., and Giansanti, J. S.: Benign fibro-osseous lesions of the jaw: a clinical-radiologic-histologic review of sixty-five cases. II. Benign fibro-osseous lesions of periodontal ligament origin, Oral Surg. **35:**340-350, 1973b.

GENERAL REFERENCES

Anderson, L., Fejerskov, O., and Philipsen, H. P.: Calcifying fibroblastic granuloma, J. Oral Surg. **31:**196-200, 1973.

Beasley, W. R., Ziffren, S. E., and Hale, M. L.: Osteogenic sarcoma involving the mandible: report of case, J. Oral Surg. **23:**254-260, 1965.

Bertelli, A. P., Costa, F. Q., and Miziara, J. E. A.: Metastatic tumors of the mandible, Oral Surg. **30:**21-28, 1970.

Beumer, J., Curtis, T. A., and Morrish, R. B.: Radiation complications in edentulous patients, J. Prosthet. Dent. **36:**193-203, 1976.

Bhaskar, S. N., and Jacoway, J. R.: Peripheral fibroma and peripheral fibroma with calcification: report of 376 cases, J. Am. Dent. Assoc. **73:**1312-1320, 1966.

Bhatt, A. P., Dholakia, H. M., and Bhoweer, A. L.: Chondrosarcoma of maxilla (report of case), J. Oral Med. **32:**51-54, 1977.

Binnie, W. H., Brocheriou, C., De Lathoower, C., and Panders, A. K.: Symposium on maxillofacial bone pathology, Int. J. Oral Surg. **4:**80-92, 1975.

Borghelli, R. F., Barros, R. E., and Zampieri, J.: Ewing sarcoma of the mandible: report of case, J. Oral Surg. **36:**473-475, 1978.

Brady, C. L., and Browne, R. M.: Benign osteoblastoma of the mandible, Cancer **30:**329-333, 1972.

Curphey, J. E.: Chondrosarcoma of the maxilla: report of case, J. Oral Surg. **29:**285-290, 1971.

Dahlin, D. C.: Bone tumors, ed. 2, Springfield, Ill., 1973, Charles C Thomas, Publisher.

Daramola, J. O., Ajagbe, H. A., Oluwasanmi, J. O., et al.: Ameloblastic sarcoma of the mandible: report of case, J. Oral Surg. **37:**432-435, 1979.

Eller, D. J., Blakemore, J. R., Stein, M., and Byers, S. S.: Transoral resection of a condylar osteochondroma: report of case, J. Oral Surg. **35:**409-413, 1977.

Ellis, D. J., Winslow, J. R., and Indovina, A. A.: Garré's osteomyelitis of the mandible. Report of a case, Oral Surg. **44:**183-189, 1977.

Eversole, L. R., Leider, A. S., Corwin, J. O., and Karian, B. K.: Proliferative periostitis of Garré. Its differentiation from other neoperiostoses, J. Oral Surg. **37:**725-731, 1979.

Eversole, L. R., Sabes, W. R., and Rovin, S.: Fibrous dysplasia a nosologic problem in the diagnosis of fibro-osseous lesions of the jaws, J. Oral Pathol. **1:**189-220, 1972.

Fisher, A. D.: Osteomyelitis of the mandible in a child, J. Oral Surg. **35:**60-63, 1977.

Freestone, J. T., Look, F., and Caulder, S. L.: Intraoral mandibular resection for osteoradionecrosis, J. Oral Surg. **31:**861-864, 1973.

Gorlin, R. J., and Goldman, H. M.: Thoma's oral pathology, ed. 6, St. Louis, 1970, The C. V. Mosby Co.

Greer, R. O., and Berman, D. N.: Osteoblastoma of the jaws: current concepts and differential diagnosis, J. Oral Surg. **36:**304-307, 1978.

Hayward, J. R., Melarkey, D. W., and Megquier, J.: Monostotic fibrous dysplasia of the maxilla: report of cases, J. Oral Surg. **31:**625-628, 1973.

Kirby, S. W., and Robinson, M. E.: Osteitis deformans of the maxilla: report of case, J. Oral Surg. **31:**64-70, 1973.

Kusen, G. J.: Chondromatosis: report of case, J. Oral Surg. **27:**735-738, 1969.

Lichtenstein, L.: Bone tumors, ed. 5, St. Louis, 1977, The C. V. Mosby Co.

Marciani, R. D., and Bowden, C. M.: Osteoradionecrosis of the maxilla: report of case, J. Oral Surg. **31:**56-58, 1973.

Mesa, M. C.: Metastatic prostate carcinoma to the mandible; report of case, J. Oral Surg. **35:**133-135, 1977.

Payne, J. V., Dahlen, D. F., Silva, M. T., et al.: Osteomyelitis of the mandible in a child due to *Bacteroides fusiformis*, Oral Surg. **43:**44-46, 1977.

Ramon, Y., Horowitz, I., Oberman, M., et al.: Osteochondroma of the coronoid process of the mandible, Oral Surg. **43:**692-697, 1977.

Rapoport, A., Sobrinho, J. D., De Carvalho, M. B., et al.: Ewing's sarcoma of the mandible, Oral Surg. **44:**89-94, 1977.

Sanders, B., Admas, D., and Scaramello, J.: Advanced osteoradionecrosis of the mandible, J. Oral Med. **33:**73-76, 1978.

Seldin, E. B.: New hope for patients with Ewing sarcoma, J. Oral Surg. **36:**583, 1978.

25

Anatomic radiopacities of the jaws

Thomas M. Lund

Anatomic radiopacities of the jawbones include the following:

Common to both jaws
Teeth
Bone
    Cancellous bone
    Cortical plates
    Lamina dura
    Alveolar process

Peculiar to the maxilla
Nasal septum and boundaries of the nasal fossae
Anterior nasal spine
Canine eminence
Walls and floor of the maxillary sinus
Zygomatic process of the maxilla and the zygomatic bone
Maxillary tuberosity
Pterygoid plates and the pterygoid hamulus
Coronoid process

Peculiar to the mandible
External oblique ridge
Mylohyoid ridge
Internal oblique ridge
Mental ridge
Genial tubercles

Superimposed radiopacities
Soft tissue shadows
Mineralized tissue shadows

A tissue or object is radiopaque because it does not permit the unrestricted passage of x rays. On properly exposed and developed radiographs it may appear light or white, depending on differential absorption of the rays. This differential absorption is a function of the density and/or thickness of the tissue or object. Normal radiopacities, then, may be defined as the radiographic images of normal anatomic structures of sufficient density or thickness or both to appear light or white on radiographs. Normal radiopacities of the jawbones may be common to both jaws, or they may represent specific anatomic structures peculiar to one jaw.

Common to both jaws

TEETH

The radiopacities produced by teeth and bone will be common to both jaws. Tooth enamel, the most dense tissue in the body, casts the whitest shadow (i.e., is the most radiopaque). It covers the coronal portion of the tooth, tapering to a thin layer at the cervical margin. Dentin, which makes up the bulk of the tooth, is less radiopaque and thus readily distinguishable from the enamel. The density of the normally thin layer of cementum covering the root of the tooth is similar to that of dentin, so cementum is usually not distinct on the regular periapical radiograph (Fig. 25-1). Enamel and dentin are both distinguishable in the calcifying tooth germ—which is normally completely surrounded by a thin layer of cortical bone until the tooth starts to emerge through the alveolar crest (Fig. 25-2).

BONE
Cancellous bone

The jaws consist chiefly of spongy cancellous (medullary) bone made up of thin strands or trabeculae that cross each other in a seemingly irregular manner. Although irregular, these strands generally assume a network pattern in the maxilla and a parallel pattern in the mandible. There is a wide normal variation in size of the marrow spaces lying between the trabeculae.

Cortical plates

The maxilla and the mandible are covered with thin dense plates of compact bone, called cortical plates, which can be seen on occlusal radiographs of the jaws but do not produce a separate shadow on routine intraoral films. The cortical plates of the mandible are thicker than those of the maxilla, and the plates over the inferior border of the

Fig. 25-1. Dense radiopaque shadows of enamel contrast with the less dense shadows of dentin. Note the continuity of the white line (lamina dura) surrounding the periodontal ligament spaces. Note also the prominent white shadow of cortical bone delineating the alveolar crest.

Fig. 25-2. Two radiopaque linear shadows of cortical bone lining the mandibular canal inferior to the apices of the second molar. Note the thin white cortex forming the limits of the developing tooth crypt.

mandible are thickest of all, being readily discernible on radiographs.

Destruction of parts of a cortical plate will produce a more radiolucent appearance than will destruction of the cancellous portion of the bone.

Lamina dura

The tooth sockets are normally lined with a thin layer of dense compact bone, which appears on radiographs as a thin white line and is referred to as the lamina dura (Fig. 25-1).

Alveolar process

The alveolar cortical plates, the lamina dura, and the spongy bone lying between them make up the alveolar process. The gingival margin of the alveolar process is termed the "alveolar crest," which is usually a thin layer of dense cortical bone that is sometimes reproduced as a fine white line on radiographs. This line is frequently discernible on radiographs of the mandibular incisors, where it may appear as a sharply pointed crest if the teeth are close together (Fig. 25-14, *A*).

In the absence of pathoses, the alveolar crest may be seen on radiographs of other areas at right angles to the lamina dura (Fig. 25-1).

Other structures, such as the mandibular canal and large nutrient canals in the maxillary alveolus, may be bordered with a thin layer of dense compact bone that shows as a fine white line on radiographs (Fig. 25-2).

The incisive, mental, and mandibular foramina may also be delineated by these white (opaque)

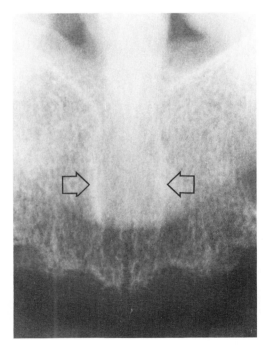

Fig. 25-3. Incisive canal. Note the two vertical thin radiopaque lines (arrows) delineating this structure.

lines, as may the edges of the maxillary bones forming the midline suture (Fig. 25-3).

Peculiar to the maxilla

The commonly seen radiopacities of the maxilla will be discussed as they are encountered, begin-

Fig. 25-4. Maxillary incisor region. The arrows denote the soft tissue outline of the tip of the nose. Note the paired radiolucencies, representing the nasal chambers, at the upper edge of the radiograph. The vertical radiopaque shadow separating them is the nasal septum. The cortical bone forming the floor of the nasal fossa shows as a broad radiopaque line.

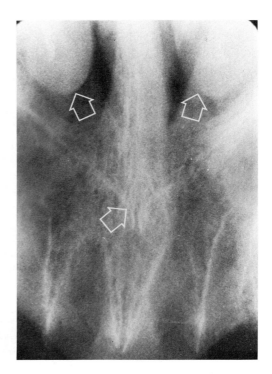

Fig. 25-5. Maxillary midline in an edentulous patient. The two arrows at the upper half of the radiograph identify the inferior turbinates. The lower arrow indicates the anterior nasal spine.

ning in the anterior region and moving posteriorly.

NASAL SEPTUM AND BOUNDARIES OF THE NASAL FOSSAE

The nasal septum may be seen on films of the central incisors positioned superiorly to the apices of these teeth (Fig. 25-4). It appears as a wide vertical radiopaque shadow and frequently deviates slightly from the midline.

The nasal fossae are lined with compact cortical bone; their floors may be seen extending bilaterally from the inferior limit of the septum as linear radiopacities that curve superiorly when the lateral walls of the fossae are approached (Fig. 25-4).

ANTERIOR NASAL SPINE

The anterior nasal spine is a projection of the maxilla at the lower borders of the nasal fossae. It is seen as a small white V-shaped opaque shadow below the nasal septum (Fig. 25-5). The bottom of the V is usually open.

CANINE EMINENCE

Frequently a bulge, sometimes referred to as the canine eminence, is present on the labial alveolar plate over the maxillary canine. It is produced by deflection of the alveolar plate over the thick root of the canine.

Since the alveolar bone covering the root is usually of normal thickness, a canine eminence is seldom discernible on radiographs of the area.

WALLS AND FLOOR OF THE MAXILLARY SINUS (ANTRUM)

The margins or walls of the maxillary sinus are formed by thin layers of dense cortical bone that appear as fine white lines on radiographs of the maxillary teeth. The outline of the sinus can be seen extending from the area of the canine to the tuberosity. When the tube and the film are occasionally fortuitously positioned, an X or an inverted Y is produced on the superior aspect of the canine and first premolar area where the anterior

Fig. 25-6. Maxillary sinus Y.

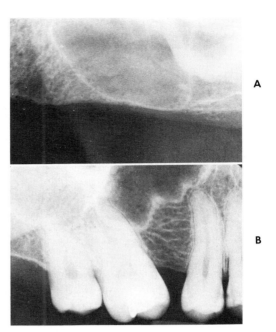

Fig. 25-7. Maxillary sinus. **A,** The radiopaque cortical line in this edentulous patient delineates a flat sinus floor. **B,** Note the scalloped floor in a dentulous patient.

medial wall of the sinus meets the lateral wall of the nasal chamber (Fig. 25-6). The X is produced when the lines are seen to cross; the inverted Y is produced when the superior portion of the anterior wall of the sinus is indistinguishable.

The floor of the sinus lies above the apices of the maxillary teeth but varies widely as to extent and contour. It is frequently scalloped as it dips between the roots to varying depths or it may be smoothly curved or flat, especially in edentulous jaws (Fig. 25-7). Sinus septa may or may not be present; and when present, they may exhibit many variations in number and location.

ZYGOMATIC PROCESS OF THE MAXILLA AND THE ZYGOMATIC BONE

The zygomatic process of the maxilla, which arises above the alveolar process of the first molar, is usually seen on periapical radiographs as a U-shaped radiopaque shadow above the roots of the maxillary first molar. The sinus may extend into this structure, making the borders appear more radiopaque and further emphasizing the U shape (Fig. 25-8).

The inferior border of the zygomatic (malar) bone may appear on the superior aspect of the maxillary molar area as a dense more or less horizontal radiopacity extending from the zygomatic process posteriorly; it may be mistaken for patho-

Fig. 25-8. Maxillary molar region. The larger white arrow identifies the zygomatic process of the maxilla. The black arrow indicates the zygomatic bone. The smaller white arrow, *1*, marks the fibrous tuberosity shadow.

sis. When a greater portion of this structure appears on the radiograph, it is readily identified (Fig. 25-8).

MAXILLARY TUBEROSITY

The maxillary tuberosity forms the posterior boundary of the maxillary alveolus. It is a rounded projection, normally of cancellous bone, usually

Fig. 25-9. Posterior maxillary region. Note the hamular process (lower arrow) and the lateral pterygoid plate (upper arrow).

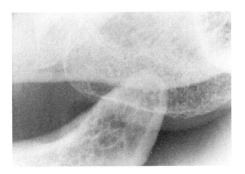

Fig. 25-10. Coronoid process in the posterior maxillary region.

outlined by a thin layer of compact bone (which is a continuation of the alveolar crest). Cancellous bone may extend into the tuberosity, causing this structure to appear on radiographs as a thin shell of cortical bone. On the radiograph the pterygoid plates of the sphenoid bone lie immediately behind the maxillary tuberosity.

PTERYGOID PLATES AND THE PTERYGOID HAMULUS

The lateral pterygoid plate is wider than the medial plate and may be seen on radiographs of the maxillary third molar region (Fig. 25-9).

The medial pterygoid plate, although thinner and rarely seen, gives rise to the hamular process (Fig. 25-9).

The pterygoid hamular process varies in length, thickness, and density; and its tip may be seen lying above or below the level of the alveolar crest on periapical films. It may also be seen on bite-wing radiographs of the molar regions.

CORONOID PROCESS

The coronoid process of the mandible often appears on radiographs of the maxillary third molar region, but it may extend as far forward as the second molar. Although generally cone shaped with its apex pointing upward and forward, it may have varied contours and positions (Fig. 25-10).

Sometimes the radiopaque shadow of the coronoid process has been mistaken for a root fragment in the maxilla.

Peculiar to the mandible

This discussion of radiopacities of the mandible will commence with the description of those in

Fig. 25-11. Edentulous right mandibular molar region. The external oblique ridge (black arrow) and the mylohyoid ridge (open arrow) can be seen.

the most posterior regions and proceed to those located more anteriorly.

The coronoid process of the mandible has already been discussed as a maxillary radiopaque structure since it is frequently visible on films of the maxillary third molar region.

EXTERNAL OBLIQUE RIDGE

The external oblique ridge is a continuation of the anterior border of the ramus, which passes forward and downward over the outer surface of the body of the mandible. It is often clearly seen as a prominent radiopaque line passing across the molar region (Fig. 25-11).

In the edentulous mandible, after resorption of the alveolar process, the external oblique ridge may delineate the superior border of the mandibular body in the molar region.

Fig. 25-12. Mandibular third molar region. Note the external oblique ridge (white arrow) and the internal oblique ridge (open arrow).

MYLOHYOID RIDGE

The mylohyoid ridge originates on the medial portion of the ramus and passes forward and downward over the lingual surface of the mandible, serving as the attachment of the mylohyoid muscle. It is most clearly seen in its posterior portion, where it is most prominent, crossing the retromolar and molar region inferior to and running approximately parallel with the external oblique ridge (Fig. 25-11).

Sometimes the mylohyoid ridge will extend along the entire lingual surface of the body of the mandible to the lower border of the symphysis; and in such cases it may be visualized as a faint narrow radiopaque line extending from the apices of the molars forward to the region below the apices of the incisors.

INTERNAL OBLIQUE RIDGE

The internal oblique ridge is the subject of some controversy. Some authors regard it as being superior to the mylohyoid ridge and consisting of a shelf of thickened lingual alveolar crest bone in the mandibular molar region. Others believe that it is a portion of the mylohyoid ridge and contend that, without a mylohyoid muscle, there would be no internal oblique ridge. In any case it may be observed as a radiopaque line crossing the mandibular molars and, because of the usual direction of the x rays, lying inferior to the external oblique ridge (Fig. 25-12).

MENTAL RIDGE

The mental ridge or mental triangle (mental protuberance) is located on the lower external aspect of the anterior portion of the body of the

Fig. 25-13. Mental ridge (arrows).

mandible (which is usually thickened to provide additional strength to the bone). It extends from the premolar region on each side to the symphysis and sweeps incisally, forming a thick inverted V-shaped radiopacity, inferior to or superimposed over the apices of the mandibular anterior teeth (Fig. 25-13).

The size and prominence of the mental ridge vary from person to person; and the differentiation of the ridge from the anterior limits of the mylohyoid ridge may at times be problematic.

GENIAL TUBERCLES

The genial tubercles, as many as four in number, surround the lingual foramen, which is situated on the internal surface of the mandible at the symphysis midway between the superior and inferior borders. They vary in size but usually appear on periapical radiographs as an approximate radiopaque ring (Fig. 25-14).

On mandibular occlusal films the genial tubercles will be seen as single or multiple protuberances on the medial surface of the mandible in the symphysial region (Fig. 25-14).

Fig. 25-14. Genial tubercles. **A,** Note the lingual foramen encircled by a radiopaque ring (arrow), which is produced by the genial tubercles. Note also the lamina dura interdentally forming the pointed alveolar crests. **B,** Occlusal view of the genial tubercles (arrow).

Fig. 25-15. Ala of the nose (arrows). **A,** Positioned over the apex of the lateral incisor. **B,** In an edentulous patient.

Fig. 25-16. Maxillary premolar region. The nasolabial fold (arrow) delineates the anterior border of the cheek.

Superimposed radiopacities

SOFT TISSUE SHADOWS

Soft tissue, because of its thickness or density, also casts radiographic shadows that must be identified. As a general rule the thicker or redder the tissue, the whiter will be its shadow.

The outline of the lip is often superimposed on the crowns of the teeth in both maxillary and mandibular anterior projections. On radiographs of the maxillary anterior teeth, shadows produced by the soft tissue of the tip of the nose (Fig. 25-4) and the nasal and alar cartilages are often present and may confuse the examiner if they are not recognized (Fig. 25-15).

The cheeks absorb and scatter x rays, and their outlines may be found on radiographs of the canines and premolars (Fig. 25-16).

Gingival tissue is evident on many routinely exposed films, especially when the soft tissues of the lips and cheeks are superimposed. Fibrous tissue, especially in the tuberosity area, is readily seen (Fig. 25-8).

MINERALIZED TISSUE SHADOWS

The radiopaque superimpositions of mineralized tissues, either normal structures or pathologic lesions, must be considered. For example, although not seen on periapical films, the radiopaque outline of the hyoid bone is commonly projected over the body of the mandible on lateral oblique views.

• • •

The foregoing discussion of the many normal anatomic radiopacities illustrates the problem that confronts the uninitiated clinician when he attempts to identify specific radiopaque shadows. It also emphasizes that he must have a thorough knowledge of the anatomic structures, their relative locations, and the limits of their normal variations in shape and size if he is going to identify and intelligently interpret the pathologic variations of these structures.

GENERAL REFERENCES

Bhaskar, S. N.: Radiographic interpretation for the dentist, ed. 3, St. Louis, 1979, The C. V. Mosby Co.

Chiles, J. L., and Gores, R. J.: Anatomic interpretation of the orthopantomogram, Oral Surg. **35:**564-574, 1973.

Ennis, L. M., Berry, H. M., and Phillips, J. E.: Dental roentgenology, ed. 6, Philadelphia, 1967, Lea & Febiger.

Knight, N.: Anatomic structures as visualized on the Panorex radiograph, Oral Surg. **26:**326-331, 1968.

Manson, J. D.: The lamina dura, Oral Surg. **16:**432-438, 1963.

Shoha, R. R., Dowson, J., and Richards, A. G.: Radiographic interpretation of experimentally produced bony lesions, Oral Surg. **38:**294-303, 1974.

Sicher, H., and DuBrul, E.: Oral anatomy, ed. 6, St. Louis, 1975, The C. V. Mosby Co.

Smith, C. J., and Fleming, R. D.: A comprehensive review of normal anatomic landmarks and artifacts as visualized on panorex radiographs, Oral Surg. **37:**291-304, 1974.

Stafne, E. C.: Oral roentgenographic diagnosis, ed. 3, Philadelphia, 1969, W. B. Saunders Co.

Worth, H. M.: Principles and practice of oral radiologic interpretation, Chicago, 1963, Year Book Medical Publishers.

Wuehrmann, A. H., and Manson-Hing, L. R.: Dental radiology, ed. 4, St. Louis, 1977, The C. V. Mosby Co.

26

Periapical radiopacities

Norman K. Wood
Paul W. Goaz

The following entities are periapical radiopacities:

True periapical radiopacities
Condensing or sclerosing osteitis
Periapical idiopathic osteosclerosis
Mature periapical cementoma
Unerupted succedaneous teeth
Foreign bodies
Hypercementosis
Rarities
    Cementifying and ossifying fibromas
    Chondroma and chondrosarcoma
    Hamartoma
    Mature cementoblastoma
    Mature complex odontoma
    Mature osteoblastoma
    Metastatic osteoblastic carcinoma
    Osteogenic sarcoma
    Paget's disease—intermediate and mature stages

False periapical radiopacities
Anatomic structures
Impacted teeth, supernumerary teeth, and compound odontomas
Tori, exostoses, and peripheral osteomas
Retained root tips
Foreign bodies
Mucosal cyst of the maxillary sinus
Ectopic calcifications
    Sialoliths
    Rhinoliths and antroliths
    Calcified lymph nodes
    Phleboliths
    Arterial calcifications
Rarities
    Calcified acne lesions
    Calcified hematoma
    Calcinosis cutis
    Cysticercosis
    Hamartomas
    Multiple osteomas of the skin
    Myositis ossificans
    Osteoma cutis
    Pathologic soft tissue masses
    Pilomatrixoma (calcifying epithelioma of Malherbe)
    Tonsillolith

SCLEROSING AND SCLEROSED CONDITIONS IN BONE

Since there is some confusion with regard to terminology and to the etiology of sclerosis in bone, a discussion of these aspects is appropriate before the individual periapical lesions are considered. The nomenclature found in the current literature for this spectrum of lesions includes the following terms: *condensing osteitis, sclerosing osteitis, osteosclerosis, enostosis, bone whorls, bone eburnations, hyperostosis, focal sclerosing osteomyelitis,* and *sclerosing tumors.*

We prefer to use the following to describe specific sclerotic lesions of the jaws:
    Condensing or sclerosing osteitis
    Idiopathic osteosclerosis
    Sclerosing osteomyelitis
    Hyperostotic border
    Osteosclerosing tumor

The term *condensing* or *sclerosing osteitis* is used when an inflammation (either present or recently past) is likely the initiating factor for the sclerosing process: the most frequent example of this condition is encountered in the periapex of a tooth with an infected root canal.

An *idiopathic osteosclerosis* develops during a healing process and is not caused by inflammation: the most frequent example of this type of sclerosis is found in the periapex of a healthy vital mandibular premolar or molar.

A *sclerosing osteomyelitis* is a chronic osteomyelitis in which there is a sclerosis of either a sequestrum or the surrounding bone. The majority of these lesions will show a combination of radiolucent and radiopaque areas.

A *hyperostotic border* is uniformly thin and radiopaque. It frequently surrounds a benign osteolytic process within bone (e.g., a cyst, a granuloma, a benign tumor, occasionally a slowly expanding malignancy). It is usually produced in response to the minimal pressures created by a slowly expanding lesion.

An *osteosclerosing tumor* produces an irregular sclerosis. It may result from a primary or a secondary malignancy involving bone or from an aggressive benign bone lesion (e.g., an ameloblastoma, another type of odontogenic epithelial tumor, a chondroma, a myxoma, a hemangioma).

Several different mechanisms have been proposed to account for the osteosclerosis that develops about nests of tumor cells:

1. Chronic inflammation, present in the tissue surrounding malignant tumor cells, is produced by the reaction of the tissue to the foreign antigens from the tumor cells; and the resultant sclerosis is essentially a condensing or sclerosing osteitis.
2. The pressure of an expanding tumor or of blood pulsations (as in an arteriovenous shunt or a hemangioma) initiates a sclerosis similar to the hyperostotic border about a cyst but usually less uniform.
3. Certain tumors possess the inherent ability to induce osteoblastic activity with resultant dense bone formation, for example, an osteogenic sarcoma, a chondrosarcoma, or a metastatic prostatic carcinoma.

Sclerotic bone may be considered an endpoint of the osseous tissue reaction to a mild chronic mechanical or chemical irritation (it probably represents the bony counterpart of cicatrization in soft tissue).

SCLEROSING OSTEITIS AND IDIOPATHIC OSTEOSCLEROSIS

An area of bony sclerosis is termed "sclerosing or condensing osteitis" if its cause can be associated with an inflammatory process and "idiopathic osteosclerosis" if its cause cannot be readily explained.

Sclerosing and sclerosed lesions of these two types are commonly seen on radiographs of patients over 12 years of age. Approximately 22% of the patients in this age group will have such a sclerotic area in their jaws. Overall incidence is equal in male and female whites and blacks (Farman et al., 1978). Basically the lesion will be a mass of compact bone within the spongiosa (medullary portion). Its density will approximate that of cortical bone. It may be totally enclosed in the medullary portion of the bone or it may be continuous with one or both of the cortical plates.

Sclerosing osteitis and idiopathic osteosclerosis share a number of characteristics:

1. They are almost invariably painless and do not produce expansion of the cortex.
2. The covering mucosa is normal in appearance.
3. Sinuses are not present, and regional lymph nodes are characteristically asymptomatic.
4. Approximately 85% of the sclerosing and sclerosed areas occur in the mandible of whites, where the first molar region is the predominant site (Farman et al., 1978). In blacks approximately 71.6% of focal bony sclerotic areas were in the mandible.
5. These sclerotic areas may remain unchanged for years (even after successful treatment of associated infected teeth), they may partially resolve, or they may completely disappear (and the region become radiographically normal again). Serial radiographs showing any increase in size will be indicative of an active lesion.

Identifying the specific types of sclerosis may not always be possible because the sclerotic area may have been induced by a previous disturbance that is no longer present. In such instances the clinician will be unable to relate the lesion to any disorder currently apparent; and he will then diagnose the lesion as an idiopathic osteosclerosis.

Radiographically the regions of sclerosis will vary in size from a few millimeters to 2 or 3 cm in diameter. Shape may also vary from irregular to round to almost linear. The appearance of the lesions will range generally from a slight or prominent accentuation of the normal trabecular pattern in milder cases to a dense homogeneous radiopacity in more pronounced cases.

Different areas of a sclerotic lesion may also demonstrate variations in density. Margins may be smoothly contoured or ragged, well defined or vague, and the radiodensity of the lesion may tend to blend with that of the adjacent normal bone. Even borders of the same lesion may have variable definition. Bony sclerosis and resorption (rarefaction) may be active in the same lesion and appear radiographically as a combined radiolucent-radiopaque image (Fig. 26-1).

Histologically the sclerosing and sclerosed lesions will consist of notably thickened trabeculae with a concomitant decrease in size and number of marrow spaces (Fig. 26-2). Vascularity and the number of lacunae present will be reduced whereas incremental lines will be numerous and prominent. Chronic inflammation may be present at the periphery of the area, depend-

Fig. 26-1. Combined periapical rarefying and condensing osteitis. **A,** At the apex of the distal root of the first molar. Note the condensing osteitis only at the apex of the mesial root of this molar. **B,** At the apices of the second molar.

ing on the cause and stage of the lesion's development.

• • •

Periapical radiopacities are a common finding on radiographic surveys of dentulous patients. These entities may be grouped into two divisions:

1. *True* periapical radiopacities are produced by lesions that actually surround the apex or are located in the periapex.
2. *False* (projected) periapical radiopacities are produced by entities that are situated buccally or lingually to the apex and whose radiopaque images lie over the apical region.

Lesions producing false radiopacities are usually situated either at the periphery of the bone (e.g., a torus) or in the soft tissues adjacent to the bone (a sialolith). False radiopaque shadows may be projected away from the apex by changing the horizontal or vertical angulation of the beam (the Clark tube-shift technique, Clark, 1910). This procedure will usually differentiate the false from the true periapical radiopacity—the image of the latter cannot be shifted from the periapex by altering the angle of exposure.

Fig. 26-2. Sclerosis of bone. This high-magnification photomicrograph reveals very dense bone with a few small fibrovascular spaces and few lacunae; some of the lacunae are empty.

True periapical radiopacities

True periapical radiopacities are a group of lesions in the immediate region of the periapex comprised of dense bone, cartilage, hard dental tissues, or foreign material.

CONDENSING OR SCLEROSING OSTEITIS

Condensing or sclerosing osteitis is a sclerosis of bone induced by inflammation. It most often occurs as a pulpoperiapical lesion and is the most common periapical radiopacity observed in adults (about 8%). In direct contrast to the reaction seen in rarefying osteitis (in which bone resorption is the predominant process), the reaction in this lesion is a proliferation of bone tissue.

Both the condensing and the rarefying lesions occur chiefly at the apex of a pulpless tooth or a tooth with an infected pulp(s) and are produced by an extension of the inflammatory process into the periapical area.

The highly concentrated products of infection are thought to act as an irritant and produce bone resorption whereas the diluted irritants may induce bone proliferation such as that seen in condensing osteitis. This concept is illustrated occasionally when a periapical area of rarefying osteitis is surrounded by a radiopaque halo of condensing osteitis (Fig. 26-1). In such instances bone is resorbed near the apex, where the toxic products from the infected canal are most concentrated; and bone proliferation is stimulated at the periphery of the rarefied area, where because of their diffusion through the tissue the products from the infected canal are more dilute.

Fig. 26-3. Periapical condensing osteitis (arrows). The pulps of all four teeth tested nonvital.

FEATURES

The clinical features of condensing or sclerosing osteitis are discussed under sclerosing osteitis and idiopathic osteosclerosis. The pulps of the involved teeth are nonvital—although the sclerosing may have commenced before the complete pulp became nonvital, in which case the tooth may react positively to electrical pulp testing procedures. In an interesting study, Jordan and co-workers (1978) showed that if these carious molar teeth were treated with indirect pulp capping, some of these periapical lesions would disappear and the pulps remain vital. Also, since the process is of such a low grade, there is usually no pain, swelling, drainage, or associated lymphadenitis. The radiographic image will vary greatly as to size, shape, contours, and discreteness of margins (Fig. 26-3).

The vast majority of these lesions are found in the mandible. The teeth most frequently involved are the mandibular premolars and molars. If the lesion is in an active stage, careful selection and examination of biopsy material from the periphery will show the presence of chronic inflammation.

DIFFERENTIAL DIAGNOSIS

Condensing or sclerosing osteitis must be differentiated from all the other true periapical radiopacities: periapical idiopathic osteosclerosis, periapical cementoma, an unerupted tooth, a foreign body introduced during root canal therapy, hypercementosis, and the rare lesions. In addition, the clinician must rule out the false periapical radiopacities by using the Clark tube-shift technique when exposing additional films.

Hypercementosis can be differentiated from the other true periapical radiopaque lesions by the fact that it is the only common lesion which is an integral (hyperplastic) part of the tooth root. Thus on the radiograph it will be completely separated from the periapical bone by the periodontal ligament shadow.

The radiographic image of a *foreign body* introduced during root canal therapy, along with the history of its insertion, should be diagnostic. The material—whether amalgam, cement, root canal points, or some other substance—will usually be recognizable on the radiograph by virtue of its shape and density. Thus it will seldom be confused with other radiopaque entities that appear in the periapex.

Condensing or sclerosing osteitis may be differentiated from the remaining periapical radiopaque lesions and from *periapical idiopathic osteosclerosis* by the fact that in the osteitis the tooth pulp will usually be nonvital whereas in the other associated lesions it will be vital (except

Fig. 26-4. A to **D,** Periapical idiopathic osteosclerosis (arrows). The pulps of these teeth tested vital. **E,** Dense trabeculation surrounding the roots of a vital molar due to heavy occlusal function.

rarely when there is concomitant but unrelated pulp death).

In addition, *periapical cementoma* will always have a thin uniform radiolucent rim in the mature radiopaque stage. This feature differentiates this lesion from condensing osteitis and idiopathic osteosclerosis.

MANAGEMENT

Extraction of the infected tooth or treatment of its root canal is indicated. Approximately 30% of these sclerotic areas will not resolve to normal-appearing bone after adequate treatment.

PERIAPICAL IDIOPATHIC OSTEOSCLEROSIS (ENOSTOSIS, BONE WHORLS, BONE EBURNATION)

Periapical idiopathic osteosclerosis is a relatively common finding on full-mouth radiographs of dentulous patients over 12 years of age. Approximately 4.3% of the patients within this age group will have at least one such periapical osteosclerotic lesion (Farman et al., 1978). It is second only to condensing osteitis as the most frequently seen periapical radiopacity. The term "idiopathic" is used to emphasize the fact that the cause of the lesion is not readily apparent or understood.

FEATURES

Most periapical radiopacities of this type, as is true of condensing osteitis, are located in the periapex of the mandibular first premolar and canine (Farman et al., 1978). The associated teeth are invariably healthy, have vital pulps, and are asymptomatic (Figs. 26-4 and 26-5). Since the patient does not complain, the region is usually discovered on routine radiographs. There is no associated pain, cortical change, softness, expansion, drainage, or lymphadenitis. The overlying alveolar mucosa appears normal.

The radiopacity of periapical idiopathic osteosclerosis may vary from a few millimeters to 2 cm

Fig. 26-5. Idiopathic osteosclerotic lesions at the apices of teeth with healthy pulps.

in diameter. Its shape may range from generally round to very irregular, and sometimes a triangular configuration will be observed. The degree of density may vary from a slight accentuation of the trabecular pattern to a dense homogeneous radiopaque mass. Borders may be well defined or vague, well contoured or ragged (Figs. 26-4 and 26-5). Multiple and bilateral periapical lesions are also occasionally discovered.

DIFFERENTIAL DIAGNOSIS

The entities most frequently confused with idiopathic periapical osteosclerosis and which must be distinguished from it are condensing osteitis, mature fibro-osseous lesions (PDLO), hypercementosis, and abnormally dense alveolar bone induced by heavy occlusal stress.

Periapical idiopathic osteosclerosis should be differentiated from the dense trabecular pattern in *alveolar bone induced by heavy masticatory function.* Frequently an isolated tooth is subjected to occlusal trauma, and the sclerosis induced by the abnormal stresses will have a more diffuse outline. It is usually not localized to the periapical region but involves the entire alveolar process about the tooth (Fig. 26-4, *D*). When forces are not directed in the long axis of the tooth, the reactive sclerosis may develop on the side of the root in line with the direction of the excessive force.

Hypercementosis is recognized by the club-shaped appearance of the affected root and by the fact that it is separated from the adjacent normal bone by the periodontal ligament.

In contrast to periapical idiopathic osteosclerosis, the *mature periapical cementoma* will be a characteristically rounded radiopacity with a well-defined border and will be separated from normal bone and the root by a thin radiolucent halo. If earlier radiographs of the area are available, they may reveal the radiolucent and radiolucent-radiopaque stages of the cementoma.

Because the periapical idiopathic osteosclerosis and *periapical condensing osteitis* are so similar clinically, radiographically, and sometimes histologically, they may be difficult to differentiate. The former entity develops in the periapex of a tooth with a healthy vital pulp, however, whereas the latter occurs at the apex of a tooth with an infected or nonvital pulp.

The following rarities may also be mistaken for idiopathic periapical osteosclerosis: complex odontoma, Paget's disease, cementoblastoma, osteoblastoma, osteogenic sarcoma, chondrosar-

coma, metastatic prostatic carcinoma, and hamartoma.

If the lesion were a *metastatic prostatic carcinoma,* the clinician would expect to find some symptoms or obtain a history of treatment for primary tumor along with a report of increased serum acid phosphatase.

If it were a *chondrosarcoma* or an *osteogenic sarcoma,* he would find ragged radiolucent areas along with the radiopacities. A mixed radiolucent-radiopaque appearance is not seen in idiopathic periapical osteosclerosis.

The *osteoblastoma* and *cementoblastoma* begin as radiolucent lesions, progress through a mixed radiolucent-radiopaque stage, and are mature as radiopaque images. If earlier radiographs of the area in question are available, they will help establish the entity's course of development. Also the cementoblastoma is usually very round whereas areas of osteosclerosis are less regular in form and outline. (In addition, the former lesion is attached to the root apex but the latter is not.)

If it were located in the periapex, the *complex odontoma,* especially a small lesion, might be difficult to distinguish from an idiopathic periapical osteosclerosis. The complex odontoma, however, occurs much less frequently than idiopathic osteosclerosis and usually is seen over the crown of an unerupted (impacted) tooth or between the roots of teeth. Also it is infrequently situated periapically. Furthermore, the denser sharper radiopacities caused by the deposits of enamel will usually produce greater variations in the degree of radio-density and thus aid the clinician in differentiating the odontoma from a periapical idiopathic osteosclerosis. Finally, a radiolucent line of more or less uniform width (corresponding to the PDL space), which rims the odontoma and separates it from the adjacent normal bone, is usually apparent; and this feature is not characteristic of idiopathic osteosclerosis.

MANAGEMENT

Areas of periapical idiopathic osteosclerosis are not of clinical significance except that they should be distinguished from condensing osteitis since teeth associated with the latter lesion require endodontic treatment.

Periodic reexamination of lesions suspected of being periapical idiopathic osteosclerosis is recommended to ensure that this clinical impression is correct. In rare cases when there is associated root resorption, the affected tooth may require endodontic care or extraction.

MATURE PERIAPICAL CEMENTOMA

The periapical cementoma undergoes maturation from an early radiolucent, osteolytic, fibroblastic stage (Chapter 16), through an intermediate radiolucent stage with radiopaque foci (Chapter 23), to a mature radiopaque stage. In this chapter the mature stage of the lesion will be emphasized as a periapical radiopacity.

FEATURES

The features of the cementoma are described in detail in Chapter 16, so only a brief summary will be given here. Ninety percent of cementomas occur in the mandible, and approximately 80% occur in women (with a definite predilection for blacks). This lesion is not commonly found in patients under 30 years of age.

The cementoma occurs at the apex of a vital tooth and is completely asymptomatic except for rare cases when the lesion reaches a size sufficient to produce an expansion of the cortical plates with possible subsequent ulceration of the mucosa.

Radiographically the completely mature periapical cementoma is predominantly round or ovoid with smoothly contoured borders. It varies in size from 0.5 to 2 cm and in rare instances may be larger. The mature lesion will be uniformly dense and devoid of trabecular pattern, and it will have a thin radiolucent border (Fig. 26-6).

Histologically the lesion will be made up of a mass of cementum containing few cells (Fig. 26-6). A mixture of cementum or bone may be present, or in some instances the calcified material will be entirely bone.

The mature cementoma is particularly interesting because its radiographic features correlate so well with the histologic picture:

1. Very little fibrous or vascular tissue is present, except at the periphery, and this produces the thin radiolucent rim about the radiopaque mass on the radiograph.
2. A hyperostotic line may be present in the bone adjacent to, and delineating, the radiolucent rim. Histologically this line is osteosclerotic bone.
3. Root resorption is not characteristic, but on occasion the adjacent root shows hypercementosis.

DIFFERENTIAL DIAGNOSIS

In the mature stage the periapical cementoma must be differentiated from periapical idiopathic osteosclerosis, condensing osteitis, and hypercementosis.

The periapical spherical type of *hypercementosis*, which sometimes involves the anterior teeth, may be confused with the cementoma by the unwary examiner. Careful study of the radiograph, however, will reveal that the hypercementosis is attached to a part of the root and is separated from the periapical bone by the radiolucent periodontal ligament space, which surrounds the entire root.

Condensing osteitis may generally be ruled out because it occurs in the periapex of a nonvital tooth whereas a cementoma usually does not. The tooth that has a cementoma at its apex, however, is equally susceptible to pulp injury by the usual agents; thus the alert clinician may (rarely) find a periapical cementoma at the apex of a pulpless tooth. In addition, condensing osteitis does not have a radiolucent rim but fibro-osseous lesions (PDLO) do.

Periapical idiopathic osteosclerosis and mature periapical cementomas may be difficult to differentiate because both occur in the periapex of healthy teeth with vital pulps. The cementoma, however, is smoothly contoured and almost always round or ovoid whereas periapical idiopathic osteosclerosis is usually quite irregular in shape. Also the uniformly thin radiolucent border that can be recognized surrounding the cementoma is not present in idiopathic osteosclerosis.

The rare periapical radiopacities (p. 551) and the false (projected) radiopacities may also be mistaken for mature fibro-osseous lesions (PDLO). The projected group, however, may be immediately eliminated if the clinician cannot shift the radiographic image from the periapex on additional films by altering the angle of exposure.

The *cementoblastoma* affects the periapices of the premolars and molars almost exclusively whereas 80% of cementomas are seen in the mandibular incisor region.

When systemic symptoms are absent, *Paget's disease* and *metastatic osteoblastic prostatic carcinoma* can be assigned a low rank in the differential diagnosis. Also many such radiopaque areas would be seen scattered throughout the jaws of most patients afflicted with Paget's disease.

Osteosarcoma, chondroma, and *chondrosarcoma* do not characteristically produce such a solid uniform radiopaque pattern.

The density of the *complex odontoma* generally is not uniform. The more opaque images of the enamel contrasting with the less opaque dentin enable the clinician to differentiate between this lesion and the more homogeneously opaque ce-

Fig. 26-6. A to **D,** Mature periapical cementomas (arrows). The pulps of these teeth tested vital. (Note the horseshoe-shaped lesion in **D.**) **E,** Microscopy of a mature cementoma. (**A** courtesy M. Smulson, D.D.S., Maywood, Ill.)

mentoma. Also the complex odontoma seldom occurs periapically.

MANAGEMENT

The proper management of a periapical cementoma requires continued observation and subsequent verification through periodic radiographic examination. Surgical enucleation and microscopic examination are indicated for the larger lesions that cause expansion of the cortical plate or when the clinician is unsure of the working diagnosis.

UNERUPTED SUCCEDANEOUS TEETH

When the permanent crowns of succedaneous teeth are completely formed and the resorption of

Fig. 26-7. Unerupted second premolar.

the root ends of the corresponding deciduous teeth is initiated, the images of the permanent tooth crowns represent periapical radiopacities (Fig. 26-7). Obviously such shadows will be seen only on radiographs of persons less than 12 or 13 years of age. Since these teeth will undoubtedly be recognized for what they are, however, this entity is included in the present discussion only for completeness and does not require any additional consideration.

Impacted teeth are not included in the discussion of true periapical radiopacities; they rarely occur at the apices of other teeth. Although they may appear at these locations, the clinician can usually shift their images in the periapical region by making another radiograph with a different angle of exposure. Impacted teeth are discussed later in this chapter with the false periapical radiolucencies.

FOREIGN BODIES (ROOT CANAL–FILLING MATERIALS)

Radiopaque foreign bodies in the periapex are almost always root canal—filling materials. The images produced by extruded gutta percha, silver points, sealer, or a retrograde amalgam restoration and the filled root canal (Fig. 26-8), coupled with the history of a related procedure, contributes to the easy recognition of these periapical radiopacities. Consequently they require no further description.

Fig. 26-8. Periapical foreign bodies (endodontic materials). **A,** Gutta percha. **B,** Retrograde amalgam filling. (**B** courtesy F. Weine, D.D.S., Chicago.)

Fig. 26-9. Hypercementosis. **A,** In a mandibular premolar. **B,** In a mandibular molar.

HYPERCEMENTOSIS (CEMENTAL HYPERPLASIA)

Hypercementosis has been defined by Stafne (1969, p. 25) as "excessive formation of cementum on the surface of the root of the tooth." The early stages are only microscopically detectable; but as additional layers of cementum are added, the accumulation becomes apparent on the radiograph (Fig. 26-9).

The etiology of hypercementosis is not well understood; but repeated observations seem to indicate that this lesion is sometimes associated with the development of periapical inflammatory conditions, periapical cementoma, and systemic disease (e.g., Paget's disease, acromegaly, giantism).

FEATURES

Hypercementosis is completely asymptomatic and is usually discovered on routine radiographic surveys. The premolars are more often affected than are the remaining teeth (6:1), and the first molars are next in order of involvement. The hypercementosis may be confined to just a small region on the root, producing a nodule on the surface, or the whole root may be involved. In multirooted teeth, one or two or all roots may show hypercementosis. Often teeth are bilaterally involved, and a generalized form with hyperplasia of cementum on all root surfaces has been reported. The teeth affected are usually vital and are not sensitive to percussion.

Radiographically the altered shape of the root is apparent if there has been a reasonable amount of cemental hyperplasia. An isolated nodule or the characteristic club-shaped root may be seen. In either case the root is surrounded by a normal periodontal ligament space* and lamina dura. The different densities of the excess cementum and root dentin are such that the original outline of the dentin root is discernible on the radiograph (Fig. 26-9). Hypercementosis on anterior teeth may appear as a spherical mass of cementum attached to the root end.

Histologically the cementum may be acellular (primary) or cellualar (secondary). It is usually deposited in layers but may be arranged in an irregular fashion with fibrovascular inclusions.

DIFFERENTIAL DIAGNOSIS

Hypercementosis may be differentiated from the *false radiopaque images* that are projected over the apex by two features:

1. The projected radiopacities will not be delineated by a periodontal ligament space and lamina dura as will the hypercementosis.
2. The projected images may be shifted in relation to the apex by altering the angle at which additional radiographs are exposed.

The true periapical radiopacities are more difficult to differentiate from hypercementosis. They include the following: cementomas, condensing osteitis, periapical idiopathic osteosclerosis, and such developmental anomalies as fused roots,

---

*Hypercementosis may well be a response to the elongation of a tooth or the loss of supporting bone and is initiated by an inherent tendency for maintenance of the normal width of the periodontal ligament (Shafer et al., 1974, p. 302).

dilacerations, and similar images caused by multirooted teeth.

The club-shaped images cast by *multirooted teeth* and the shadows of *dilacerated roots* can be identified by making successive radiographs exposed from different angles.

Sometimes the *fused roots* of multirooted teeth will have a bulbous shape, but these can be recognized by the fact that the apparently expanded region of the root will not have the relatively lower radiodensity of hyperplastic cementum.

Periapical idiopathic osteosclerosis, condensing osteitis, and *cementomas* can be differentiated from hypercementosis by the fact that all these entities lie outside the shadow of the periodontal ligament and lamina dura whereas hypercementosis forms an integral part of the root surface and is therefore enclosed by a normal periodontal ligament space and lamina dura. Nevertheless, there may be difficulty when the periodontal ligament space and lamina dura are indistinct. Also differentiation may be a problem when the clinician is confronted by the spherical type of hypercementosis occasionally seen on the anterior teeth. In hypercementosis, continuity with the root surface will be discernible if the radiograph is carefully examined.

MANAGEMENT

Hypercementosis does not require special treatment except for the obvious surgical problem encountered during the removal of the involved tooth. When many teeth show hypercementosis, the patient should be examined for diseases such as Paget's, acromegaly, and giantism.

RARITIES

A number of entities may cause true periapical radiopacities; but since they are rare or are only rarely homogeneous and radiopaque, they have been placed in the following list and are given no further attention (Fig. 26-10):

Cementifying and ossifying fibroma
Chondroma and chondrosarcoma
Hamartoma
Mature cementoblastoma
Mature complex odontoma
Mature osteoblastoma
Metastatic osteoblastic carcinoma
Osteogenic sarcoma
Paget's disease—intermediate and mature stages

The reader is directed to the general reference list at the end of the chapter for sources of further information concerning these disorders.

Fig. 26-10. Paget's disease. (**A** courtesy R. Goepp, D.D.S., Zoller Clinic, University of Chicago.)

The complex odontoma is included in this list of rarities because it usually occurs supracoronally or between the roots of adjacent teeth so it only rarely produces a periapical radiopacity. It is listed under true periapical radiopacities because its image cannot usually be shifted from the apex since its buccolingual dimension is relatively large.

False periapical radiopacities

False (projected) periapical radiopacities are produced by a large number of entities. These entities may be categorized into two groups, however:

1. Radiodense bodies within the bone situated either buccally or lingually to the apex
2. Hard or soft tissue situated on the periphery of the bone or in the adjacent soft tissue

It is important to emphasize that a normal or pathologic soft tissue mass projected over bone may impart a considerably denser quality to the shadow of the bone.

False periapical radiopacities have a characteristic that is diagnostically useful. Their relation to the apex is such that the radiopaque images can be shifted from the apex by altering the angle of exposure. Additional views (e.g., occlusal, lateral

Fig. 26-11. Projected anatomic periapical radiopacities. **A,** Ala of the nose (arrow). **B,** Mylohyoid ridge (arrow).

Fig. 26-12. Impacted supernumerary teeth as projected periapical radiopacities.

oblique, posteroanterior, Waters, panographic) may be necessary to establish the true location of these entities.

ANATOMIC STRUCTURES

Either soft tissue or bony anatomic structures may be projected as radiopaque shadows over tooth apices. Examples of such configurations include the anterior nasal spine, the ala of the nose, the malar process of the maxilla, the external oblique ridge, the mylohyoid ridge, the mental protuberance, and the hyoid bone (Fig. 26-11).

Identification of these structures will hinge on an awareness of the regional anatomy, a general understanding of the geometry required to radiographically visualize the area, and usually at least two different radiographic projections of the area.

IMPACTED TEETH, SUPERNUMERARY TEETH, AND COMPOUND ODONTOMAS

Since it is unusual for impacted or supernumerary teeth or those in a compound odontoma to be situated directly at the apex of an erupted tooth, these entities are classified as false periapical radiopacities.

The periapical radiopaque images produced by an impacted or supernumerary tooth or by an odontoma will be readily identified by their density and shape (Fig. 26-12). In most cases the images can be shifted from the apex by the Clark tubeshift technique.

TORI, EXOSTOSES, AND PERIPHERAL OSTEOMAS

Tori, exostoses, and, less frequently, osteomas are situated at the periphery of the jaws and may vary greatly in size, shape, and location. Although the true nature of these bony protuberances is still a matter of debate, the tori and exostoses are usually considered to be developmental lesions and the osteoma a benign neoplasm. They are all discussed in detail in Chapter 7 as examples of exophytic lesions. Because they originate deep to the surface epithelium and are slow growing, they have a smoothly contoured surface.

Radiographically tori, exostoses, and periosteal osteomas may appear as single or multiple, smoothly contoured, somewhat rounded, dense radiopaque masses (Fig. 26-13). Since they are peripheral, if their shadows happen to fall in an apical area on the radiograph, shifting the tube on a subsequent exposure (Clark tubeshift technique) will readily demonstrate that these images are false periapical radiolucencies.

Fig. 26-13. A, Maxillary torus (arrow) as a projected periapical radiopacity. **B,** Microscopy of the torus.

Such information from the radiographs and corroborated by clinically apparent intraoral bony protuberances will make the diagnosis obvious. In addition, these radiopaque images are not circumscribed by a periodontal ligament space and lamina dura.

RETAINED ROOT TIPS

Retained root tips, especially in the molar regions, may be so situated that their radiopaque shadows are projected over the apex of an adjacent tooth (Fig. 26-14). When this happens, the root tip's position relative to the apex in question can be demonstrated on subsequent films by the Clark tube-shift technique. If the shapes of the root, its root canal, the surrounding periodontal ligament, and the lamina dura remain unaltered,

Fig. 26-14. Retained root tip of the mesial root of the third molar (arrow) projected into the periapex of the second molar.

Fig. 26-15. Metal fragments projected as periapical radiopacities. **A,** This foreign body proved to be in the buccal cortical plate. **B,** This foreign body proved to be in the upper lip.

the identification is relatively easy; if these features are obliterated, however, the nature of the radiopacity may not be so obvious. Furthermore, a condensing osteitis may develop about the root tip and obscure it on the radiograph.

FOREIGN BODIES

A variety of foreign materials within the jawbone or in the surrounding soft tissue may be projected over apices and cause periapical radiopacities on the radiograph (Fig. 26-15). A list of such objects would include metal fragments, buttons, zippers, hooks, other metal dress accessories and jewelry, and various dental materials and fragments of instruments. Usually the images cast by such items are distinctive and readily identifiable. If there is a history of trauma to the region, the clinician may anticipate finding a foreign body embedded in the tissue and even look for its appearance on the radiograph.

MUCOSAL CYST OF THE MAXILLARY SINUS

The mucosal cyst of the maxillary sinus affects about 2% of the population. This entity represents a retention cyst in the lining mucosa of the maxillary sinus.

FEATURES

The incidence of mucosal cyst of the maxillary sinus, which affects men and women equally and may be bilateral, peaks during the third decade. Although the majority are symptomless, a significant number will produce accompanying symptoms of a sinusitis.

Radiographically the cyst usually appears as a relatively dense dome-shaped mass with its base on the floor of the maxillary sinus; and the apices of the maxillary first and second molars may appear to be within the opaque image of the cyst (Fig. 26-16).

Fig. 26-16. Tentative diagnosis of benign mucosal cyst (arrow) of the maxillary sinus projected as a radiopacity over the molar roots.

The location and appearance of the dome-shaped radiopaque structure of a maxillary sinus mucosal cyst are almost diagnostic. Although the cyst may remain constant in size for a long time, it also may spontaneously empty either slowly or rapidly; thus periodic radiographic examinations will frequently reveal a radiopacity of varying dimensions.

DIFFERENTIAL DIAGNOSIS

When a mucosal cyst of the maxillary sinus appears as a periapical radiopacity, it must be differentiated from the true radiopacities—a condensing or sclerosing osteitis, a periapical idiopathic osteosclerosis, a cementoma. Additional views (e.g., panographic, Waters, posteroanterior) will usually identify it as a mass situated in the maxillary sinus.

Its smooth dome shape often differentiates a mucosal cyst of the maxillary sinus from a *malignant tumor of the sinus.*

Occasionally *fibrous dysplasia* originating on the floor of the maxillary sinus will mimic a maxillary sinus retention phenomenon; but the ground-glass appearance of the former entity will help to distinguish this lesion from the mucosal cyst.

MANAGEMENT

When the clinician discovers what appears to be a mucous retention cyst in the maxillary sinus, he may refer the patient to an otolaryngologist for an opinion. If the mass appears to be of odontogenic origin, an oral surgeon should be consulted for evaluation and management.

ECTOPIC CALCIFICATIONS

Ectopic calcifications* in the soft tissues surrounding the jaw may be mistaken on radiographs for calcified odontogenic structures. Such deposits of abnormal calcific salts may be readily distinguished from calcified odontogenic structures and lesions by the fact that the latter are almost always surrounded by a periodontal ligament type of space and a lamina dura whereas the former radiopacities do not have such characteristic borders. Also the location of these ectopic calcifications can be shown to be some distance from the teeth by Clark's tube-shift technique.

Sialoliths (salivary gland calculi)

Sialoliths are calcareous (radiopaque) deposits in the ducts of the major or minor salivary glands or within the glands themselves. They are thought to form from a slowly calcifying nidus of tissue or bacterial debris (organic matrix).

In their early stages the sialoliths may be either too small or insufficiently mineralized to be visualized on radiographs. If they are not expelled from the duct, however, they will eventually assume sufficient proportions to become apparent as radiopacities (Fig. 26-17).

FEATURES

When they reach a critical size or position, sialoliths effect a partial or complete obstruction of the duct.

This obstruction results in a sialadenitis, which is manifested as a painful swelling of the gland that is most pronounced just before, during, and immediately after meals. The enlargement will usually be minimal when the patient awakes in the morning. Often several episodes of sialadenitis will be experienced by the patient before he seeks professional help. Since the major or collecting ducts are generally completely occluded, milking the gland and duct will be nonproductive.

The submaxillary salivary gland and duct are the most frequent sites of sialoliths. Some clinicians believe this is because the oral terminus of the duct is superior to the gland and gravity tends to cause secretions to the pool in the gland and duct system. Sialoliths vary greatly in size, shape, density, contour, and position and they may be solitary or multiple (Fig. 26-17). They are frequently seen within the substance of the submaxillary gland and may be one solid mass or many smaller masses.

---

*Pathologic deposits of calcium salts in tissues that are normally uncalcified.

Fig. 26-17. Sialolith. **A,** In the submandibular salivary gland projected over the apex of the mandibular second molar (arrow). **B,** Note the shift in the image of the stone caused by altered angle of exposure. **C,** Photomicrograph.

Although sialoliths in the submaxillary gland and duct may be seen on periapical films, they are best visualized on occlusal, lateral oblique, and panographic radiographs. They are rarely found in the parotid gland or its duct but, when present in the duct, may be seen on periapical films superimposed over the maxillary molars or the posterior maxillary alveoli.

Histologically a sialolith resembles calculus, showing concentric rings of alternating lighter and darker bands (Fig. 26-17).

DIFFERENTIAL DIAGNOSIS

The first step in the diagnostic procedure is to obtain another radiographic view of the stone taken at a different angle from the first. This will ensure that the radiopacity in question is actually a false (projected) periapical radiopacity.

Once the radiopacity is established as a projected radiopacity, the sialolith must be distinguished from several similar entities—a calcified lymph node, an avulsed or embedded tooth, a foreign body, a phlebolith (calcified thrombus), calcification in the facial artery, myositis ossificans, an anatomic structure (e.g., the hyoid bone).

The radiopaque image of the *hyoid bone* is frequently projected over the region of the submaxillary gland, duct, and mandible on lateral oblique radiographs but is bilaterally visualized on panoramic films. Thus, if the mass is single on both the lateral oblique and the panographic radiographs, it is not likely to be the hyoid bone.

The shape of the hyoid bone (v) is actually so diagnostic that the clinician will not mistake this structure for pathosis.

Myositis ossificans is a rare disturbance characterized by the formation of bone in the interstitial tissue of muscle. It has also been observed in the superficial tissues away from muscle, however, even in the skin. When muscles about the face are involved, the masseter muscle is most frequently affected. This results in a restriction of mandibular movements, which should alert the clinician to the possibility of myositis ossificans.

Calcification in the walls of the facial artery may also be projected over the suspicious area. If a significant length of the artery is involved, the resultant serpentinelike calcified image will be diagnostic; but if there are calcific deposits in just a short section of the vessel, the resultant image may be mistaken for a sialolith, especially if the section of facial artery that courses through the submandibular space is involved.

A *phlebolith* sometimes occurs in the floor of the mouth and may be seen on an occlusal radiograph; it usually accompanies a clinically discernible varicosity. If the clinician finds a radiopacity in the floor of the mouth and there is no sialadenitis, he should be inclined to favor phlebolith as a diagnosis. The final differentiation between these two entities may have to await surgery.

A *foreign body* is usually readily diagnosed by its characteristic shape and by the history of a traumatic incident to the region.

An *avulsed tooth* lying in the soft tissues should also be recognizable by its shape and relative density. In addition, the clinician should be able to obtain a history of a traumatic incident.

A *calcified submandibular lymph node* may be difficult to distinguish from a sialolith occurring within the submandibular gland since some of the lymph nodes in the submandibular space rest on the surface of the submandibular gland (some are even inside the capsule of the gland). Also a calcified lymph node and a sialolith would be projected into the same general region on the radiograph. The relative incidences of the two entities, however, would favor the diagnosis of sialolith; and, furthermore, if a painful swelling accompanied a calcified mass in the submandibular space, this would be strongly indicative of a sialolith since a calcified node represents an old burned-out asymptomatic lesion. On the contrary, if the calcified mass has a smooth rounded contour, it is more apt to be a calcified lymph node than a sialolith. A sialogram may help to distinguish between these entities. When painful swelling is not present, the examiner may be able to determine by careful bimanual palpation whether or not the firm mass is within the submaxillary salivary gland.

MANAGEMENT

When a stone is discovered in the duct or in the gland proper, it should always be removed.

If the sialolith is impacted in the duct and the case is complicated by secondary infection, the infection should be eliminated before the stone is surgically removed. If the stone is in Wharton's duct, it may be approached and removed intraorally.

When the sialolith is small and located within the gland, it can ordinarily be removed by simple incision. If it is large, however, the gland will have to be excised; also when a sialolith is in the gland, the surgery may have to be performed even though there is a concurrent sialadenitis.

Rhinoliths and antroliths

Rhinoliths and antroliths are calcified masses occurring in the nasal cavity and maxillary sinus, respectively. Their development is similar to that of a sialolith—commencing with the calcification of a nidus of tissue debris or concentrated mucus, which continues to grow because of the precipitation of calcium salts in concentric layers.

Rhinoliths and antroliths are included in this chapter because their images on periapical radiographs may be cast over the apices of adjacent maxillary teeth.

FEATURES

Usually no symptoms accompany the smaller rhinoliths or antroliths, but the larger stones may be associated with a sinusitis or a nasal obstruction.

These calcifications are usually found on routine radiographs of the region and are of various shapes from round to ovoid to irregular with outlines that may be smooth or ragged (Fig. 26-18). They may appear as a dense homogeneous radiopacity or may show concentric rings of radiopaque and radiolucent material. In some instances small radiolucent areas are distributed haphazardly throughout the radiopaque mass.

Rhinoliths and antroliths may contain so little mineral that their image is quite faint. Microscopically they resemble sialoliths and calculus.

DIFFERENTIAL DIAGNOSIS

When solitary radiopacities are seen in the superior aspect of a maxillary periapical film, an-

Fig. 26-18. A, Large antrolith projected over the roots of a molar. **B,** Lens of the patient's eyeglasses projected as a radiopacity.

troliths and rhinoliths must be considered as possible diagnoses. It is then particularly important to obtain additional maxillary views (e.g., panoramic, occlusal, Waters, posteroanterior) as well as several additional periapical views to facilitate the differential diagnosis since these projections will show the complete lesion or structure and will demonstrate whether the mass is in the sinus, nasal cavity, or adjacent maxillary alveolar bone.

Different projections will further enable the clinician to determine the relative location of the object as he compares its apparent shift in position on the varying angles of exposure.

A knowledge of the anatomy of the area coupled with the information obtained from a complete radiographic examination will enable the clinician to identify and differentiate the following entities, which can be confused with antroliths and sialoliths: the malar process of the maxilla, the ala of the nose, an impacted tooth, a palatal torus, a buccal exostosis, a periapical condensing osteitis, a mature cementoma, a complex odontoma, eyeglasses, and a cone cut.

A *cone cut* in the superior aspect of a periapical film will appear as a homogeneous radiopacity containing no detail. Its contour will be concave rather than convex like that of the rhinolith. Hopefully such cone cuts will not be present or similarly positioned on additional films.

Eyeglasses will occasionally show on radiographs as a solid homogeneous radiopacity rather than a radiopaque rim (Fig. 26-18). Although antroliths would not be likely to occur bilaterally and with such symmetry, additional films should be taken after the removal of the eyeglasses to reveal the true identity of the opacities.

The radiopaque images of a *complex odontoma* and a *mature cementoma* may mimic those produced by an antrolith, but they will have characteristically radiolucent borders. When these odontogenic tumors become large enough to cause a bulge in the floor of the antrum, differentiation from an antrolith may be difficult; but fortunately the complex odontoma and the mature cementoma rarely reach such a size in this location.

Periapical condensing osteitis at the apices of a maxillary premolar may simulate an antrolith on periapical films. The fact that the adjacent teeth test nonvital, however, and also that additional films show the mass not encroaching on the antrum will help to identify the radiopacity as a periapical condensing osteitis.

The dense rounded radiopacity produced by a *buccal exostosis* or a *palatal torus* is frequently seen in the superior aspect of a maxillary periapical radiograph and may closely resemble the image produced by an antrolith or a sialolith. Clinical detection of the torus or the exostosis, however, will provide the correct diagnosis.

An *impacted tooth* may be confused with an antrolith or a rhinolith, especially when it is projected high on the film or when it is positioned in the jaw so that its image is not characteristic of a tooth. Good-quality films properly positioned will show the typical clear outlines of the impacted tooth.

The *ala of the nose* may be projected over the periapices of the upper incisors or canines and appear as a partially mineralized rhinolith (Fig. 26-11, *A*). Again additional films and a familiarity with the regional anatomy will suggest the correct diagnosis.

The inferior portion of the *malar process of the maxilla* or the zygomatic bone on some periapical films appears to be identical to an antrolith (Fig. 27-20). Additional projections will enable the clinician to correctly identify this structure.

When a mature cementoma or a complex odontoma produces a bulge in the floor of the maxillary sinus, differentiating it from an antrolith or some other pathosis of the maxillary sinus (e.g., a mucosal retention cyst, fibrous dysplasia, a tumor, root tips) will be more difficult.

Root tips in the maxillary sinus may be difficult to differentiate from a small antrolith unless the root canal is evident.

Except for the rare osteoma, a *tumor* of the maxillary sinus will usually be less radiopaque than an antrolith.

Although possibly quite opaque on a Waters projection, *fibrous dysplasia* will usually have a ground-glass appearance on periapical films.

The dome-shaped appearance of a *mucosal retention cyst* will usually distinguish this phenomenon from the more spherical-appearing antroliths.

MANAGEMENT

Patients with antroliths and rhinoliths should be referred to an otolaryngologist for evaluation and management.

CALCIFIED LYMPH NODES

Calcified lymph nodes occur in the cervical and submaxillary regions (Fig. 26-19). The majority are calcified tuberculous nodes. On certain radiographic views their images will be projected over the mandibular bone and occasionally over the apex of a mandibular tooth.

FEATURES

Calcified lymph nodes are asymptomatic and are usually found on a routine radiographic survey.

The patient may have a history of successful treatment for tuberculosis. Any of the cervical and submandibular nodes may be involved. In some cases just an isolated node has been calcified whereas in others several nodes or perhaps a whole chain of nodes became calcified.

If the nodes are superficial, they may be palpated as bony, hard, round or linear masses with variable mobility.

Radiographically a single round, ovoid, or linear calcified radiopaque mass may be seen (Fig. 26-19). Frequently the outlines are well contoured and well defined, depending on whether the original inflammatory process was contained within the capsule of the lymph node.

DIFFERENTIAL DIAGNOSIS

The differential diagnosis of calcified lymph nodes is discussed with the differential diagnosis of the sialolith (p. 556).

A calcified lymph node is classified as a false periapical radiopacity, and its image may be projected over a wide range of views. One helpful feature differentiating it from a sialolith is that the calcified node is invariably asymptomatic whereas the sialolith is frequently accompanied by a painful sialadenitis of the associated gland. Also the sialolith usually has an irregular outline whereas the calcified node is most often smoothly contoured.

MANAGEMENT

Calcified lymph nodes do not require treatment.

Phleboliths

Phleboliths are calcified thrombi occurring in venules, veins, or sinusoidal vessels of hemangiomas. They may occur singly or as multiple calcifications, are usually small radiopacities, may be round or ovoid, and may show concentric light and dark rings (Fig. 27-22). When they are projected over the mandibular bone or the periapices of mandibular teeth, they may easily be confused with sialoliths.

Arterial calcifications

Calcification frequently accompanies arteriosclerosis, and the facial artery is sometimes affected. When a considerable length of this artery is involved, the serpentine outline and the position of the faint radiopacity are pathognomonic. When just a small segment of the artery is involved, however, and the radiopaque image of this segment is cast over the body of the mandible

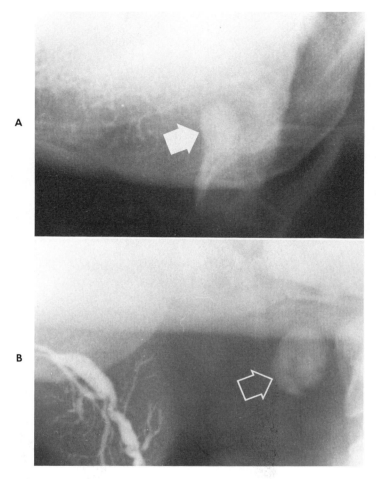

Fig. 26-19. Solitary calcified cervical lymph node (arrow). **A,** Projected over the mandible as a radiopacity. **B,** Another view of the same node showing the image shifted away from the mandible. A sialogram of the submandibular salivary gland proved the calcified lesion was not a sialolith. (Courtesy R. Goepp, D.D.S., Zoller Clinic, University of Chicago.)

near the inferior border, the artery may simulate a sialolith within the submaxillary gland or duct or a small calcified lymph node.

RARITIES

Included among the rarities are soft tissue calcifications that occur as single or multiple entities:

Calcified acne lesions
Calcified hematoma
Calcinosis cutis
Cysticercosis
Hamartomas
Multiple osteomas of the skin
Myositis ossificans
Osteoma cutis
Pathologic soft tissue masses

Pilomatrixoma (calcifying epithelioma of Malherbe)
Tonsillolith

SPECIFIC REFERENCES

Clark, C. A.: A method of ascertaining the relative position of unerupted teeth by means of film radiographs, Proc. R. Soc. Med. **3:**87-90, 1910.
Farman, A. G., Joubert, J. J., and Nortje, C. J.: Focal osteosclerosis and apical periodontal pathosis in "European" and Cape Colored dental outpatients, Int. J. Oral Surg. **7:**549-557, 1978.
Jordan, R. E., Suzuki, M., and Skinner, D. H.: Indirect pulp-capping of carious teeth with periapical lesions, J. Am. Dent. Assoc. **97:**37-43, 1978.
Shafer, W. G., Hine, M. K., and Levy, B. M.: A textbook of oral pathology, ed. 3, Philadelphia, 1974, W. B. Saunders Co.
Stafne, E. C.: Oral roentgenographic diagnosis, ed. 3, Philadelphia, 1969, W. B. Sauders Co.

GENERAL REFERENCES

Allan, J. J., Finch, L. D., and Chippendale, I.: Sialolithiasis of the minor salivary glands, Oral Surg. **27:**780-785, 1969.

Bahn, S. C.: Sialolithiasis of minor salivary glands, Oral Surg. **32:**371-377, 1971.

Bosshardt, L., Gordon, R. C., Westerberg, M., and Morgan, A.: Recurrent peripheral osteoma of mandible: report of case, J. Oral Surg. **29:**446-450, 1971.

Boyne, P. J.: Incidence of osteosclerotic areas in the mandible and maxilla, J. Oral Surg. **18:**486-491, 1960.

Brusati, R.: Large calculus of the submandibular gland: report of case, J. Oral Surg. **31:**710-711, 1973.

Cherrick, H. M., King, O. H., Lucatorto, F. M., and Sugs, D. M.: Benign cementoblastoma, a clinicopathologic evaluation, Oral Surg. **37:**54-63, 1974.

Chiles, J. L., and Gores, R. L.: Anatomic interpretation of the orthopantomogram, Oral Surg. **36:**564-574, 1973.

Curran, J. B., and Collins, A. P.: Abbreviated case report: benign (true) cementoblastoma of the mandible, Oral Surg. **35:**168-172, 1973.

DeGregori, G., and Pippen, R.: Sialolithiasis with sialadenitis of a minor salivary gland, Oral Surg. **30:**320-324, 1970.

Dutta, A.: Rhinolith, J. Oral Surg. **31:**876-877, 1973.

Eliasson, S. T., and Holte, N. O.: Rubber base impression material as a foreign body: report of case, Oral Surg. **47:**379-380, 1979.

Elmostehy, M. R.: Parotid salivary calculus: report of case, Oral Surg. **26:**18-21, 1968.

Farhood, V. W.: Osteoma cutis: cutaneous ossification with oral manifestations, Oral Surg. **45:**98-103, 1978.

Greer, R. O., and Berman, D. N.: Osteoblastoma of the jaws: current concepts and differential diagnosis, J. Oral Surg. **36:** 304-307, 1978.

Halsted, C. L.: Mucosal cysts of the maxillary sinus: report of 75 cases, J. Am. Dent. Assoc. **87:**1435-1441, 1973.

Hays, J. B., Gibilisco, J. A., and Juergens, J. L.: Calcification of vessels in cheek of patient with medial arteriosclerosis, Oral Surg. **21:**299-302, 1966.

Hayward, J. R.: The consultant, J. Oral Surg. **22:**278, 1964.

Hedin, M., and Polhagen, L.: Follow-up study of periradicular bone condensation, Scand. J. Dent. Res. **79:**436-440, 1971.

Hoffman, H.: Tonsillolith-roentgeno-oddities, Oral Surg. **45:** 657-658, 1978.

Karges, M. A., Eversole, L. R., and Poindexter, B. J.: Antrolith: report of case and review of literature, J. Oral Surg. **29:**812-814, 1971.

Kenneth, S.: Bilateral submandibular sialolithiasis, Oral Surg. **27:**445-450, 1969.

King, D. R., and Moore, G. E.: An analysis of torus palatinus in a transatlantic study, J. Oral Med. **31:**44-46, 1976.

Knight, N.: Anatomic structures as visualized on the Panorex radiograph, Oral Surg. **26:**326-331, 1968.

Knight, W. O.: Sialolithiasis and sialadenitis of a minor salivary gland: report of case, J. Oral Surg. **30:**370-372, 1972.

Kwapis, B. W., and Whitten, J. B.: Mucosal cysts of the maxillary sinus, J. Oral Surg. **29:**561-566, 1971.

Marano, P. D., Smart, E. A., and Kolodny, S. C.: Rhinolith simulating osseous lesion: report of case, J. Oral Surg. **28:**615-616, 1970.

Mesa, M. L.: Metastatic prostate carcinoma to the mandible: report of case, J. Oral Surg. **35:**133-135, 1977.

Meyer, R. A.: Osteochondroma of coronoid process of mandible: report of case, J. Oral Surg. **30:**279-300, 1972.

Miller, A. S., and Pullon, P. A.: Case of the month: hard, raised lesion in the right buccal mucosa, Dent. Survey **55:**28, 1979.

Morris, C. R., Marano, P. D., Swinley, D. C., and Runco, J. G.: Abnormalities noted on panoramic radiographs, Oral Surg. **28:**772-782, 1969.

Mourshed, F.: A radiographic survey of 1,000 Egyptian edentulous patients, Oral Surg. **28:**844-853, 1969.

Nelson, D. F., Gross, B. D., and Miller, F. E.: Osteoma of the mandibular condyle: report of case, J. Oral Surg. **30:**761-763, 1972.

Noren, G. D., and Roche, W. C.: Huge osteoma of the mandible: report of case, J. Oral Surg. **36:**375-379, 1978.

Northrop, P. M.: Complex composite odontoma: report of three cases, J. Oral Surg. **21:**492-499, 1963.

Panders, A. K., and Hadders, H. N.: Chronic sclerosing inflammations of the jaw, Oral Surg. **30:**396-412, 1970.

Parker, L. A., and Frommer, H. H.:Phleboliths, Oral Surg. **18:** 476-480, 1964.

Pullon, P. A., and Miller, A. S.: Sialolithiasis of accessory salivary glands: review of 55 cases, J. Oral Surg. **30:**832-834, 1972.

Rust, T. H., and Messerly, C. D.: Oddities of salivary calculi, Oral Surg. **28:**862-865, 1969.

Sammartino, F. J.: Radiographic appearance of a mucoid retention cyst, Oral Surg. **20:**454-455, 1965.

Scandret, F. R., Tebo, H. G., Quigley, M. B., and Miller, J. T.: Radiographic examination of the edentulous patient, Oral Surg. **35:**872-875, 1973.

Snyder, S. R., Merkow, L. P., and White, N. S.: Prostatic carcinoma metastatic to the mandible, J. Oral Surg. **29:**205-207, 1971.

Van Der Wall, I., Beemster, G., Kraaijenhagen, H. A., and Van Der Kwast, W. A. M.: Pilomatrixoma in the differential diagnosis of pathological calcification of the paraoral soft tissue, Int. J. Oral Surg. **6:**283-286, 1977.

Wells, T. J., Hooker, S. P., and Roche, W. C.: Osteochondroma cutis: report of case, J. Oral Surg. **35:**144-145, 1977.

Worth, H. M.: Principles and practice of oral radiologic interpretation, Chicago, 1963, Year Book Medical Publishers.

Youmans, R. D., Caulder, S. L., and Hays, L. L.: Peripheral osteoma of the mandible, Oral Surg. **25:**785-791, 1968.

Zegarelli, E. V., Kutscher, A. H., Budowski, J., and Hoffman, P. J.: The progressive calcification of the cementoma, Oral Surg. **18:**180-183, 1964.

Zegarelli, E. V., Kutscher, A. H., Napoli, N., et al.: The cementoma, Oral Surg. **17:**219-224, 1964.

27

Solitary radiopacities not necessarily contacting teeth

Norman K. Wood
Paul W. Goaz

Following is a list of radiopacities that may not be in contact with the roots of teeth:

True intrabony radiopacities
Tori, exostoses, and peripheral osteomas
Unerupted, impacted, and supernumerary teeth
Retained roots
Idiopathic osteosclerosis
Condensing or sclerosing osteitis
Mature cementoma
Fibrous dysplasia
Sclerosing ostemyelitis
Garré's osteomyelitis
Mature complex odontoma
Ossifying subperiosteal hematoma
Rarities
    Cementifying and ossifying fibroma
    Chondroma and chondrosarcoma—radiopaque variety
    Mature osteoblastoma
    Metastatic osteoblastic carcinoma—radiopaque variety
    Osteoblastoma
    Osteogenic sarcoma—radiopaque variety

Projected radiopacities
Anatomic structures
Foreign bodies
Pathologic soft tissue masses
Ectopic calcifications
    Sialoliths of major and minor salivary glands
    Rhinoliths and antroliths
    Calcified lymph nodes
    Tonsillolith
    Phleboliths
    Arterial calcifications
Rarities
    Calcified acne lesion
    Calcified hematoma (soft tissue)
    Calcinosis cutis
    Hamartoma
    Myositis ossificans
    Peripheral fibroma with calcification
    Pilomatrixoma

Well-defined borders

Ill-defined borders

Many of the radiopacities included in this chapter are discussed in Chapter 26. It seems expedient, however, to repeat the listing of these entities in the present chapter and to reconsider some of them in light of the fact that they may also occur as solitary radiopacities not contacting the roots of teeth. Such an arrangement is appropriate since there is a difference in the incidence of these entities, which correlates with their contacting the roots of teeth.

Consequently this consideration will attach a great deal of importance to the development of a valid differential diagnosis. Condensing or sclerosing osteitis is a good case in point: as a periapical radiopacity, it is quite a common lesion; but its occurrence as a solitary radiopacity not contacting the roots of teeth is uncommon. Thus

Fig. 27-1. A, A palatal torus (arrows) appears as bilateral radiopacities in this panograph. **B,** Palatal torus (arrow) projected superior to the apex of the canine. **C,** Small lingual mandibular torus (arrow) appearing as a rounded radiopacity.

the two entities are discussed in Chapter 26 and in this chapter.

In this chapter solitary radiolucencies not contacting the roots of teeth will be discussed as two groups: true intrabony radiopacities and projected radiopacities.

True intrabony radiopacities

TORI, EXOSTOSES, AND PERIPHERAL OSTEOMAS

Tori, exostoses, and peripheral osteomas are discussed in Chapter 7 as exophytic lesions and in Chapter 27 as projected (false) periapical radiopacities.

Some authors contend that tori and exostoses are developmental lesions, in contrast to osteomas (which they describe as a neoplasm). From the standpoint of clinical diagnosis, however, we prefer to consider that these three lesions probably represent the same pathologic process and arise on a hereditary basis. This inference is based on the limited information currently available relating to the incidence of osteoma and is coupled with the fact that all three entities pro-

duce similar clinical and radiographic pictures and have almost identical microstructures.

Consequently, although the clinical differentiation of tori, exostoses, and osteomas may be quite arbitrary, those that occur in the midline of the palate or on the lingual aspect of the mandibular ridge (usually in the region of the premolars) will be termed palatal and mandibular "tori," respectively; those that occur in other alveolar sites will be referred to as "exostoses"; and when a torus or an exostosis becomes unusually large, it will be called on "osteoma." The tori, exostoses, and osteomas usually become discernible after 16 years of age.

FEATURES

Whether the well-defined radiopaque shadows of these bony protuberances are projected over the images of tooth roots on periapical films depends on which jaw the radiograph is of and whether the segment of the jaw most proximal to the bone lesion is dentulous (Fig. 27-1). A torus on the mandible, an exostosis, and sometimes an osteoma (in either jaw) will usually cast radiopaque shadows over the images of tooth roots if

Fig. 27-2. Ossifying fibroma in an 8-year-old boy, which resembled an exostosis both clinically, **A,** and in the occlusal radiograph, **B. C,** Orthopantograph showing that the radiopaque lesion has blocked the eruption of the lower right permanent incisor and canine tooth. (Courtesy N. Choukas, D.D.S., Maywood, Ill.)

the jaw segments in which they occur are bearing teeth.

King and Moore (1976) compared the incidence of tori in London, England, and Lexington, Kentucky, and found that the percentage and size of maxillary tori were higher and larger in the Kentucky sample than in the English sample.

DIFFERENTIAL DIAGNOSIS

Correlating the clinical finding of a smooth, nodular, hard protuberance with the radiographic finding of a smoothly contoured radiopacity establishes the correct diagnosis and eliminates the need for additional radiographs or an extensive differential diagnosis. Nevertheless, Fig. 27-2 shows a case of a mature ossifying fibroma that

mimics an exostosis. However, periapical films showed a thin radiolucent rim surrounding the mature fibro-osseous lesion. In addition, an early osteogenic sarcoma or a small chondrosarcoma can mimic a torus or exostosis.

MANAGEMENT

Tori, exostoses, and peripheral osteomas may not have to be treated; but they may be removed surgically for phonetic, psychologic, or prosthetic reasons or if they are being chronically irritated.

UNERUPTED, IMPACTED, AND SUPERNUMERARY TEETH

Unerupted permanent molars and impacted and supernumerary teeth are the next most com-

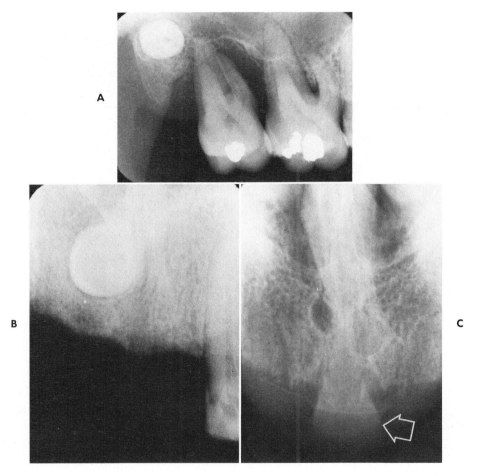

Fig. 27-3. A and **B,** Impacted teeth. **C,** Cartilage of the nasal septum (arrow) resembling the crown of a developing incisor.

men solitary radiopacities after tori, exostoses, and osteomas whose images may not overlap the roots of other teeth. If good-quality radiographs are obtained, the recognizable outline of a tooth plus the radiolucent shadows of the pulp canal, periodontal ligament, and follicular space will establish the identity of these entities (Fig. 27-3). Bizarre shapes of malformed teeth coupled with technically poor films may complicate the identification of the entities.

RETAINED ROOTS

Retained roots are a common finding in edentulous regions of the jaws where they are not associated with roots of other teeth. Ennis and Berry's survey of edentulous patients (1949) disclosed that approximately 25% of these patients had retained roots and 80% of the roots were located in the posterior regions of the alveolar processes. Approximately 6% of the retained roots had an accompanying radiolucency. This last group would be classified as mixed radiolucent-radiopaque lesions, which are discussed in Chapter 23.

In a recent study completed in London, Ritchie and Fletcher (1979) found that approximately 50% of edentulous patients had a retained root. Interestingly, the vast majority were seen in the upper jaw.

FEATURES

The majority of retained roots are quiescent, asymptomatic, and found on routine radiographs. If they are unaltered, their identification is relatively easy; but if chronic infection has caused the root canals to be obliterated or has resulted

Fig. 27-4. Retained roots. The periodontal ligament space and lamina dura cannot be clearly detected around some of the root fragments. The root canal shadows are not apparent.

in some peripheral resorption and/or enveloping condensing osteitis, their recognition may be difficult (Fig. 27-4). A careful study of the radiograph, however, will usually disclose the homogeneous quality of the root tip's shadow—in contrast to the more or less obscure trabecular character of the sclerotic bone. Thus the differentiation is possible.

On occasion, either retained roots become infected or long-standing chronic infection is exacerbated and local swelling, pain, regional lymphadenitis, space infections, and even osteomyelitis ensue.

DIFFERENTIAL DIAGNOSIS

The differential diagnosis for retained roots is discussed under the differential diagnosis section of condensing osteitis (p. 568).

MANAGEMENT

The management of a retained root tip depends on the circumstances of the individual case. If the root tip is small, asymptomatic, and situated relatively deep so that its removal would require removing a good deal of bone or if it is so close to an important structure that the structure could be severely damaged during the root's removal, it should not be removed. The patient should merely be apprised of its presence, and its status should be periodically evaluated by serial radiographs.

Roots that are near the surface and will be beneath a proposed artificial denture or bridge, are associated with a pathologic lesion, or are causing pain should be removed.

IDIOPATHIC OSTEOSCLEROSIS

Idiopathic osteosclerosis is discussed in Chapter 26 as a periapical radiopacity. The objective of the present chapter is to emphasize and illustrate that this entity is not always found in association with the roots of teeth.

FEATURES

Idiopathic osteosclerotic lesions may occur in the alveolus, between the roots of teeth, just below the crest of the ridge, or in the body of the mandible (Fig. 27-5).

Usually the cause is obscure. When the lesion is present in the alveolus between the first and second premolars or between the second premolar and the first molar, its occurrence is generally described as a sequela of retained decidu-

Fig. 27-5. A to **C,** Idiopathic osteosclerosis. The second premolar pulp in **B** was vital. **D,** Socket sclerosis (arrow). Note the central linear radiolucent shadow, which resembles a root canal.

ous molar roots. These retained roots are resorbed and replaced by sclerotic bone, or fragments of the roots are completely surrounded and obliterated by the condensed bone.

Because the radiopaque areas of periapical condensing osteitis frequently do not resolve after extraction of a tooth, many such residual areas may be diagnosed as idiopathic osteosclerosis if the clinician is unaware that teeth with infected or nonvital pulps have been removed from the area. This possibility should be considered when a suspicious-looking area is encountered. Post-extraction wounds and other surgical defects may be the site of idiopathic osteosclerosis (Fig. 27-5, *D*).

The sclerotic lesion is usually solitary but may be multiple or even bilateral; however, its bilateral occurrence would be only incidental and should not be considered a significant diagnostic feature.

Microscopically, thickened trabeculae with few lacunae and greatly reduced marrow and fibrovascular spaces are seen.

DIFFERENTIAL DIAGNOSIS

The differential diagnosis of idiopathic osteosclerosis is discussed under condensing osteitis (p. 568).

MANAGEMENT

The identification of idiopathic osteosclerosis is all that is necessary. The clinician should observe the course of the lesion with serial radiographs, however.

CONDENSING OR SCLEROSING OSTEITIS

Condensing or sclerosing osteitis is an osteosclerosis that can be explained as a sequela of an inflammatory process.

It occurs much less frequently in edentulous regions, of course, than as a periapical radiopacity. In edentulous regions, it is almost always a residual lesion or limited to reactions around retained roots or root tips. Its appearance as a periapical radiopacity is described in Chapter 26.

FEATURES

Radiographically condensing or sclerosing osteitis resembles the radiopacity of idiopathic osteosclerosis except that root tips are usually identifiable within the radiopaque lesion or there may be a history or some presumptive evidence that an infected tooth was previously removed from the area. The borders may be ragged or smoothly contoured, vague or well defined (Fig. 27-6).

Fig. 27-6. Condensing osteitis. **A,** Surrounding a small round root tip (arrow). **B,** Surrounding the mesial root of a grossly decayed molar.

The microscopic picture will be identical with that of idiopathic osteosclerosis except that, if the lesion is still active, an extensive examination of the specimen will disclose restricted areas of chronic inflammation. If the source of infection was removed some time before the specimen was taken, the inflammatory reaction may have completely subsided with only the dense mass of trabeculae remaining.

DIFFERENTIAL DIAGNOSIS

Many of the entities discussed in this chapter must be included in the differential diagnosis. The lesions most frequently confused with condensing or sclerosing osteitis are idiopathic osteosclerosis, tori, exostoses, and peripheral osteomas, sclerosing osteomyelitis, osteoblastic malignant tumor, mature complex odontoma, unerupted tooth, retained roots, cementoma, and a variety of the projected radiopacities that are not attached to or within the alveoli or jawbone under scrutiny.

As discussed in Chapter 26, the *projected radiopacities* can be readily identified by obtaining additional radiographs of the area using Clark's tube-shift technique.

The opacities produced by hard odontogenic tissue—including the *mature cementoma, retained roots, unerupted tooth,* and *mature complex odontoma*—may be recognized by their distinctive shapes and densities and their radiolucent borders. A partially resorbed root tip or root fragment is usually relatively small and if not surrounded by condensing osteitis will, in most cases, retain enough of its shape to be recognizable. It should be found only in tooth-bearing areas of the jaws.

Although an *osteoblastic malignancy* producing a completely radiopaque lesion in this area would be very rare, in the event of such an occurrence, the examining clinician must consider osteogenic sarcoma, metastatic prostatic carcinoma, or metastatic mammary carcinoma. In addition to the symptoms of the primary tumor or history of its treatment, pain, swelling, and frequently paresthesia would usually accompany the tumor. Paresthesia, if present, would strongly suggest that the lesion was malignant.

Sclerosing osteomyelitis is a moderate proliferative reaction of the bone to a mild type of infection. The patient will usually give a history of a prolonged tender swelling with, in some cases, intermittent drainage through a sinus from the body of the mandible. A helpful feature is the fact that osteomyelitis seldom becomes established in healthy persons without a history of jaw fracture. Condensing osteitis, by comparison, is usually asymptomatic.

The opacities produced by the *tori, exostoses,* and *peripheral osteomas* will be promptly identified if the characteristic painless smooth nodular swelling on the jaws is detected during the clinical examination.

Differentiating between condensing or sclerosing osteitis and *idiopathic osteosclerosis* is often very difficult if not impossible when the suspicious-looking lesion is in an edentulous region and cannot be related to a specific tooth. Of course, if a root tip can be observed within the region of sclerotic bone, the diagnosis is condensing osteitis. Thus, if the sclerotic area does not contain root tips and the lesion did not form at the apex of a tooth with an infected or nonvital pulp, then the diagnosis of idiopathic osteosclerosis is appropriate.

MANAGEMENT

The treatment of condensing of sclerosing osteitis surrounding a root tip must be tailored to the individual situation.

As with root tips, lesions that are in the superficial alveolar crest should be removed as a step in preprosthetic preparation and to prevent the occurrence of active infection.

Deeper lesions that are asymptomatic are usually not disturbed but are observed with serial radiographs.

Lesions complicated by acute or chronic infection should be enucleated, and the patient should receive appropriate presurgical and postsurgical antibiotic therapy.

MATURE CEMENTOMA

The cementoma that develops from cells of the periodontal ligament is discussed in Chapter 16 as a periapical radiolucency, in Chapter 23 as a mixed radiolucent-radiopaque lesion, and in Chapter 26 as a periapical radiopacity. In the present chapter its occurrence as a solitary radiopaque mass in edentulous regions of the jaws will be discussed.

FEATURES

The following comments relative to the features of this mature fibro-osseous lesion relate to the occurrence of these lesions without apparent relation to teeth:

1. They are ordinarily found at the apices of vital teeth but also occur with significant frequency in edentulous regions. Many of these latter lesions are undoubtedly residual (i.e., they were left in place when the involved tooth was removed).
2. They may be solitary or multiple, and their radiographic appearance is similar to that of the periapical variety. The mature lesions are uniformly radiopaque and almost invariably have a radiolucent border. Most of the lesions are round to ovoid but occasionally will have an irregular shape (Fig. 27-7).
3. Histologically they consist almost entirely of varying proportions of dense cementum and bone with few lacunae or vascular spaces. Polarizing microscopy is usually required to differentiate cementum from sclerotic bone.

DIFFERENTIAL DIAGNOSIS

The differential diagnosis of a mature cementoma is discussed under the differential diagnosis section of condensing osteitis (p. 568).

MANAGEMENT

The proper treatment of a mature cementoma entails only its recognition and periodic observa-

Fig. 27-7. **A** to **C,** Mature cementomas. **D,** Mature ossifying fibroma. (Courtesy N. Barakat, D.D.S., Beirut, Lebanon.)

A

B

C

D

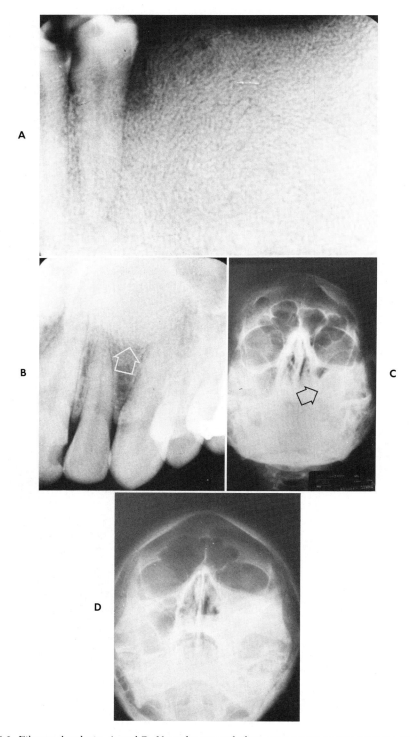

Fig. 27-8. Fibrous dysplasia. **A** and **B,** Note the ground-glass appearance in two patients. **C** and **D,** Waters views of two other patients with fibrous dysplasia of the left maxillary sinus. A ground-glass appearance was seen on periapical films. (**D** courtesy E. Palacios, M.D., Maywood, Ill.)

tion by serial radiographs. Its identification is important so that surgical removal will not be mistakenly undertaken.

Lesions situated in the crest of the ridge, however, are usually removed if a denture is to be placed over the area (Fig. 27-7, D). Lesions that continue to enlarge may produce an expansion of the mandible and cause pain or numbness in the area, so these should be enucleated. This procedure will enable the clinician to establish the correct diagnosis by microscopic examination of the tissue removed.

FIBROUS DYSPLASIA (FIBRO-OSSEOUS LESIONS NOT OF PERIODONTAL LIGAMENT ORIGIN)

Much confusion and disagreement have persisted over the years concerning the fibro-osseous lesions. More recently, however, pathologists have recognized that this group should be subdivided, on the basis of a number of features, into fibro-osseous lesions arising from cells of the periodontal ligament (PDLO) and fibro-osseous lesions not derived from elements of the periodontal ligament.

The cementomas, cemento-ossfying fibromas, and ossifying fibromas are examples of the former type whereas fibrous dysplasia of the facial bones is an example of the latter.

Fibrous dysplasia is included under ill-defined radiolucencies in Chapter 20 and is discussed in Chapter 24 as a mixed radiolucent-radiopaque lesion. In the present chapter its more radiopaque classic ground-glass appearance will be emphasized.

FEATURES

Fibrous dysplasia is basically a bone lesion of children, adolescents, and young adults, which may involve the jawbones. Males and females are equally afflicted. It occurs in the maxilla only slightly more often than in the mandible. When it occurs in the maxilla, it may extend into the maxillary sinus, floor of the orbit, and zygomatic process and backward toward the base of the skull (Fig. 27-8).

The lesion is a painless expansion of the jawbone, which grows slowly for some years and then becomes arrested. The jawbone expansion will usually be fusiform (low plateau) rather than nodular or dome-like and is firm, smoothly contoured, and covered with normal-appearing mucosa.

The majority of the enlargements measure between 2 and 8 cm in length.

The radiographic picture cast by these lesions is generally uniform and of the classic ground-glass* type (Fig. 27-8). In an earlier stage there may be a mixed pattern with irregular radiodense foci distributed throughout a ground-glass lesion or through a radiolucent area. As the lesion matures, the foci will become more radiopaque. The margins of the lesion are vague because there is a gradual transition between the pathosis and the surrounding normal bone.

Mature lesions on extraoral radiographs often appear to be completely radiopaque, but usually on periapical films the region will show the ground-glass feature.

Histologically bony spicules of woven bone appearing in Chinese letter–like (reteform) patterns are seen scattered throughout a fibrous tissue stroma. Osteoblastic rimming of the bony spicules is usually missing. More mature lesions will show a larger proportion of bone to fibrous tissue and will frequently contain some lamellar-type bone with osteoblastic rimming.

DIFFERENTIAL DIAGNOSIS

A solitary painless fusiform enlargement—which is firm, smooth, and covered with normal mucosa and has a radiopaque ground-glass appearance—in the jawbone of a relatively young person is almost certainly fibrous dysplasia.

Other diseases such as *Paget's disease* in the radiolucent stage and *hyperparathyroidism* may produce a ground-glass appearance of the bone, but the overall effect is one of rarefaction and not of radiopacity. Also the radiographic pattern in these two diseases will be generalized rather than localized and solitary as in fibrous dysplasia. Occasionally radiopaque ground-glass patterns may be seen in both Paget's disease and hyperparathyroidism (Fig. 27-9).

Although several bones may be involved with fibrous dysplasia in *Albright's syndrome*, which affects young girls, this syndrome is readily identified by its accompanying features of precocious puberty and the café-au-lait spots on the skin.

Occasionally mature cementifying and ossifying fibromas may assume a radiopaque ground-glass appearance as may also calcifying post-surgical bone defects (Fig. 27-9).

MANAGEMENT

Patients with fibrous dysplasia should be closely observed clinically and radiographically since

---

*The terms "orange peel," "stippled," and "salt-and-pepper" are also used synonymously with "ground-glass" to describe the image produced by many closely arranged small trabeculae.

Fig. 27-9. Ground-glass lesions. **A** and **B,** Fibrous dysplasia. **C,** Paget's disease. **D,** Secondary hyperparathyroidism. **E,** Resolving traumatic bone cyst. (**D** courtesy P. O'Flaherty, D.D.S., Chicago.)

the lesions may undergo surges of growth during hormonal changes. Recontouring of the bone is occasionally necessary to correct a deformity for esthetic or prosthetic reasons, but block resection is seldom if ever indicated. Radiation therapy is not recommended because of the possibility of radiation-induced sarcomas.

SCLEROSING OSTEOMYELITIS

Osteomyelitis is discussed in Chapter 16 as a periapical radiolucency, in Chapter 20 as a ragged radiolucency, and in Chapter 23 as a mixed radiolucent-radiopaque lesion. The sclerosing variety of osteomyelitis, which represents a reaction to a low-grade infection, is included in this chapter

because it sometimes occurs as a totally radiopaque lesion.

FEATURES

The borders of the radiopaque lesions may be ragged or smooth, well defined or vague (Fig. 27-10).

Identification of a diffuse sclerosing osteomyelitis in the bone is usually dependent on detecting some symptoms of chronic infection: tenderness, pain, local swelling. A regional lymphadenitis is a frequent complaint, and a draining sinus may accompany some cases.

Microscopically dense sclerotic nonvital bone will be seen. Acute inflammation will be present

Fig. 27-10. Sclerosing osteomyelitis after a jaw fracture. **A,** Radiopaque lesion (arrow) in the ramus. **B,** Photomicrograph. (**A** courtesy O. H. Stuteville, D.D.S., M.D., St. Joe, Ark.)

in some areas, and occasionally focal collections of pus will be found (Fig. 27-10).

DIFFERENTIAL DIAGNOSIS

The lesions that would necessarily be included in the differential diagnosis for such a solitary intrabony area of sclerosis would be a condensing osteitis, fibrous dysplasia, diffuse cementosis, and an osteoblastic or sclerosing malignancy.

A totally radiopaque *osteoblastic or sclerosing malignancy* would be rare—possibly an osteogenic sarcoma or a metastatic osteoblastic prostatic, bronchogenic, or mammary carcinoma. Should one occur, however, rapid growth, frequent pain without symptoms of infection, and paresthesia (frequently produced by malignant lesions of bone) would help distinguish it from the more common sclerosing osteomyelitis. Nevertheless, a malignant tumor with a superimposed osteomyelitis may be difficult to identify because of the overlapping signs and symptoms. Lesions occurring after radiation may also present a problem in differentiating between a sclerosing osteoradionecrosis and a recurrent tumor.

Condensing osteitis can usually be eliminated from the differential diagnosis by the presence of the more subjective symptoms of infection that frequently accompany a chronic osteomyelitis and are not a feature of condensing osteitis.

MANAGEMENT

The first step in managing sclerosing osteomyelitis is to control the contributing systemic disease that is usually present. A protracted course of antibiotics, judiciously selected and administered, will usually be effective; however, some cases will require incision and drainage and possibly enucleation and saucerization if the antibiotic therapy fails to eliminate the bone infec-

tion. The use of hyperbaric oxygen may be beneficial.

GARRÉ'S OSTEOMYELITIS (PERIOSTITIS OSSIFICANS, NONSUPPURATIVE OSTEOMYELITIS)

Garré's osteomyelitis is a particular type of osteomyelitis, which is so distinctive that it is considered a separate entity. It is characterized by the formation of new bone on the periphery of the cortex over an infected area of spongiosa. The new bone formation is a response of the inner surface of the periosteum to stimulation by a low-grade infection that has spread through the bone and penetrated the cortex.

Strains of staphylococci and streptococci are the most common microorganisms cultured. Periapical odontogenic infection is a frequent cause of Garré's osteomyelitis of the jaws although an occasional case can be traced to a pericoronitis.

The paucity of reports in the dental literature recounting the occurrence of this disease, coupled with our own experience, tends toward the conclusion that Garré's osteomyelitis of the jaws is not a frequent dental complication.

For this lesion to develop, a peculiar combination of circumstances must coexist:

1. The periosteum must possess a high potential for osteoblastic activity (this requirement is satisfied in young patients).
2. A chronic infection must be present.
3. A fine balance between the resistance of the host and the number and virulence of organisms present must be maintained so the infection can continue at a low chronic stage—adequate to stimulate new periosteal bone formation but not enough to reach a level of severity that will induce bone resorption.

Garré's osteomyelitis is included in this chapter because it may produce a solitary radiopacity that does not contact the roots of teeth.

FEATURES

Garré's osteomyelitis is seen almost exclusively in children and rarely occurs in patients over 30 years of age.

The patient may complain of pain due to odontogenic infection before the intermittent, usually nontender, swelling at the inferior border or other peripheries of the mandible develops. The most frequent site is the inferior border of the mandible below the first molar (Fig. 27-11). The maxilla is seldom affected.

If the chronic infection becomes established just beneath the periosteum and is not treated, the swelling will persist and soon become hard as new bone is laid down. After the infection has been eliminated the hard elevation will usually slowly disappear as the bone is recontoured by the functional forces.

The swelling is characteristically convex, varying in length and depth of bone deposits. It may range from 2 cm to involve the whole length of the body of the mandible on the affected side. The covering skin or overlying mucosa may appear normal or be moderately inflamed. Occasionally fever and a leukocytosis will be present.

Radiographically a smoothly contoured, mod-

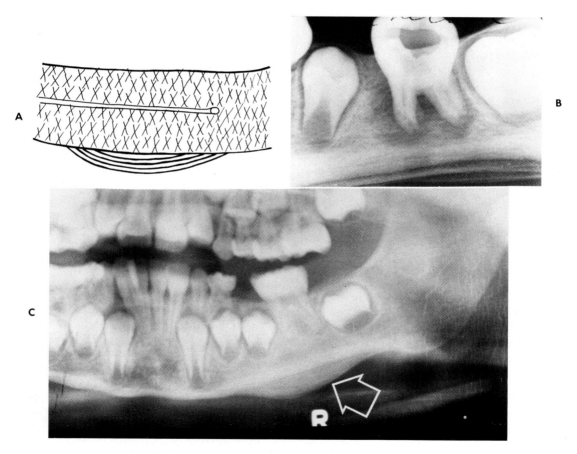

Fig. 27-11. Garré's osteomyelitis. **A,** Diagram of periosteal new bone formation in a layered or "onion-skin" appearance. The integrity of the original cortex is usually maintained. **B** and **C,** Two cases of Garré's osteomyelitis in the first molar region of the mandible. **B,** Note the definite layering effect and the rarefying osteitis at the apex of the pulpless molar. **C,** The layering effect is not so noticeable in this more radiopaque periostitis, which was caused by a chronically infected second deciduous molar tooth that had been extracted recently. (**B** courtesy N. Barakat, D.D.S., Beirut, Lebanon. **C** courtesy J. Baird, D.D.S., Evanston, Ill.)

erately convex, bone shadow will be seen extending from the preserved cortex of the jaw (Fig. 27-11). The space between this new thin shell of bone and the cortex will usually be quite radiolucent without images of trabeculae. Later an alternating light and dark laminated appearance may be seen; and when the whole lesion mineralizes, the lesion will be completely radiopaque (Fig. 27-11).

In most cases the adjacent jawbone appears normal on the radiograph, but sometimes there may be accompanying radiolucent and/or osteosclerotic osteomyelitic changes.

Histologically dense new bone is seen with minimal vascular spaces. The periosteum will be thickened and shown an overactive osteoblastic layer. Scattered regions of chronic inflammation may be present.

DIFFERENTIAL DIAGNOSIS

A list of the lesions that would necessarily be included in the differential diagnosis for a condition that resembles Garré's osteomyelitis would include the following: tori, exostoses, and peripheral osteomas, ossifying hematoma, callus, infantile cortical hyperostosis, osteogenic sarcoma, fibrous dysplasia, and Ewing's sarcoma.

Ewing's sarcoma may produce a convex peripheral radiopaque lesion quite similar to that of Garré's osteomyelitis; and indeed its classic onion-ring appearance mimics the laminated radiopacity frequently observed in the osteomyelitis (Fig. 27-12). This characteristic, plus the shared predilection for children and the fact that both entities may produce tender swellings, often makes distinguishing between a case of Ewing's sarcoma and one of Garré's osteomyelitis quite difficult. Their recognition is further complicated by the fact that in both diseases the adjacent bone may show osteolytic changes, although a moth-eaten type of destruction is more typical of Ewing's sarcoma (Eversole et al., 1979). Ewing's sarcoma also will have rapid unrestricted growth and often produce a paresthesia of the lip.

Fibrous dysplasia may appear to be located on the periphery, but a careful inspection of the radiograph will usually reveal that the complete thickness of bone is altered and has the ground-glass appearance.

Osteogenic sarcoma may cause a peripheral radiopacity, and it occurs predominantly in somewhat the same age group as Garré's osteomyelitis. The radiographic image of this tumor, however, will usually appear more irregular and the sunburst effect (if present) will be so characteristic

that the two entities are not likely to be confused.

Although it occurs in the same age group of children, *infantile cortical hyperostosis* differs from Garré's osteomyelitis in that it is a generalized expansion of the cortices of several bones (Fig. 27-12), usually including the mandible, whereas the osteomyelitis is a single local expansion.

A *callus* developing around a healing fracture may also appear as a peripheral radiopacity, but it is usually not very radiodense. A history of trauma and radiographic evidence of the fracture line will help identify the callus.

A *hematoma* may develop subperiosteally after trauma to a bone. This collection of extravasated blood occasionally will ossify, resulting in a peripheral radiopaque enlargement of the bone. It may then be confused with Garré's osteomyelitis, but its radiopacity will not be so uniform; rather, there will be a more mottled appearance, which, coupled with a history of trauma to the suspicious area, should identify the ossifying hematoma.

Since they also occur at peripheral borders of the mandibular body, *tori, exostoses,* and *peripheral osteomas* might be confused with Garré's osteomyelitis. These entities are distinguishable from Garré's osteomyelitis, however, since they do not show a predilection for patients under 20 years of age; they are more nodular (even polypoid in some cases); and they require months and years to appreciably increase in size.

Eversole and co-workers (1979) reviewed six new cases of Garré's osteomyelitis and outlined criteria for its differentiation from the other neoperiostoses.

MANAGEMENT

In most cases Garré's osteomyelitis can be successfully treated by simply removing the source of infection (usually an infected tooth) and administering an appropriate antibiotic. The periosteal lesion will then gradually regress until the original bone contour has been reestablished.

Sometimes the projecting mass will be extensive, and surgical contouring for esthetics may be in order. This, in turn, will provide a specimen for microscopic study and establishment of a final diagnosis.

MATURE COMPLEX ODONTOMA

The complex odontoma is a developmental anomaly of tooth tissue that, like teeth, is completely radiolucent in the initial stage, passes into a mixed radiolucent-radiopaque stage, and may mature as a completely radiopaque lesion sur-

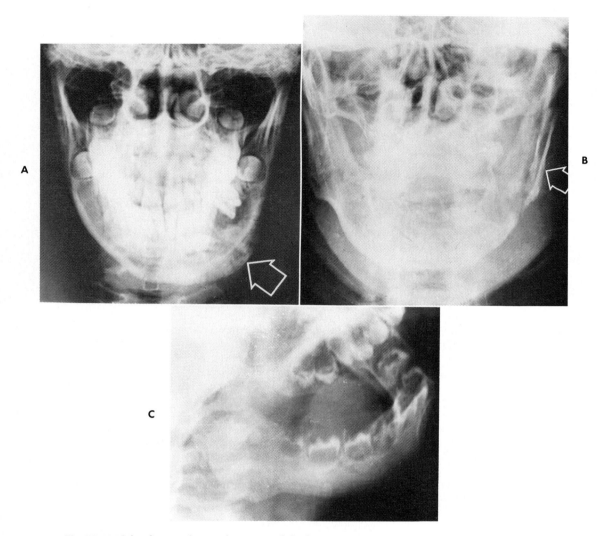

Fig. 27-12. Other lesions that produce cortical duplication. **A,** Posteroanterior radiograph of Ewing's sarcoma in the left mandible of a young girl. Note the cortical redundancy and layering effect (arrow) at the inferior border of the mandible. (Fig. 20-15 shows the extent of bone destruction in a lateral view.) **B,** Posteroanterior radiograph showing a cortical redundancy in the left ramus. This appearance was produced by a large segment of bone being fractured and displaced to the buccal during a traumatic episode to a 56-year-old man. A chronic osteomyelitis had become established here by the time this radiograph was taken and so the segment became a large sequestrum. **C,** Redundancy of inferior border of the mandible in a case of cortical infantile hyperostosis. (**A** courtesy N. Barakat, D.D.S., Beirut, Lebanon. **C** courtesy R. Moncada, M.D., Maywood, Ill.)

rounded by a radiolucent halo of varying width. The tumor is made up of the three calcified dental tissues, but these are laid down in a disorganized irregular mass without any normal morphologic relationships of one tissue to another.

Odontomas are discussed in detail in Chapter 23, which describes their radiolucent images containing radiopaque foci.

FEATURES

The mature complex odontoma is seldom seen in patients under 6 years of age. When it occurs, it most commonly affects the first and second permanent mandibular molars, often forming in the alveoli just superior to the crowns of these teeth and effectively preventing their eruption (Fig. 27-13).

Fig. 27-13. Complex odontoma. **A,** Causing impaction of a mandibular molar. **B,** In the maxillary third molar region (arrows). (**A** courtesy V. Barresi, D.D.S., DeKalb, Ill., and D. Bonomo, D.D.S., Flossmoor, Ill. **B** courtesy B. Saunders, D.D.S., Los Angeles.)

Fig. 27-14. Calcified subperiosteal hematoma (arrow) after tooth extraction with primary closure of the mucosa. **A,** Clinical appearance. **B,** Periapical radiograph.

Pain or paresthesia is not characteristic of these tumors, which may vary in size from 1 to approximately 6 cm and may produce a bulge on the mandible.

Radiographically the mature lesion, of considerable buccolingual width, will appear as a homogeneously dense radiopacity; the earlier lesion, of less width, may show irregular radiodense patterns throughout and may even cast a cottonwool image on the radiograph. Although the outline of the calcified mass within the odontoma may be quite irregular, the radiolucent rim surrounding the lesion will have a well-defined and smooth outer periphery.

Histologically the lesion is composed of varying proportions of enamel, dentin, cementum, and pulp tissue in a disorganized arrangement.

DIFFERENTIAL DIAGNOSIS

Because they are solitary dense radiopacities with radiolucent rims, *mature fibro-osseous lesions (PDLO)* (e.g., cementomas) are the entities most frequently confused with the mature complex odontoma. Usually, however, a cementoma will form in persons who are over 30 years of age whereas an odontoma will develop in much

younger patients (although both lesions may persist and be found in late adulthood). A cementoma may be situated deep in the alveolar bone whereas the complex odontoma will extend high into the alveolus, even to the crest of the ridge.

MANAGEMENT

Surgical enucleation of the odontoma is the treatment of choice, and the excised material should be microscopically examined.

OSSIFYING SUBPERIOSTEAL HEMATOMA

Occasionally a subperiosteal hematoma sustained as the result of trauma will ossify instead of resolving. Early in the course of its ossification, it will appear as a mixed radioucent-radiopaque lesion; but as ossification is completed, it will become a dense radiopaque smoothly contoured convex expansion on the periphery of the bone (Fig. 27-14). The swelling is nontender.

DIFFERENTIAL DIAGNOSIS

The differential diagnosis of the ossifying subperiosteal hematoma is discussed in the differential diagnosis section under Garré's osteomyelitis (p. 575).

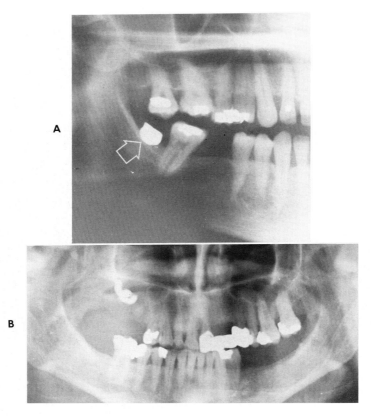

Fig. 27-15. Foreign bodies. **A,** Bullet in the cheek (arrow). **B,** Endodontic filling material in the right maxillary sinus. (**B** courtesy N. Barakat, D.D.S., Beirut, Lebanon.)

Fig. 27-16. Soft tissue shadows. **A,** Fibrous tuberosity (arrow) superimposed over the coronoid process. **B** and **C,** Retention cysts of the maxillary sinus (arrows). (**C** courtesy E. Palacios, M.D., Maywood, Ill.)

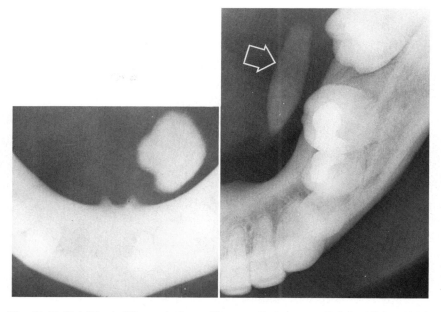

Fig. 27-17. Sialoliths in Wharton's ducts. (Courtesy R. Latronica, D.D.S., Albany, N.Y.)

MANAGEMENT

Functional forces will reshape the deformed bone and reestablish normal contour if the lesion is subjected to the vectors of these forces. If the bone enlargement persists for a few months, recontouring may be necessary for improved function and esthetics and in preparation for the construction of a prosthetic appliance.

RARITIES

The following entities rarely occur as solitary completely radiopaque lesions:

Cementifying and ossifying fibromas
Chondroma and chondrosarcoma—radiopaque variety
Mature osteoblastoma
Metastatic osteoblastic carcinoma—radiopaque variety
Osteoblastoma
Osteogenic sarcoma—radiopaque variety

Projected radiopacities

Radiopaque shadows that may be projected over the roots of teeth are discussed on consider-able detail in Chapter 26. The radiopacities that may be projected over the jawbone but not necessarily over a periapex are essentially the same. Consequently illustrations of these entities will be included in this chapter without further discussion (Figs. 27-15 to 27-25). They include the following:

Anatomic structures
Foreign bodies
Pathologic soft tissue masses
Ectopic calcifications
  Sialoliths of major and minor salivary glands
  Rhinoliths and antroliths
  Calcified lymph nodes
  Tonsillolith
  Phleboliths
  Arterial calcifications
Rarities
  Calcified acne lesion
  Calcified hematoma (soft tissue)
  Calcinosis cutis
  Hamartoma
  Myositis ossificans
  Peripheral fibroma with calcification
  Pilomatrixoma

Fig. 27-18. Sialolith. **A** and **D,** In the submaxillary glands. **E,** Resembling an impacted tooth (arrow). (**B** and **C** courtesy O. H. Stuteville, D.D.S., M.D., St. Joe, Ark. **D** courtesy R. Goepp, D.D.S., Zoller Clinic, University of Chicago. **E** courtesy D. Bonomo, D.D.S., Flossmoor, Ill.)

Fig. 27-19. Calcified cervical nodes (arrows) projected over the angles of the mandible. Both patients had a history of tuberculosis. (Courtesy O. H. Stuteville, D.D.S., M.D., St. Joe, Ark.)

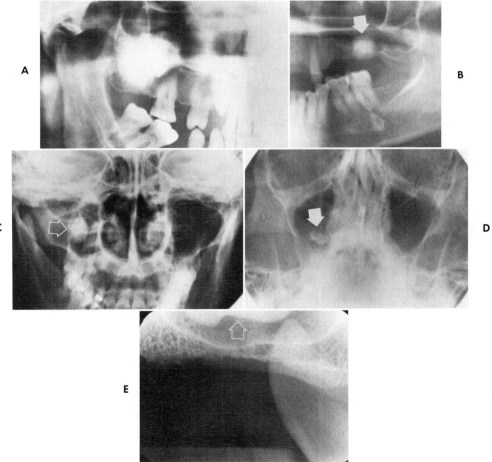

Fig. 27-20. Antrolith. A, In the maxillary sinus above the third molar. B, In the left maxillary sinus (arrow). C, In the maxillary sinus (arrow) above the premolar. D, Resembling a developing crown of a tooth or a complex odontoma. E, The inferior aspect of the radiopaque zygomatic bone (arrow) could be mistaken for an antrolith. (B courtesy M. Kaminski, D.D.S., and S. Atsaves, D.D.S., Chicago.)

Fig. 27-21. Calcified arteries. **A** to **C,** Three arteriosclerotic facial arteries. **D,** Calcified inferior labial artery projected over the alveolar bone in the anterior mandible. (**A** to **C** courtesy R. Latronica, D.D.S., Albany, N.Y. **D** courtesy R. Goepp, D.D.S., Zoller Clinic, University of Chicago.)

Fig. 27-22. Phlebolith just below the inferior border of the mandible. (Courtesy E. Palacios, M.D., Maywood, Ill.)

Fig. 27-23. Foreign metallic object in the cheek. Note the shifting of the image in the two periapical radiographs, which were taken at different angles.

Fig. 27-24. Sialolith of minor salivary gland of the lip near the angle. **A,** Clinical picture showing the small nodular mass in the soft tissue, which was very firm to palpation. **B,** Soft tissue radiograph of the lip showing round radiopaque sialolith, which appears to be less dense in the center. (Courtesy J. Jensen, D.D.S., Long Beach, Calif.)

Fig. 27-25. Round radiopacity situated in the soft tissue on the crest of the ridge in the mandibular canine region. Biopsy proved the lesion to be a peripheral fibroma with ossification, which probably developed in the interdental papilla when the patient still had teeth in the region. (Courtesy P. D. Toto, D.D.S., Maywood, Ill.)

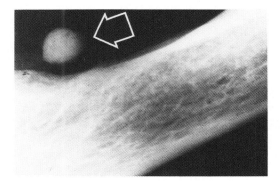

SPECIFIC REFERENCES

Ennis, L. M., and Berry, H. M., Jr.: The necessity for routine roentgenographic examination of the edentulous patient, J. Oral Surg. **7:**3-19, 1949.

Eversole, L. R., Leider, A. S., Corwin, J. O., and Karian, B. K.: Proliferative periostitis of Garré's: its differentiation from other neoperiostoses, J. Oral Surg. **37:**725-731, 1979.

King, D. R., and Moore, G. E.: An analysis of torus palatinus in a transatlantic study, J. Oral Med. **31:**44-46, 1976.

Ritchie, G. M., and Fletcher, A. M.: A radiographic investigation of edentulous jaws, Oral Surg. **47:**563-567, 1979.

GENERAL REFERENCES

Allan, J. H., Finch, L. D., and Chippendale, I.: Sialolithiasis of the minor salivary glands, Oral Surg. **27:**780-785, 1969.

Bakry, N. S.: An ectopic odontoma in the cheek, Oral Surg. **43:** 583-584, 1977.

Batcheldor, G. D., Giansanti, J. S., and Hibbard, E. D.: Garré's osteomyelitis of the jaws: review and report of two cases, J. Am. Dent. Assoc. **87:**892-897, 1973.

Binnie, W. H., DeLathouwer, C., Brocheriou, C., and Panders, A. K.: Symposium on maxillofacial bone pathology, Int. J. Oral Surg. **4:**80-92, 1975.

Borghelli, R. F., Barros, R. E., and Zampieri, J.: Ewing sarcoma of the mandible: report of case, J. Oral Surg. **36:**473-475, 1978.

Bosshardt, L., Gordon, R. C., Weterberg, M., and Morgan, A.: Recurrent peripheral osteoma of mandible: report of case, J. Oral Surg. **29:**450-466, 1971.

Boyne, P. J.: Incidence of osteosclerotic areas in the mandible and maxilla, J. Oral Surg. **18:**486-491, 1960.

Brusati, R., and Fiamminghi, L.: Large calculus of the submandibular gland: report of case, J. Oral Surg. **31:**710-711, 1973.

Chiles, J. L., and Gores, R. J.: Anatomic interpretation of the orthopantomogram, Oral Surg. **35:**564-574, 1973.

DeGregori, G., and Pippen, R.: Sialolithiasis with sialadenitis of a minor salivary gland, Oral Surg. **30:**320-324, 1970.

Eliasson, S. T., and Holte, N. O.: Rubber-base impression material as a foreign body, Oral Surg. **47:**379-380, 1979.

Ellis, D. J., Winslow, J. R., and Indovina, A. A.: Garré's osteomyelitis of the mandible, Oral Surg. **44:**183-189, 1977.

Elmostehy, M. R.: Parotid salivary calculus: report of case, Oral Surg. **26:**18-21, 1968.

Eversole, L. R., Sabes, W. R., and Rovin, S.: Fibrous dysplasia: a nosologic problem in the diagnosis of fibro-osseous lesions of the jaws, J. Oral Pathol. **1:**189-220, 1972.

Farhood, V. W., Steed, D. L., and Krolls, S. O.: Osteoma cutis: cutaneous ossification with oral manifestations, Oral Surg. **45:**98-103, 1978.

Farman, A. G., Joubert, J. J., and Nortje, C. J.: Focal osteosclerosis and apical periodontal pathosis in "European" and Cape Colored dental outpatients, Int. J. Oral Surg. **7:**549-557, 1978.

Fisher, A. D.: Osteomyelitis of the mandible in a child, J. Oral Surg. **35:**60-64, 1977.

Goldstein, B. H., Byrne, J. E., and Miller, A. S.: Clinical-pathological conference. Case 27. Part 2. Chronic sclerosing osteomyelitis, J. Oral Surg. **37:**101-102, 1979.

Greer, R. O., and Berman, D. N.: Osteoblastoma of the jaws: current concepts and differential diagnosis, J. Oral Surg. **36:**304-307, 1978.

Halstead, C. L.: Mucosal cysts of the maxillary sinus: report of 75 cases, J. Am. Dent. Assoc. **87:**1435-1441, 1973.

Hoffman, H.: Tonsillolith, Oral Surg. **45:**657-658, 1978.

James, R. B., Alexander, R. W., and Traver, J. G.: Osteochondroma of the mandibular coronoid process, Oral Surg. **37:**189-195, 1974.

Kennett, S.: Bilateral submandibular sialolithiasis, Oral Surg. **27:**445-450, 1969.

King, R. E., Altini, M., and Shear, M.: Basal cell extensions in human oral mucosa, Oral Pathol. **8:**140-146, 1979.

Knight, W. O.: Sialolithiasis and sialadenitis of a minor salivary gland: report of case, J. Oral Surg. **30:**370-372, 1972.

Mesa, M. C.: Metastatic prostatic carcinoma to the mandible: report of case, J. Oral Surg. **35:**133-135, 1977.

Meyer, R. A.: Osteochondroma of coronoid process of mandible: report of case, J. Oral Surg. **30:**297-300, 1972.

Miller, A. S., and Pullon, P. A.: Case of the month: hard, raised lesion in the right buccal mucosa, Dent. Survey **55:**28, 1979.

Nelson, D. F., Gross, B. D., and Miller, F. E.: Osteoma of the mandibular condyle: report of case, J. Oral Surg. **30:**761-763, 1972.

Noren, G. D., and Roche, W. C.: Huge osteoma of the mandible: report of a case, J. Oral Surg. **36:**375-379, 1978.

Payne, J. V., Dahlen, D. F., Silva, M. T., et al.: Osteomyelitis of the mandible in a child due to *Bacteroides fusiformis,* Oral Surg. **43:**44-46, 1977.

Pullon, P. A., and Miller, A. S.: Sialolithiasis of accessory salivary glands: review of 55 cases, J. Oral Surg. **30:**832-834, 1972.

Rapoport, A., Sobrinho, J. D., DeCarvalho, M. B., et al.: Ewing's sarcoma of the mandible, Oral Surg. **44:**89-94, 1977.

Riesner, N. R., and Woolridge, E. D.: Supernumerary premolars: a summary and case report, J. Oral Med. **32:**79-82, 1977.

Sammartino, F. J., Miller, A. S., Mohmac, A. M., and White, D. K.: Sclerotic mandibular bone lesion, Oral Surg. **43:**643-646, 1977.

Seldin, E. B.: New hope for patients with Ewing sarcoma, J. Oral Surg. **36:**583, 1978.

Smith, C. J., and Fleming, R. D.: A comprehensive review of normal anatomic landmarks and artifacts as visualized on Panorex radiographs, Oral Surg. **37:**291-304, 1974.

Smith, S. N., and Farman, A. G.: Osteomyelitis with proliferative periostitis (Garré's osteomyelitis). Report of case affecting the mandible, Oral Surg. **43:**315-318, 1977.

Stafne, E. C.: Oral roentgenographic diagnosis, ed. 3, Philadelphia, 1969, W. B. Saunders Co.

Van Der Wall, I., Beemster, G., Kraaijenhagen, H. A., and Van Der Kwast, W. A. M.: Pilomatrixoma in the differential diagnosis of pathologic calcification of the paraoral soft tissue, Int. J. Oral Surg. **6:**283-286, 1977.

Waldron, C. A., and Giansanti, J. S.: Benign fibro-osseous lesions of the jaws: a clinical-radiologic-histologic review of sixty-five cases. I. Fibrous dysplasia of the jaws, Oral Surg. **35:**190-201, 1973.

Waldron, C. A., and Giansanti, J. S.: Benign fibro-osseous lesions of the jaws: a clinical-radiologic-histologic review of sixty-five cases. II. Benign fibro-osseous lesions of periodontal ligament origin, Oral Surg. **35:**340-350, 1973.

Weinberg, S.: Osteoma of the mandibular condyle: report of case, J. Oral Surg. **35:**929-932, 1977.

Wells, T. J., Hooker, S. P., and Roche, W. C.: Osteochondroma cutis: report of case, J. Oral Surg. **35:**144-145, 1977.

Worth, H. M.: Principles and practice of oral radiologic interpretation, Chicago, 1963, Year Book Medical Publishers.

28

Multiple separate radiopacities

Norman K. Wood
Paul W. Goaz

Most of the lesions that appear as multiple but separate radiopacities occur more frequently as solitary radiopacities.

Tori and exostoses
Multiple retained roots
Multiple socket sclerosis
Multiple mature cementomas
Multiple idiopathic osteosclerosis
Multiple periapical condensing
  osteitis
Multiple embedded or impacted
  teeth
Cleidocranial dysostosis
Rarities
    Calcinosis cutis
    Cretinism (unerupted teeth)
    Cysticercosis
    Gardner's syndrome (osteomas)
    Idiopathic hypoparathyroidism
    Maffucci's syndrome
    Multiple calcified acne lesions
    Multiple calcified nodes
    Multiple chondromas (Ollier's
      disease)
    Multiple odontomas
    Multiple osteochondromas
    Multiple osteomas of skin
    Multiple phleboliths
    Multiple sialoliths
    Myositis ossificans
    Oral contraceptive sclerosis
    Paget's disease—intermediate stage
    Sickle cell sclerosis

The majority of the entities included here are discussed in Chapter 26 as periapical radiopacities or in Chapter 27 as solitary radiopacities not contacting the roots of teeth. As described in those two chapters, radiopaque lesions that appear to be within the jaw may actually be in or on the periphery (cortex) of the jawbone or in the adjacent soft tissues.

TORI AND EXOSTOSES

Tori and exostoses are described as exophytic lesions in Chapter 7 and as single radiopacities in Chapters 26 and 27. In the context of this chapter, therefore, it remains only to note that tori (especially the lingual mandibular type) frequently develop as multiple nodules that may be contiguous or separate. Exostoses may also be multiple, especially those occurring on the buccal surfaces of the jaws. In either case they will appear as relatively dense, smoothly contoured, multiple radiopacities on radiographs of the jaws (Fig. 28-1).

DIFFERENTIAL DIAGNOSIS

Multiple tori or exostoses must be differentiated from any of the other similar-appearing entities included in the present chapter. If multiple smoothly contoured radiopacities are present on periapical radiographs and the typical peripheral nodules are palpable on the buccal or lingual alveolar surfaces, the diagnosis is clear-cut.

Rare diseases such as *Maffucci's syndrome, Ollier's disease,* and *multiple osteochondromas* should sometimes be considered, but a detailed discussion of these entities is beyond the scope of this text.

Fig. 28-1. Multiple large tori. **A** and **B,** Clinical and radiographic appearances in one patient. **C,** Periapical radiograph of another patient. (**A** and **B** courtesy P. Akers, D.D.S., Chicago.)

Fig. 28-2. Multiple root fragments. **A,** Readily identified. **B,** Not so readily identified (arrows).

MANAGEMENT

Multiple tori and exostoses require surgical exicision (1) for psychologic reasons, (2) if they are continually being traumatized, (3) if they are interfering with speech or mastication, or (4) if they will interfere with the fabrication of a prosthetic appliance.

MULTIPLE RETAINED ROOTS

Solitary retained roots are discussed in Chapter 27. Multiple retained roots are usually asymptomatic but may cause pain if they become infected.

A painful ulcer on the crest of a ridge may be the first sign of retained roots, especially if a relatively large root fragment has been present under a denture for a number of years. A periapical radiograph will reveal the cause of the ulcer.

Since some patients' roots seem to be prone to fracture during extraction, the clinician will occasionally find several retained root fragments on the radiographs of one person. If the shapes of the roots, pulp canals, and periodontal ligaments have persisted, these multiple well-defined radiopacities will be easily identified as root fragments (Fig. 28-2). A low-grade infection and accom-

Fig. 28-3. Multiple socket sclerosis. (**A** courtesy R. Goepp, D.D.S., Zoller Clinic, University of Chicago.)

panying resorption and/or condensing osteitis, however, may obscure the diagnosis. Nevertheless, careful study of the radiograph will enable the clinician to distinguish a root tip from an area of sclerotic bone on the basis of the texture of the radiopacity: the root fragment will have a homogeneous density, whereas the trabeculated nature of the sclerotic bone will usually be detectable.

DIFFERENTIAL DIAGNOSIS

The radiographic appearance of multiple retained roots is diagnostic. If the root fragments have been fractured at the level of the alveolar crest and the radiolucent images of the periodontal ligaments are indistinct, however, multiple retained roots may be difficult to distinguish from *multiple sclerosed sockets*. The study of available radiographs taken soon after the extractions were done will enable the clinician to distinguish between retained roots and sclerosed sockets.

Another incidence in which retained root tips may not be readily recognized is when the root tips are chronically infected and *condensing osteitis* has developed about them. Where there are multiple retained roots, however, all the roots would not likely be involved with sclerosed bone; one or two fragments would retain their typical appearance, and these would suggest the correct diagnosis. A more detailed discussion of the dif-

ferentiation of retained root fragments may be found under the differential diagnosis section of condensing osteitis in Chapter 27 (p. 568).

MANAGEMENT

Since it is not safe to assume on the basis of radiographic evidence alone that retained roots are free of infection, removal of every root should always be considered. If the root tips are small, asymptomatic, and apparently free of pathosis, however, and if a relatively large amount of alveolar bone will probably have to be removed, it is best to leave them undisturbed. Periodic radiographic surveillance will be required.

MULTIPLE SOCKET SCLEROSIS

Tooth socket sclerosis is a special form of osteosclerosis that occasionally develops in a socket after tooth removal. Examples of the sclerosis of solitary sockets are described in Chapter 27; but such multiple sclerotic lesions may also occur when a number of tooth sockets are healing after multiple extraction, so this entity is included in the present discussion as well (Fig. 28-3).

Although the specific cause is unknown, socket sclerosis is believed to be the result of a sudden disturbance of the osteogenic-osteolytic balance in bone metabolism. Burrell and Goepp (1973) reported an increased incidence of socket sclerosis among patients with gastrointestinal malabsorption problems or kidney disease. In their study, which included both inpatients and out-patients, 2.7% had one or more sclerosed tooth sockets. They calculated that this incidence was much higher than would be found in the general population.

FEATURES

Since the development of sclerosed bone in healing sockets is not accompanied by local symptoms, the radiopaque lesion is discovered on routine radiographs. Sclerosis of tooth sockets is found more often in older adults and seldom if ever in persons under 16 years of age. Sequential radiographs made when the sclerosis is active will reveal the successive stages of development.

When a socket is healing normally, the lamina dura usually disappears within 4 months and the socket is completely obliterated by 8 months. When socket sclerosis is developing, however, the lamina dura fails to resorb. The deposition of sclerotic bone begins in the depth of the socket and continues along the socket walls. As the lateral walls of sclerotic bone approximate each other, the thin vertical radiolucent shadow of the void between them resembles the image of a pulp canal on periapical radiographs (Fig. 28-3). At this stage the sclerosed socket can be easily mistaken for a retained ankylosed root.

Histologically socket sclerosis is identical with osteosclerosis in other locations. Dense broad trabeculae of bone with few lacunae and few vascular marrow spaces are characteristic of the microscopic picture.

DIFFERENTIAL DIAGNOSIS

Socket sclerosis may be mistaken for *retained roots* because both have identical shapes. Differentiating between the two is especially difficult when the socket has not yet completely calcified and a thin central core resembles a root canal. Since osteosclerosis of a tooth socket usually involves the length of the socket, however, the radiopaque images of roots fractured well below the alveolar crest will not be confused with this dense remodeling of the socket. If the periodontal ligament space is not apparent, the radiopacity should be identified as socket sclerosis. Unusual exceptions would be ankylosed roots. If radiographs of the area are available and were made soon after the extractions, the identity of the opaque material in the sockets will not be in doubt; the retained root tips would be apparent from the time of the extractions, whereas the osteosclerotic healing of the sockets would require months to become obvious.

MANAGEMENT

Once the diagnosis of socket sclerosis has been established (biopsy may be necessary in some cases), consultation with the patient's physician is recommended since there is reason to suspect that the patient may have a gastrointestinal malabsorption problem or a kidney malady (Burrell and Goepp, 1973).

The sclerosed tooth socket does not require definitive treatment.

MULTIPLE MATURE CEMENTOMAS

Variations in the appearance and nature of cementomas have been discussed in other chapters (16, 18, 23, 24, 26). In the present chapter multiple mature cementomas occurring in the jaws will be emphasized (Fig. 28-4).

Although multiple cementomas are most frequently found in the periapices of mandibular incisors, they may occur in the periapices of any of the mandibular teeth and (less frequently) in the maxilla. Multiple mature cementomas have also been found in edentulous regions; these probably represent residual cementomas that persisted after the removal of the associated teeth. The features of multiple cementomas are similar to those of the solitary cementoma (Chapter 16).

DIFFERENTIAL DIAGNOSIS

Multiple mature cementomas must be differentiated from multiple retained root fragments, tori, exostoses, and osteomas, idiopathic osteosclerosis, the complex odontoma, diffuse cementosis, and the intermediate stage of Paget's disease as well as some of the rare lesions noted in the introductory list of this chapter.

In some cases of intermediate-stage *Paget's disease,* separate round radiopaque areas will be seen scattered throughout the jaws. The margins of these radiopaque osteoblastic areas are not so well defined as the margins of mature cementomas, however, nor do they have uniform radiolucent rims. Further examination of the patient will reveal the deformation of the skull as well as of other bones, and these findings will aid in recognizing Paget's disease.

The features of *diffuse cementosis* are quite different from those of mature multiple cementomas. The lesions of diffuse cementosis are much less common, relatively large, and multiple—merging together and occupying much of the body of the mandible and maxilla. They appear as large radiopaque masses usually with radiolucent borders and have the cotton-wool appearance often seen in the late stages of Paget's

Fig. 28-4. A and **B,** Multiple cementomas in two patients. **C,** Two mature cementomas in the mandibular incisor region of another patient. Note that mature cementomas have radiolucent rims.

disease. The occurrence of diffuse cementosis in families suggests that these tumors are inherited as an autosomal dominant trait. The lesions are most common in black women over 35 years of age.

The *complex odontoma* may resemble a mature cementoma in that it will often be a dense radiopacity surrounded by a radiolucent border; but it will usually be larger and will occur almost invariably as a solitary lesion. Furthermore, most complex odontomas do not show a homogeneous opacity as the mature cementomas do but instead show varying degrees of opacity corresponding to the various densities of enamel, dentin, cementum, and pulp tissue present.

Idiopathic osteosclerotic lesions are frequently solitary; but they may occur bilaterally, usually in the mandibular molar regions. Unlike multiple mature cementomas they are often irregularly shaped radiopacities without radiolucent rims. In addition, the opacity of the mature cementomas is more homogeneous. Although the images of the osteosclerotic lesions may be dense, a trabecular quality will usually be apparent; and in some areas there will be a branching continuity with the adjacent normal trabeculae.

Tori, exostoses, and *osteomas,* like multiple mature cementomas, are radiopaque; but they do not have radiolucent perimeters. Also their identi-

ty can be clinically substantiated by the presence of bony hard exophytic nodules.

In contrasting the radiographic images of *multiple retained root fragments* and multiple mature cementomas, the clinician will often note that one or more of the fragments are root shaped and have the shadows of root canals. In addition, most of the root fragments will have some of the radiolucent periodontal ligament still present; and the cementomas will be separated from the adjacent normal bone by a thin radiolucent space. Furthermore, the cementomas will usually be more rounded than the root fragments and will not have a radiolucent feature suggesting a root canal.

MANAGEMENT

It is not usually necessary to remove multiple mature cementomas unless a rare lesion grows large enough to expand the cortex. Radiographs of cementomas should be taken periodically to observe their course and verify the working diagnosis.

MULTIPLE IDIOPATHIC OSTEOSCLEROSIS

Idiopathic osteosclerosis is discussed in detail in Chapter 26 as a periapical radiopacity and in Chapter 27 as a solitary radiopacity not contacting

Fig. 28-5. Multiple idiopathic osteosclerosis.

Fig. 28-6. Multiple periapical condensing osteitis. Note that the lesions are present in the periapices of both roots of the first molar.

teeth. Because this entity sometimes occurs bilaterally and in multiple separate areas in the mandibular molar or premolar region (Fig. 28-5), it is included in the present chapter. The lesions are quite dense irregularly shaped radiopacities, varying from 0.5 to about 2.0 cm in diameter. They are most often found at the periapices of vital teeth.

MULTIPLE PERIAPICAL CONDENSING OSTEITIS

Condensing osteitis is discussed in Chapter 26 as a periapical radiopacity and in Chapter 27 as a solitary radiopacity not contacting the roots of teeth. Since a patient may readily develop pulp pathosis in more than one tooth and since the lesions of condensing osteitis may be found in more than one periapex, it is appropriate to include condensing osteitis in this chapter (Fig. 28-6). Periapical idiopathic osteosclerosis is differentiated from periapical condensing osteitis in that the pulps of the teeth involved with the former are vital whereas those of the teeth involved with the latter are degenerating or nonvital. Also, multiple lesions of condensing osteitis may be found surrounding multiple root fragments.

Fig. 28-7. Multiple impacted teeth (no syndrome). **B,** Note the impacted canine and several other teeth in a compound odontoma. (**A** courtesy W. Schoenheider, D.D.S., Oak Lawn, Ill.)

MULTIPLE EMBEDDED OR IMPACTED TEETH (NO SYNDROME)

Occasionally the clinical and radiographic examinations of a patient will reveal several embedded* or impacted teeth. The particular entity being considered here is not the usual impacted third molar or canine but is the more unusual circumstance of failure of eruption of a number of permanent teeth. Sometimes this failure to erupt results from crowding by supernumerary teeth. Other times the normal number of permanent teeth will be present and there will be no apparent mechanical explanation for the lack of eruption.

The inexplicable failure to erupt is caused by a loss or lack of the eruptive force. In contrast to cleidocranial dysostosis, which is characterized by a number of other defects in addition to impacted teeth, this entity is not accompanied by a fixed complex of symptoms. Lateral oblique and posteroanterior radiographs of the jaws of these patients will reveal the multiple radiopacities scattered throughout the jaws (Fig. 28-7).

Good-quality periapical films will enable the clinician to readily identify the radiopacities as unerupted and/or impacted teeth.

FEATURES

When during a clinical examination the clinician encounters one or more edentulous areas in conjunction with malposition and malocclusion of the permanent teeth that are present and there is no history of tooth extraction, then he should

---

*In the present discussion the term "embedded" is used to describe a tooth that has failed to erupt because of some imbalance in the coordinated forces responsible for the axial movement of teeth. This is in contrast to the "impacted" tooth, which is prevented from erupting by a physical barrier in the path of eruption.

anticipate finding embedded or impacted teeth on the patient's radiographs.

DIFFERENTIAL DIAGNOSIS

When there is a clinical absence of a number of teeth, three diseases should be included in the differential diagnosis: cleidocranial dysostosis, cretinism, and partial anodontia.

Partial anodontia may be considered during the initial oral screening examination when certain permanent teeth are observed not to be present and the history indicates they have not been extracted. When radiographs are available, however, and reveal that the missing teeth are in reality present as embedded or impacted teeth, then partial anodontia can be rejected.

In some instances *cretinism* (hypothyroidism in young children) causes crowding, delayed eruption, and impaction of permanent teeth. The short stature of the patient, however, combined with a history of hypothyroidism and low serum thyroxine levels, should guide the clinician to the correct diagnosis.

The radiographic pictures of a patient with *cleidocranial dysostosis* will demonstrate similar problems of multiple supernumerary and impacted teeth. The accompanying features of cranial and clavicular abnormalities, however, will enable the clinician to recognize this entity. It is helpful to remember that multiple embedded or impacted teeth more commonly occur as isolated events than as part of a syndrome.

MANAGEMENT

Impacted teeth should be removed because of the danger of pathologic fracture, odontogenic infection, or development of a follicular cyst. Another indication for removal would be to prepare for a prosthetic appliance. A careful clinical examination of these patients should be performed

to eliminate the possibility of their having cleidocranial dysostosis.

CLEIDOCRANIAL DYSOSTOSIS

Cleidocranial dysostosis is a syndrome of unknown cause. It is usually transmitted as an autosomal dominant trait. The fact that one of the features characterizing it is multiple supernumerary and impacted teeth explains the inclusion of the disease in the present chapter.

FEATURES

Usually the stature of persons with cleidocranial dysostosis is shorter than average. The syndrome derives its name from the fact that the two bones that are always involved are the skull and the clavicles.

The skull is enlarged but has a shorter than normal anteroposterior dimension (brachycephaly). Frontoparietal bossing is usually present. There is delayed closing of the fontanelles, and occasionally they will remain open throughout life. Secondary centers of ossification develop in the suture lines, so an unusual number of wormian bones are formed.

The clavicles are either partially or completely absent (Fig. 28-8), which permits the patient an unusual range of shoulder movements; some patients are able to approximate their shoulders in front of their chests.

The jaws are also involved. The maxilla is often small and the mandible is usually normal in size, so a pseudoprognathism results. The palate frequently has a high arch and may be cleft. There is a delayed eruption of the permanent dentition because of the presence of many supernumerary teeth, most of which resemble premolars. Thus multiple impactions occur (Fig. 28-8). Follicular cysts may be associated with the impacted teeth.

Often the multiple impactions are the first

Fig. 28-8. Cleidocranial dysostosis. **A,** Note the numerous impacted teeth on this lateral oblique radiograph of the mandible. **B,** Note the complete absence of clavicles. (**A** courtesy R. Goepp, D.D.S., Zoller Clinic, University of Chicago. **B** courtesy R. Kallal, D.D.S., Chicago.)

manifestation of the syndrome to be recognized; and as a result of this discovery, the clinician is prompted to look for other features. The air sinuses may be underdeveloped or absent. The zygoma and lacrimal and nasal bones may show hypoplasia. The nasal bridge may be depressed and its base broad. Additional bones (e.g., vertebrae, long bones, pubic bone, hands) may show faulty development.

DIFFERENTIAL DIAGNOSIS

The differential diagnosis of the multiple impaction feature of cleidocranial dysostosis is dis-

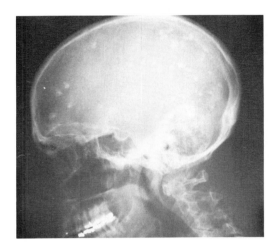

Fig. 28-9. Cysticercosis. Note the many small radiopaque foci scattered within the cranium. One small faint radiopacity is present over the mandibular third mclar region. (Courtesy E. Palacios, M.D., Maywood, Ill.)

Fig. 28-10. Multiple calcified cervical nodes projected over the ramus. Other radiographic views showed the radiopacities in different positions. The patient had a history of tuberculosis. (Courtesy O. H. Stuteville, D.D.S., M.D., St. Joe, Ark.)

cussed under the differential diagnosis section of embedded and impacted teeth (p. 592). The differentiation of the remaining features of cleidocranial dysostosis from other craniofacial syndromes is beyond the scope of this discussion.

MANAGEMENT

When the clinician encounters multiple embedded or impacted teeth other than third molars or canines, he should pursue the patient's history and clinical examination—paying special attention to any of the other features of cleidocranial dysostosis that may be present. The syndrome must be managed by a team of health professionals so all the ramifications of the disease will receive adequate treatment. The impacted teeth should be removed in most cases.

RARITIES

Multiple soft tissue calcifications may be projected over the jawbones on radiographs. In addition, rare tumors of teeth, bone, and cartilage as well as the intermediate stage of Paget's disease may show multiple radiopacities of the jaws. Following is a list of these rarities:

Calcinosis cutis
Cretinism (unerupted teeth)
Cysticerosis (Fig. 28-9)
Gardner's syndrome (osteomas)
Idiopathic hypoparathyroidism
Maffucci's syndrome
Multiple calcified acne lesions
Multiple calcified nodes (Fig. 28-10)
Multiple chondromas (Ollier's disease)
Multiple odontomas
Multiple osteochondromas
Multiple osteomas of skin
Multiple phleboliths (Fig. 28-11)

Fig. 28-11. Multiple phleboliths in a patient with large hemangiomas of the face. Note the short radiopaque rods, which are radon seeds. (Courtesy E. Palacios, M.D., Maywood, Ill.)

Fig. 28-12. Multiple sialoliths. **A,** Bilateral occurrence. **B,** Two stones in Wharton's duct (arrows). **C,** Multiple occurrence (arrow) in the submaxillary gland. (**A** and **B** courtesy R. Latronica, D.D.S., Albany, N.Y. **C** courtesy E. Palacios, M.D., Maywood, Ill.)

Multiple sialoliths (Fig. 28-12)
Myositis ossificans
Oral contraceptive sclerosis
Paget's disease—intermediate stage (Fig. 28-13)
Sickle cell sclerosis

SPECIFIC REFERENCE

Burrell, K. H., and Goepp, R. A.: Abnormal bone repair in jaws, socket sclerosis: a sign of systemic disease, J. Am. Dent. Assoc. **87:**1206-1215, 1973.

GENERAL REFERENCES

Alling, C. C., Martinez, M. G., Ballard, J. B., and Small, E. W.: Clinical-pathological conference case 5. Part 1, J. Oral Surg. **32:**114-116, 1974.

Alling, C. C., Martinez, M. G., Ballard, J. B., and Small, E. W.: Clinical-pathological conference case 5. Part 2. Osteoma cutis, J. Oral Surg. **32:**195-197, 1974.

Darzenta, N. C., and Giunta, J. L.: Radiographic changes of the mandible related to oral contraceptives, Oral Surg. **43:**478-481, 1977.

Douglas, B. L., and Greene, H. J.: Cleidocranial dysostosis: report of case, J. Oral Surg. **27:**42-43, 1969.

Ennis, L. M.: Roentgenographic appearance of calcified acne lesions, J. Am. Dent. Assoc. **68:**351-357, 1964.

Halse, A., Roed-Petersen, B., and Lund, K.: Gardner's syndrome, J. Oral Surg. **33:**673-676, 1975.

Maw, R. B.: Cleidocranial dysostosis: report of case, J. Am. Dent. Assoc. **96:**306-309, 1978.

McFarland, P. H., Scheetz, W. L., and Kinisley, R. E.: Gardner's

Fig. 28-13. Multiple radiopacities in the maxillary premolar region caused by Paget's disease.

syndrome: report of two families, J. Oral Surg. **26:**632-638, 1968.

Miller, R., Sakamoto, E., Zell, A., et al.: Cleidocranial dysostosis: a multidisciplinary approach to treatment, J. Am. Dent. Assoc. **96:**296-300, 1978.

Neal, C. J.: Multiple osteomas of the mandible associated with polyposis of the colon (Gardner's syndrome), Oral Surg. **28:** 628-631, 1969.

Ruhlman, D. C.: Multiple impacted and erupted supernumerary teeth, Oral Surg. **17:**199-203, 1964.

Thompson, R. D., Hale, M. L., and McLeran, J. H.: Multiple compound composite odontomas of maxilla and mandible: report of case, J. Oral Surg. **26:**478-480, 1968.

Timosca, G., and Gaurilita, L.: Cysticercosis of the maxillofacial region: a clinicopathologic study of five cases, Oral Surg. **37:**390-399, 1974.

Witkop, C. J.: Gardner's syndrome and other osteognathodermal disorders with defects in parathyroid functions, J. Oral Surg. **26:**639-642, 1968.

29

Generalized radiopacities

Thomas E. Emmering

A multitude of diseases are capable of causing osseous changes in the jaws and skull. Discussion in this chapter is limited primarily to those that at one stage or another in their progression appear as generalized radiopacities of the jawbones.

Diffuse cementosis
Paget's disease—mature stage
Osteopetrosis
Rarities
    Albright's syndrome
    Caffey's disease (infantile cortical hyperostosis)
    Camurati-Engelmann's disease
    Craniometaphyseal dysplasia
    Craniodiaphyseal dysplasia
    Fluorosis
    Gardner's syndrome
    Hyperostosis deformans juvenilis
    Metastatic carcinoma of prostate
    Multiple large exostoses and tori
    Osteogenesis imperfecta
    Pyknodysostosis
    van Buchem's disease

Diseases of bone that can produce generalized radiopacities are not frequently encountered in the general population. Diffuse cementosis, Paget's disease, and osteopetrosis are the most common of these and are listed in order of diminishing frequency. They will be discussed in some detail, whereas the rarer disorders will be only listed.

DIFFUSE CEMENTOSIS (SCLEROSING CEMENTAL MASSES OF THE JAWS, GIGANTIFORM CEMENTOMAS, MULTIPLE ENOSTOSES, CHRONIC DIFFUSE SCLEROSING OSTEOMYELITIS, FLORID OSSEOUS DYSPLASIA)

Diffuse cementosis, sclerosing cemental masses of the jaws, gigantiform cementomas, multiple enostoses, chronic diffuse sclerosing osteomyelitis, and florid osseous dysplasia very possibly refer to the same disease process. Although such a grouping is not accepted by all pathologists, Waldron and co-workers (1975) prefer to combine these entities under one heading—"sclerotic cemental masses of the jaws"—because of their obvious similarities. Melrose and co-workers (1976) suggest the term "florid osseous dysplasia" for this group of lesions. Wood and Goaz prefer to use the term "diffuse cementosis," although it seems to us that there are two different appearances. One appearance would best be described as "nodular" (Fig. 29-1) while the other appearance would better be described as "diffuse" (Fig. 29-2).

The large radiopaque masses (cementum)* in diffuse cementosis frequently become so disseminated that the complete body of the mandible and tooth-bearing regions of the maxilla show a generalized radiopacity (Figs. 29-1 and 29-2).

My experience is that diffuse cementosis represents the most common cause of pathologic generalized radiopacities of the jaws.

FEATURES

Diffuse cementosis is apparently inherited as an autosomal dominant trait (Winer et al., 1972)

---

*If one considers this condition to be basically a benign fibro-osseous lesion of periodontal ligament origin, one would expect to find cementum or bone or a mixture of these two tissues. In any event the presence of the large aggregations of densely calcified tissues predisposes to a secondary osteomyelitis.

Fig. 29-1. Diffuse cementosis. **A,** Note the nodular, rather well-circumscribed, radiopaque masses distributed throughout the maxilla and mandible. This panograph is of a 45-year-old black woman. **B,** A panograph of nodular masses in another black woman, 42 years of age, showing greater involvement of the mandible than of the maxilla. (**B** courtesy R. Kallal, D.D.S., Chicago.)

Fig. 29-2. Diffuse cementosis in a middle-aged black woman who was asymptomatic. The particular pattern that is prevalent in this case is more diffuse, less nodular, and less well defined.

although a good statistical evaluation is precluded by the paucity of reported cases.

Bhaskar and Cutright (1968) summarized the characteristics of this disorder as follows:

1. The lesions are restricted to the jawbones.
2. The vast majority of the patients are past 30 years of age.
3. There is a marked predilection for women, and the disease is more common in blacks.
4. Mandibular involvement is much more common than maxillary involvement.

Early or mild cases are detected on routine radiographic surveys. More advanced or severe cases, however, may be detected by a painless expansion of the alveolar process of the mandible and less frequently of the maxilla. If the patient is wearing dentures, he will complain of the constant need for adjustment of his prosthesis. In extreme cases the surface mucosa over the expanded alveolar process may become ulcerated and a superimposed osteomyelitis may develop. Patients with this complication usually experience tenderness, pain, and possibly purulent drainage from the region. Serum chemistry levels will characteristically be within normal limits because of the insidious nature of the bone changes.

Radiographs, at first glance, seem to demonstrate a pagetoid cotton-wool appearance with multiple irregularly shaped radiopaque areas. On closer examination well-defined radiolucent rims will be seen surrounding most of the radiopaque areas (Bhaskar and Cutright, 1968; Winer et al., 1972) (Fig. 29-1). The radiopaque patterns vary in size but will usually be large and may be multiple or else diffuse and continuous throughout the jaw (Figs. 29-1 and 29-2). As with most odontogenic hard tissue lesions, diffuse cementosis commences as a radiolucency and matures through the mixed stage into the radiopaque stage.

Using polarizing microscopy, Waldron and co-workers (1975) demonstrated that the radiopacities in 34 of 38 cases were cementum whereas in the remaining four cases the radiopacities were bone.

DIFFERENTIAL DIAGNOSIS

The differentiating features of diffuse cementosis are discussed in the differential diagnosis section at the end of the chapter (p. 605).

MANAGEMENT

Patients with asymptomatic mild cases of diffuse cementosis do not require treatment. The disease must be correctly identified and observed annually with radiographs, however; and if the

natural dentition is present, every effort must be made to preserve it since patients with this disease exhibit poor healing and osteomyelitis may develop after tooth loss.

Patients with more severe cases or cases in which there are superficial lesions located near the crest of the alveolar ridge may require recontouring to accommodate dentures or prevent ulceration.

The management of a superimposed or primary osteomyelitis is discussed in Chapter 20.

PAGET'S DISEASE—MATURE STAGE

Paget's disease is a chronic disease of bone that may occur in three stages:

1. The early osteoclastic stage (generalized rarefaction)
2. The intermediate stage, which demonstrates both osteoclastic and osteoblastic activity (a mixed radiolucent-radiopaque appearance)
3. The mature stage, in which osteoblastic activity predominates (a generalized cotton-wool radiopacity)

The osteoclastic stage is described in Chapter 22 as a generalized rarefaction, and the intermediate stage is described in Chapter 24 as a mixed radiolucent-radiopaque image. The mature cotton-wool appearance will be emphasized in the present chapter.

FEATURES

True Paget's disease occurs most often in patients over 40 years of age and may present many clinical signs and symptoms, which are not always obvious until the disease becomes relatively far advanced. The notable features may be enlargement of the skull and jaws (Fig. 29-3), usually the maxilla, although there have been incidences of mandibular involvement only (Gee et al., 1972). Prominent involvement of the facial bones (occasionally seen) may produce a leonine appearance sometimes referred to as a leontiasis ossea.

Additional clinical features will depend on which other bones are involved. Deformities of the spine, femurs, and tibiae result in shortened stature, broadening of the chest, spinal curvature, and a waddling gait. Involved bones are more easily subject to fracture; some authors claim an incidence of up to 30% as evidenced by the appearances of bone callus on radiographs.

Dental problems become notable as osteoblastic activity creates expansion and progressive enlargement of the maxilla. The alveolar ridge is widened, the palate is flattened, and any teeth present undergo migration, tipping, possible

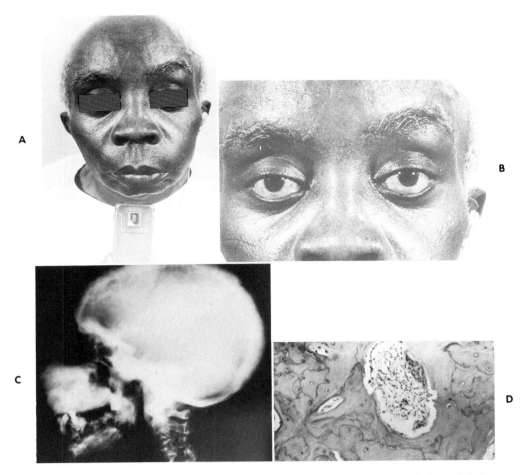

Fig. 29-3. Paget's disease. **A** and **B,** Note the enlarged skull and maxilla, the marked exophthalmos, and the hearing aid in the left ear. **C,** Lateral radiograph reveals a dense cotton-wool appearance throughout the skull and maxilla. **D,** Photomicrograph depicts the classic mosaic pattern within the bone, which resembles finger painting. Note the presence of osteoblasts and osteoclasts at the bone margins.

loosening, and increased interproximal spacing. Edentulous patients experience great difficulty wearing removable prostheses, which must be periodically remade to accommodate alveolar expansion.

Although many authorities believe osteoclastic and osteoblastic activites continue throughout, the radiographic picture will vary, depending on the stage of the disease. The osteoblastic phase eventually becomes predominant. Osteoblastic areas initially show as small radiopaque foci but coalesce as the disease matures into large radiopaque patches with minimal residual radiolucent areas (Figs. 29-4 and 29-5). This image is often referred to as the cotton-wool appearance.

In patients with jaw involvement, generally the skull is also affected; and sometimes osteolytic activity will continue intermittently in these bones even after the predominant activity in the jaws has become osteoblastic. Dental radiographs of later stages of Paget's disease will demonstrate proliferation of bone and hypercementosis of tooth roots; and the hypercementosis may become quite exaggerated. Frequently there is loss of definite lamina dura around the teeth and rarely some root resorption. On occasion, local areas of the jaw will continue to grow at an accelerated rate.

The dental practitioner must be alert to the presence of areas of bone resorption and apposi-

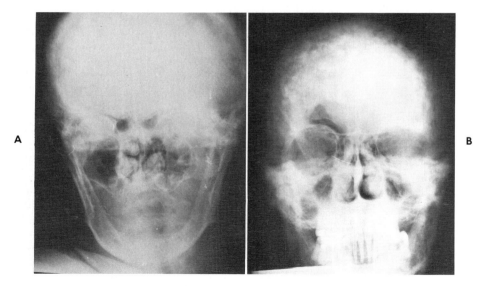

Fig. 29-4. Paget's disease. Note the cotton-wool appearance in the edentulous maxillary molar region, **A,** and in the canine and premolar region, **B.** (Courtesy R. Goepp, D.D.S., Zoller Clinic, University of Chicago.)

Fig. 29-5. Paget's disease in two patients. **A,** Note the dense cotton-wool pattern in the skull. The maxilla and mandible are not involved in this patient. **B,** Note the cotton-wool radiopacities throughout the maxilla, zygoma, and skull. The mandible is not involved in this patient. (**A** courtesy E. Palacios, M.D., Maywood, Ill. **B** courtesy O. H. Stuteville, D.D.S., M.D., St. Joe, Ark.)

tion since these areas may signal the development of osteogenic sarcoma, which has an increased incidence in Paget's disease.

Serum alkaline phosphatase values are characteristically markedly elevated whereas serum calcium and phosphorus levels are usually within normal limits.

The mature stage of Paget's disease produces some distinct microscopic features:

1. The bone is very dense with a few small fibrovascular spaces appearing between massive trabeculae that have resulted from the fusion of smaller trabeculae.
2. The classic mosaic pattern is usually present in the trabeculae and is produced by the many reversal lines that are a result of the increased resorption and apposition of bone.
3. Osteoblasts and some osteoclasts are seen rimming the trabeculae (Fig. 29-3, *D*).

DIFFERENTIAL DIAGNOSIS

The differentiating aspects of generalized radiopacities of the jawbones are discussed in the differential diagnosis section at the end of the chapter (p. 605).

MANAGEMENT

The management of patients with Paget's disease is discussed in Chapters 22 and 24. The clinician must be especially watchful for the development of osteosarcoma in bones affected with Paget's disease.

OSTEOPETROSIS (ALBERS-SCHÖNBERG DISEASE, MARBLE BONE DISEASE)

Osteopetrosis, characterized by overgrowth and sclerosis of bone with resultant thickening of the bony cortices and narrowing of the marrow cavities throughout the skeleton, is an uncommon disease of unknown etiology (Figs. 29-6 and 29-7). The resultant generalized radiopacity of the skeleton explains why this disease is included in the present chapter. The disease was first described in 1907 by Albers-Schönberg. A survey of the literature by Cangiano and co-workers (1972) revealed approximately 300 reported cases.

FEATURES

Osteopetrosis is generally subdivided into two main types: the clinically benign dominantly inherited form and the clinically malignant recessively inherited form (Shafer et al., 1974, p. 631).

Benign osteopetrosis usually develops later in

Fig. 29-6. Malignant osteopetrosis of the skull and jaws in a 4-year-old boy. Note the uniformly dense radiopaque involvement of the bones. (Courtesy R. Moncada, M.D., Maywood, Ill.)

life than the malignant form of the disease and is considerably less severe, a few cases not being diagnosed until middle age. Although the patient may sustain fractures after minor trauma, the marked symptoms of the malignant form are not characteristic of the benign disorder. Usually benign osteopetrosis is discovered incidentally on routine radiographs. The serum chemistry levels characteristically show normal values in both forms of the disease.

The malignant form of osteopetrosis is present at birth or develops in early childhood. The disease is severe and debilitating, with no known survivals beyond the age of 20 years. Patients with malignant osteopetrosis experience symptoms indicative of neurologic and hematologic derangements, which are direct results of the primary bone disorder—severe anemia, blindness, deafness, multiple fractures of the long bones with resulting deformity, hepatosplenomegaly, hydrocephalus, possible mental retardation, and osteomyelitis.

Fig. 29-7. A, Osteopetrosis of the lower extremities in an 8-year-old boy. Note the almost complete obliteration of the medullary portions of the femurs and tibiae as well as the cast on the left leg. **B,** Upper extremities of an infant with malignant osteopetrosis. (Courtesy R. Moncada, M.D., Maywood, Ill.)

Radiographically osteopetrosis is characterized by an increased density of the entire skeleton, resulting in a diffuse homogeneous symmetrically sclerotic appearance of all bones (Cangiano et al., 1972). Pathologic fractures are the most common clinical sign to occur (40%).

Marked changes in the radiographic appearance of the skull are evidenced in osteopetrosis: the normal landmarks are lost in the dense diffuse radiopacity; the diploës are effaced (Fig. 29-6); there is encroachment and narrowing of the cranial foramina, which results in nerve and vessel compression. Hearing loss, impariment of vision, and facial palsy ensue.

The bone may appear so dense on a dental radiograph that the roots of the teeth are obscured. Density is generally homogeneous with greatly increased thickening of the trabeculae and corresponding reduction of the marrow spaces. The radiographic appearance of the lamina dura is often lost in the overall density, and the presence of possible periapical pathosis is extremely difficult to discern (Fig. 29-6). This factor, coupled with the reduction of marrow spaces, causes a predilection toward osteomyelitis.

Fig. 29-8. Jaws and arms of a 6-month-old infant with infantile cortical hyperostosis. Proliferation of the cortices has almost completely obliterated the shadows of the medullary cavities. (Courtesy R. Moncada, M.D., Maywood, Ill.)

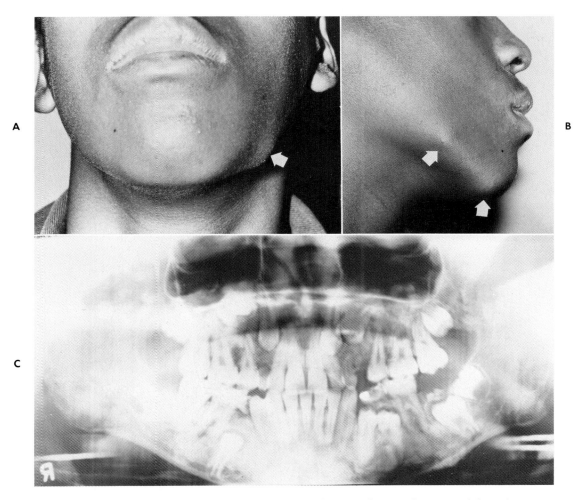

Fig. 29-9. Gardner's syndrome in a young man. **A** and **B,** Facial views showing nodular enlargements (arrows) on the inferior aspect of the mandible caused by the multiple osteomas. **C,** Panograph showing the diffuse and nodular radiopacities in the jaws that are produced by the multiple osteomas. (Courtesy W. Heaton, D.D.S., Chicago.)

DIFFERENTIAL DIAGNOSIS

The differentiating aspects of generalized radiopacities of the jawbones are discussed in the differential diagnosis section on p. 605.

MANAGEMENT

There is at present no cure for the primary defect in osteopetrosis. Palliative measures are instituted to alleviate the secondary symptoms of the disease. The teeth and periodontal structures should be maintained in good health to minimize the possibility of superimposed osteomyelitis of the jaws.

RARITIES

A considerable number of rare diseases, some of which are syndromes, may manifest generalized radiopacities of a few or many bones of the skeleton. A list includes the following:

Albright's syndrome
Caffey's disease (infantile cortical hyperostosis) (Fig. 29-8)
Camurati-Engelmann's disease
Craniometaphyseal dysplasia
Craniodiaphyseal dysplasia
Fluorosis
Gardner's syndrome (Fig. 29-9)

Fig. 29-10. Unusually large and numerous exostoses and tori in a 56-year-old black man. **A** and **B,** Intraoral clinical views. **C** to **E,** Panographic and periapical radiographs showing the dense radiopaque pattern throughout the body of the mandible.

Hyperostosis deformans juvenilis
Metastatic carcinoma of prostate
Multiple large exostoses and tori (Fig. 29-10)
Osteogenesis imperfecta
Pyknodysostosis
van Buchem's disease

DIFFERENTIAL DIAGNOSIS OF GENERALIZED RADIOPACITIES OF THE JAWBONES

When a clinician detects a generalized radiopacity of the jaws, he must consider especially these conditions in the differential diagnosis: normal variations in form and density, diffuse cementosis, Paget's disease, osteopetrosis, and polyostotic fibrous dysplasia.

Polyostotic fibrous dysplasia may be confused with Paget's disease because several bones will occasionally be involved; however, fibrous dysplasia usually involves a section of a bone rather than the complete bone. Hence the involved bones will generally exhibit asymmetric enlargement. Furthermore, serum chemistry changes in fibrous dysplasia if present will be slight.

Malignant osteopetrosis cannot be confused with Paget's disease and diffuse cementosis because it is almost invariably fatal by age 20 years whereas the other entities occur predominantly in patients beyond the fourth decade of life. *Benign osteopetrosis,* however, may be seen in older persons. The fact that osteopetrosis usually involves all the skeletal bones helps to differentiate it from Paget's disease, which commonly involves five or six bones at most. Diffuse cementosis involves only the mandible and the maxilla.

Paget's disease can be differentiated from diffuse cementosis and malignant osteopetrosis by the classic bones it most often involves: skull, pelvis, vertebrae, femurs, maxilla, and mandible. Also the serum chemistry measurements will show markedly elevated alkaline phosphatase values, which, in combination with diffuse radiopacities for some bones, is practically pathognomonic for Paget's disease. Likewise, advanced hypercementosis of the teeth, in combination with generalized radiopacities of several bones, is often considered pathognomonic.

Diffuse cementosis has a strong predilection for black women over 30 years of age. The most salient features of this disease are that (1) only the jaws are affected and (2) radiographs of the jaws reveal radiopaque masses frequently rimmed by a radiolucent border. These two features are unique to diffuse cementosis and clearly differentiate it from Paget's disease and osteopetrosis.

Normal variations in form and radiodensity of the jawbones must be considered in the differential diagnosis, and this aspect is discussed in detail in Chapter 22 (p. 467). Dense radiographic images of the jawbones may be seen in patients who have heavy jawbones and ruddy complexions or who are overweight. Such an image may also be related to incorrectly exposed or processed radiographs, however.

The clinician should also bear in mind the rarer diseases that are capable of causing this condition, but a detailed discussion of these is beyond the scope of this text.

SPECIFIC REFERENCES

Albers-Schönberg, H.: Ein bisher nicht beschriebene Allgemeinerkrankung des Skelettes im Röntgenbild, Fortschr. Geb. Roentgenstr. **11:**261, 1907; cited in Thoma, K. H.: Oral pathology, ed. 2, St. Louis, 1944, The C. V. Mosby Co., chapter 7.

Bhaskar, S. N., and Cutright, D. E.: Multiple exostosis: report of cases, J. Oral Surg. **26:**321-326, 1968.

Cangiano, R., Mooney, J., and Stratigos, G. T.: Osteopetrosis: report of case, J. Oral Surg. **30:**217-222, 1972.

Gee, J. K., Zambito, R. F., Argentieri, G. W., et al.: Paget's disease (osteitis deformans) of the mandible, J. Oral Surg. **30:** 223-227, 1972.

Melrose, R. J., Abrams, A. M., and Mills, B. G.: Florid osseous dysplasia. A clinical, pathologic study of 34 cases, Oral Surg. **41:**62-82, 1976.

Shafer, W. G., Hine, M. K., and Levy, B. M.: A textbook of oral pathology, ed. 3, Philadelphia, 1974, W. B. Saunders Co.

Waldron, C. A., Giansanti, J. S., and Browand, B. C.: Sclerotic cemental masses of the jaws (so-called chronic sclerosing osteomyelitis, sclerosing osteitis, multiple enostosis, and gigantiform cementoma), Oral Surg. **39:**590-604, 1975.

Winer, H. J., Goepp, R. A., and Olson, R. E.: Gigantiform cementoma resembling Paget's disease: report of case, J. Oral Surg. **30:**517-519, 1972.

GENERAL REFERENCES

Brady, F. A., Roser, S. M., and Sapp, J. P.: Osteomyelitis of the mandible as a complicating factor in Paget's disease of bone, Br. J. Oral Surg. **17:**33-42, 1979.

Dick, H. M., and Simpson, W. J.: Dental changes in osteopetrosis, Oral Surg. **34:**408-416, 1972.

El-Mofty, S.: Chronic diffuse sclerosing osteomyelitis, Oral Surg. **36:**898-904, 1973.

Feig, H. I., Edmunds, W. R., Beaubien, R., and Finkleman, A. A.: Chronic osteomyelitis of the maxilla secondary to Paget's disease, Oral Surg. **28:**320-325, 1969.

Gigliotti, R.: Paget's disease of prolonged chronicity, Oral Surg. **28:**499-504, 1969.

Gomez, L. S. A., Taylor, R., Cohen, M. M., and Shklar, G.: The jaws in osteopetrosis (Albers-Schönberg disease): report of case, J. Oral Surg. **24:**67-74, 1966.

Gorlin, R. J., and Goldman, H. M.: Thoma's oral pathology, ed. 6, St. Louis, 1970, The C. V. Mosby Co.

Haddad, J. G.: Paget's disease of bone: problems and management. Symposium on metabolic bone disease, Orthop. Clin. North Am. **3:**775-786, 1972.

Halse, A., Roed-Petersen, B., and Lund, K.: Gardner's syndrome, J. Oral Surg. **33:**673-675, 1975.

Jolly, D. E., and Harris, T. B.: Osteitis deformans—a case of late involvement of the maxilla, J. Oral Med. **34:**54-59, 1979.

Jacobsson, S., and Heyden, G.: Chronic sclerosing osteomyelitis of the mandible: histologic and histochemical findings, Oral Surg. **43:**357-364, 1977.

Jacobsson, S., Hollender, L., Lindberg, S., and Larsson, A.: Chronic sclerosing osteomyelitis of the mandible, Oral Surg. **45:**167-174, 1978.

Kawahara, K., Nishikiori, M., Imai, K., et al.: Radiographic observations of pyknodysostosis, Oral Surg. **44:**476-482, 1977.

Kirby, J. W., and Robinson, M. E.: Osteitis deformans of the maxilla: report of atypical case, J. Oral Surg. **31:**64-70, 1973.

Mincer, H. H., McGinnis, J. P., and Wyatt, J. R.: Ultrastructure of sclerotic cemental masses, Oral Surg. **43:**70-81, 1977.

Morgan, G. A., and Morgan, P. R.: Oral and skull manifestations of Paget's disease, J. Can. Dent. Assoc. **35:**208-212, 1969.

Ramon, Y., and Buchner, A.: Camurati-Engelmann's disease affecting the jaws, Oral Surg. **22:**592-599, 1966.

Rosenmertz, S. K., and Schare, H. J.: Osteogenic sarcoma arising in Paget's disease of the mandible, Oral Surg. **28:**304-309, 1968.

Smith, N. H.: Albers-Schönberg disease (osteopetrosis): report of case and review of the literature, Oral Surg. **22:**699-710, 1966.

Thompson, R. D., Hale, M. L., Montgomery, J. C., and Montana-Villamizar, E.: Manifestations of osteopetrosis, J. Oral Surg. **27:**63-71, 1969.

Towns, T. M.: Chronic sclerosing osteomyelitis of maxilla and mandible: review of the literature and report of case, J. Oral Surg. **30:**903-905, 1972.

Uthman, A. A., and al-Shawaff, M.: Paget's disease of the mandible: report of case, Oral Surg. **28:**866-870, 1969.

Wade, G. W., Hayes, R. L., and Griffiths, N. H. G.: Osteitis deformans: a systemic disease with oral manifestations: report of case, J. Am. Dent. Assoc. **71:**43-49, 1965.

Welborn, J. F., and Molnar, R. W.: Gardner's syndrome with concomitant tertiary lues: report of case, J. Oral Surg. **28:**131-133, 1970.

30

Diseases of the maxillary sinus

Norman K. Wood
Paul W. Goaz

The diseases that affect the maxillary sinus are many in kind and number and varied in complexity, and the skill and success demonstrated by the clinician will depend on the nature of his training and experience as well as the type of practice pursued. For instance, the general medical practitioner sees and successfully treats many cases of acute sinusitis that are complications of the common cold or allergic rhinitis. The resistant cases of sinusitis, including those of dental origin, will usually be referred to the otolaryngologist for treatment. As a result the otolaryngologist may well see a greater percentage of sinusitis cases of dental origin than will the general medical practitioner. Also the otolaryngologist or oral surgeon managing a trauma-type practice will treat a considerable number of fractures that involve the sinus walls, as well as any resulting complications arising as the result of injury to the sinus(es). In addition, the oral surgeon may see and treat a significant number of roots in the sinus and oroantral fistulas referred by the general dental practitioner.

In spite of this interest and attention focused on the maxillary sinus by the allied healing groups it is still essential that the general dental practitioner also be well informed about the anatomy and pathology of the maxillary sinus. After all, the alveolar process that supports the posterior maxillary teeth forms the floor of the sinus. The dentist must daily recognize and evaluate the image of an inferior portion of the maxillary sinus that is a regular feature of the radiographs of these maxillary teeth. It must also be of concern to him that many of the pathoses that involve the maxillary sinus may refer pain to the dental structures; so they must be distinguished from frank dental disease.

The following is a list of the pathologic entities that involve the maxillary sinus. An attempt has been made to rank them according to their frequency of occurrence in the general population of the United States.

Maxillary sinusitis
Benign mucosal cysts
Local hyperplasia from odontogenic infection
Fractures involving the sinus
Foreign bodies
    Teeth and roots
    Antrolith
Bony cysts
Fibrous dysplasia
Oroantral fistulas
Odontomas
Malignant tumors
Other odontogenic tumors
Other osseous conditions and tumors
Rarities
    Aplasia
    Burkitt's lymphoma
    Cholesteatoma
    Emphysema
    Encephalocele
    Enostosis and osteoma
    Hemangioma
    Inverted schneiderian papilloma
    Juvenile angiofibroma
    Leprosy
    Lethal midline granuloma
    Meningocele
    Mucocele
    Mycoses
    Neurogenic tumors
    Osteomyelitis
    Osteopetrosis
    Paget's disease
    Pyocele
    Rare odontogenic tumors
    Rhinosporidiosis
    Sarcoidosis
    Systemic disease (rarefaction)
    Tuberculosis

The four paranasal sinuses are a group of air cavities that surround the nasal chambers and take their names from the bones in which they are located: the maxillary, the frontal, the ethmoid, and the sphenoid sinuses. The maxillary sinus is the largest of the group and is proximate to the dental oral complex. It originates as an outpouching of the nasal mucosa during fetal life or early childhood. Nathaniel Highmore is thought to be the first to recognize the anatomic and clinical significance of the maxillary sinus; hence it is sometimes referred to as the antrum of Highmore (Waite, 1971).

ANATOMIC CONSIDERATIONS

The maxillary sinuses are paired structures located within the maxillary bones just lateral to the nasal chambers. Each cavity is in the shape of a three-sided pyramid, the apex being located in the zygomatic process of the maxilla, which with age and loss of function may extend into the zygomatic bone. The base of the pyramid (or medial wall of the sinus) is formed by part of the lateral bony wall of the nose. The floor of the orbit that forms the roof of the sinus is a side of the pyramid. The maxillary alveolar process forms the inferior boundary. A third side of the pyramid, the posterior wall of the sinus, is represented by the protruding wall of the posterior aspect of the maxilla. In most adults the inferior extension of the sinus lies below the level of the floor of the nose (Kelly and Strothers, 1974).

The infraorbital nerve courses through a canal within the bony roof of the antrum and exits onto the face through the infraorbital foramen. This nerve is sensory and originates from the maxillary branch of the trigeminal nerve. The posterior superior alveolar nerve branches from the infraorbital nerve just before it enters the canal. It passes anteriorly and inferiorly in a canal in the sinus wall to be directed along the floor of the sinus. Along with the middle and anterior superior branches that also reach the floor through canals in the sinus walls, it provides innervation to the maxillary bone, teeth, and periodontal ligaments and mucosa, as well as the mucus membrane of the sinus (Sicher, 1960, p. 368). The images of these canals frequently appear on periapical radiographs that include a portion of the sinus. They are recognized as radiolucent lines of usually uniform width, traversing the sinus wall.

The average volume of the adult maxillary sinus is said to be approximately 15 ml, but not only is there considerable variation in the size of the antra between individuals but also between the two sides of the same individual.

Fig. 30-1. Diagram showing relationship of maxillary sinuses, *MC*, to nasal chambers, *N*. Note the position of the ostium, *O*, in the superior aspect of the medial wall and its relationship to the middle turbinate bone, *M*.

The three molar and two premolar teeth are the teeth most closely associated with the sinus but in unusual cases the sinus may extend anteriorly to the lateral incisor (Fireman and Noyek, 1976).

The maxillary sinus communicates with the nasal cavity by the ostium, a short channel in the nasal wall about 4 mm in diameter and 5 to 10 mm in length. The sinus end of this channel is on the anterior superior aspect of the sinus wall and on the nasal surface it opens into the middle meatus, under the overlapping middle turbinate. An accessory ostium occurs with some regularity below the posterior end of the middle turbinate (Fig. 30-1). One's first impression is that the position of the ostium is a "mistake of nature" for it would seem much more functional if it were located on a level with the floor and not with the roof of the sinus so that gravity might aid rather than hinder drainage. On the other hand, the accessory ostium is lower and slightly more advantageously placed for drainage than the principal ostium.

However, consideration of the anatomic relationships that develop during fetal and postnatal growth illustrates how the ostium occurs in its seemingly disadvantageous position. Late in fetal life the nasal mucosa invaginates into the maxillary bones forming bilateral horizontal pouches in the lateral nasal walls smaller than peas (Fig. 30-2). These pouches deepen by extending laterally into the shallow maxilla. As the maxilla grows anteriorly and inferiorly the deciduous and permanent teeth develop and fill the body of the bone. However, as these teeth erupt the maxillary sinus expands and hollows out the space initially occupied by the developing teeth. It is apparent then that when the sinus expands it must be down-

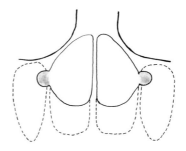

Fig. 30-2. Diagram showing the bilateral, small, horizontal invaginations (gray) in the lateral walls of the nose during fetal life. During childhood and adolescence these primitive maxillary sinuses will expand by following the growth of the maxilla in an inferior and anterior direction (broken lines). The sites of the original invaginations persist as the ostia.

Fig. 30-3. Photomicrograph of pseudostratified columnar ciliated epithelium that lines the sinus.

ward, away from its original position into the maxillary bone and into the alveolar process (Ritter, 1978, p. 6). The ostium necessarily remains in its original position, that is, high on the medial wall of the enlarged cavity.

In spite of this apparent inefficient arrangement the normal sinus drains satisfactorily as the result of the action of the cilia of the pseudostratified columnar epithelium (Fig. 30-3) that beat toward the ostium. Thus a thin film of mucus is moved along with any contaminants to the ostium, through which it is eliminated, and the antrum remains sterile under normal conditions.

Contrary to what must appear to be obvious, the supine position during sleep, with the individual's head on one side and then the other, does not facilitate the drainage of normal sinuses. In reality any benefit that might accrue from the improved position of the ostium during sleep is more than offset by congestion of the nasal mucosa that occurs when the body is supine. Such congestion will narrow and possibly close the ostium and is due to increased central venous pressure in the head, which occurs when it is lowered as it is in the supine position (Aust and Drittner, 1975).

Microscopic anatomy

Like the other air cavities the antrum is lined with pseudostratified columnar ciliated epithelium with many goblet cells* (Fig. 30-3). This respiratory epithelium is continuous through the ostium with the nasal mucosa but is much thinner and more delicate within the sinus. It is usually not over 1 mm in thickness and is covered with a thin film of mucus. In addition to the goblet cells in the epithelium, scattered seromucinous glands lie in the thin submucosal tissue, but these are restricted mainly to the medial wall near the ostium.†

---

*The goblet cells secrete the mucus that is very important to the maintenance of the membrane lining.
†However, as the result of the repeated or chronic infection there is proliferation of these seromucinous glands and they occur in large numbers on the floor and lateral wall of the sinus (Van Norstrand and Goodman, 1976).

PHYSIOLOGY

The functions of the maxillary sinus are not well understood. The following possibilities have been suggested: (1) to lighten the skull, (2) as resonators for the voice, and (3) and (4) to warm and moisten the inspired air. However, not one of these proposed functions has been accepted to be the essential purpose. The most probable explanation of the development of the maxillary sinus relates to the elimination of nonfunctioning bone that has lost its mechanical requirement as the jaw develops and the trajectories of stress change.

The normal functioning mucosal lining is covered by a thin blanket of mucus that is produced by both the glands in the mucosa and the goblet cells of the epithelium. The mucus blanket is carried to the ostium by the action of the cilia on the mucosal surface that beat in that direction. When the mucus is discharged into the nose it is moved, again by cilia, to the pharyngeal end of the esophagus where it is swallowed or expectorated. The mucus blanket is a thin, sticky, tenacious, and adhesive sheet that is also bacteriostatic and shields the underlying cells from infection by protecting them from the deleterious effects of bacteria, particulate matter, noxious pollutants, and drying of the surface. It is observed that on occasion scar tissue forms in the mucosa after traumatic incidents or surgery. Such scar tissue may prevent the movement of mucus to the ostium, and this may cause a pooling and septic effect in the distal segment.

EXAMINATION OF THE SINUS
History

Although Fascenelli (1969) has reported that some 26% of the asymptomatic population will have radiographic evidence of maxillary sinus abnormalities, the diagnosis of maxillary sinus disease is usually reserved for those conditions that cause significant subjective symptoms (complaints).

Symptoms produced by maxillary sinus disease may relate to the face, the eye, the nasal and oral cavities, and to the superior aspect of the head. Pain is the most frequent symptom and may be manifested as a deep-seated pain of the maxillary bone on the involved side, or else, it may be referred to the face, eye, nose, or premolar-molar teeth. In some instances the patient will describe a vague headache or poorly localized facial pain.

Facial manifestations involve the skin of the infraorbital region, the upper lip, and the lateral aspect of the nose. Complaints such as unilateral paresthesia, anesthesia, and the feeling of fullness or pain is common in maxillary sinus disease.

Ophthalmologic complaints include epiphora, diplopia, a feeling of fullness, unilateral decrease in vision, pain, or change in the position of the eyeball, as well as paresthesia or anesthesia of the inferior eyelid.

Nasal symptoms include obstruction, epistaxis, drainage, postnasal drip, and cacosmia (sensation or hallucination of a stench). The patient will frequently relate a history of a recent nose cold or allergic rhinitis or that he has a deviated septum. The history may reveal that a mouth-breathing habit has recently developed. The description of food and liquid discharging through the nose during meals suggests an oroantral communication. Further questioning of the latter patient usually reveals that a maxillary posterior tooth has been removed recently.

Intraorally the majority of complaints focus on the maxillary premolar-molar region, although paresthesia or anesthesia, usually unilateral, of the complete facial gingiva and mucosa may be experienced. Intraoral pain characteristically manifests itself in most or all of the maxillary premolar-molar teeth on the involved side. Occasionally the patient will discover a recent bite problem or an expansion of the alveolar process, the adjacent vestibule, or the posterolateral hard palate.

Clinical examination

The visual examination should initially be directed toward evaluating the skin in the infraorbital region, checking for unusual redness, malposition of an eyeball, asymmetry of the face due to a swelling over the sinus, or a unilateral swelling in the posterior maxilla.

The intranasal examination should be carried out using a good light and a suitable speculum to open the nose and must include a careful examination of the ostium and the surrounding nasal mucosa. The size and proximity of the middle turbinate bone and septum relative to the ostium should be observed for they may obstruct free drainage. Presence or absence of drainage from the ostium should be noted, and the discharge should be described as clear mucus, mucopus, frank pus, or blood.

All the maxillary teeth should be percussed to determine if there is a unilateral difference in the sensitivity of the posterior group. The maxillary teeth on the side in question should also be subjected to a battery of pulp tests.

All swellings should be palpated to determine whether they are soft tissue or bone, as well as to identify the various other features that characterize masses. If the expansion proves to be bone then moderate digital pressure should be applied in an effort to detect crepitus. Crepitus would indicate the presence of a disease process that has produced a significant thinning of the bone walls. Thinning may or may not be accompanied by expansion of the sinus walls. In checking for changes in sensation of the face it is helpful to draw a finger slowly over the skin in each infraorbital region simultaneously (bilaterally) to see if the patient is able to detect a difference in the degree of or nature of the feeling on one side. If paresthesia or anesthesia is demonstrated its extent can be mapped by gentle use of a sharp sterile hypodermic needle.

Transillumination of the maxillary sinus is usually not diagnostic but may yield useful ancillary information. For this procedure, conducted in a darkened room, a bright fiber optics light is placed in the patient's mouth and directed toward the palate. (Prostheses with palatal coverage must be removed.) The patient's lips are closed tightly around the probe and the eyes are open. Uniform crescents of light will be observed bilaterally just above the infraorbital rims, at the position of the eyelids, and the pupils will both glow if both sinuses are healthy (Waite, 1971). The principle of the test is as follows: a sinus of normal size and aeration will readily permit passage of light but if pathosis is present in the form of a soft tissue mass, calcified material, or fluid such as pus or blood then the transmitted light will be duller or perhaps the sinus will be completely opaque on the affected side. It is instructive that certain cysts that contain thin fluid will not significantly interfere with the passage of light and will not be detected by transillumination. Clinicians do not solely depend on transillumination but use it to supplement historical, clinical, and radiographic findings. Evans and co-workers (1975) demonstrated by aspiration that acute symptoms coupled with an opaque antrum strongly suggested sinus infection.

Radiographic considerations

Frequently disease of the maxillary sinus is relatively clinically occult. Thus radiographs of the structures are frequently revealing and are especially helpful in completing an examination of the maxillary sinuses. However, the usefulness of a radiographic examination of the maxillary sinus is dependent on the clinician's ability to correctly interpret the images on the various projections and his awareness of their limitations. An excellent review and illustration of the radiographic appearance of the maxillary sinus in health and disease has been published by Poyton (1972).

PERIAPICAL FILMS

Since the peripical films provide better definition than any of the other types of radiographs employed they also give the best detail of the maxillary sinuses, but unfortunately only the floor and inferior portion of these cavities are included on the film. The various images of the sinus have been discussed in Chapters 15, 16, 18, 19, and 25. Fireman and Noyek (1976) and many authors of dental radiology textbooks have described in detail the appearance of the maxillary sinus on periapical radiographs.

OCCLUSAL FILMS

Although the images on the maxillary occlusal films are almost as well defined as those on periapical projections, they are also limited because only the anterior portions of the maxillary sinuses are included on this radiograph. *Oblique maxillary occlusal* films made by shifting the film and tube to the side of interest and directing the central beam through the infraorbital foramen are much superior to the midline projection since they often include the whole sinus. The disadvantage of this projection is that only one sinus appears on the film, so interfilm variables preclude a completely convincing comparison of the sinuses.

PANOGRAPHIC FILMS

Panographic radiographs have proved to be very useful for demonstrating the maxillary sinuses. Ohba and Katayama (1975) have described the panoramic reoentgenographic anatomy of the maxillary sinus in detail. Shramek and Rappaport (1969) encouraged the use of the panoramic radiograph as a screening device for maxillary sinus pathosis and as a guide for surgical planning. Lyon (1973) reported that the Panorex radiograph may be as useful as the Waters' film for the study of the maxillary sinus. Also Ohba (1977) contends that panographic radiography is superior to the Waters' projection for the detection of malignancies in the maxillary sinus and cystlike lesions near the floor of the sinus. Pathosis of the posterior wall of the sinus would also be much more readily detected in the panoramic view.

In contrast, Ohba and Katayama (1976) maintain that the Waters' film is much better than the panoramic radiograph for the comparison of the opacity of the left and right sinus. We in part corroborate this opinion as it is not possible to ensure that the two sides of the panoramic radiograph have been exposed at the same angle and that some shifting of the patient has not occurred. Slight variations in the panographic technique produce a marked difference in the images of the left and right maxillary sinus in the same patient.

THE WATERS FILM

Since its development by Waters and Waldron in 1915 the Waters' film has proved to be one of the most useful for the demonstration of the maxillary sinus. It is a variation of the posteroanterior projection with the midsaggital plane perpendicular to the plane of the film, but with the chin touching the film, the nose about 2.5 cm off the cassette, and the central ray projected in the midsaggital plane and perpendicular to the film. Yanagisawa and Smith (1976) have described the appearance and landmarks of the normal maxillary sinus as seen on the Waters' film in detail.

Killey and Kay (1975, p. 15) described a useful technique to conclusively substantiate the impression of an air-fluid level in the sinus by taking a second Waters' view with the head held at a slight lateral tilt. If the line of demarcation between the more translucent and more opaque portions of the sinus shifts to remain horizontal it is diagnostic of a fluid level.

The advantages of the Waters' film over the panoramic film are as follows: (1) all the major sinuses can be seen on one film, which is very helpful in cases of generalized sinus disease; (2) it is an excellent film for comparing the opacification of the right and left antrum; (3) it gives a much better image of the lateral, medial, and orbital walls of the antrum (also roof and superior aspects of the maxillary sinuses are much more readily visualized); (4) Le Fort I, II, and III fractures can be more clearly visualized. A comparative evaluation of these two films clearly indicates that the panoramic and Waters' views are complementary for the study of the maxillary sinuses. Ohba and Katayama (1976) in a comparison reported that both should be used in order to obtain more accurate diagnoses of maxillary sinus disease.

CALDWELL VIEW

Basically the Caldwell view is a slight modification of the posteroanterior view of the maxillary sinuses. It is taken in a manner similar to the posteroanterior view of the skull and jaws with the forehead and nose resting on the film and the central ray directed parallel to the sinus floor and perpendicular to the film. Because the beam is directed parallel to the antral floor, small pathologic masses situated on the posterior aspect of the antral floor are more likely to be seen. Such masses are hidden in the usual Waters' film because of the 15° tilt of the head for this view to raise the chin off the film. The Caldwell film also gives an excellent view of the medial wall and the roof of the sinus. Excellent illustrations of this view in both health and disease appear in the report by Yanagisawa and Smith (1976).

LATERAL VIEW

The lateral view is made with the head touching the film and the midsaggital plane parallel to the film. Although the images of the maxillary sinuses are superimposed on other structures, some useful information can frequently be obtained from this view. Specifically this film will help to pinpoint the anteroposterior position of a small mass in the sinus.

TOMOGRAM

Tomography is a technique by which a sharp radiographic image of a layer of tissue below the surface can be achieved by blurring the images of the structures that lie above and below it. Tomography radiographs in either a saggital or frontal plane will yield considerable information about sinus disease that has involved bone. They may not indicate the presence of inflammatory disease. They are particularly helpful in identifying blowout fractures of the orbit (see below) and also in delineating the extent of bony sinus lesions. The presence of calcified bodies in the maxillary sinus is easily detected by tomograms.

OTHER RADIOGRAPHIC TECHNIQUES

The evaluation of relatively new diagnostic techniques has also focused on their application in the areas of the oral and perioral structures. For example, Olsen and co-workers (1976) described the use of xeroradiography for the study of malar fractures, while Binnie and co-workers (1979) considered its general utilization in dentistry. Also the use of thermography for the detection of maxillary sinus disease has not escaped consideration (Wortzman and Holgate, 1976); and angiography, isotope scanning, and opacification by the injection of radiopaque fluid have also been used in special situations for the demonstration of, and the extension of, information about these pathoses.

Proof puncture

"Proof puncture" is an investigative procedure that may be used to demonstrate whether the sinus contains a fluid such as pus, exudate, blood, soft tissue, or a combination of any of these. It is accomplished with local anesthesia by passing a trocar through the bony wall of the antrum and aspirating the contents of the cavity. The entry is preferably made in the lateral wall of the nose just under the anterior end of the inferior turbinate, but it can also be made intraorally over the apices of the premolar teeth. The sample obtained using this technique also provides material for bacteriologic study.

Endoscopy

Endoscopy or sinoscopy is a procedure that has been introduced recently. Basically this procedure involves the insertion of a cannula either via the canine fossa or the inferior meatus (below and lateral to the inferior nasal concha). A Hopkins optic system is then used to examine the interior of the maxillary sinus (Illum and Jeppesen, 1972). Kreidler and Koch (1975) used this technique to study sinus conditions following middle-face fractures, and Illum and co-workers (1972) compared sinoscopic findings with radiographic findings in maxillary sinus disease. These investigators reported that sinoscopy is more suitable than x-ray examination in the diagnosis of many conditions and was especially effective for detecting early cancer.

PATHOSES OF THE MAXILLARY SINUS
An overview

The pathologic conditions of the maxillary sinus may be conveniently characterized according to the tissue of origin: (1) sinus mucosa, (2) bone walls, (3) odontogenic tissues, and (4) foreign bodies. A useful classification that is based on the fundamental nature of the disease processes and one that facilitates their presentation is given in the following outline:

1. Inflammatory process
   a. Acute sinusitis
   b. Chronic sinusitis
   c. Osteomyelitis
2. Cysts
   a. Intrinsic
   b. Extrinsic

3. Tumors
   a. Odontogenic
   b. Nonodontogenic
4. Trauma
   a. Fractures
   b. Foreign bodies
5. Other local osseous pathology
6. Systemic disease

Many of the lesions of the maxillary sinus and especially those that are localized in the inferior portion are clinically and subjectively occult. This is the case since they do not block the free flow of fluid or gas through the ostium and pressure does not increase within the sinus. Conversely when disease conditions block the ostium the stage is set for considerable discomfort and pain. When maxillary sinus pathoses encroach on neighboring tissue, then symptoms may be referred to such structures as the nose, eye, face, maxillary posterior teeth, alveolus, and posterolateral hard palate.

Radiographic considerations in maxillary sinus disease

As with diseases of other organs, radiographic findings from the maxillary sinus must be correlated with those obtained by the other modes of examination in order to formulate a valid working diagnosis.

In contrast to the jawbones, in which disease is recognized as either areas of increased, decreased, or mixed radiodensity, almost all the pathologic conditions that occur within the sinus increase the radiopacity of the chambers that are normally filled with air. The rare exception to this is the pneumocele that is the result of air being trapped in the maxillary sinus. At times it becomes enlarged, and being filled with air it may appear even more radiolucent than the unaffected side. In contrast, any space-occupying lesion, whether it be soft or hard tissue, or liquids will appear as a relative radiopacity when compared with the normal sinus.

As a general rule with experience it is possible to differentiate the homogeneous, less radiopaque shadow of fluid or soft tissue proliferation from the much more dense, radiopaque, calcified or ossified lesion.

The spectrum of radiographic appearances that may result from maxillary sinus disease is detailed in the following list (modified from Zizmor and Noyek, 1973):

1. Generalized luminal opacification
2. Generalized mucosal thickening

3. Discrete soft tissue mass
4. Fluid level
5. Localized calcification or ossification
6. Teeth and roots
7. Foreign bodies
8. Alterations in bone walls
   a. Dehiscence
   b. Fractures
   c. Decalcifications and lysis
   d. Hyperostosis
   e. Expansion of bone walls
   f. Decreased luminal volume

Maxillary sinusitis

Because at least 25% of the population apparently have inflamed maxillary sinus membranes (Fascenelli, 1969) that are radiographically detectable, it is customary to reserve the term "sinusitis" for those conditions causing subjective symptoms as well as the apparent thickened and hyperplastic lining.

For our purposes here the term "sinusitis" is used to describe an inflamed condition of most or all of the lining of the maxillary sinus. This excludes the many smaller localized areas of inflamed hyperplastic lining that are predominantly seen on the floor of the sinus and are frequently the result of chronic dental infection but that rarely cause symptoms associated with the sinus. Sinusitis, on the other hand, usually gives rise to many and varied troublesome symptoms.

Sinusitis may occur in acute, subacute, and chronic forms. Subacute suppurative sinusitis will develop in those patients who are not cured of acute sinusitis by conservative management. Chronic suppurative sinusitis is usually a sequel to negligent management of either acute or subacute sinusitis (Waite, 1971).

One or several or all of the paranasal sinuses may be involved simultaneously (parasinusitis), but the maxillary sinus is probably more frequently infected. Maxillary sinusitis is usually a direct result of a blocked ostium, which is in turn caused by a swelling of the nasal mucosa. The inflammation is generally caused by a nose cold or an allergic rhinitis; less frequently, nasal polyps and deviated septa may occlude the opening.

Other predisposing causes of a maxillary sinusitis are cleft palate and invasion of the maxillary sinus during dental procedures. Although infected teeth have been considered a significant cause of sinusitis, the current consensus is that this is a rare occurrence in the absence of surgical violation of the sinus.

Haemophilus influenzae and *Diplococcus pneu-*

moniae are the most frequent bacteria associated with acute sinusitis. Streptococci, staphylococci, and various fungi are occasionally found (Axelsson and Brorson, 1972), as are the adenoviruses (Evans et al., 1975).

FEATURES

Usually the patient has experienced a nose cold. After 3 or 4 days, instead of recuperating, the patient's stuffiness and nasal discharge increases. The discharge is a yellowish mucopus or frank pus and it may be blood stained. The patient's sense of smell is altered, and cacosmia may be experienced. Headache and facial and intraoral paresthesia may be symptoms. The patient usually complains of malaise and has an elevated temperature.

A sense of fullness may be experienced over the cheek, especially on bending forward, and the patient may experience pain of varying intensity deep in the upper jaw* or over the malar bone, the eye, or the posterior maxillary teeth. All the maxillary premolar and molar teeth on the affected side may be sensitive or painful to percussion. A proof puncture will usually yield mucopus or frank pus.

The Waters' film is the best radiographic projection to use in a suspected case of sinusitis (Axelsson and Jensen, 1974), and the following changes may be observed: (1) mucous membrane thickening only, (2) mucous membrane thickening and a fluid level, (3) a fluid level only, and (4) complete opacity of the antrum (Fig. 30-4). Occasionally it is difficult to differentiate between a soft tissue shadow and a fluid level. This can be readily accomplished by taking a second Waters' film with the patient's head tilted (see p. 617). In cases where the sinus floor has been violated during dental procedures, the bony defect will usually be evident on periapical films (Fig. 30-20). Likewise, teeth or segments of teeth that have been pushed into the sinus should be readily discernible as characteristic radiopacities without a periodontal ligament shadow (Fig. 30-11).

Complications of acute sinusitis include the following: (1) production of antral polyps, (2) subacute or chronic sinusitis, (3) osteomyelitis, (4) orbital cellulitis, (5) development of fistula, (6) meningitis, (7) cavernous sinus thrombosis, and (8) abscesses of the brain (Zizmor and Noyek, 1973).

---

*This pain is usually described by the patient as dull and nagging in nature.

Fig. 30-4. Acute sinusitis. **A,** Note the fluid-air level in the right maxillary sinus. The fluid in this case was pus and caused the opacification of the inferior half of the sinus. There appears to be a generalized even thickening of the mucosa lining the sinus segment that remains aerated. **B,** Tomogram of another case showing a generalized opacification of the left sinus, which is filled with exudate.

DIFFERENTIAL DIAGNOSIS

Acute sinusitis accompanied by the characteristic dull nagging pain, purulent discharge, paresthesia, and characteristic radiographic change of fluid level or generalized opacification is easily differentiated from all other sinus conditions. However, it is important to realize that it is possible that the picture of acute sinusitis is superimposed over a preexisting condition such as malignancy.

Differentiating the pain of sinusitis from odontogenic pain may be a very difficult task since the maxillary premolar and molar teeth may seem to ache and are actually painful to percussion in many cases of acute sinusitis. Usually a complete examination of the teeth in question, which includes a history, clinical and radiographic examination, and extensive pulp testing will identify or rule out a dental problem. Also if the patient has recently experienced a paresthesia of the facial gingiva and mucosa then it is most likely that he has a sinusitis; however, facture and malignancy must be ruled out.

Chronic sinusitis with its milder symptoms and less dramatic radiographic changes may be easily confused with other disease conditions such as a malignancy. Both of these pathoses may cause pain, bone destruction, and unilateral epistaxis (Towers and McAndrew, 1975). If a malignancy is expected after an appropriate suitable radiographic examination, sinoscopy or surgical exploration and biopsy should be done.

MANAGEMENT

Specimens of the discharge from the sinus should be collected on the initial visit for the purpose of culture and sensitivity testing of the isolated microorganisms. Initial therapy of acute sinusitis, which can be initiated before the data from the cultures is at hand, includes the administering of antibacterial agents, decongestants, and analgesics. Broad-spectrum antibiotics such as ampicillin, erythromycin, tetracyclines, and sulfonamides are used. The dosage of antibiotics utilized must be reatively high because the organisms are in the sinus fluid and thus outside the tissue (body) and more difficult to reach.

Decongestants are used in attempts to open the ostium and thus to reestablish normal evacuation of the sinus. Ephedrine nose drops (0.5%) are recommended t.i.d. (Alberti, 1976). Antihistamine-decongestant combination capsules may also be adminstered orally. Some patients' symptoms are greatly relieved by inhalation of steam.

Varying opinions are held regarding whether antral lavage or intranasal antrostomy should be done in acute sinusitis (Alberti, 1976; Kelly and Strothers, 1974) or postponed for use in case the condition becomes subacute or chronic.

In chronic sinusitis surgical intervention is indicated, and a Caldwell-Luc procedure is the initial treatment. In this procedure part or all of the mucosal lining of the sinus is removed through a surgical incision in the canine fossa.

Frequently an intranasal window is established

Fig. 30-5. Benign asymptomatic mucosal cysts. **A** and **B,** Panorex radiographs. **C** and **D,** Periapical radiographs.

in the medial wall, much inferior to the ostium, to facilitate drainage. If a tooth root is in the sinus it should be removed and if an oroantral fistula is present it may be repaired at the time of the surgical procedure.

Benign mucosal cysts

Benign mucosal cysts are referred to in the literature by a plethora of names: nonsecreting cyst, mucosal cyst, mucus cyst, mesothelial cyst, polyp, retention cyst, mucocele,* serous cyst, inclusion cyst, pseudocyst, lymphangiectatic cyst, and cyst of McGregor (Killey and Kay, 1975, p. 95; Mattila and Westerholm, 1968).

The majority of benign mucosal cysts are false cysts that occur predominantly on the floor of the maxillary sinus and occasionally on the lateral wall. Although their cause is uncertain chronic sinus infection and dental infection have been suggested. Most of the cases are detected on routine radiographic surveys.

---

*In the discipline of otolaryngology, at least, this term is reserved for the retention cysts that occur in the sinus and become destructive.

FEATURES

The benign mucosal cysts are common lesions that are usually asymptomatic and occur in from 2% to 9.6% of the general population (Myall et al., 1974). The symptoms that have been described as rare include vague or localized pain as well as unilateral nasal discharge. While benign mucosal cysts may be observed on periapical radiographs they are best seen on panoramic films. Radiographically the mucosal cyst is a curved homogeneous radiopaque area that is spherical, ovoid, or dome shaped (Figs. 30-5 and 30-6). It has a smooth uniform outline, and the base of the attachment may be narrow or broad (Kwapis and Whitten, 1971). Although lesions are usually single, Halstead (1973) reported multiple cases in the sinus and also bilateral lesions. The images of mucosal cysts vary greatly in size, ranging from fingertip size to 25 × 19 mm. The lesions are found in patients of all ages, and reported sexual preference varies from study to study.

Periodic radiographic studies have shown that benign mucosal cysts may remain stationary in size, completely disappear, decrease in size, or in-

Fig. 30-6. Benign mucosal cysts. **A,** Interesting bosselated contour. **B,** Two cysts in the same sinus.

crease in size over an interval of months. Gothberg and co-workers (1976) suggested that the majority of these cysts will eventually regress spontaneously.

Surgical explorations have produced the following clinical picture: a round, distended, translucent mass with a light bluish or yellowish color. The walls are thin and rupture readily, yielding a watery fluid or a thicker sticky mucoid fluid. Fixation to the antral floor is reasonably firm (Kwapis and Whitten, 1971; Mattila and Westerholm, 1968).

Microscopic study shows that the vast majority of these are false cysts (the lumens are not lined with epithelium) and that glandular elements are not associated with these cysts. The rounded sinus surface is covered with respiratory epithelium, which may show areas of metaplasia. The lumen is filled with an amorphous material that contains a few inflammatory cells. Flat, elongated fibroblasts line the lumen. The cyst wall is composed of interwoven collagen fiber bundles and fibroblasts. This layer is sometimes edematous and contains varying numbers of round cells.

DIFFERENTIAL DIAGNOSIS

Benign mucosal cysts of the sinus must be differentiated from other soft tissue lesions of the sinus such as polyps, hyperplasia of dental infection, extrinsic cysts, sinusitis, and malignant soft tissue tumors. Calcified entities such as condensing osteitis, root tips, other foreign bodies, antroliths, odontomas, and bone-producing tumors generally have a much denser image and can usually be ruled out rather quickly because the benign mucosal cyst has a homogeneous, slightly radiopaque appearance, which gives the impression that the image is of soft tissue.

Occasionally in patients who have a *prominent ala* and when the periapical radiograph has been angled from an anterior direction the shadow of the ala may be cast over the inferoanterior image of the sinus. This image can be shifted from the sinus and recognized by taking a second periapical film with the proper angulation.

Antral polyps are much less common than benign mucosal cysts. Unlike the latter entity they do not have a predilection for the floor or inferolateral aspect of the sinus, and they are commonly associated with a thickened mucosa. Also polyps are usually multiple whereas benign mucosal cysts are usually solitary.

Hyperplasia as a result of chronic dental infection is frequently seen on radiographs of the antral floor, adjacent to teeth with obvious pulpoperiapical problems or advanced periodontal disease (Figs. 30-7 and 30-8). Both lesions may show similar convex, homogeneous, faintly opaque shadows, the differentiating feature of hyperplasia of dental infection being the juxtaposed chronically infected tooth. Usually dental infection is not seen in association with benign mucosal cysts or if present it is not construed as the etiologic agent. It is worthwhile noting that some investigators, such as Halstead (1973), feel that perhaps there is a causative relationship between dental infection and benign mucosal cysts especially because odontogenic pathosis was noted in 89% of his cases.

Extrinsic cysts such as radicular, dentigerous, primordial, and globulomaxillary may encroach on the sinus but are rather easily identified either by their characteristic location in the jaws or their relationship to a tooth. Also most extrinsic cysts will retain a thin curved radiopaque rim of bone, which separates the cyst from the antral

Fig. 30-7. Local hyperplasia of mucosal floor of sinus produced by periodontal disease.

Fig. 30-8. A to **C,** Local hyperplasia of mucosal floor of sinus produced by pulpoperiapical lesions. The pulps of all teeth were nonvital. **D,** The nonvital second premolar tooth was recently extracted.

shadow (Figs. 30-15 to 30-17). In addition, the shadows produced by the benign mucosal cysts are usually a shade or two more radiopaque than those produced by extrinsic cysts. An extensive discussion of the differential diagnosis of cystlike lesions of the jaws may be found in Chapter 18.

Hyperplasia of the antral lining caused by an *acute* or *chronic sinusitis* is usually seen as a generalized rather than localized thickening of the lining and is frequenlty accompanied by an overall sinus opacification.

Malignant tumors will not usually appear as symmetric or as smoothly contoured as the be-

nign mucosal cysts but in some cases may look quite similar. Both of these lesions share a predilection for the inferior aspect of the antrum. Ominous evidence of bone destruction of the sinus walls accompanied by a paresthesia would prompt a greater suspicion of malignancy.

MANAGEMENT

The majority of benign mucosal cysts will regress spontaneously. However, it is advisable to observe the patients with periodic radiographs in order to certify the diagnosis. If the patient is symptomatic, consultation should be sought with an otolaryngologist. If any doubt exists concerning the benignity of the lesion, surgical exploration and biopsy should be done as soon as possible.

Local hyperplasia from odontogenic infection

Local inflammatory hyperplasia of the floor of the sinus caused by dental infection is a common occurrence. For our purposes here we differentiate such a local change from "sinusitis" or "antritis," which implies that the whole mucosa lining of the sinus is inflamed and is accompanied by syptoms. Specifically, pulpoperiapical and periodontal disease are the two odontogenic entities that will produce this local hyperplasia. The lesion is almost always asymptomatic for periapical disease and seldom produces a full-blown sinusitis (Maloney and Doku, 1968).

It is important to note that the association between the benign mucosal cyst and chronic dental infection has not been satisfactorily established. Halstead suggests that even the presence of benign mucosal cysts above edentulous segments of an arch does not necessarily eliminate dental infection as the cause since presumably the majority of the preexisting teeth were extracted for reasons of pulpoperiapical pathosis (gross caries) or advanced periodontal disease.

FEATURES

Local mucosal hyperplasia of dental origin occurs on the floor of the maxillary sinus juxtaposed to a tooth root or roots of teeth that have an obvious bone lesion either of the pulpoperiapical or periodontal disease type (Figs. 30-7 and 30-8). Occasionally a lesion might develop on a lateral or medial wall of the sinus, especially where the apices are buccal or lingual to the sinus floor. The offending causative teeth may or may not be painful. The lesions may be single, multiple, or bilateral and are usually found during a routine radiographic survey. They are best observed on pantograph-type radiographs, but their images also occur on periapical radiographs. These lesions, like large benign mucosal cysts, may be overlooked on periapical films because their slightly radiopaque shadow may cover the image of the sinus so there will not be a portion of the unaffected cavity for comparison. Thus the usual contrast between cyst and involved sinus is not present to prompt the recognition of the hyperplastic tissue on casual observation.

Size of the lesions varies considerably and if two or more bone lesions are present then the hyperplastic lesion is correspondingly larger (Mattilla, 1965). The lesion may be flat and ribbonlike, hemispheric or corrugated with two or more arcs (Worth and Stoneman, 1972), and the soft tissue shadow will show varying degrees of grayness. The free margin of the soft tissue shadow is usually smoothly contoured and definite but may be indistinct, merging imperceptibly with the darker air shadow.

The roots of the contributing teeth may be situated at various distances from the sinus floor and soft tissue bulge but usually are directly beneath it. Such teeth will generally show the reason for the pulpoperiapical defect, for example, gross caries, deep restorations, calcified canals, or fractures, or else will have sustained periodontal bone loss. In unusual cases calculus isolated in the tissues can produce a local hyperplasia of the sinus floor (Worth and Stoneman, 1972).

Various bone changes may be observed in the region between the root of the offending tooth and the antral floor (the region directly beneath the local hyperplasia): (1) a periodontal disease type of bone loss (Fig. 30-7), (2) widening of the periodontal ligament shadow, particularly at the root end in the periapex, (3) discontinuity of the lamina dura, (4) presence of a radiolucent pulpoperiapical lesion (Fig. 30-8), (5) pulpoperiapical lesion showing a mixed radiolucent-radiopaque shadow (rarefying and condensing osteitis), (6) a completely radiopaque image (condensing osteitis), and (7) minimal sclerosis of a small segment of the antral cortex (Powell, 1965).

Mattila's extensive study of the local mucosal hyperplasia (1965) yielded the following observations: (1) a distinct correlation exists between the number of hyperplastic lesions and the number of periapical lesions; (2) there is an increased risk of patients developing a sinusitis who have dental foci of infection and hyperplastic lesions; (3) the closer the bone lesion is to the sinus floor the greater the chance of observable changes in the sinus lining; and (4) painful teeth did not produce more sinus changes than did symptomless teeth.

Worth and Stoneman (1972) reported that most often the soft tissue shadow disappears in a few days once treatment is initiated, especially in the case of lesions of short duration. Also Ericson and Welander (1966) reported that of their cases of local hyperplasia that were caused by periapical osteitis, 78% had disappeared completely after 11 to 20 months following treatment. However, in chronic cases more fibrous tissue would develop, and thus the degree of regression would vary in an inverse manner with the amount of fibrosis that had prevailed in the inflamed lining membrane. Thus some of these local mucosal hyperplasias will become very dense and "fibromalike," undergoing stages similar to the inflammatory hyperplastic lesions of the oral cavity.

In an interesting study using monkeys Valderhaug (1973) demonstrated that 10 to 14 cases of local antral tissue shadows that were induced experimentally by opening pulp chambers were cysts. The remainder proved to be granulomas.

DIFFERENTIAL DIAGNOSIS

The differential diagnosis for a local hyperplasia of the sinus lining (of the maxillary sinus) would require that it be distinguished from the benign mucosal cysts, anatomic variations, malignant tumors, generalized antritis, buccal exostosis, and ala of the nose.

Although the shadow of the *ala* of the nose in some patients may be cast over the shadow of the sinus in periapical radiographs the sinus shadow can be readily cleared by exposing the radiograph with the horizontal angulation of the tube reduced.

Buccal exostoses may also be cast over the inferior aspect of the sinus as radiopaque shadows. However, these radiopacities are more dense and their presence is also readily detected during the clinical examination.

In case of an *antritis* the thickened lining mucosa may be thrown up in an irregular fold. A panoramic radiograph or a Waters film will show the generalized thickening and most likely a cloudiness of the involved sinus, indicating the true nature of the condition. However, if the altered sinus is detected in a periapical radiograph the clinician may misinterpret the restricted image of the tissue reaction as representing localized hyperplasia. In addition, this film may be especially misleading if dental pathosis is also apparent in the limited view of the area. By contrast, the bone changes that are a distinguishing feature of the local hyperplasia from dental infection would be missing in antritis. Images of malignant tumors at relatively early stages of development may mimic the slightly radiographic appearance of a local hyperplasia: a mildly dense radiopaque soft tissue shadow that may be accompanied by some limited bone destruction in the floor of the sinus. However, incidence alone prompts the ranking of malignant tumors considerably below that of local hyperplasia, especially if dental pathosis is or has been recently present in the quadrant in question.

Worth and Stoneman (1972) explained that the inner surfaces of the normal antrum are uneven with localized bulges or depressions, which are covered with varying thicknesses of mucosa. These authors state that if such a shadow is demarcated by a vascular groove then the associated radiopacity is likely anatomic.

In view of the fact that some investigators suspect that dental infection may well be the cause of benign mucosal cyst, a distinction between them and local hyperplasia may not be possible. However, if dental pathosis is present and convincing evidence that definite periapical bone changes are pulpoperiapical in origin then a working diagnosis of local hyperplasia due to dental infection is appropriate.

MANAGEMENT

Treatment is directed toward eradication of the infection through such measures as extraction, root canal therapy, or periodontal surgery. The lesion should be kept under radiographic surveillance to ensure that it is regressing. In cases where the patient has concomitant sinus symptoms, consultation with an otolaryngologist is in order.

Fractures involving the sinus

The maxillary sinus is involved by the Le Fort types I, II, and III fractures, and its inferior portion may be compromised by inferior fractures of the tuberosity. Since this subject is traditionally well detailed in oral surgery textbooks the following discussion will be limited to the differential diagnosis of the unilateral opaque sinus on films from patients who have sustained facial trauma.

Obviously in such a case the cloudiness of the sinus could be due to preexisting pathosis. If the opacity of the sinus is related to the traumatic incident it could be simply the result of gross edema or a hematoma in the overlying cheek and facial tissue. Also when the films have been taken a few days after the traumatic incident the increased density of the sinus could be caused by a large abscess in the overlying facial tissue. In all these cases a clinical examination would readily identify the overlying soft tissue pathosis that is projected over the sinus and is responsible for its relative opacity.

In the case of a fracture the sinus will generally appear more radiopaque, which is caused by either generalized inflammation and thickening of the mucosal lining or by the sinus being full of exudate, pus, or blood. Careful examination of its bone walls will disclose the characteris-

Fig. 30-9. Two cases of zygomaticomaxillary fractures involving the left maxillary sinus. Note the opacification of the involved sinus and the discontinuity of the sinus walls in the fracture lines. **A,** Classic "four point" fracture of the zygomaticomaxillary complex. **B,** Unusual fracture across body of the zygoma as well as the infraorbital rim.

Fig. 30-10. Waters' view showing a premolar tooth apparently within the right maxillary sinus. Panograph and periapical films revealed the presence of lamina dura and pericoronal cortex around this impacted premolar tooth. (Courtesy M. V. Kaminski, D.D.S., Chicago.)

tic discontinuity caused by the fracture (Fig. 30-9).

FOREIGN BODIES

Although the complete list of foreign bodies that have been discovered in the sinus is too lengthy for presentation, the most common are avulsed teeth, roots, dental instruments, endodontic and restorative materials, foodstuffs, and antroliths. Identification of the foreign body as it appears on the radiograph is usually relatively easy. It is often much more difficult to determine

whether or not the object is actually situated within the sinus. The following discussion is limited to teeth, roots, and antroliths.

Teeth and roots
FEATURES

History, symptomatology, and radiographic evidence provide the most effective clues for the identification of teeth or tooth roots within the maxillary sinus. Occasionally whole teeth are evulsed into the maxillary sinus during an accident or by a careless exodontist. Postincident radiographs will show the tooth lying within the shadow of the maxillary sinus. However, it is important that the surgeon determine that the "lost" tooth is actually within the antrum for it may have slipped into the infratemporal space. Although such a tooth may appear on a radiograph to be in the maxillary sinus, a Caldwell view in combination with a lateral sinus view will usually clearly indicate its actual location. Also unerupted and malposed teeth will occasionally appear on a radiograph to be within the sinus (Fig. 30-10). However, the presence of a lamina dura, as well as the pericoronal cortex, will clearly identify the tooth's position in bone rather than within the maxillary sinus. The combination of a history of the recent "loss" of a maxillary posterior tooth, the shadow of the tooth in a cloudy antrum, and the clinical features of a sinusitis leaves little doubt about the situation.

Because of the extremely thin bone separating

root apices from the sinus, it is not surprising that at the time of extraction root tips are frequently pushed up into the sinus. Jones and Steel (1969) reported that the order of frequency in which apices are forced into the sinus are as follows: first molar, 60%; second molar, 16.1% third molar, 8.9%; first premolar, 7.8%; second premolar, 6.7%; and canine, 0.5%. While tooth roots and root fragments are usually readily identified by their characteristic shape and root canal shadows, there are occasions when it is very difficult to determine whether they are lying within the maxillary sinus or are actually within the overlying alveolar bone. Should the surgeon experience the upward loss of a root tip of one of the teeth near the sinus, this is not a certainty that the root is in the sinus. The fragment may have been pushed up into a cystic space, which may have been mistakenly identified as a portion of the maxillary sinus shadow on the presurgical radiographs. Also the root tip may be pushed through the buccal bone to lie between the oral mucosa and the alveolar bone. Radiographically a root in such a position would appear on certain films to be within the sinus.

A general but useful criterion is that if a tooth root does not have a periodontal ligament space and the shadow of a lamina dura, it is very likely within the maxillary sinus (Fig. 30-11). Unfortunately there are exceptions to this guideline. For instance, the case of the tooth root lying between the oral mucosa and bone surface would not be associated with a lamina dura or periodontal ligament space. Another example would be a root embedded in bone, surrounded by a *slight* rarefying osteitis. A radiograph of such a retained root segment would fail to show a periodontal ligament or lamina dura shadow so it

might be presumed that the root was within the sinus. Additional radiographic views will help clarify these situations. The Caldwell view gives a straight posteroanterior projection and, when combined with the information provided by a lateral view, will indicate whether the root is actually within the sinus.

A change in the position of the root fragment after the patient shakes his head will be apparent on subsequent radiographs and indicate that the tooth is within the sinus cavity. If the root is trapped between the sinus mucosa and the sinus floor the fragment will not change position when the head is shaken. Van Wowern (1971) reported that 13% of his cases had root tips trapped below the sinus mucosa, and the remainder were lying loose within the maxillary sinus. A Waters' view is usually not helpful in detecting root tips in the sinus, because the majority lie near their alveolae (on the floor) and the tilted image of the sinus floor that is inherent to the Waters' view will usually obscure the images of the root tips. Nevertheless, the Waters' view will reveal the cloudiness of a generalized sinusitis, which may result from the contamination or prolonged presence of a tooth or root in the maxillary sinus.

Complications following the avulsion of a tooth or root fragment into the sinus include the significant possibility of developing a persistent oroantral fistula or an acute bacterial sinusitis.

DIFFERENTIAL DIAGNOSIS

The diagnosis of a tooth or tooth root within the sinus is not easily confused with other antral pathoses. However, small radiopacities of the bone that project over the shadow of the antrum must be differentiated from root fragments actually lying within the sinus. Such entities would

Fig. 30-11. Root tips in the sinus. Both are semi-inverted molar root segments without a periodontal ligament or lamina dura shadow. Root tip in **B** was asymptomatic and had been present for many years.

include retained root segments in bone, small mature cementomas, small odontomas, condensing osteitis, and socket sclerosis.

MANAGEMENT

Prevention is always the best approach. Detailed study of high-quality preoperative radiographs combined with careful surgical manipulation will prevent many of these iatrogenic situations. Whole teeth or larger root fragments should be removed as soon as possible after the evulsion (immediately if possible) because of the high incidence of bacterial sinusitis when their removal is delayed. Smaller fragments pose the additional threat of passing through the ostium and being inhaled by the patient.

If the sinus perforation is large, careful aspiration, irrigation, ensnaring the fragment in iodoform gauze, and having the patient sneeze are simple methods that may recover the fragment. If larger access is required the procedure may be done either at the local site or through a Caldwell-Luc approach (Lee, 1970); these two procedures have been reported to be equally successful (Van Wowern, 1971). Herd (1974) advised that if a small fragment has been present for some time beneath an apparently healthy sinus lining and the patient is asymptomatic, immediate removal is not necessary, but the fragments "may be placed on probation."

Antrolith

An antrolith is a relatively rare lesion that is similar to the rhinolith in the nose. It is produced by the calcification of a nidus, which may be a blood clot, inspissated pus or mucus, or exogenous foreign bodies such as cherry pits or gauze (Bowerman, 1969; Evans, 1975). Crist and Johnson (1972) classified antroliths as true and false. The true variety forms on an endogenous nucleus whereas the false variety deposits on or around a foreign body.

FEATURES

Antroliths are usually grayish-black in color. They vary considerably in size, ranging from a small pea to large examples that completely obliterate the sinus. They may be asymptomatic, and they are found on routine radiographic films, but some are detected during the examination of a patient with a sinusitis.

Shapes and external contour, as well as degree of calcification, vary considerably. Some antroliths are round, while others have a very irregular shape (Fig. 30-12). They may have smoothly contoured surfaces, or they may be rough. The extent of calcification varies from those that have a dense homogeneous radiopacity to those with a mottled appearance to those that are minimally calcified and faintly radiopaque.

The microscopic appearance of an antrolith would show concentric laminations similar to the pattern seen in sialoliths, kidney stones, gallstones, and so on.

DIFFERENTIAL DIAGNOSIS

The differential diagnosis of antroliths should include tooth and root fragments in the sinus, radiopaque bony pathoses such as odontomas, cementomas, condensing osteitis, tori, exostoses,

A   B

Fig. 30-12. Antrolith in left maxillary sinus, which had produced a sinusitis. Note the less densely calcified center. **A,** Waters' film. **B,** Tomogram. (**A** and **B** from Blaschke, D. D., and Brady, F. A.: Oral Surg. **48:**187-189, 1979.)

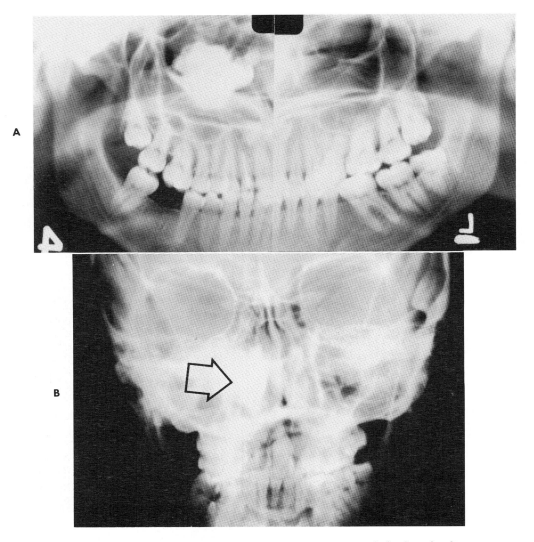

Fig. 30-13. Rhinolith. **A,** Panorex film showing an interesting irregularly shaped radiopaque mass that appears to be in the right maxillary sinus. **B,** Posteroanterior view shows that the calcified lesion is actually in the right nasal chamber. (**A** and **B** from Allan, G. A., and Liston, S. L.: J. Oral Surg. **37:**54-55, 1979. Copyright by the American Dental Association. Reprinted by permission.)

osteomas, osteoblastic tumors, and rhinoliths, as well as bone cysts. Adequate radiographic views will usually reveal whether the radiopaque lesion is in the sinus or not (Fig. 30-13). Of the radiopaque lesions that are demonstrated to lie completely within the antrum, only the tooth or root fragment could be easily confused with an antrolith. One may expect that the patient will recall the traumatic incident when a tooth or root was pushed into the sinus. However, in the absence of such a history and after ruling out bone pathoses then the diagnosis of antrolith is relevant.

MANAGEMENT

Antroliths should be removed, preferably through a Caldwell-Luc approach (Killey and Kay, 1975, p. 94).

Bony cysts

Odontogenic and nonodontogenic cysts of the maxilla may slowly expand into the antrum. Dentigerous and radicular cysts represent 85.22% of cysts that occur in the maxilla (Killey and Kay, 1975, p. 103), while primordial cysts, odontogenic keratocysts, and globulomaxillary cysts may en-

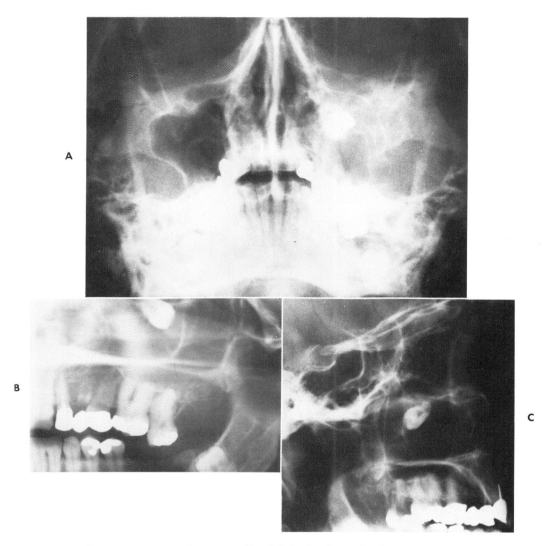

Fig. 30-14. Dentigerous cyst involving a maxillary left third molar tooth, which has obliterated most of the left maxillary sinus. **A,** Waters' view. **B,** Panorex radiograph showing the marked superior position of the third molar. Note that the cyst itself cannot be seen in this view. **C,** Lateral radiograph showing the anteroposterior location of the tooth. (Courtesy J. Ireland, D.D.S., and J. Dolce, D.D.S., Mundelein, Ill.)

croach on the antral space with much less frequency (Johnson and Stoopack, 1966).

FEATURES

Intrabony cysts with the potential to intrude into the sinus usually grow slowly and may produce a rounded smooth-surfaced bony expansion of the buccal surface of the alveolar process in the premolar-molar region of the maxilla. Dentigerous cysts usually involve impacted third molar teeth, and the tooth is malposed in a superior direction (Figs. 30-14 and 30-15). In some instances the cyst is easily detected as a gray radiopacity associated with the crown of the unerupted tooth and it perhaps has a thin radiopaque rim, which is the image of a thin layer of cortical bone separating the cyst from the antrum. Occasionally the cyst may not be apparent in a radiograph of the area (Fig. 30-16). However, if the unerupted maxillary third molar on one side of the maxilla is at a significantly higher level than the contralateral tooth and it is not im-

Fig. 30-15. Dentigerous cyst. **A,** Orthopantograph showing the faint radiopaque shadow surrounding the impacted right maxillary third molar tooth, which is in a superior position. **B,** Waters' view of another dentigerous cyst. The cyst has almost completely filled the sinus. Note the smooth thin radiopaque margin of the cyst. **C,** Waters' view of bilateral dentigerous cysts in the basal cell nevus syndrome, which have encroached on both antral cavities. (**A** and **B** courtesy N. Barakat, D.D.S., Beirut, Lebanon. **C** courtesy W. N. Smith, D.D.S., M.D., San Diego.)

Fig. 30-16. Orthopantograph showing bilaterally unerupted third maxillary molar teeth. Note that the one on the right (arrow) is in a more superior position than its counterpart on the other side. Note also that it is not impacted against another tooth. Such a finding is highly suggestive that there is pericoronal pathosis present, which has forced the tooth into a more superior position. Such pathosis is not evident on this film, but additional radiographs showed pericoronal pathosis that proved to be a dentigerous cyst through surgery and biopsy.

pacted against another tooth then it is almost certain that a pericoronal pathologic process is present and has pushed the tooth into a superior malposition (Fig. 30-16). Additional radiographs should be taken in an effort to actually demonstrate the pathologic process.

Radicular cysts have been discussed in detail in Chapter 16. In this context of sinus involvement the cyst will be associated with a pulpless premolar or molar tooth, which has a periapical radiolucency with smooth borders and which extends superiorly into the sinus. It will be roundish and slightly radiopaque, and its image will often have a thin radiopaque rim separating it from the sinus (Fig. 30-17).

Fig. 30-18 shows an example of a primordial cyst that proved to be an odontogenic keratocyst on microscopic study.

DIFFERENTIAL DIAGNOSIS

The differential diagnosis of the pathologic process associated with the crown of an impacted tooth includes dentigerous cyst, ameloblastoma, adenomatoid odontogenic tumor, immature odontoma, ameloblastic fibroma, and epithelial odonto-

genic tumor. Refer to Chapter 17, "Pericoronal Radiolucencies," for a more detailed discussion.

The differential diagnosis of radicular cyst in the maxillary posterior quadrant includes dental granuloma, local hyperplasia of the sinus floor, benign mucosal cyst, and unusual antrolith.

In many cases it may be difficult to differentiate a cyst from a sinus although Killey and Kay (1975, p. 104) and Berry and Beideman (1973) have detailed how this may be done. Aspiration will frequently yield results that will permit the clinician to differentiate between a cyst and the antrum.

MANAGEMENT

If a bony separation from the sinus still remains, enucleation of the cyst is usually a simple matter. If just the soft tissue linings separate the two large cavities complications should be anticipated.

Fibrous dysplasia

Fibrous dysplasia has been discussed in detail in Chapters 20 and 24. This disease commonly affects the maxilla and zygoma of young individuals. Fig. 30-19 demonstrates its characteris-

Fig. 30-17. Radicular cysts. **A** and **B,** Note the thin cortical rims in each case. **C,** Waters' view showing a ringlike radiopacity in left maxillary sinus. **D,** Waters view showing opacification of left maxillary sinus as well as unusual faintness of lateral wall near the alveolus where bone has been destroyed by the cyst. The indistinct appearance of the wall in this location suggests the possibility of malignancy. (**C** courtesy N. Barakat, D.D.S., Beirut, Lebanon. **D** courtesy O. H. Stuteville, D.D.S., M.D., St. Joe, Ark.)

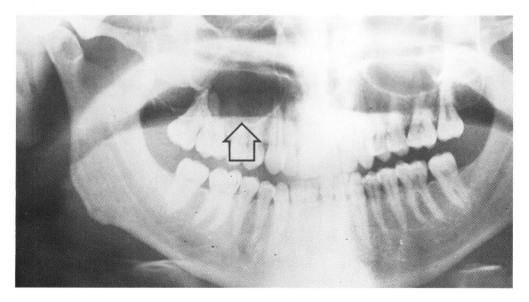

Fig. 30-18. Odontogenic keratocyst (arrow) in right maxilla, which has occupied most of the antrum on that side as well as resorbing the roots of several of the teeth. Casual inspection might produce the error of considering the cyst to be the sinus cavity although bilateral comparison would show considerable dissimilarity. (Courtesy N. Barakat, D.D.S., Beirut, Lebanon.)

Fig. 30-19. Fibrous dysplasia of the zygoma and maxilla. **A,** Uniform ground-glass expansion has obliterated the left maxillary sinus. **B,** A similar case where only the superiomedial aspect of the sinus has been preserved.

tic densely homogeneous, ground-glass, radiopaque appearance and the greatly reduced antral space of the maxillary sinus on the involved side. Patients are usually free of sinus-related symptoms.

DIFFERENTIAL DIAGNOSIS

The uniformly dense, smoothly contoured expansion of the zygoma and maxilla is quite classic for fibrous dysplasia of the facial bones. Cases of fibrous dysplasia may also have a mottled radiographic image and must then be differentiated from osteosarcoma, chondrosarcoma, Paget's disease, and other radiolucent-radiopaque lesions. It is interesting that, although more than one bone is involved, the patients do not often demonstrate the characteristic triad of Albright's syndrome.*

MANAGEMENT

In fibrous dysplasia surgical recontouring may be necessary for cosmetic purposes and restoring the occlusion. The patient should be examined periodically during the course of the disease.

Oroantral fistulas

A fistula may be defined as a pathologic tract that joins two body cavities or surfaces. The frequency of oroantral fistulas varies according to the type and location of the reporting clinician's practice. Haanaes (1974) studied 150 chronic oroantral fistulas and reported that 105 resulted from simple extractions, 29 from the surgical removal of impacted teeth, 11 from cystectomies, 7 from periapical surgery, and 1 from the removal of a foreign body. Fistulas have also been reported

*(1) Polyostotic fibrous dysplasia, (2) café-au-lait spots on the skin, and (3) precocious puberty in young girls.

after facial fractures and rarely as a result of periodontal diseases and pulpoperiapical pathosis (Selden and August, 1970).

FEATURES

The first molar was the most frequent tooth to be involved when fistula development followed extraction and the second molar was the next most frequent (Haanaes, 1974). Usually the surgeon becomes aware of the opening in the sinus floor during the surgical procedure, but this is not always the case. Also it is possible that a communication may develop a few days after the procedure, while some of the smaller openings created during surgery will heal spontaneously.

A patient with a patent communication will be aware that air is entering his mouth from his nose during eating and smoking. Frequently complaints will include regurgitation of food through the nose while eating, and mild sinus infection will manifest as postnasal drip. Acute infection may follow and produce an unpleasant discharge into the mouth or the nose. If blockage of both fistula and ostium occurs the stage is set for a severe attack of bacterial sinusitis.

Radiographic changes will be apparent in a significant number of cases. These include a bony defect in the sinus floor (Fig. 30-20), local hyperplasia of the sinus mucosa, and generalized swelling of the mucosa with opacification and fluid level (Haanaes, 1974).

DIFFERENTIAL DIAGNOSIS

Detection of an oroantral fistula is usually not difficult especially if the characteristic complaints are evoked. However, it is necessary to establish the cause, because occasionally a fistula will be

A ·   B

Fig. 30-20. Oroantral fistula. Two cases where the bone defect in the sinus floor is apparent radiographically.

produced by a malignant tumor of the antrum. Also a sinus tract from a chronic alveolar abscess or osteomyelitis in this area could be mistaken for an oroantral fistula. A radiograph taken with a gutta-percha cone placed in the tract will yield differential information.

MANAGEMENT

Management of the fistula immediately following its creation should include the following procedures. If the opening is small, instrumentation should be avoided and the mucosa sutured closed if possible. Broad-spectrum antibiotics and nose drops should be prescribed, and the patient should be advised to refrain from blowing his nose or smoking for at least 1 week. If a communication exists for 14 days it is unlikely to heal spontaneously and should be regarded as a chronic fistula (Killey and Kay, 1975, p. 50).

If a chronic oroantral fistula develops, successful closure will depend on how well the three basic surgical goals are achieved: (1) adequate mucosal closure, (2) eliminating the defect in the alveolar bone, and (3) eradication of the sinus pathosis at the time of closure.

Buccal or palatal flaps are utilized for mucosal closure. Bone grafting, gold plate, and reduction of the alveolar bone are used to eliminate the bone defect (Cockerham and Wood, 1976; Frederics et al., 1965; Goodman and Fenton, 1972). Eradication of antral pathology is usually accomplished through a surgical opening, which is maintained as an oral or nasal antrostomy (Goodman and Fenton, 1972; Haanaes et al., 1975), although some surgeons advise against an antrostomy.

Fig. 30-21. A large complex odontoma of the posterior maxilla, which has caused the impaction of the third molar tooth and has expanded into the sinus, producing a marked reduction in the size of the maxillary sinus. (Courtesy N. Barakat, D.D.S., Beirut, Lebanon.)

Odontomas

Virtually any odontogenic tumor or hamartoma may arise in the maxilla and encroach upon the antral space. However, the radiopaque odontoma occurring in the posterior portion of the maxilla frequently seems to lie within the sinus on radiographs (Fig. 30-21). Thus the odontoma may be quite troublesome from a differential diagnosis standpoint. The odontoma has been described in detail in Chapters 23 and 26.

FEATURES

Both the complex variety and the compound type may occur in the posterior maxilla. The odontoma develops and matures at the same time as the dentition and passes through the same stages of maturity: radiolucent, mixed, and radiopaque. Odontomas are usually detected during routine radiographic surveys, unless they precipitate symptoms such as jaw expansion or delayed eruption of teeth. Occasionally they will cause an attack of acute sinusitis (Dunn et al., 1976; Griffith and Imperato, 1977; Sanders et al., 1976).

Radiographically the mature compound odontoma will be easily recognized because of the characteristic appearance of its complement of many small teeth. In contradistinction, the mature complex odontoma will usually be a homogeneously dense radiopacity varying greatly in shape and size and will be surrounded by a radiolucent rim (border). Those occurring in the posterior maxilla frequently project into the antrum (Fig. 30-21). Radiographic views at various angles of projection will aid the clinician in establishing that the lesion is indeed partly contained within the maxillary bone and thus extending into the sinus.

DIFFERENTIAL DIAGNOSIS

In formulating the differential diagnosis an initial distinction must be established between radiopaque lesions in the sinus and radiopaque lesions of the surrounding maxilla and alveolus. Examples of the former would be an antrolith, an osteoma, an enostosis, and foreign bodies. Examples of those arising in bone would be mature cementoma, condensing osteitis, mature ossifying or cementifying fibroma, tori, osteogenic malignancies, exostosis, or the shadow of the malar bone.

A careful study of various good-quality radiographs will usually permit the examiner to determine that the radiopaque lesion under study has primarily arisen in the bone. Then the fact that under usual circumstances all the hard dental tissue lesions are surrounded by a radiolucent rim greatly aids in eliminating many of the possible lesions that arise in bone. If the radiopaque lesion has prevented the eruption of a tooth it is much more likely to be an odontoma than a cementoma. Also the posterior maxilla is a rare location for a cementifying or ossifying fibroma.

Tori, buccal exostoses, and the malar bone can be projected as radiopacities over the image of the sinus. However, they are readily observable clinically and also their images may be separated from the antral shadow by changing the angulation of a subsequent radiograph.

MANAGEMENT

Surgical removal is generally advised as soon as the odontoma is found so that the eruption of teeth will be interfered with as little as possible and also to hopefully prevent the development of a sinus infection.

Malignant tumors

Malignant tumors arising in the paranasal sinuses are quite uncommon, accounting for 0.2% of all the malignant tumors (Birt and Briant, 1976). Approximately 80% occur in the maxillary antrum, and the vast majority are squamous cell carcinomas, while adenoid cystic carcinomas and adenocarcinomas form the second and third most common groups (Figs. 30-22 to 30-25). The following types also occur but more rarely: melanoma, lymphoma, olfactory neuroepithelioma, osteosarcoma, chondrosarcoma, plasmacytoma, and metastatic tumors (Figs. 30-26 and 30-27). Malignant disease of the antrum may arise within the sinus lining proper, in the surrounding bone, or in the nasal and oral cavities secondarily invading the sinus.

FEATURES

Jackson and co-workers (1977) reported the following statistics from their study of 115 malignant tumors of the antrum: (1) age ranged from 19 to 94 years; (2) mean age was 61.5 years; (3) male:female ratio was 4:3; and (4) 5-year survival rate was 32%.

Because cancer of the maxillary sinus characteristically arises in the soft tissue lining, the tumor usually fills the sinus cavity before specific symptoms occur. In the early stages mild symptoms similar to those of chronic sinusitis may be present. When the advancing tumor erodes through the bony walls the swelling may be manifested in various locations: intranasally, on the face, intraorally, and orbitally. Jackson and co-workers (1977) reported the following frequency of symptoms in their cases: nasal obstruction, 61%; local pain, 43%; epistaxis, 40%; swelling, 29%; nasal discharge, 26%; epiphora, 19%; exophytic palatal lesion, 10%; diplopia, 8%; decreased cheek sensitivity, 8%; decreased vision in one eye, 8%; neck mass, 4%; proptosis, 3%; and trismus, 2%. Pearlman and Abadir (1974) stated that 80% of their cases were first seen in a stage of advanced destruction.

Radiographically the antrum will be partly or completely filled with a soft tissue shadow. In advanced tumors the ominous sign of bone wall destruction will be evident coupled with gen-

Fig. 30-22. Case of squamous cell carcinoma of the left maxillary sinus in a 58-year-old man. **A,** Full-face view. Note the moderate expansion in the left infraorbital region. **B,** Intraoral view showing tumorous expansion in vestibule. **C,** Waters' view showing opacification of the left antrum and loss of definition of its walls.

Fig. 30-23. Another case of squamous cell carcinoma of the left maxillary sinus in a 63-year-old man. **A,** Full-face view; the tumor has eroded through the facial aspect of the maxilla and is seen as a firm reddish exophytic mass in the infraorbital region. **B,** Waters' projection, which shows the opacified left sinus with some discontinuity of its walls. Note the small radon seed that has been placed to treat the carcinoma that has spread to the ethmoid sinus.

Fig. 30-24. Adenoid cystic carcinoma involving the right maxillary sinus. Waters' view showing the tumor that has opacified the inferior aspect of the sinus. The tumor had originated on the right posterolateral hard palate and had infiltrated through the palatal and alveolar bone into the sinus.

Fig. 30-25. Squamous cell carcinoma of the maxillary sinus. Periapical film showing the ragged moth-eaten destruction of the alveolar bone that forms the floor of the sinus. (Courtesy E. Zegarelli, School of Dental and Oral Surgery, Columbia University, New York.)

Fig. 30-26. Osteogenic sarcoma. **A,** Waters' projection showing dense radiopacity of right maxillary sinus. Note the complete radiographic loss of the lateral wall and the irregular image of the infraorbital margins. **B,** Osteogenic sarcoma occurring in a case of fibrous dysplasia of the left maxillary sinus, which had been previously radiated. Note the rather uniform ground-glass appearance of the fibrous dysplasia, which has obliterated the inferior aspect of the sinus. The oblique superior margin (arrow) marks the area of malignant change. (**A** courtesy E. Palacios, M.D., Maywood, Ill. **B** courtesy O. H. Stuteville, D.D.S., M.D., St. Joe, Ark.)

Fig. 30-27. Plasmacytoma. **A,** Extraoral view showing tumor within the right nostril. The tumor had originated in the right antrum and had extended into the right nasal chamber. **B,** Modified Waters' view showing the opacification of the right maxillary sinus as well as the right nasal chamber.

eralized sinus opacity. The bone destruction of the sinus floor and superior portion of the alveolar process will usually appear as a ragged radiolucency (Fig. 30-25).

Malignant salivary gland tumors arising in the characteristic posterolateral location of the hard palate may erode through into the sinus floor and show as a unilateral blunting of the apex portion of the sinus unilaterally (Fig. 30-24). These tumors will usually be clinically obvious when the hard palate is examined (Chapter 7). Occasionally a squamous cell carcinoma will arise on the posterior alveolar process and erode superiorly into the sinus.

DIFFERENTIAL DIAGNOSIS

In its early stages before bone destruction occurs it is not possible to differentiate between a

Fig. 30-28. Odontogenic tumors. **A,** Myxoma that had produced a divergence of the maxillary lateral incisor and canine teeth on the right side of this patient has almost obliterated the right antrum. **B,** Adenomatoid odontogenic tumor of the left sinus. Note the circular radiopaque line (arrow), which marks the thin bony rim of this tumor, which has occupied all of the sinus. An impacted and displaced maxillary canine tooth is undiscernible at the superior edge of the tumor. (**A** courtesy M. Lehnert, D.D.S., Minneapolis. **B** courtesy P. Akers, D.D.S., Evanston, Ill.)

malignancy and chronic sinusitis on a symptomatic basis. Radiographically one would not expect the early soft tissue shadow of a malignant tumor to be as smoothly contoured as benign soft tissue lesions such as a benign mucosal cyst, local hypertrophy from dental infection, bone cysts, and polyps. Evidence of bone wall destruction, except for pulpoperiapical lesions, in the floor should alert the clinician to the probable diagnosis of malignancy, provided recent fracture and osteomyelitis have been ruled out.

Osteoblastic malignancies will combine destruction of the antral walls with dense irregular radiopaque patterns. Osteogenic sarcoma, chondrosarcoma, and osteoblastic metastatic carcinoma also would have to be considered here as would osteomyelitis and the mottled stage of fibrous dysplasia.

MANAGEMENT

It now seems to be the consensus that a combination of radiotherapy and surgery is the management of choice for squamous cell carcinoma of the maxillary antrum (Birt and Briant, 1976). The prognosis is not encouraging as illustrated by the low 5-year survival rate, namely, between 20% and 32%. Late detection is usually the reason given for the high mortality rate.

Other odontogenic tumors

Theoretically any of the odontogenic tumors may arise in the posterior aspect of the upper jaw and thus encroach on the maxillary sinus. Cementomas, ameloblastomas, cementifying and/or ossifying fibromas, adenomatoid odontogenic tumors, calcifying epithelial odontogenic tumors, ameloblastic odontomas, and other variants such as myxomas and fibromas have been reported from time to time (Fig. 30-28).

Other osseous conditions and tumors

Like the odontogenic tumors virtually any osseous lesion can occur in the posterior maxilla and compromise the antral space by expansion or invasion. Giant cell granulomas, brown giant cell tumors, aneurysmal bone cysts, Paget's disease, cherubism, and intrabony hemangiomas have all been described (Figs. 30-29 and 30-30).

RARITIES

The following is a list of rarities involving the maxillary sinus:

Aplasia
Burkitt's lymphoma
Cholesteatoma
Emphysema
Encephalocele

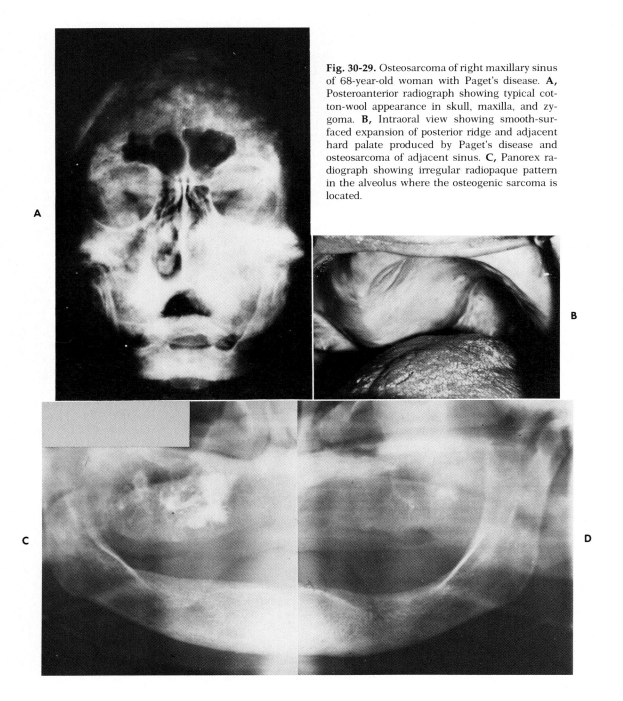

Fig. 30-29. Osteosarcoma of right maxillary sinus of 68-year-old woman with Paget's disease. **A,** Posteroanterior radiograph showing typical cotton-wool appearance in skull, maxilla, and zygoma. **B,** Intraoral view showing smooth-surfaced expansion of posterior ridge and adjacent hard palate produced by Paget's disease and osteosarcoma of adjacent sinus. **C,** Panorex radiograph showing irregular radiopaque pattern in the alveolus where the osteogenic sarcoma is located.

Fig. 30-30. Rare lesions of the maxillary sinus. **A,** Waters' projection of a central giant cell granuloma of the right maxillary sinus. Note the moderate degree of opacification and some loss in definition of the bone walls. **B,** Aneurysmal bone cyst of left maxillary sinus. Note the general opacification with a faint soap-bubble pattern. (**A** courtesy N. Barakat, D.D.S., Beirut, Lebanon. **B** courtesy M. Karakourtis, D.D.S., Naperville, Ill.)

Enostosis and osteoma
Hemangioma
Inverted schneiderian papilloma
Juvenile angiofibroma
Leprosy
Lethal midline granuloma
Meningocele
Mucocele
Mycoses
Neurogenic tumor
Osteomyelitis
Osteopetrosis
Paget's disease
Pyocele
Rare odontogenic tumors
Rhinosporidiosis
Sarcoidosis
Systemic disease (rarefaction)
Tuberculosis

SPECIFIC REFERENCES

Alberti, P. W.: Applied surgical anatomy of the maxillary sinus: symposium on maxillary sinus, Otolaryngol. Clin. North Am. **9**(1):3-20, 1976.

Allen, G. A., and Liston, S. L.: Rhinolith: unusual appearance on panoramic radiograph, J. Oral Surg. **37**:54-55, 1979.

Aust, R., and Drittner, B.: The patency of the maxillary ostium in relation to body posture, Acta Otolaryngol. **80**:443-446, 1975.

Axelsson, A., and Brorson, J. E.: Bacteriological findings in acute maxillary sinusitis, O.R.L. **34**:1-9, 1972.

Axelsson, A., and Jensen, C.: The roentgenologic demonstration of sinusitis, Am. J. Roentgenol. **122**(3):621-627, 1974.

Berry, H. M., and Beideman, R. W.: Radiographic visualization of the bone wall between cysts and the antrum, J. Oral Surg. **31**:878-880, 1973.

Binnie, W. H., Cawson, R. A., Davis, R., and Stacey, A. J.: Applications of xeroradiography in dentistry—a review, Int. Dent. J. **29**:34-40, 1979.

Birt, B. D., and Briant, T. D. R.: Management of malignant tumors of the maxillary sinus. Symposium on the maxillary sinus, Otolaryngol. Clin. North Am. **9**(1):242-254, 1976.

Blaschke, D. D., and Brady, F. A.: The maxillary antrolith, Oral Surg. **48**:187-189, 1979.

Bowerman, J. E.: The maxillary antrolith, J. Laryngol. **83**:873-882, 1969.

Cockerham, S., and Wood, W. H.: Closure of a large oroantral communication, J. Oral Surg. **34**:1098-1100, 1976.

Crist, R. D., and Johnson, R. L.: Antrolith: report of case, J. Oral Surg. **30**:694-695, 1972.

Dunn, W. P., Bollinger, T. E., Messer, E. J., and Bass, A.: Clinical-pathological conference case 15: large complex odontoma of the maxilla, J. Oral Surg. **34**:448-449, 547-550, 1976.

Ericson, S., and Welander, N.: Local hyperplasia of maxillary sinus mucosa after elimination of adjacent periapical osteitis, Odont. Rev. (Malmo) **17**:153-159, 1966.

Evans, J.: Maxillary antrolith: a case report, Br. J. Oral Surg. **13**:73-77, 1975.

Evans, O. F., et al.: Sinusitis of the maxillary antrum, N. Engl. J. Med. **293**(15):735-739, 1975.

Fascenelli, F. W.: Maxillary sinus abnormalities, Arch Otolaryngol. (Chicago) **90**:190-193, 1969.

Fireman, S. M., and Noyek, A. M.: Dental anatomy and radiology of the maxillary sinus: symposium on the maxillary sinus, Otolaryngol. Clin. North Am. **9**(1):83-92, 1976.

Fredrics, H. J., Scopp, I. W., Gerstman, E., and Morgan, F. H.: Closure of oroantral fistula with gold plate: report of case, J. Oral Surg. **23**:650-654, 1965.

Goodman, W. S., and Fenton, R. S.: The treatment of established antro-alveolar fistula, Can. J. Otolaryngol. **1**(2):97-101, 1972.

Gothberg, T. K. A., Little, J. W., King, D. R., and Bean, L. R.: A clinical study of cysts arising from mucosa of the maxillary sinus, Oral Surg. **41**:52-58, 1976.

Griffith, C. R., and Imperato, A. A.: Large antral odontoma as the cause of acute maxillary sinusitis: report of case, J. Am. Dent. Assoc. **94**:107-110, 1977.

Haanaes, H. R.: A radiographic and clinical follow-up study of 150 oroantral communications, Int. J. Oral Surg. **3**:412-421, 1974.

Haanaes, H. R., Pedersen, N. K., and Eigil, A.: Oral antrostomy, Int. J. Oral Surg. **4**:55-60, 1975.

Hall, I. S.: Diseases of the nose, throat and ear; a handbook for students and practitioners, ed. 10, Baltimore, 1973, The Williams & Wilkins Co.

Halstead, C. L.: Mucosal cysts of the maxillary sinus: report of 75 cases, J. Am. Dent. Assoc. **87:**1435-1441, 1973.

Herd, J. R.: The tooth root within the maxillary sinus, Aust. Dent. J. **19:**77-83, 1974.

Illum, R., and Jeppesen, F.: Sinoscopy: endoscopy of the maxillary sinus, Acta Otolaryngol. **73:**506-512, 1972.

Illum, P., Jeppesen, F., and Langeback, E.: X-ray examination and sinoscopy in maxillary sinus disease, Acta Otolaryngol. **74:**287-292, 1972.

Jackson, R. T., Firtz-Hugh, G. S., and Constable, W. C.: Malignant neoplasms of the nasal cavities and paranasal sinuses (a retrospective study), Laryngoscope **87:**726-736, 1977.

Johnson, W. C., and Stoopack, J. C.: Globulomaxillary cyst invading the maxillary antrum, Oral Surg. **22:**675-681, 1966.

Jones, E. H., and Steel, J. S.: Roots in the maxillary sinus, Aust. Dent. J. **14:**8-11, 1969.

Kelly, J. C., and Strothers, G.: Monograph 1. Sinusitis. In American Academy of Family Physicians, New York, 1974, Pfizer Laboratory, pp. 5-93.

Killey, H. C., and Kay, L. W.: The maxillary sinus and its dental implications. Dental practitioner handbook no. 18, Bristol, England, 1975, John Wright & Sons Limited.

Kreidler, J. H., and Koch, H.: Endoscopic findings of maxillary sinus after middle face fractures, J. Maxillofac. Surg. **3:**10-14, 1975.

Kwapis, B. W., and Whitten, J. B.: Mucosal cysts of the maxillary sinus, J. Oral Surg. **29:**561-566, 1971.

Lee, F. M. S.: The displaced root in the maxillary sinus, Oral Surg. **29:**491-504, 1970.

Lyon, H. E.: Reliability of panoramic radiography in the diagnosis of maxillary sinus pathosis, Oral Surg. **35:**124-128, 1973.

Maloney, P. L., and Doku, H. C.: Maxillary sinusitis of odontogenic origin, J. Can. Dent. Assoc. **34:**591-603, 1968.

Mattila, K.: Roentgenological investigations into the relation between periapical lesions and conditions of the mucous membrane of the maxillary sinus, Acta Odontol. **23:**5-77, 1965.

Mattila, K., and Westerholm, N.: Round shadows in maxillary sinus, Odont. Tidskr. **76:**121-136, 1968.

Myall, R. W. T., Eastep, P. B., and Silver, J. B.: Mucous retention cysts of the maxillary antrum, J. Am. Dent. Assoc. **89:**1338-1342, 1974.

Ohba, T.: Value and limitation of panoramic radiography in the diagnosis of maxillary sinus pathosis, Int. J. Oral Surg. **6:**211-214, 1977.

Ohba, T., and Katayama, H.: Panoramic roentgen anatomy of the maxillary sinus, Oral Surg. **39:**658-664, 1975.

Ohba, T., and Katayama, H.: Comparison of panoramic radiography and Water's projection in the diagnosis of maxillary sinus disease, Oral Surg. **42:**534-538, 1976.

Olson, D. J., Guralnick, W., Kalisher, L., and Donoff, B. R.: The application of xeroradiography in oral surgery, J. Oral Surg. **34:**438-441, 1976.

Pearlman, A. W., and Abadir, R.: Carcinoma of maxillary antrum: the role of pre-operative irradiation, Laryngoscope **84:**400-409, 1974.

Powell, R. N.: Periodontal disease and the maxillary sinus, Oral Surg. **19:**24-27, 1965.

Poyton, G. H.: Maxillary sinus and the oral radiologist, Dent. Radiogr. Photogr. **45**(3):43-50, 54-59, 1972.

Ritter, F. N.: The paranasal sinuses: anatomy and surgical technique, ed. 2, St. Louis, 1978, The C. V. Mosby Co.

Sanders, B., Halliday, R., and McKelvey, B.: Odontoma of the antrum presenting as a maxillary sinusitis, J. Oral Med. **31:**60-62, 1976.

Selden, H. S., and August, D. S.: Maxillary sinus involvement: an endodontic complication, Oral Surg. **30:**117-122, 1970.

Shramek, J. M., and Rappaport, I.: Panoramic x-ray screening for early detection of maxillary sinus malignancy, Arch Otolaryngol. **90:**347-351, 1969.

Sicher, H.: Oral anatomy, ed. 3, St. Louis, 1960, The C. V. Mosby Co.

Towers, J. F., and McAndrew, P. G.: Maxillary sinusitis mimicking malignant disease, Oral Surg. **39:**718-723, 1975.

Valderhaug, J.: Reaction of mucous membranes of the maxillary sinus and the nasal cavity to experimental periapical inflammation in monkeys, Int. J. Oral Surg. **2:**107-114, 1973.

Van Norstrand, A. W., and Goodman, W. S.: Pathological aspects of mucosal lesions of the maxillary sinus, Otolaryngol. Clin. North Am. **9**(1):21-34, 1976.

Van Wowern, N.: Oroantral communications and displacements of roots into the maxillary sinus: a follow-up of 231 cases, J. Oral Surg. **29:**622-627, 1971.

Waite, D. E.: Maxillary sinus, Dent. Clin. North Am. **15**(2):349-368, 1971.

Waters, C. A., and Waldron, C. W.: Roentgenology of the accessory nasal sinuses describing a modification of the occipito-mental position, Am. J. Roentgenol. Detroit New Series **2:**633-639, 1915.

Worth, H. M., and Stoneman, D. W.: Radiographic interpretation of antral mucosal changes due to localized dental infection, J. Can. Dent. Assoc. **38:**111-116, 1972.

Wortzman, G., and Holgate, R. C.: Special radiological technique in maxillary sinus disease. Symposium on the maxillary sinus, Otolaryngol. Clin. North Am. **9**(1):117-133, 1976.

Yanagisawa, E., and Smith, H. W.: Radiology of the normal maxillary sinus and related structures. Symposium on the maxillary sinus, Otolaryngol. Clin. North Am. **9**(1):55-81, 1976.

Zizmor, J., and Noyek, A. M.: Inflammatory disease of the paranasal sinuses. Symposium on radiology in otolaryngology, Otolaryngol. Clin. North Am. **6**(2):459-472, 1973.

GENERAL REFERENCES

Abadir, R.: Carcinoma of maxillary antrum, The Eye, Ear, Nose and Throat Monthly **52:**443-448, 1973.

Afshin, H., and Sharmin, R.: Hemangioma involving the maxillary sinus, Oral Surg. **38:**204-208, 1974.

Albright, C. R., and Hannig, G. H.: Large dentigerous cyst of the maxilla near the maxillary sinus, J. Am. Dent. Assoc. **83:**1112-1115, 1971.

Alder, P.: Age- and sex-dependence of the risk of intruding a root into the maxillary sinus, J. Oral Surg. **1:**185-189, 1972.

Atterbury, R. A., and Vazirani, S. J.: Maxillary sinus perforations and closures, J. Oral Surg. **25**(4):534-539, 1968.

Axelsson, A., Chidekel, N., Grebelius, N., and Jensen, C.: Treatment of acute maxillary sinusitis, Acta Otolaryngol. **70:**71-76, 1970.

Baumann, M., and Pajarola, G.: Experiences on the sequela of maxillary sinusitis following closure of the causative oroantral fistula, J. Maxillofac. Surg. **3**(3):164-169, 1975.

Berthrong, M.: Pathologic spectrum of neoplasms of the nasal cavity and paranasal sinuses, J.A.M.A. **219**(3):339-345, 1972.

Blaschke, D. D., and Brady, F. A.: The maxillary antrolith, Oral Surg. **48:**187-189, 1979.

Boies, L. R., Hilger, J. A., and Priest, R. E.: Acute and chronic sinus disease. In Fundamentals of otolaryngology, ed. 4, Philadelphia, 1964, W. B. Saunders Co., pp. 264-289.

Bosch, A., Vallecillo, L., and Frias, Z.: Cancer of the nasal cavity, Cancer **37**(3):1458-1463, 1976.

Brennom, E. F.: Case report: cancer of the antrum, Dent. Surgery **46:**24-26, 1970.

Caldwell, R. D. Morrow, L., and Gold, L.: Clinicopathologic conference. Case 6. Part 2. Carcinoma of the maxillary antrum in an 8-year-old child, J. Oral Surg. **32:**367-369, 1974.

Carenfelt, C., Eneroth, C-M., Lundberg, C., and Wretlind, B.: Evaluation of the antibiotic effect of treatment of maxillary sinusitis, Scand. Infect. Dis. **7:**259-264, 1975.

Caton, R. B., Marble, H. B., Jr., and Topazian, R. G.: Complex odontoma in the maxillary sinus, J. Oral Surg. **36**(5):658-662, 1973.

Chidekel, N., Jensen, C. C., Axelsson, A., and Grebelius, N.: Diagnosis of fluid in the maxillary sinus, Acta Radiol. [Diagn.] Stockh.) **10:**433-440, 1970.

Curreri, R. C., Messer, J. E., and Abramson, A. L.: Complex odontoma of the maxillary sinus: report of case, J. Oral Surg. **33:**45-48, 1975.

Davis, A.: The emergence of American dental medicine: the relation of the maxillary antrum to focal infection, Tex. Rep. Biol. Med. **32**(1):141-156, 1974.

D'mont, G.: Les ostéomas du sinus maxillaire, Acta Otorhinolaryngol. Belg. **27:**464-470, 1975.

Douek, E.: Acute sinusitis: disease of the ear, nose and throat. Vol. 3. The nose, ed. 3, Philadelphia, 1971, J. B. Lippincott Co., p. 183.

Dutta, A.: Rhinolith, J. Oral Surg. **31:**876-877, 1973.

Eichel, B. S.: The medical and surgical approach in management of the unilateral opacified antrum, Laryngoscope **87:**737-750, 1977.

El-Deiry, A.: Maxillary sinus carcinoma, Can. J. Otolaryngol. **2:**101-106, 1973.

Esquirel, J. L.: Nasal polyps in maxillary sinus, Oral Surg. **26:**585-687, 1968.

Fondo, J. J., and De Granges, G.: Clinical aspect of hypertrophied lesions of the sinusal mucosa, Acta Otorhinolaryngol. Belg. **29**(4):621-626, 1975.

Francis, F. H., and Bosshardt, L. L.: Roentgeno-oddities (unusual extension of the maxillary sinus), Oral Surg. **28**(6):854, 1969.

Fu, Y. S., and Perzin, K. H.: Nonepithelial tumors of the nasal cavity, paranasal sinuses and nasopharynx, Cancer **43:**611, 1979.

Galil, K. A.: Dentigerous cyst of the maxillary sinus (case report), J. Oral Med. **32**(2):56-58, 1977.

Galil, K. A.: An unusual complex odontoma (case report), J. Oral Med. **33:**32-34, 1978.

Gonty, A. A., and Page, L. R.: Aspergillosis of the maxillary sinus, Oral Surg. **43**(3):350-356, 1977.

Haanaes, H. R., and Gilhuss-moe, O.: A histologic study of experimental oroparanasal communications in monkeys, Int. J. Oral Surg. **1:**250-257, 1972.

Hames, R. S., and Rakoff, S. J.: Diseases of the maxillary sinus, J. Oral Med. **27**(4):90-95, 1972.

Hartenian, K. M., and Stenger, T. G.: Carcinoma of the maxillary sinus (report of case), J. Oral Surg. **36:**898-901, 1978.

Herd, J. R.: Exostoses of the sinus wall: a diagnostic problem, Aust. Dent. J. **19:**269-273, 1974.

Iwamoto, H., Katsura, M., and Fujimaki, T.: Mycosis of the maxillary sinuses, Laryngoscope **82:**903-909, 1972.

Januska, J. R., and Leban, S. G.: Improved visualization of the maxillary sinus, J. Oral Surg. **35:**74, 1977.

Kalm, O., Kamme, C., Bergstrom, B., et al.: Erythromycin stearate in acute maxillary sinusitis, Scand. J. Infect. Dis. **7:**209-217, 1975.

Karmody, C. S.: Osteoma of maxillary sinus, Laryngoscope **79:**427-434, 1969.

Kiley, C. H., and Kay, L. W.: Benign mucosal cysts. In Kay, L. W.: Oral surgical transactions of the Fourth International Conference on Oral Surgery, Copenhagen, 1973, Munksgaard, pp. 169-174.

Kimura, T., and Kataura, A.: Clinical and histological study of cyst forming maxillary sinusitis, J. Otolaryngol. Jpn. **78:**721-728, 1976.

Larsson, L., Gunnar, L., and Martensson, G.: Maxillary antral cancers. In Cancer of the head and neck, New York, 1971, American Cancer Society, pp. 65-68.

Lavelle, J. R., and Harrison, S. P.: Infection of the maxillary sinus: the case for the middle meatal antrostomy, Laryngoscope **81:**90-106, 1971.

Lehtinen, R., and Aitasalo, K.: An orthopantomographic study of the incidence of pathological changes in the jaws outside the dento-alveolar area, Proc. Finn. Dent. Soc. **69:**13-16, 1973.

Leopard, J. P.: Osteoma of the maxillary antrum, Br. J. Oral Surg. **10:**73-77, 1972.

Lilly, G. E., Cutcher, J. L., and Steiner, M.: Spherical shadows within the maxillary antrum, J. Oral Med. **23**(1):19-21, 1968.

Liston, L. S., Barker, B. F., and Cocayne, D. R.: Multiple osteomas of the maxillary sinus, J. Oral Surg. **37:**113, 114, 1979.

Moore, M. S.: An original procedure for closing large oroantral openings where conventional procedures have failed. In Kay, L. W.: Oral surgical transactions of the Fourth International Conference in Oral Surgery, Copenhagen, 1973, Munksgaard, pp. 175-178.

Nortjé, C. J., Farman, A. G., and Joubert, J.: Pathological conditions involving the maxillary sinus: their appearance on panoramic dental radiographs, Br. J. Oral Surg. **17:**27-32, 1979.

Noyek, A., M., Zizmor, J., and Wortzman, G.: Osteoma of the maxillary sinus—its occurrence following surgery, Can. J. Otolaryngol. **3:**90-92, 1974.

Osborne, T. P., Park, J. K., Levy, B. A., and Tewes, D. W.: Odontoma containing ghost cells in the maxillary sinus, Oral Surg. **38**(5):819-823, 1974.

Pissiotis, L.: Removal of root fragment from maxillary sinus, Dent. Digest **73:**110-112, 1967.

Polakow, S.: The treatment of chronic maxillary sinusitis by inhalation therapy with Bisolvon, S. Afr. Med. J. **47:**985-987, 1973.

Porter, J., Miller, R., and Stratigos, G. T.: Ameloblastoma of the maxilla, Oral Surg. **44**(1):34-38, 1977.

Prasanna, N. M., and Mendelsohn, M.: Maxillary sinus sarcomas, Can. J. Otolaryngol. **4:**704-711, 1975.

Raley, L. L., and Granite, E. L.: Plasmacytoma of the maxilla (report of case), J. Oral Surg. **35:**497-500, 1977.

Rhea, R. L.: A readily available intraoral catheter for irrigation of the maxillary sinus, J. Oral Surg. **34:**747, 1976.

Sako, K.: Management of cancer of the maxillary sinus, J. Surg. Oncol. **6:**325-333, 1974.

Schaeffer, J. P.: The embryology, development and anatomy of the nose, paranasal sinuses, naso-lacrimal passageways and olfactory organ in man, Philadelphia, 1920, P. Blaston's and Son Co.

Schechter, G. L.: Maxillary sinuses malignancy, Laryngoscope **82:**796-806, 1972.

Tabb, H. G.: Cancer of the maxillary sinus, Laryngoscope **81:** 818-827, 1971.

Van Alyea, O. E.: Nasal polyps and sinusitis, Ann. Otol. **75:**881-887, 1966.

Virabec, D. P.: The inverted Schneiderian papilloma: a clinical and pathological study, Laryngoscope **85:**186-200, 1975.

Williams, P. E.: Disease of the maxillary sinus of dental origin. In Kruger, G. O.: Textbook of oral surgery, ed. 4, St. Louis, 1974, The C. V. Mosby Co.

Winkler, T., von Wowern, N., and Bittmann, S.: Retrieval of an upper third molar from the infratemporal space, J. Oral Surg. **35:**130-132, 1977.

Zizmor, J., and Noyek, A. M.: Benign tumors. In Symposium on radiology in otolaryngology, Otolaryngol. Clin. North Am. **6**(2):497-503, 1973.

Zizmor, J., and Noyek, A. M.: In Paparella, M. M., and Shumrick, D. A.: Otolaryngology, vol. 1, Philadelphia, 1973, W. B. Saunders Co., chap. 46, pp. 1053-1095.

Zizmor, J., and Noyek, A. M.: Tumors of the paranasal sinuses. In Symposium on radiology in otolaryngology, Otolaryngol. Clin. North Am. **6**(2):493-496, 1973.

Lesions of bone that may have two or more major radiographic appearances

	Completely radiolucent	Radiolucent and radiopaque	Completely radiopaque
Adenomatoid odontogenic tumor	Yes	Yes	No
Ameloblastoma and variants	Yes	Yes	No
Calcifying epithelial odonto-genic tumor	Yes	Yes	No
Cementoblastoma	Yes	Yes	Yes
Chondroma	Yes	Yes	No
Chondrosarcoma	Yes	Yes	No
Ewing's sarcoma	Yes	Yes	No
Fibro-osseous lesions (PDLO)	Yes	Yes	Yes
Fibrous dysplasia	Yes	Yes	Yes
Garré's osteomyelitis	Yes	Yes	Yes
Giant cell granuloma	Yes	Yes	No
Hemangioma	Yes	Yes	No
Lymphosarcoma	Yes	Yes	No
Metastatic carcinoma	Yes	Yes	Yes
Odontogenic fibroma	Yes	Yes	No
Odontoma	Yes	Yes	Yes
Osteitis	Yes	Yes	Yes
Osteoblastoma	Yes	Yes	Yes
Osteomyelitis	Yes	Yes	Yes
Osteosarcoma	Yes	Yes	Yes
Paget's disease	Yes	Yes	Yes
Postsurgical bone defect	Yes	Yes	Yes
Reticulum cell sarcoma	Yes	Yes	No
Subperiosteal hematoma	Yes	Yes	Yes
Teeth	Yes	Yes	Yes

Normal values for laboratory procedures*

Hematology

Hemoglobin (Hgb)	
Men	14-18 g/dl
Women	12-16 g/dl
Hematocrit (PCV)	
Men	40-54 ml/dl
Women	37-47 ml/dl
Erythrocytes (RBC)	
Men	5.0-5.5 million/cu mm
Women	4.5-5.0 million/cu mm
Leukocytes (WBC)	5,000-10,000/cu mm
Differential	
Polymorphonuclear neutrophils	54%-62%
Lymphocytes	25%-33%
Monocytes	3%-7%
Eosinophils	1%-3%
Basophils	0%-1%
Platelets	150,000-450,000/cu mm
Reticulocyte count	0.5%-1.5%
Bleeding time (Ivy)	7-8 minutes
Coagulation time (Lee-White)	6-17 minutes
Prothrombin time	11-16 seconds (control, 12 seconds)
Partial thromboplastin time	Less than 100 seconds
Sedimentation rate (Wintrobe)	
Men	0-10 mm/hr
Women	0-25 mm/hr

Blood chemistry levels

Glucose (fasting)	50-150 mg/dl
Bromsulphalein (BSP)	5% or less retention in 45 minutes
Urea nitrogen (BUN)	9.0-20.0 mg/dl
Total protein	6.5-8.0 g/dl
Albumin	4.0-5.2 g/dl
Globulin	1.3-2.7 g/dl
Calcium (serum)	9-11 mg/dl or 4.5-5.5 mEq/liter
Phosphorus (inorganic)	3.0-4.5 mg/dl or 1-1.5 mEq/liter
Alkaline phosphatase (serum)	0.5-2.0 Bodansky units

Urinalysis

Specific gravity	1.015-1.025
Albumin	Negative
Acetone	Negative
Sugar	Negative
pH	6 (4.5-8.2)

*It is necessary for each laboratory to establish a range of normal values because of variations in technique and local conditions. This appendix was prepared by Charles C. Alling.

Index

Boldface—Main discussion.
Italics—Rarities list.
Asterisk (*)—Listing of entities.